PHARMACEUTICAL WATER SYSTEMS

THEODORE H. MELTZER

TALL OAKS PUBLISHING, INC.
Littleton, Colorado

Library of Congress Catalog Card Number: 96-061415

ISBN 0-927188-06-6

FIRST PRINTING

TALL OAKS PUBLISHING, INC.
P.O. Box 621669
Littleton, CO 80162-1669
U.S.A.
303/973-6700
fax: 303-973-5327

PRINTED IN THE UNITED STATES OF AMERICA

To my wife and companion
Xavier Magdalene Meltzer

Blessed art thou who endows mortalman with understanding.
--The morning liturgy

PREFACE

The subject of pharmaceutical water systems and the waters products they produce should be of profound interest in that they impact upon societal well being. The intention of this writing is to set forth the important changes now pending in the pharmaceutical water field and to make plain the current trends and their implications for future design constructions.

The examination of pharmaceutical water purification system designs are approached from a non-engineering point of view based on the analyses of unit process operations. The process validation requirements are considered on the bases of the purposes and performances of the several unit operations of which the various systems are composed. Each unit process utilized in pharmaceutical water preparations is detailed separately in its respective chapter.

This work is an outgrowth of the information gathered during the compilation of *"High Purity Water Preparation for the Semiconductor, Pharmaceutical and Power Industries"*, now three years old. Consequently, much of the acquirement contained in that volume is here expanded and updated.

As stated, the chapter on Pharmaceutical Waters reflects the important changes and trends that are now pending. The chapter on Validation discusses current thinking at the FDA; it attempts to anticipate logical progressions in the field of pharmaceutical water preparation. The views on the validation requirements inevitably come to mirror the subjectivity of the author's personal outlook. Hopefully, this may prove a guide, not an impediment to further thinking on the subject.■

Theodore H. Meltzer, Ph. D.
Arlington, Virginia

ACKNOWLEDGEMENTS

The complexities of pharmaceutical water system design and validation obliges a dependence on many sources. The information herein presented was furnished by many individuals over a very considerable time. It is, regrettably, simply impossible for me to make proper attribution in many cases; memory dims, notations are lost, and names, unlike gratitude, are overlooked. For this error of omission I offer my sincerest apologies. There are, however, those who contributed most directly to this book and whose names are remembered.

I do wish especially to thank Gary V. Zoccolante of the U.S. Filter Corporation for the profusion of papers, lecture notes, and technical conversations that he provided, particularly on the subjects of reverse osmosis and pretreatments. His views on the subject of ozone applications, and on electrically-driven demineralization devices were most enlightening. His assistance and encouragement were vital to this endeavor. I prize his collegiality and friendship.

I acknowledge my heavy dependence on Dr. Frank L. Slejko and the *Ultrapure Water Expo* and *Watertech* Conferences, and to the publications forthcoming therefrom. They are central to following the progression of pharmaceutical water system developments on an ongoing basis. The assistance of Marjorie K. Balazs, is recognized with gratitude. The papers forthcoming from her *Semiconductor Pure Water and Chemical Conferences* (SPWCC) are indispensable, as are the conferences themselves. The Balazs Analytical Laboratory of Sunnyvale, CA has, in its analytical operations, contributed significantly to the scientific development of pharmaceutical waters.

In matters microbiological, my special thanks to Dr. Murray S. Cooper of the Microbiological Update, Islamorada, FL, to Dr. Marc W. Mittelman of the University of Toronto, and to Gary R. Husted of MicroTeco, Hinesburg, VT.

Information on the subject of ion-exchange was especially forthcoming from Brian J. Hoffman of the Rohm and Haas Company of Philadelphia, PA; from Frank X. McGarvey of Sybron Chemicals Inc. of Birmingham, NJ; and from Dr. Robert J. Kunin, consultant, of West Trenton, NJ. These contributors were also kind enough to review the chapter on ion exchange.

A significant review and much pertinent information was furnished on the subject of filtration by Maik W. Jornitz of the Sartorius AG organization of Goettingen, Germany. I truly thank this valued colleague for his helpful assistance.

Henry C. Kuhlman of Kuhlman Technologies, Inc. of Kirkland, WA, Dr.

Deborah Jackman of the Milwaukee School of Engineering, Milwaukee, WI, and Verity Smith of Verity Consultants, Dedham, MA kindly supplied much information on stills and distillation, and furnished reviews of the chapter on the subject. Mr. Kuhlman was especially supportive of this effort. Both he and Dr. Jackman were each most generous with their course notes on the subject.

Information on materials of construction was liberally supplied by Reinhard Hanselka of Advanced Industrial Design, Danville, CA and by Thomas Sixsmith of the same organization but then with George Fischer Signet, Inc. of Tustin, CA. Joseph Manfredi of GMP Systems, Pine Brook, NJ was also exceedingly helpful in this regard. Messrs. Manfredi and Sixsmith also provided appreciated reviews on the subject.

Robert W. Powitz of R.W. Powitz and Associates, Detroit, MI is thanked for his helpful review of and his useful information on ultraviolet light systems. Eric Petersen of the Aquafine Corporation, Valencia, CA supplied needed information concerning the validation of such systems. Thomas Veloz, formerly also of that organization but now of UV Devices Incorporated of Valencia, CA furnished much information on the subject of UV applications and provided a much appreciated review of the relevant chapter.

Dr. Rip G. Rice of Rip Rice Associates of Ashton, MD supplied material information on ozone, and in a separate endeavor coauthored with me a chapter on ozone and ultraviolet light. I am very grateful to Dr. Marc W. Mittelman of the University of Toronto and to Dr. Gill G. Geesey of Montana State University for permitting liberal use of material from that chapter and from others in their book, *"Biological Fouling of Industrial Water Systems: A Problem Solving Approach"*. Information concerning the validation of ozone systems was forthcoming from Gaspar Lesznik of Ozonia North America of Lodi, NJ.

Mrs. Marilyn J. Gould and Michael E. Dawson of Cape Cod Associates, Falmouth, MA, assisted greatly with articles and discussions on the bacterial endotoxins and on the practical implications of lipopolysaccharide assays.

Peter S. Cartwright of the Cartwright Consulting Company, Minneapolis, MN, and Lee Comb of Osmonics, Minnetonka, MN separately reviewed the chapter on reverse osmosis, as did also Gory Zoccolante. These reviews were very much appreciated.

My deep appreciation is extended to Dr. Paris M. Allen of Paris M. Allen & Associates of Decatur, IL for his friendship and for his helpful technical assistance.

George Laird of Water and Power Technology of Salt Lake City, UT is thanked most sincerely for his especially helpful and enlightening contributions. Both his expertise and knowledge helped sustain this endeavor.

Hugh Eggborn, Engineering Field Director of the Environmental Field Office of the Virginia State Health Department, Culpeper, VA, not only supplied most of the information pertaining to potable water, but was kind enough to review the relevant write-up. His patience was endless, as is also my gratitude for his efforts.

On the general subject of pharmaceutical water I owe much to information from Dr. Murray S. Cooper of the Microbiological Update, Islamorada, FL; to Dr. Roger Dabbah of the USP Convention of Rockville, MD; to Dr. Aubrey S. Outschoorn of the Pharmaceutic Advisory Corporation of Bethesda, MD; to Dr. Ronald F. Tetzlaff, then of the FDA but now with Kemper-Masterson of Atlanta, GA; and to Terry E. Munson, then of the FDA but now with Kemper-Masterson of Rockville, MD.

For discussions and views on the validation of water systems, and for much useful information on the matter, I am profoundly indebted to Daniel Meshnick of Foster-Wheeler USA, Clinton, NJ; to John Lee of PSA Pharmaceutical Compliance of North Massapequa, NY; and especially to Terry E. Munson whose patient reviews were central to the selected approach.

The enabling assistance of the United States Pharmacopeial Convention in permitting so generous a use of materials from its various publications is sincerely acknowledged.

There is a talmudic tradition stating that the world stands on three foundations: knowledge, benevolence and service to others. The many contributors to this book demonstrated by their participation that this is indeed so. The debts owed by me to these colleagues are clear and unmistakable. I acknowledge the same with my sincerest thanks.

Reviews by experts in the relevant fields of the several chapters were essential to support the author's vaulting efforts to deal with subjects beyond his expertise. Yet none of the reviewers saw the chapters in final form, none knew whether their advices were wisely dealt with or not. Much is obviously owed the reviewers, especially the acknowledgment that the errors inherent in this presentation were not of their making.

This project could not have been realized without the work of the production staff and the meticulous copy editing by Johanna Staton. The publisher and I are both grateful for their dedicated commitment to this undertaking.

Yet, the assistance and collaboration detailed above could not have availed had not my companion and wife, Xavier, been ever present to sustain my endeavors and smooth my path. The attributes of the worthy wife as described in Proverbs 31 aptly characterize her and her actions. May the Good Lord bless her.

For all this assistance I am profoundly grateful. I hope to have justified the confidence of my many colleagues, and to have augmented their generous efforts.■

Theodore H. Meltzer
Arlington, VA

CONTENTS

CHAPTER 1

PHARMACEUTICAL WATERS

Water is a singular substance, with high versatility as a solvent. The phenomenon of wetting, often a prelude to solution formation, usually stems from the hydrogen bonding of water molecules to solid surfaces. The ability of water to form hydrogen bonds with oxygenated molecules suits it to the dissolution of covalently bonded matter, and to the hydration of such structures and of ions. The high dielectric constant of water causes the solubilization of ionic materials, separating their ionic lattices by the attenuation of their mutually attracting charges.

For all these reasons, the waters encountered in nature are hardly of pristine purity. Having had contact with their surroundings, they have variously leached and dissolved minerals and salts from the components of the earth and rocks they have encountered. Falling as rain, they have scrubbed various gases from the atmosphere. As runoff or streams they have picked up and carried a wide variety of impurities such as organic materials, salts, colloids, and various other soil constituents, whether in solution or suspension, into the lakes, ponds, aquifers, and such that serve as their collection areas.

Natural waters serve also to nurture organisms such as bacteria and viruses. Algae, diatoms, and other growths often find natural waters hospitable. The source waters that one encounters are, therefore, never water *qua* water, but are always aqueous solutions or suspensions of various compositions. These require purification into the high-purity waters of applicational interest in this book.

The chemical and physical makeup of a natural water tends to be very site-specific. It reflects the local geology and/or topography as modified by human activities such as housing, agriculture, and industry. It is thus difficult to generalize regarding raw water constituents. By the same token, there is no single water purification scheme that will fit all raw water. The treatment and equipment necessary to convert a natural water into its high-purity counterpart will also be site-specific. It will reflect the nature and concentrations of the water's components; the usage requirements in terms of volumes, rates, and peak rates; and the purity requirements of the particular application.

Surface waters—rivers, lakes, ponds, and streams—exhibit compositional variations over a period of time because of such factors as seasonal changes, locations, neighboring land managements, and rainfall densities. Farm runoffs may involve pesticides, fertilizers, and animal excrement; industrial pollutants may add their contributions; and everywhere vegetation may be present in its various stages of decay. Surface water collection areas such as lakes and ponds are subject to seasonal turnovers occasioned by density changes in their upper and lower layers as caused by seasonal temperature changes. In the temperate zone, there are two water inversions: autumn and spring. The autumn event is the more profound, with the chilled top water layers slipping to the bottom, roiling the waters and stirring sediments. This results in higher readings of total suspended solids (TSS) and total organic carbon (TOC). It is interesting that vegetative contamination is more enduring in the temperate zone than in the tropics because its oxidative destruction is slower at more moderate temperatures.

Surface waters usually contain lower mineral contents than groundwaters, but they more plentifully contain oxygen, organisms, and suspended solids; and thus

Table 1-1
Well Water
(expressed in ppm as $CaCO_3$ unless otherwise stated)

Calcium	49.5 ppm
Magnesium	13.6 ppm
Sodium	156.6 ppm
Potassium	3.59 ppm
Bicarbonate alkalinity	35.0 ppm
Sulfate	22.06 ppm
Chloride	62.75 ppm
Phosphate	0.01 ppm
Nitrate	3.46 ppm
Free CO_2	23.59 ppm
Silica	9.71 ppm
Iron, as Fe	0.03 ppm
Manganese, as Mn	0.01 ppm
pH	6.4
TDS, as NaCl	128.26 ppm
Turbidity, NTU	0.46
Color, Pt-Co units	11.80
Organics, as O_2 consumed	8.1

Table 1-2
Surface Water
(expressed in ppm as $CaCO_3$ unless otherwise stated)

Calcium	15.75 ppm
Magnesium	2.47 ppm
Sodium	10.9 ppm
Potassium	2.30 ppm
Bicarbonate alkalinity	10.0 ppm
Sulfate	7.49 ppm
Chloride	12.84 ppm
Phosphate	0.68 ppm
Nitrate	0.45 ppm
Free CO_2	3.53 ppm
Silica	3.18 ppm
Iron, as Fe	0.10 ppm
Manganese, as Mn	0.01 ppm
pH	6.8
TDS, as NaCl	34.70 ppm
Turbidity, NTU	1.35
Color, Pt-Co units	21.0
Organics, as O_2 consumed	8.1

Gagnon et al. (1991); Courtesy, Ultrapure Water Expo '91 East

exhibit lower clarities (Bates et al., 1988; also Gagnon et al., 1991). (See Tables 1-1, 1-2.) At least one water drawn from a well, 600 feet into a large freshwater aquifer, was found to contain a high organic content, 5 to 11 parts per million (ppm) of TOC (Arseneaux et al., 1990).

Groundwaters from wells do exhibit compositional differences caused by different geologies, yet on the whole they remain remarkably constant. In Virginia, well depths are usually from 100 to 1,000 feet. There, in sinking a well, the concern is to avoid if possible the aquifers bearing hydrogen sulfide and soluble iron or manganese. These impurities can be dealt with, of course, but their avoidance may be more economical. Soluble iron and manganese are prevalent over much of the Midwest, as are also the hard-water components derived from limestone deposits. The iron and manganese may be present as the soluble ferrous and manganous ions. Tables 1-3 and 1-4 present analytical data of one such well water containing iron. Usually, iron and manganese are present in only minimal amounts.

Source Water Characteristics

There are broad regional differences among the source waters utilized in the United States. Climatic differences with regard to rainfalls exert influences. Even within restricted geographical locations, however, local geologies can cause marked variations in the raw water quality.

Starting waters in the Northeast, despite their largely surface origins, may have low TSS, usually having been processed by some water authority, municipal or otherwise. Often being the product of land runoffs, however, they can be high in organic matter, with TOC seasonally as high as 10 ppm. Their hardness is generally not too high, some 6 to 7 grains. Their total dissolved solids (TDS) content is often below 300 ppm.

Midwestern waters are often drawn from wells. They may have a high hardness, often approaching 20 grains. Their TDS content of 300 to 400 ppm may consist of about 75% hardness and alkalinity. By alkalinity is meant the sum of the bicarbonate, carbonate, and hydroxide moieties. Essentially, however, alkalinity is an indication of the bicarbonate (temporary hardness) content. Interestingly, certain Detroit waters of high calcium and magnesium content do not deposit mineral scale on pipe surfaces. Being usually of groundwater origins, midwestern source waters may contain dissolved iron and manganese, but are low in organics.

Western waters are often characterized by a high silica content. Certain well waters may contain up to 60 ppm of silica. They may include in excess of 1,000 ppm of TDS, but are usually below 1 ppm in organic components. There are exceptions, however. Many Santa Clara Valley water sources have low TDS but high organic contents. One California pharmaceutical company using sources originating in snow melts from the Sierras has starting water that is very low in

TDS and contains only 2 ppm of sodium ions.

The part of the Northwest within which rainfall is plentiful has surface run-off waters roughly similar to those found in the Northeast. The TDS is generally low, at about 50 to 100 ppm. It may contain 3 ppm of sodium and about 9 ppm of silica.

A generalized characterization of various source waters was made by Crits (1989) with regard to the impurities they may contain.

Water Impurities

Ionic and organic contaminants. Sodium and potassium ions are almost always among the species that are present. If their combined amount in a water is from 5 to 10 ppm, they are likely present in approximately equal amounts. With higher concentrations, sodium predominates. Calcium and magnesium ions are apt to be present. These, leached from limestone, are the causes of permanent water hardness, along with barium and strontium that are less frequently analyzed for. Actually, the entire cation content is expressed by conversion to its equivalence in terms of calcium carbonate. As the molecular weight of calcium carbonate is 100, and its equivalent weight is 50, a convenient unit of exchange is at hand for expressing the total of all the ions present, instead of more arduously summing the individual ions, each with its particular equivalence.

Table 1-3
Case 1: An Iron Profile*

Sample Point	*Fe(II) (ppb)*	*Fe(total) (ppb)*
Well water**	49	37
Before filter	18	21
After filter	21	16
Skid #1		
Feedwater	16	16
Permeate	ND	ND
Reject	52	48
Skid #2		
Feedwater	16	
Permeate	ND	ND
Reject	54	50
Skid #3		
Feedwater	17	21
Permeate	ND	ND
Reject	51	48

ND: Nondetectable (<2 ppb)
* Accuracy of samples collected on site is not greater than ± 5 ppb
** Variations in well water iron concentrations are consistant with the presence of particulate iron in the sample stream. Zeiher et al; (1991), Courtesy ULTRAPURE WATER Expo '91 East.

Total hardness is the sum of the calcium and magnesium ions. Carbonate hardness, more frequently referred to as *temporary hardness* or *bicarbonate hardness*, is that portion of the total hardness represented by the calcium and magnesium associated with bicarbonate. The remainder of the total hardness is the calcium and magnesium associated with sulfates, chlorides, and nitrates. This remainder is called *noncarbonate hardness*.

The exigencies of electrical neutrality of solutions ensure the presence of like quantities of anions. Bicarbonate, carbonate, and hydroxide ions collectively constitute water alkalinity. As will subsequently be discussed, they relate to one another by a connection involving carbon dioxide and considerations to pH. This relationship governs temporary water hardness. Chloride and sulfate ions are usually present. The topical setting can be important. Chloride ions may result from seawater incursions, and sulfate ions derive from gypsum rock or from sodium sulfate (Glauber's salt) deposits. Nitrate ions are usually the vestigial remains of nitrogenous substances, and in high quantities therefore often bespeak contamination by sewage or other organic matter. The total anion concentration is referred to as the total mineral acidity (TMA).

Total dissolved solids is the sum of all that is soluble in the water—chiefly, its mineral constituents. The TDS is performed by an evaporation to dryness at 103 to 105 °C. Bicarbonates are converted to carbonates, with a corresponding loss in weight. For instance, if bicarbonates were reported as 164 ppm as bicarbonate, then when they are evaporated to dryness there would be 100 ppm of carbonate. An alternative is to evaporate at a higher temperature, at 180 °C. Here, all water of crystallization is driven off, and carbonates may be partially

Table 1-4
Case : First Water Analysis
Bacterial counts are given in cfu/mL. All other concentrations are given in ppm.

Component	*Feed*	*Product*	*Reject*	*% Injection*	*% Recovery*
				(based on concentration)	
Boron	0.70	0.30	1.60	57.14	69.23
Calcium	160.00	1.50	500.00	99.06	68.20
Chloride	64.00	0.70	220.00	98.91	71.14
Iron	0.20	0.00	.80	100.00	75.00
Magnesium	90.00	0.50	270.00	99.44	66.79
Phosphorus	0.20	0.10	.50	50.00	75.00
Potassium	17.00	0.70	51.00	95.88	67.59
Silicon (SiO_2)	7.10	0.00	23.00	100.00	69.13
Sodium	180.00	5.70	580.00	96.83	69.65
Strontium	2.40	0.00	7.20	100.00	66.67
Sulfate	230.00	0.50	730.00	99.78	68.54
Total aerobic bacterial counts	200.00	100.00	500.00	50.00	75.00
Antiscalant	5.78	0.00	19.26	100.00	69.99
Permeate flow	78.00				
Reject flow	34.00				
Feed flow	112.00				
% Recovery flow	69.64				

Zeiher et al., (1991); Courtesy, Ultrapure Water Expo '91 East decomposed to oxides or other basic salts.

The specific electrical resistance, expressed in microohms-cm (μΩ-cm), and its reciprocal, specific conductance, expressed in microsiemens per centimeter, μS-cm, formerly in micromhos/cm, are a very convenient, rapid determination used to estimate the total amount of dissolved solids in water. For most natural waters, it has been found that when the specific conductance is multiplied by a factor within the range of 0.55 to 0.7, the product is equal to the total residue. The conductance can be computed directly from the chemical analysis by multiplying the concentration of each constituent by its appropriate specific conductance.

Ions arise principally from the solubilization of dissociative inorganic molecules. However, organic molecules bearing polar functional groups may also be ionizable.

The soluble organic impurities present in water sources are usually derivative of the vegetative contamination common to surface waters. This organic pollution may include the complexities of farm runoff. It may even contain trihalomethanes, which are suspected carcinogens, not originally present in the water, but generated from organics that were present by the degradative action of the chlorine added to the water to control bacterial growth.

The organic entities may be nonionic. However, weakly ionic functionality may also characterize relatively large, otherwise nonpolar organic moieties. The ionized organic molecules may be amenable to ion-exchange removal. Nonionic organics can be adsorbed to the surfaces of activated carbon. However accomplished, the removal from the water supply of organic impurities optimizes the further purification of the water and permits the ultimate manufacture of the compendial waters.

There are industrial applications of purified waters, such as of semiconductor rinsewaters, wherein the prohibition against the presence of any ions is total. In the case of pharmaceutical waters, the concentrations of calcium, sulfate, and chloride ions are permissible to given limits. Acceptable concentrations of ammonia and carbon dioxide gases, generators of the ammonium and bicarbonate/carbonate ions, respectively, have been stipulated. Additionally, the upper concentration limits of the heavy metals, determined as copper, have also been regulated.

Water purification concerns transcend considerations of final, permissible concentrations, however. For instance, if ion-exchange resin columns are being used to remove ions, access to the exchange sites must not be preempted or blocked by depositions of undissociated organic material, whether stipulated or not. Such organic entities as fulvic or humic acids, originating usually from vegetative matter, must be removed. Otherwise the manufacture of the highly purified water may be interfered with.

Likewise, the presence of ions such as barium, calcium, and strontium in the water source may necessitate their early management in such a way as to prevent the irreversible fouling, by scale precipitation, of reverse osmosis (RO) membranes. Water pretreatments are thus required to protect the means whereby ions may be removed from the water sources to accord, ultimately, with the high-purity water specifications required for the particular application.

Bicarbonate and scaling. Reference has been made to the bicarbonate ion. There is an equilibrium among carbon dioxide and the bicarbonate and carbonate ions. Shortly to be treated in greater detail, this equilibrium reflects the influence of pH. High concentrations of hydrogen ions (the hydronium ion, H_3O^+) predispose to the existence of carbonic acid (H_2CO_3), of which the first and principal dissociation is into the bicarbonate ion (HCO_3^-). Secondary dissociation of the bicarbonate ion to yield the carbonate ion (CO_3^{2-}) is dependent upon higher pH (i.e., lower hydrogen ion concentrations).

The existence of the bicarbonate ion, the product of carbonic acid dissociation, is dependent upon carbon dioxide concentrations as well as upon pH. The removal of carbon dioxide from an aqueous system is tantamount to a pH shift to higher values. It results in the transformation of bicarbonate ions into carbonate ions. This occurrence is very important to water purification protocols, as it reflects also on the presence of calcium ions. Calcium bicarbonate is soluble; calcium carbonate is quite insoluble. Calcium ions may remain in solution, given a sufficiency of hydrogen ions and carbon dioxide. Diminishing the concentration of either risks the precipitation of calcium carbonate. The untoward consequences are scale formation, and the compromise of membrane and still surfaces, along with blockage of pipes and other equipment. To avoid such undesirable occurrences, carbon dioxide and/or bicarbonate ions are removed in the water purification process under controlled conditions, and the precipitated calcium is dealt with at a time and place of one's choosing.

The Langelier Saturation Index, which will receive further discussion, is a method of predicting the scale-forming tendencies of water. In order to calculate the index, it is necessary to know the methyl orange alkalinity, the calcium hardness, the TDS, the pH value, and the temperature. From these, an index can be calculated by subtracting the pH of saturation, that of the water saturated with calcium carbonate, from the actual pH. If the measured pH exceeds the pH of saturation, the index is positive and, being saturated with calcium carbonate, the water is likely to form scale. This index is employed commonly when considering a water to be treated with RO techniques.

Suspended matter. Suspended solids, whether of inorganic or organic origin (the latter possibly from seasonal vegetative sources) may clog filters as well as carbon and ion-exchange beds. Colloids may do the same, or may more perniciously escape removal by filters or ion exchange. Silica often exists in colloidal form. The silt density index (SDI) test is a useful measure of the filter-clogging propensity of a water.

Difficult to remove from suspension are particles of clays whose ionic charges repel one another. The particles, as a result, do not agglomerate to sizes large enough to be responsive to the sedimentation induced by gravitational forces. Colloids are extreme examples of the latter. The separating out of suspended colloidal particles may involve the neutralization of mutually repulsive electrical charges, followed by agglomeration and flocculation of the suspended particles.

The colloids usually encountered in water sources can be filtered out by ultrafilters having molecular-weight cutoffs (MWCOs) of 100,000 or less. Colloids can also be retained by charge-modified filters. Unless removed from the water stream undergoing processing, colloids may come to foul reverse osmosis membranes, stills, and deionizing resin beds, thus interfering with the manufacture of the pharmaceutical waters.

Silica. Silica often appears as one component of a complex colloid that also commonly includes organic material and heavy metal ions. It may well be that the organic material exhibits weak ion-exchange properties that bind the heavy metal ions to it, and that the silica/organic matter in combination form a complex colloidal system. In any case, silica chemistry is notoriously obscure; and silica, existing in both weakly ionic and nonionic forms, is difficult to detect analytically.

The ionized form of silica is subject to ion-exchange reactions involving strong anion-exchange resins. It can also be removed by charge-modified filters. Silica in its colloidal form can be removed by ultrafilters of 100,000 MWCO or lower. Silica is particularly to be avoided in water distillation contexts, as in pharmaceuticals, or in steam generation for turbine operations in the power-generating industry. Silica may volatilize with steam to condense into vitreous coatings that interfere with the heat transference properties of condenser surfaces, and that can cause serious imbalances in spinning turbines, with potentially serious consequences.

Dissolved gases. Gases can be solubilized in water, and their presence may be deemed an impurity. Hence in pharmaceuticals there are upper concentration limits for ammonia and for carbon dioxide. Less frequently, hydrogen sulfide (H_2S) and even sulfur dioxide (SO_2) may emerge from deep wells as water impurities. In the power-generating industry, even oxygen may be considered an undesirable impurity because of its corrosive influence, especially at elevated temperatures. Then too, chlorine gas added to water supplies to control bacterial growth must ultimately be removed before its strong oxidative forces cause the corrosion of stainless steel stills or the degradation of the membranes used in the various water-purification processes.

Henry's Law describes the extent of a gas solubility as being an expression of its partial pressure above the solution. One can thus aid the removal of a gas from

Table 1-5
An Analysis of a Source Water

		Analysis (ppm as such)	*Conv. factor (x)*	*Analysis (ppm as $CaCO_3$)*	*meq/L*
Cations					
Calcium	(Ca^{2+})	60.0	2.50	150	3.00
Magnesium	(Mg^{2+})	7.3	4.12	30	0.60
Sodium	(Na^{+})	50.5	2.18	110	2.19
Potassium	(K^{+})	7.8	1.28	10	0.20
Hydrogen = FMA*	(H^{+})		—		
Total Cations				300	5.99
Anions					
Bicarbonate	(HCO_3^-)	183.0	0.82	150	3.00
Carbonate	(CO_3^{2-})	—	*0.5	—	—
Hydroxide	(OH^-)	—	2.94	—	—
Sulfate	(SO_4^{2-})	53.8	1.04	56	1.12
Chloride	(Cl^-)	63.8	1.41	90	1.79
Nitrate	(NO_3^-)	2.5	0.81	2	0.04
Phosphate(ortho)	(PO_4^{3-})	1.3	1.58	2	0.04
Total Anions				300	5.99
Total hardness	($CaCO_3$)	—	—	180	
M.O. alkalinity	($CaCO_3$)	—	—	150	
pH alkalinity	($CaCO_3$)	—	—	—	
Carbon dioxide	(CO_2)	211	*1.15	2.4	
Silica (reactive)	(SiO_2)	30	0.83	24.9	
Silica (nonreactive)		5			
Iron	(Fe)	2			
Manganese	(Mn)	0.1			
Chlorine, free	(Cl)	0.5			
Total dissolved solids		360			
COD by permanganate		5			
TOC		8			
Turbidity		2			
Color		—			
Specific conductance (μmho/cm @ 25 °C)		660			
Specific resistance (ohm-cm @ 25 °C)		1,520			
Temperature -°F		55-68			
pH		8.1			
pH*		7.62			
Langelier index		0.48			

* Free mineral acidity
Courtesy, Continental Penfield Water

its solution by several methods of deaeration. The solution may be trickled through a packed column, where widespread exposure to air helps to remove the offending gas. Vacuum deaeration, using expensive devices, is effective. Use of a sparging stream of air risks infecting the solution with airborne microbes. Traditionally, activated carbon beds have been utilized to remove gases, especially chlorine, by adsorption. Noncondensed gases (e.g., nitrogen, or those that unlike carbon dioxide or ammonia do not dissolve in or react with water) can be removed by the venturi action of air eductors.

Microorganisms. Natural waters, perhaps with some very few exceptions, are not sterile. Both Gram-negative and Gram-positive organisms of many species flourish in natural waters, for these normally contain plenty of nutrients. It should be noted, however, that while Gram-negative organisms find nutritional sources even in extremely pure waters, they are far less indifferent to elevated temperatures, being killed at temperatures above 60 °C. From the catabolism of the outer membranes of Gram-negative organisms such as *Pseudomonas* arise the lipopolysaccharides that are the most common bacterial endotoxins, pyrogenic factors when injected into the blood stream.

The containment and eventual elimination of organisms is of paramount concern in water purification endeavors. It is a chief preoccupation of point-of-use purification activities. Microbes can multiply and proliferate even from a single, individual organism; and even when sterile waters have been prepared, they are prone to bacterial recontamination from their surroundings. Bacterial assays are thus an important part of the water purification protocol. Indeed, for each and every contaminant whose removal is sought, analysis is central to the

Table 1-6
City Water Analysis

Sanger, CA

Calcium	32.5 mg/L as $CaCO_3$
Magnesium	79.1 mg/L as $CaCO_3$
Sodium	58.7 mg/L as $CaCO_3$
Potassium	5.1 mg/L as $CaCO_3$
Alkalinity	111.0 mg/L as $CaCO_3$
Sulfate	25.9 mg/L as $CaCO_3$
Chloride	38.5 mg/L as $CaCO_3$
TDS	175.4 mg/L as $CaCO_3$
Conductivity	334.0 mg/L as $CaCO_3$
Silica	31.7 mg/L as SiO_2
pH	7.4
Carbon dioxide	8.0 mg/L as CO_2

Comb and Fulford (1991); Courtesy, Ultrapure Water Expo '91 East

purification effort, guiding the attainment and certifying the achievement.

There is, of course, no standard water source, no universal purified water, nor any single analytical protocol adequate to represent the problems of water purification. Each source water is site-specific. Table 1-5 is an example of one water analysis performed to characterize one source water. Table 1-6 represents the analytical data obtained for another source. Table 1-7 illustrates a feedwater as characterized by a third investigator. All these analytical profiles share certain contaminants in common, but all reveal, nevertheless, differences in the attempts by the analysts to characterize source waters.

Applicational Requirements

The use of waters for a given purpose requires the removal of the objectionable impurities they contain. The various waterborne impurities may or may not be tolerable in specific applications. It may be unnecessarily expensive to remove an impurity whose presence would not be unacceptable in a given application. As a consequence, different classes of water eventuate. Each is defined by the concentration limits of specific ingredients, as required for particular applications.

Examples of Analytical Approaches

Martyak et al. (1991a, b) reviewed the analytical techniques used for the characterization of a deionized water, albeit for semiconductor usage. The water was measured for its resistivity at 25 °C, for its TOC in terms of parts per billion

Table 1-7
Results of a Water Analysis

	City Water	*RO I Feed*	*RO I Permeate*	*RO II Feed*	*RO II Permeate*
Calcium	13.0	12.0	0.2	0.2	0.05
Magnesium	19.0	19.0	0.5	0.5	0.05
Sodium	27.0	22.0	2.8	3.6	0.30
Potassium	7.0	4.0	0.3	0.3	0.00
Sulfate	27.0	71.0	0.4	1.9	0.01
Chloride	27.0	22.0	0.8	1.0	0.01
Alkalinity	111.0	40.0	8.0	8.0	0.80
pH	7.4	5.8	5.1	6.2	5.8
Carbon dioxide	8.0	79.0	78.0	2.0	2.0
Chlorine	0.0	0.4	0.0	0.0	0.00
Silica	31.7	32.0	6.1	6.2	0.035
Conductivity	334.0	335.0	21.0	23.0	1.5

All results are as mg/L, which is expressed as the ion (or molecule), except for alkalinity, which is expressed as $CaCO_3$. Conductivity is expressed as µS/cm.
Comb and Fulford (1991); Courtesy, Ultrapure Water Expo '91 East

Table 1-8
Design Spec and Contaminant Characterization Procedures

Charcterization Parameter	*Specification*	*Limit*	*Analytical Procedures*
Resistivity	18.0 MΩ-cm		Thornton
Dissolved oxygen	< 75.0 ppb		Orbisphere
Bacteria	< 1 cfu/100 mL		ASTM F60-68
SEM bacteria	8/L	8 ± 10	SEM
TOC	<10 ppb	10 ppb	Anatel A100
Silicon	< 5 ppb	5 ppb	Hach, Colormetric (molybdosilicate)
Chloride	< 0.2 ppb	0.5 ppb	Ion chromatography
Sodium	< 0.2 ppb	0.2 ppb	ICP/MS
Calcium	< 1 ppb	1.0 ppb	ICP/MS
Potassium	< 3.0 ppb	3.0 ppb	ICP/MS
Lithium	< 1 ppb	1.0 ppb	ICP/MS
Nitrate/nitrite	< 0.1 ppb	0.5 ppb	Ion chromatography
Sulfate	< 0.3 ppb	0.3 ppb	Ion chromatography
Phosphate	< 0.2 ppb	0.5 ppb	Ion chromatography
Iron	< 0.1 ppb	1.0 ppb	ICP/MS
Copper	< 0.1 ppb	0.1 ppb	ICP/MS
Aluminum	< 0.5 ppb	0.5 ppb	ICP/MS
Nickel	< 0.1 ppb	1.0 ppb	ICP/MS
Chromium	< 0.1 ppb	0.1 ppb	ICP/MS
Zinc	< 1 ppb	1.0 ppb	ICP/MS
Magnesium	< 0.5 ppb	0.5 ppb	ICP/MS
Lead	< 1 ppb	1.0 ppb	ICP/MS
Particles:			
5.0 µm	< 1/L	0 ± 120	Particle Measuring Systems (PMS) laser-based particle counter
2.0 µm	< 1/L	0 ± 120	Particle Measuring Systems (PMS) laser-based particle counter
.5 µm	< 1/L	0 ± 120	SEM
.2 µm	< 1/L	0 ± 120	SEM
>.1 µm	< 10/L	10 ± 117	SEM
Temperature	70° F		Temperature probe
Pressure	55 psig		Pressure gauge

Martyak et al. (1991); Courtesy, *Microcontamination*

(ppb), its dissolved oxygen content in ppb, and its total silica and sodium in ppb. The total number of particles present per liter and their size distribution were determined. Bacterial presences were assayed by scanning electron microscope (SEM) counts, total heterotrophic plate counts, and *Pseudomonas* plate counts, all in terms of colony-forming units (cfu) (or number) per 100 milliliters (mL).

More specifically, Martyak et al. (1991) utilized on-line meters, sensors, and probes to monitor particles, dissolved oxygen, silica, sodium, TOC, specific resistance, and temperature. The membrane filtration technique, soon to be discussed, was used in conjunction with appropriate growth media in the assaying of heterotrophic or *Pseudomonas*-type microbes. Total bacteria enumeration was also performed using epifluorescence techniques and SEM. The latter method was carried out using filters precounted to 0.1 micron (μm) to

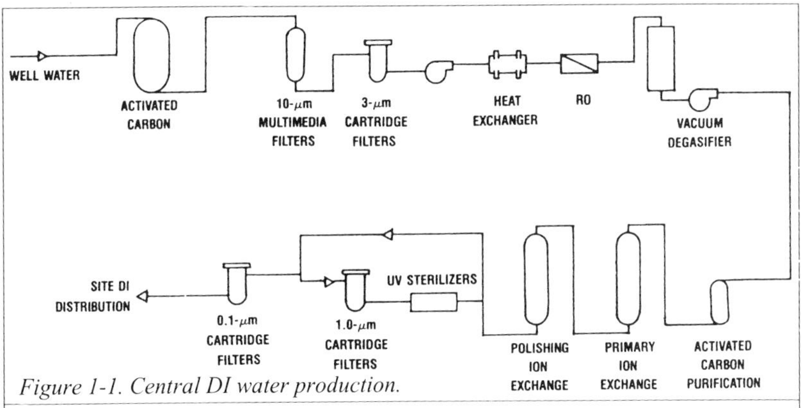

Figure 1-1. Central DI water production.

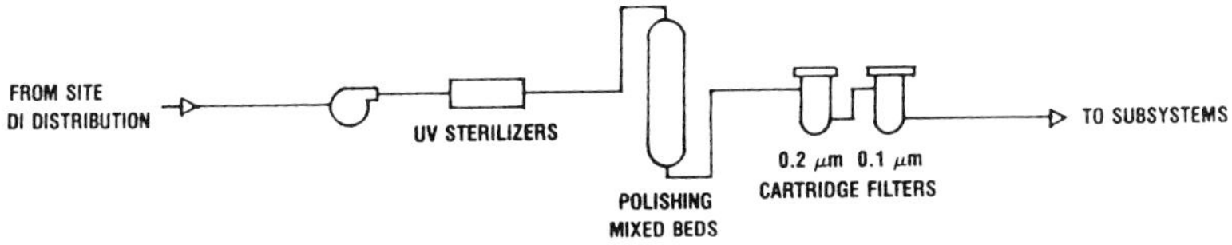

Figure 1-2. Main DI water polishing.

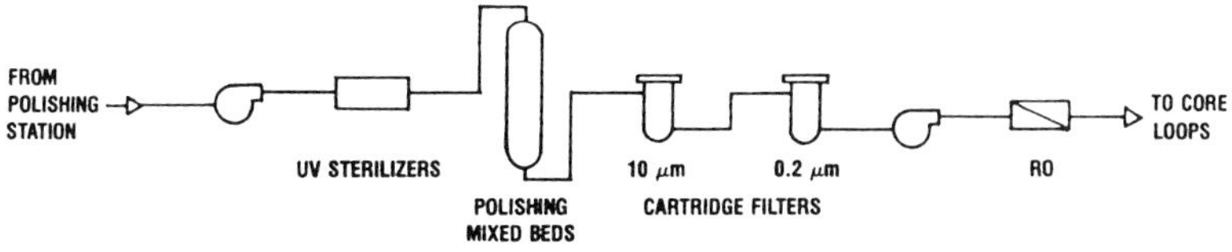

Figure 1-3. RO/DI subsystem polishing.
Martyak et al. (1991a, b); Courtesy, *Microcontamination*

ensure accuracy.

Specialized analytical tools and methods were used to identify foreign matter. Energy-dispersive X-ray (EPX) was employed for elemental analysis. Ion chromatography served for anion identification, and inductively coupled plasma/ mass spectrometry (ICP/MS) was used for cation recognitions. Table 1-8 lists design specifications by Martyak et al. (1991) for their water, along with the pertinent analytical methods. Flow diagrams of the water purification system operative at the IBM plant in East Fishkill are shown in Figures 1-1 through 1-3.

The nature and utility of such devices and installations, and the operations necessary to particular water purification efforts are, in fact, the very subject of this writing.

Different concentrations of the same type of contaminants, as characterized by analysis, can require markedly different water treatments. A study reported by Gagnon et al. (1991) is indicative of the influences that quantitative differences in analysis can exert on the purification system design. A well water having a high TDS but low TSS, turbidity, and organic material (Table 1-9) had been satisfactorily purified of its high TDS by a mixed-bed ion-exchange operation protected by an ultrafiltration prefilter. However, blending this well water with a surface water having low TDS but high turbidity, TSS, and TOC (Table 1-10) resulted in premature plugging of the ultrafilter and its succeeding mixed beds. To prepare the desired product water, it was necessary to diminish the high TSS of the blended feedwater by addition of polymeric polyelectrolyte coagulant,

Table 1-9
Well Water Analysis

Calcium	49.50
Magnesium	13.60
Sodium	156.6
Potassium	3.59
Bicarbonate alkalinity	35.00
Sulfate	22.06
Chloride	62.75
Phosphate	0.01
Nitrate	3.46
Free CO_2	23.59
Silica	9.71
Iron, as Fe	0.03
Manganese, as Mn	0.01
pH	6.4
TDS, as NaCl	128.26
Turbidity, NTU	0.46
Color, Pt-Co units	11.80
Organics, as O_2 consumed	0.0

(in ppm as $CaCO_3$ unless otherwise stated)

Gagnon et al. (1991); Courtesy, Ultrapure Water Expo '91 East

followed by a multimedia deep bed. So protected, the ultrafilter exhibited a useful service life as prefilter for the ion-removing mixed bed. The proper action of the polymeric polyelectrolyte was guided by SDI determinations. Reductions in the SDI of the feedwater were effected from the 30 to 50 range, down to the 5 to 6 level. In particular, the cited work of Gagnon et al. (1991) demonstrates the importance of quantitative differences, in this case largely in the TSS, on the requisite design of the water purification train, as evidenced by the SDI analysis of the source water.

Pharmaceutical Waters

The impurities whose removal or reduction is required for pharmaceutical compendial water manufacture can variously be grouped as inorganic ionic species; organic matter, both nonionized and ion-charge-bearing (however weakly); suspended matter, colloidal and otherwise; water hardness elements, such as the alkaline earths (e.g., calcium and magnesium) and carbon dioxide, whether in the form of carbonate or bicarbonate; soluble iron and manganese; silica; and microorganisms.

Certain impurities require removal or reduction in quantity in order to conform to the *United States Pharmacopeia (USP)* stipulations for Purified Water or Water for Injection. Others must be eliminated or managed because their uncontrolled presence could cause the dysfunction of the water purification devices.

Table 1-10
Surface Water Analysis

Calcium	15.75
Magnesium	2.47
Sodium	10.90
Potassium	2.30
Bicarbonate alkalinity	10.00
Sulfate	7.49
Chloride	12.84
Phosphate	0.68
Nitrate	0.45
Free CO_2	3.53
Silica	3.18
Iron, as Fe	0.10
Manganese, as Mn	0.01
pH	6.8
TDS, as NaCl	34.70
Turbidity, NTU	1.35
Color, Pt-Co units	21.00
Organics, as O_2 consumed	8.10

(in ppm as $CaCO_3$ unless otherwise stated)
Gagnon et al. (1991); Courtesy, Ultrapure Water Expo '91 East

It would be fair to say that the sophistication of semiconductor pure water preparation far exceeds that practiced in pharmaceutical settings. This is so because the water purity requirements of pharmaceutical manufacture are less demanding. Thus compendial waters need not achieve an almost ion-free status. Yet that is the very goal of integrated-circuit water purification: 18-megohm-cm* resistivity, a complete absence of ions other than those arising from the dissociation of water. The rigors of semiconductor pure water manufacture may be excessive for pharmaceutical purposes. Nevertheless, these more demanding practices should be studied for the teachings they extend to the needs of compendial water preparation.

USP Specifications

The United States Pharmacopoeia Convention (USPC) is a private, not-for-profit organization that sets standards for drugs, devices and diagnostics. One of its compendia, the *US Pharmacopeia*, contains the standards set for drug products as well as for other articles, such as those now in the Food, Drug and Cosmetics Act as "devices or diagnostics." Its other compendium, the *National Formulary* (*NF*), sets the standards for drug excipients. Both compendia are published within a single cover titled *US Pharmacopeia/National Formulary*, currently (as of 1995) the *USP 23* and *NF 18*. In essence, the *USP* defines what a drug is. The particulars are described in the *USP* "Official Monographs" section.

There is a legal status to the compendium of drug standards established by the *USP* as listed in its monographs. The Food, Drug and Cosmetics Act recognizes the *USP 23* and *NF 18* as Official Compendia and and their standards are enforceable by the Food and Drug Administration (FDA). Drugs not in keeping with compendial standards are judged to be adulterated, misbranded, or both, according to Section 501 of the Act, or they have to be labeled as non-USP.

The *USP 23* also contains a section on "General Information." The information imparted is not enforceable by the FDA. It is seen as not quite having the force of the USP monographs.

The USP lists monographs on four type of waters intended for finished dosage forms. In addition there are listed two waters that are prepared in bulk form, not containerized, namely Purified Water (PW), often called USP Purified Water to distinguish it from waters purified by some means or other, and Water for Injection (WFI). These are the compendial waters. Waters may also be used for other purposes in pharmaceutical manufacture—for example, cooling water and waters for washing and rinsing. The terms *compendial waters* and *pharmaceutical waters* may therefore imply different meanings.

*The theoretical maximum usually given is 18.3 ± 0.1 MΩ-cm, although some authorities insist on slightly different values. It is referenced to water at 25 °C. Higher conductivity values result when higher temperatures are referenced because water dissociates into ions more as the temperature is raised.

As of November 1996, *USP 23 Fifth Supplement, Monograph Section*, also permits the use of waters comparable by European Union or Japanese regulations.

Purified Water. Purified Water is described in the *USP 23* monograph (p. 1637) as follows: "Purified Water is water obtained by distillation, ion-exchange treatment, reverse osmosis, or other suitable process. It is prepared from water complying with the regulations of the U.S. Environmental Protection Agency (EPA) with respect to drinking water. It contains no added substances."

Inherent in this statement is the understanding that waters not of potable quality must first be brought up to comparable standards before being utilized for compendial water preparation.

Regarding the bacteriological purity of PW, the monograph states only that PW must comply with the EPA regulations for drinking water (40 CFR 141.14;141.21).

Confusion sometimes results when the stipulatory nature of the remarks in the monograph is coupled with, or is incorrectly seen as being modified by, statements in the informational chapter.

In its informational guideline dealing with "action guidelines for the microbial control of ingredient water," *USP 23* (p. 1984) says: "A total microbial (aerobic) count that may be used for source drinking water is 500 colony-forming units (cfu) per mL. A general guideline for Purified Water may be 100 cfu/mL." The language itself, as well as these numbers being omitted from the PW monograph, attests to the advisory or guideline nature of the numbers. They represent an alert/action limit, not a reject level. Actually, the limit of 500 cfu/mL is concerned not with any specific threat to health that a larger number would bring, but simply to the interference in reliably detecting coliforms.

This section also suggests that the microbial action limits for PW should be

Table 1-11*
Interpretations of USP Standards for Water Purity

Component	*Purified Water*	*Water for Injection*
pH	5.0-7.0	5.0-7.0
Chloride (mg/L)	0.2	0.2
Sulfate (mg/L)	1.0	1.0
Ammonia (mg/L)	0.1	0.1
Calcium (mg/L)	1.0	1.0
Carbon dioxide (mg/L)	5.0	5.0
Heavy metals (mg/L)	0.1 as Cu	0.1 as Cu
Oxidizable substances	Pass USP Permanganate Test	Pass USP Permanganate Test
Total solids (mg/L)	10.0	10.0
Pyrogens (EU/mL by LAL)	—	0.25

* Not a USP table

based on the intended use of the water (which may vary greatly), on the nature of the product being made, and on the effect of the manufacturing process on the resident organisms. It is thus recognized that microbial limits for PW require being defined on a case-by-case basis. Purified Water is used in the preparation of noninjectable dosage forms. What the note states is that sterile PW may be used for the preparation of sterile but nonparenteral dosage forms.

In its informational section on water for pharmaceutical purposes, *USP 23* (p. 1984) advises that although PW may be prepared sterile by distillation, the use of ion-exchange columns and RO units affords opportunities for microbial presences. Indeed, it is seldom if ever alleged that waters issuing from ion-exchange columns are organism-free, at least for any significant length of time. Reverse osmosis devices, it has been found, also cannot be relied on to produce sterile water. This is exactly why the FDA advises the use of two RO units in tandem where sterile water production is desired.

Most often, PW is prepared by the use of ion exchange. More recently, as will be discussed, there has been an advocacy for its manufacture by the use of tandem RO units—two-pass, product-staged RO. However prepared, PW is stipulated to have limitations to its ionic and other components, as shown in Tables 1-11 and 1-12.

Water for Injection. The *USP 23* (p. 1635) monograph states: "Water for Injection (WFI) is water purified by distillation or reverse osmosis." The European pharmacopoeia permits the preparation of Water for Injection only by distillation. Purified Water may, as in the United States, be manufactured by distillation or by any other suitable method. The same is being advocated both in Europe and in the USA for Water for Injection. Bacterial endotoxin limits of 0.25 EU/mL have recently been introduced.

The Japanese Pharmacopoeia allows the preparation of WFI by distillation, by reverse osmosis, and by ultrafiltration. It is required, however, that the WFI prepared by membrane processes be stored at 80 to 90 °C. Bacterial endotoxin

Table 1-12
Various Microbial Levels for Compendial Waters in Cfu/mL

	Potable	*PW*	*WFI*
EPA	500	—	—
USP XXI	—	100**	50**
GMP/LVP	—	50***	0.1*
USP23	—	100**	No stated value

*Plus a complete absence of *pseudomonads*
**Action Guidlines, not limits
***Case by case basis

testing is stipulated. Sterile Purified Water is not to be used for parenteral preparations. The chemical testing for Purified Water is similar to that expected for WFI.

The Japanese Pharmacopeial microbial requirements for tap water or well water are set at no more than 100 cfu/mL, and no coliforms in 50 mL. The source water stipulations include, in addition to pH, purity limits for odor, taste, nitrogen from both nitrates and nitrites, ammonium, cyanide, heavy metals, iron, zinc, cadmium, copper and lead. There are also concerns with total hardness, residues on evaporation, and anionic surfactants. These source water requirements are the subject of the monograph.

The *USP 23* monograph makes no references to bacterial stipulations for WFI. It does, however, specify that WFI not contain more than 0.25 *USP* endotoxin units (EU) per mL.

The designated endotoxin limit makes redundant any microbiological limit. The endotoxin arises from the Gram-negative organisms that, being native to water, could be expected to be present. Therefore, it is reasoned, the water must be of a very high microbial quality not to yield an excessive endotoxin concentration. Strictly speaking, the WFI organism level is moot. It is possible, some endotoxin experts contend, that Gram-positives could be present, even in substantial numbers.

For this reason, the appropriate Subcommittee of the *USP* Committee of Revision may come to stipulate as an informational guideline, not as a reject level, 10 cfu/100 mL, the level championed for WFI by the FDA.

The proper preparation of WFI, whether by RO or by distillation, ought to result in a sterile product. Be that as it may, WFI need not be sterile for its intended use in formulating large-volume parenterals, since these preparations will be terminally sterilized, usually by autoclaving, after being containerized. Indeed, WFI, or any other product, may not be termed sterile unless specifically subjected to treatments designed to render it such.

The WFI monograph also notes that WFI is intended as a solvent for the preparation of parenteral solutions. It is stated that the WFI purity requirements, other than microbiological and as related to endotoxin, meet those stipulated for Purified Water (Table 1-11). Actually, the limits shown in Table 1-11 are not directly stated in the *USP 23* monograph. They become defined by translation of the actual texts in terms of the referenced analytical methods. For example: "Chloride—To 20 mL in a color-comparison tube add 5 drops of nitric acid and 1 mL of silver nitrate TS, and gently mix: any turbidity formed within 10 minutes is not greater than that produced in a similarly treated control consisting of 20 mL of High Purity Water (see under Chemical Resistance) - Glass Containers (661), containing 10 mg of Cl, viewed downward over a dark surface with light entering the tubes from the sides (0.5 ppm)." And more succinctly, "Chloride—To 100 mL, add 5 drops of nitric acid and 1 mL of silver nitrate TS: no opalescence is produced."

Many of the nonmicrobiologically-related values stipulated by the *USP 23* are of uncertain origin. Many derive from inherited empirical statements, or of good manufacturing practices at the time they were implemented. Some of the values can be traced as far back as 1840, but the older confirming records have simply disappeared. The heavy metal specifications stem from the years 1880 to 1890, when concerns involved lead pipes used as water conduits. The need for the updating of these figures has been recognized; and current efforts offer the promise of newer and more pertinent numbers, designations, and methods,

Water Quality Committee Recommendations.
Some seven years ago the USP enlisted the cooperation of the Pharmaceutical Manufacturer's Association (PMA), now the Pharmaceutical Research And Manufacturing Association (PhRMA), in reviewing all USP monographs, standards and general chapters relating to water. The organization's Water Quality Committee (WQC) has over the course of this period proposed many considerations to the USP subcommit-tee in charge of water. It is likely that most, but not necessarily all, of these proposals will be adopted by the USP Committee of Revision; some after an additional period of study and consideration. The basic strategy that has evolved considers the present quality of the pharmaceutical water satisfactory. Contemplated are changes in testing procedures. It is recognized that the maintenance of USP quality standards importantly requires the validation of each water system.

Of the many propositions and suggestions offered and considered, the subcommittee of the USP Committee of Revision, in August 1993, proposed that the present tests for oxidizable substances, heavy metals, total solids, chloride, calcium, sulfate, carbon dioxide, and ammonia be dropped. Wet chemistry analyses for the latter five entities would be replaced by electrical conductivity measurement, and total organic carbon (TOC) testing would substitute for the oxidizable substances analysis.

The total solids test deletion was proposed because of its poor reproducibility and because the TOC testing could largely replace it except for the detection of high silica levels, which could, however, be managed in the validation program.

The compendial waters require being prepared from feedwaters of potable quality. In its specification of drinking water quality the Environmental Protection Agency (EPA), whose domain this is, stipulates heavy metal standards to a level lower than the present USP-required wet chemistry analysis. The need for USP specification is thereby obviated. However, pharmaceutical manufacturers should confirm that heavy metals are not reintroduced into the waters. A proposal to include testing for aluminum was not endorsed by the subcommittee.

As stated, the British Pharmacopeia and the European Pharmacopeia specify that only distillation may be used to prepare Water for Injection. The USP specifies distillation and reverse osmosis. The Japanese Pharmacopeia, permits distillation or reverse osmosis in combination with ultrafiltration. From time to time advocacy is made in the USA that Water for Injection preparation be permitted by "other suitable means" as supported by system validation. That Water for Injection quality can be obtained by means other than distillation or (two-pass product-staged) reverse osmosis is not disputed. What is questioned is whether the validation of water systems is at present being adequately performed on a sufficiently widespread basis. Absent such a necessary supporting action, the opening of Water for Injection production to "other suitable means," it is feared, offers unnecessary risks. There is some reason to believe that water system validation practices still require implementation in many production

Table 1-13
Stage 1--Temperature and Conductivity Requirements
(for non-temperature compensated conductivity measurements only)

Temperature C°	*Conductivity (μS/cm)**
0	0.6
5	0.8
10	0.9
15	1.0
20	1.1
25	1.3
30	1.4
35	1.5
40	1.7
45	1.8
50	1.9
55	2.1
60	2.2
65	2.4
70	2.5
75	2.7
80	2.7
85	2.7
90	2.7
95	2.9
100	3.1

* μS/cm (microSiemen per centimeter) = μmho/cm = reciprocal of Megohm-cm.

Courtesy, *USP Convention Water Quality Committee Pharmaceutical Forum*, Jan.-Feb. 1996 situations.

Substitution of conductivity testing for the wet chemistry analyses would also obviate the need to test the water for its pH. However, on the basis of a long experience in water system inspections, it has been found that pH testing very frequently reveals inadequacies in water systems. On the basis of its being a useful diagnostic tool, therefore, the pH test is retained, allowing time for additional consideration and study.

Conductivity measurements. Of the various molecular entities whose analyses are required for Purified Water or Water for Injection, six (pH, chloride, sulfate, ammonia, calcium, and carbon dioxide) have ionic expressions in water and can consequently each be measured by the electrical conductivity of its solution.

Table 1-14
Stage 3--pH and Conductivity Requirements
(for atmosphere and temperature equilibrated samples only)

pH	*Conductivity (µS/cm)*
5.0	4.7
5.1	4.1
5.2	3.6
5.3	3.3
5.4	3.0
5.5	2.8
5.6	2.6
5.7	2.5
5.8	2.4
5.9	2.4
6.0	2.4
6.1	2.4
6.2	2.4
6.3	2.3
6.4	2.3
6.5	2.2
6.6	2.1
6.7	2.7
6.8	3.1
6.9	3.8
7.0	4.6

* µS/cm (microSiemen per centimeter) = µmho/cm = reciprocal of Megohm-cm.

Courtesy, *USP Convention Water Quality Committee Pharmaceutical Forum*, Jan.-Feb. 1996

Such measurement can serve, therefore, as a substitute for chemical analysis.

However, each of the various ions has a different conductivity. It is impossible, therefore to quantify the different ion concentrations from a single conductivity reading of their mixtures. One can, however, ascribe the total conductivity to that ion having the lowest specific conductivity, thereby exaggerating in the calculation its actual concentration. Where limitations in ionic concentrations are sought, as in the subject water analysis, such a maximization of an ion's concentration translates to an exercise in prudence. It is to be encouraged.

It turns out that the conductivities of the several ions increase differently with pH. At pH 5.0 to 6.2, the chloride ion is the least conductive. From pH 6.3 to 7.0, it is the ammonium ion. Because the acceptable pH range for the com-pendial waters is from 5.0 to 7.0, the conductivity readings must be considered as reflecting a mixture of chloride and ammonium ions. (Figures 1-4 and 1-5)

Temperature also has an effect upon the equilibrium concentration and upon the specific conductivity of each ionic species. It becomes necessary, therefore, to couple the electrical conductivity reading with a temperature determination. The reference temperature is selected as being 25 °C. It is known how each of the ions increases in its conductivity as a function of temperature. If only a single type of ion were being measured, temperature compensation would consequently be possible. By way of suitable tables it could be learned what the conductivity of a given ion, measured at one temperature, would be at another. However, the different ions have conductivities that change differently with temperature. Therefore, for a mixture of ions, such as of chloride and ammonium, temperature compensation cannot be used. Actual conductivity readings will have to be performed at actual temperature readings.

For the chloride ion model the theoretical end point for the chloride ion in the *USP 23* silver nitrate test, 0.47 ppm, is 1.01-µS/cm conductivity. (The

Table 1-15
Levels for Carbon in Various Combined Forms at Which Water Will Still Pass the Oxidizable Substances Test.

Compound	*Maximum Level (mgC/L)*
Acetonitrile	>5000
Methanol	2500
Potassium hydrogen phthalate	500
Glucose	5
Sucrose	2.5
Sodium dodecylbenzenesulfonate	1

Crane et al. (1991); Courtesy, *J. Parenteral Science and Technology*

microsiemens-per-centimeter conductivity replaces the previous designation of 1 micromho per cm, 1 μMHO/cm, which is the reciprocal of resistivity expressed as megohms-cm). The attainment of the 1.01-μS/cm value based on the chloride (it being the lowest conductivity of the ionic species of concern) means that an acceptable level is also present for sulfate and calcium ions, ammonia, and carbon dioxide.

The pH of water containing only enough hydrogen ions to counter the 1.33×10^{-5} moles/L of chloride ions, corresponding to 1.01 μS/cm resistivity, limits the pH to below 5. Since the acceptable pH range of compendial waters is 5.0 to 7.0, such a water would thus have too low a pH. Counterions to the chloride other than hydrogen are therefore needed—for example, sodium and ammonium ions. The ammonium, sodium, and chloride ions were utilized in establishing the conductivity limits. However, carbon dioxide, ubiquitous in the atmosphere above the open water sample, also influences the water's conductivity.

Carbon dioxide in its equilibration with water yields a pH of 5.65 (some authorities give a lower value), it being the acid anhydride of carbonic acid. Carbon dioxide (CO_2) equilibrates with bicarbonate ions (HCO_3^-), carbonate ions, hydrogen ions, and thus with hydroxyl ions as well.

$$\begin{aligned} H_2O + CO_2 &\longleftrightarrow H_2CO_3 \\ H_2CO_3 &\longleftrightarrow H^+ + HCO_3^- \\ HCO_3^- &\longleftrightarrow H^+ + CO_3^{2-} \\ H_2O &\longleftrightarrow H^+ + OH^- \end{aligned} \qquad \text{Eq. 1-1}$$

Within the acceptable pH range of 5.0 to 7.0, the carbonate ion concentration is too low to be significant. Only H^+, OH^-, and HCO_3^- need be considered. The H^+ and OH^- concentrations can be obtained in terms of their equivalent conductivities from the pH. The bicarbonate ion concentration is also a function of pH.

The total conductivity attributable to dissolved carbon dioxide would be the sum of the conductivities of hydrogen ion, hydroxide ion, and bicarbonate ion. For the necessary condition of electrical neutrality, the sodium and ammonium ion would also be included. The conductivity contributed by the sodium and ammonium ion at any pH can be calculated. This value can be added to that of the chloride ion to define a maximum allowable conductivity at any specific pH level.

Similar reasoning applies to the ammonium ion model at pH 6.3 to 7.0 (WQC Jan.-Feb. 1996).

The total conductivity as a function of pH of a water exposed to the carbon dioxide of the atmosphere has been presented for both the chloride and ammonium ion models (Figure 1-5) by the Water Quality Committee of the Pharmaceutical Manufacturers Association, now the Pharmaceutical Research and

Manufacturing Association, PhRMA (WQC/PMA, Jan.-Feb. 1996). From these data upper conductivity limit specifications can be determined as a function of pH (Tables 1-13 and 1-14). These will be used to establish whether a pharmaceutical water is within its chemical and pH specifications. The pH of 5.0 in Table 1-5 has a total conductivity of 4.71 μS/cm. This value will fall to 2.38 at pH 6.0 and rises to 4.63 at pH 7.0. A correlation of pH values for waters and their acceptable corresponding upper limits of conductivity values are thus at hand as criteria against which to judge the compendial water purity.

These values apply to Water for Injection and to Purified Water but not to containerized pharmaceutical waters. The effect of the factors such as containers, leachables, time, exposure to light, and temperature over the period of storage requires assessment before those standards can be set.

Testing the suitability of the product water will be possible at each of three stages. Stage 1 will be assayed by on-line conductivity tests, a situation presumably free of the influences of carbon dioxide and its ionic pH and conductivity consequences. The temperature of the water will also be read directly, not compensated for. Comparisons will then be made of the conductivity/temperature values with those presented in an official table of acceptable levels. The conductivity at the temperature value equal to or less than the measured temperature will define the acceptable limit; ≤1.3 μS/cm at ≥25 °C (Table 1-13)..

If the conductivity is equal to or less than that tabulated value, the water quality will be acceptable. If it is greater, a Stage 2 determination will be made to see whether the higher conductivity is occasioned by the presence of carbon dioxide. In the Stage 2 assay, the water is stirred vigorously at 25 ± 1 °C to permit its complete equilibration with the atmospheric carbon dioxide. The attainment of equilibrations is measured by the leveling off of the periodically determined change in conductivity. When the net alteration becomes less than 0.1 μS/cm per

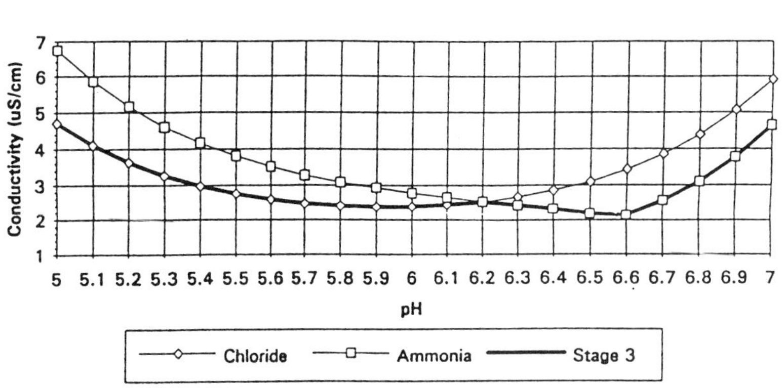

Figure 1-4. Chloride-ammonia conductivity-pH model.
Courtesy; *USP Convention Pharmaceutical Forum*, Nov.-Dec. 1965

5 minutes, the sample conductivity will be recorded. If it is no greater than 2.1 μS/cm, the water will be deemed to be acceptable. If the conductivity value is greater, the possible influence of pH will be ascertained in a Stage 3 assay.

Saturated potassium chloride will be added to the sample examined in the Stage 2 tests to enable its pH to be measured. Reference will be made to a predetermined pH/conductivity requirements (see Table 1-14) to find the acceptable conductivity limit at the measured pH level. Unless either the conductivity of the water is greater than the acceptable limit, or the pH is outside the 5.0 to 7.0 range, the water quality is judged to be proper. (See Figures 1-6 and 1-7)

By the same token, if at either of the earlier stages of testing the conductivity is found to be acceptable, then the pH, of necessity, must be within its proper range. Indeed, the original role of pH was to limit the concentration of ions not otherwise specifically identified. Therefore, the specific requirement to determine directly the pH of the water would seem to be redundant where the conductivity is suitable.

The acceptable limits were extrapolated from the old tests; it was not intended to tighten the requirements. The specified limits, with the possible exception of sodium and chloride, when these are high in quantity, can easily be met by the use of distillation, reverse osmosis, or ion exchange. Nevertheless some tightening does result. Thus, the presence of ammonia in amounts permitted by the USP chemical tests, namely 0.1 mg/L, may be too high to pass the conductivity test, 1 ppm of ammonia causing a reduction of 8 μS/cm in the resistivity of water (Disi, 1995) (see page 331).

The use of on-line conductivity instruments is advised against because of their limited functional range, their reliance upon automatic temperature compensations (previously discussed), and their insufficient appraisal of carbon dioxide concentrations. The more ready versatility of laboratory instruments is urged instead (WQC/PMA, 1991).

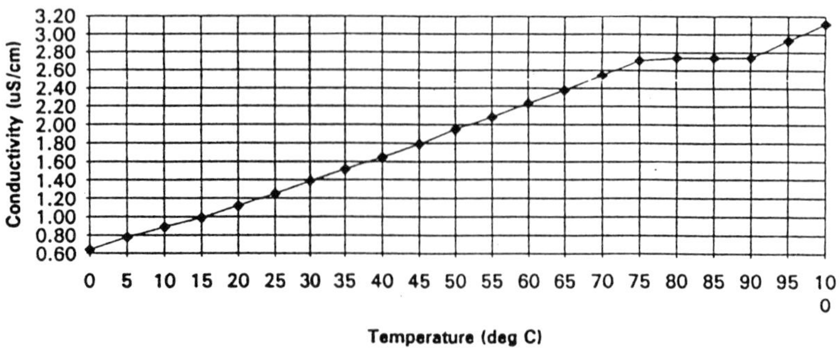

Figure 1-5. Stage 1 conductivity limit as a function of temperature.
Courtesy; *USP Convention Water Quality Committee Pharmaceutical Forum*, Jan.-Feb. 1996

The adoption of the proposed conductivity standards based on calculations involving the chloride ions will make more difficult harmonization with European practices. In Europe, chlorine is far less used than in the United States. Therefore, conductivities based on chloride ions are inappropriate. The nitrate ion is used instead. The acceptable conductivity values relative to pH are, consequently, different. A proposal to accommodate conductivity standards based on either chloride or nitrogen may enable harmonization.

Oxidizable substances/TOC measurements. The details of the Oxidizable Substance Test in the *USP 23* (p.1636) are as follows:"To 100 mL add 10 mL of 2N sulfuric acid, and heat to boiling. Add 0.1 mL N potassium permanganate, and boil for 10 minutes; the pink color does not completely disappear."

In actual operations the test may become obfuscated by suspended matter or colors other than pink. The end-point detection can be improved by the use of ultraviolet (UV)-visible spectra to detect the presence of permanganate, or by the filtrative removal of haze-forming particles of manganese dioxide and other colloids (Kenley et al., 1990) (see page 320).

The Oxidizable Substance Test is nonquantitative and lacks sensitivity. It serves as a go/no-go test, not yielding numbers whereby trend lines can be established. Crane (1989) stated that the amount of permanganate called for is sufficient to oxidize only 0.3 mg of carbon per liter in the standard 100-mL sample. The test's detection limits are about ten times grosser, however. Waters can pass the test to indicate an absence of oxidizables when they contain at least 1 mg of carbon per liter. Pharmaceutical waters and semiconductor rinsewaters may contain far less than that of carbon compounds (organics). In other words,

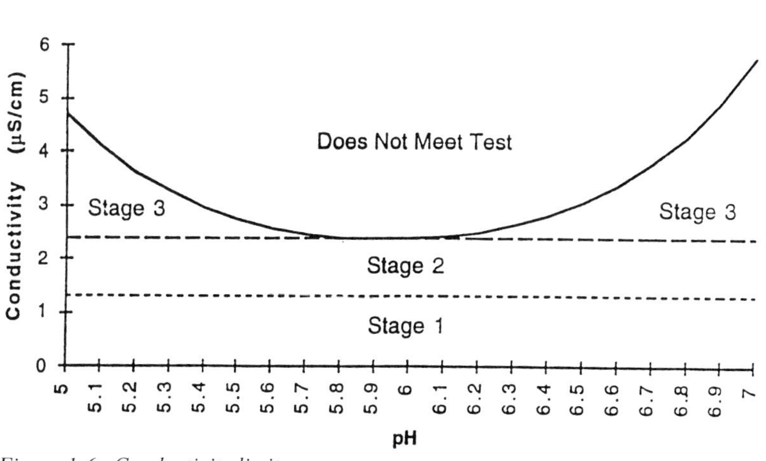

Figure 1-6. Conductivity limits.

Courtesy; *USP Convention Water Quality Committee Pharmaceutical Forum*, Jan.-Feb. 1996 the USP Oxidizable Substance Test does not function at current levels of water purity. Where the test is applicable, as shown in Table 1-15, organic compounds may give varying results because of their different susceptibilities to permanganate oxidation.

Detection of the presence of those oxidizable organics that are responsive to

Table 1-16
Some Physical Properties of the Volatile Pollutants

Systematic and Trivial Name	*Formula*	*m.w.*	*D o/rl*	*m.p. °C*	*b.p. °C*	*References*
Trichloromethane	$CHCl_3$ (chloroform)	119.38	1.446	-63	61.0	a
1,1,1-Trichloroethane	CH_3CCl_3	133.41	1.338	-50	75.0	a
Tetrachloromethane	CCl_4	153.82	1.594	-23	77.0	a
1,1,2-Trichloroethylene	$ClCH{=}CCl_2$	131.39	1.464	-87	86.9	a
Bromodichloromethane	$CHBrCl_2$	163.83	1.980	55	87.0	a
Bromotrichloromethane	$CBrCl_3$	198.28	2.012	-6	105.0	a
Chlorodibromomethane	$CHBr_2Cl$	208.29	2.451	-22	119.5	a
1,2-Dibromoethane	$BrCH_2CH_2Br$	187.64	2.160	8	131.5	a
Tetrachloroethylene	$Cl_2C{=}CCl_2$	165.83	1.623	-22	121.0	a
Tribromomethane (bromoform)	$CHBr_3$	252.75	2.894	8.3	150.5	a
Benzene		78.12	0.879	5.5	80.1	a
1,3-Dimethylbenzene		106.17	0.864	-47.9	139.1	a
1,4-Dimethylbenzene (p-xylene)		106.17	0.861	13.3	138.4	a
1,2-Dimethylbenzene (o-xylene)		106.17	0.850	-25.2	144.4	b
Methylbenzene		92.15	0.867	-95	110.6	c

a. Griesinger and Banks (1986). b. Weast (1976). c. Roller (1965).

Kroneld (1991); Courtesy, *J. Parenteral Science and Technology*.

this test is limited by the sensitivity of the test to only parts per million. In contrast, TOC analyzers utilized in the semiconductor industry are routinely used to detect 20 parts per billion of organics in semiconductor rinsewaters. Certain of these instruments are specified to detect 5 ppb, and actually measure even lower values when properly maintained (See Page 325).

TOC analysis. The use of TOC monitors will be substituted for the permanganate oxidizable substances test. The WQC/PMA found the technique capable of accurately analyzing a broad variety of organic compounds. The method is reliable and gives consistent results in interlaboratory testing. It is sensitive with a high degree of accuracy and precision.

Sucrose, an easily oxidizable specimen of TOC, is selected in a 500-ppb concentration as the standard for the TOC analysis. A more difficult to oxidize organic compound will serve as the standard for judging the suitability of the various TOC oxidizing systems and the TOC instruments themselves (see page 320). A TOC monitor will be judged adequate if it recovers at least 85% of the suitability standard in its analytical performance.

The organic compound intended to serve as the system suitability standard has undergone careful selection. The Japanese, the pioneers in this effort, use sodium dodecylbenzene sulfonate, an anionic surfactant often used in the cleaning of water systems. In order not to exclude any TOC instruments on the market, other TOC compounds were advanced for the suitability standard. One such compound is para benzoquinone.

The procedure is based upon the Japanese practice wherein 500 ppb of TOC is taken as the standard of acceptability. An examination of some 16 pharmaceutical water systems by the WQC/PMA revealed TOC levels of 50 to 200 ppb of TOC in final compendial water preparations; (an average of 107 ppb for PW, and

Table 1-17
Volatile Hydrocarbons in Some Essential Pharmaceutical Solutions as Hospital and Laboratory Solutions.

Substance n=23 µg/L	*Sodium Chlor. Isot. Rinse Sol.*	*Sodium Bicarb 7.5% Sol.*	*Sodium Citr. Rinse Sol.*	*Sodium Chlor. Physiol. Infusion Sol.*	*Aqua Sterilisata*
$CHCl_3$	4.40 ± 0.30	2.40 ± 0.20	2.10 ± 0.10	1.70 ± 0.08	5.30 ± 3.70
$CHBrCl_2$	0.07 ± 0.02	0.04 ± 0.01	0.05 ± 0.01	0.04 ± 0.02	0.03 ± 0.01
$CHBr_2Cl$	0.02 ± 0.01	0.02 ± 0.01	0.03 ± 0.01	0.02 ± 0.01	0.02 ± 0.01
$CHBr_3$	0.03 ± 0.01	0.1 ± 0.08	0.05 ± 0.01	0.02 ± 0.01	0.01 ± 0.01
CCl_4	0.02 ± 0.01	0.02 ± 0.01	0.03 ± 0.02	0.02 ± 0.01	0.01 ± 0.01
Cl_2=CCl_2	0.02 ± 0.01	0.01 ± 0.01	0.02 ± 0.01	0.03 ± 0.01	0.06 ± 0.02
CHCl-CHCl	0.02 ± 0.01	0.03 ± 0.02	0.01 ± 0.01	0.02 ± 0.01	0.03 ± 0.02

Kroneld (1991); Courtesy, *J. Parenteral Science and Technology*

an average of 87 ppb for WFI; the average plus 3 times the standard deviation equals to 450 ppb). The Japanese Pharmacopoeia establishes a limit of 500 ppb. The higher value was recommended to the USP. It would accord with the idea of international harmonization. It was felt that the 200-ppb level actually found in American water could be unnecessarily restrictive. Yet there are those who ask why the looser level of 500 ppb merits adoption when less than 200 ppb is already being achieved.

The Japanese use potassium biphthalate (potassium hydrogen phthalate) as the calibration standard for the TOC measurement. It is an easily oxidized organic compound. The WQC/PMA prefers sucrose for this purpose. An ion-containing standard was seen as possibly complicating the water conductivity measurement.

The term TOC represents a general classification. It becomes necesary to define it by way of some organic compound(s) considered typical, in terms of difficulty of oxidizability, of the organic materials that might be present in pharmaceutical waters. The chosen compound would be used to access the suitability of any TOC-measuring device proposed for application to this method.

Table 1-18
Different Methods Used in Eliminating Some Volatile Hydrocarbons from Water

Substance mg/L n = 20	*After Treatment: Tap Water*	*After Treatment: Distillation, Traditional*	*After Treatment: Water Softening*
$CHCl_3$	67.7 ± 0.6	69.1 ± 0.9	44.9 ± 0.6
$CHBrCl_2$	10.8 ± 0.5	11.1 ± 0.6	9.7 ± 0.5
$CHBr_2Cl$	2.4 ± 0.4	2.5 ± 0.3	1.6 ± 0.3

Substance mg/L n = 20	*After Treatment: Active Charcoal Filtering*	*After Treatment: Reverse Osmosis*	*After Treatment: Paper Filtering*	*After Treatment: Used Dialysis Fluid*
$CHCl_3$	47.1 ± 0.7	38.1 ± 1.2	37.9 ± 0.8	37.3 ± 1.3
$CHBrCl_2$	9.8 ± 0.5	7.8 ± 0.5	7.9 ± 0.4	7.5 ± 0.5
$CHBr_2Cl$	1.7 ± 0.4	1.4 ± 0.3	1.4 ± 0.3	1.4 ± 0.3

Crane et al., (1991); Courtesy, *J. Parenteral Science and Technology*

The intention is not to exclude any TOC instrument by the selection of an unnecessarily difficult-to-oxidize organic compound. This can also avoid restraint of trade considerations. However, the selection of the least common denominator in TOC instruments is also being avoided. A balance is being sought.

The Japanese use difficult-to-oxidize dodecylbenzene sulfonate, as ionic (anionic) surfactant, as the suitability standard. It is often used as a cleaning agent for water systems. As stated, the current preference is for an avoidance of ion-containing standards. The WQC/PMA (May-June 1994) recommended Octoxynol-9RS, a nonionic surfactant, as a substitute. The gratuitous introduction of ions, a possible complication to conductivity measurements, is thereby avoided. However, not all TOC instruments seem capable of detecting its standard concentration within the desired range of 80% to 115%. The 5% disparity in the ±15% range recognizes some loss by adsorption to glassware.

Its strong adsorption to the glassware used in the TOC procedure was found to be unnecessarily complicating. It was felt a molecularly well defined, water-soluble solid would be preferable. (Most surfactants are mixtures of multimolecular species.)

A choice was made from among 1,4-benzoquinone, α-naphthylresorcinol, and o-octyl-β-D-glucopyranoside, based on a widespread laboratory evaluation. The reference compound selected for the instrument suitability test was 1,4-benzoquinone. It has the useful properties of being a powder at room temperature, is readily available in pure form, is relatively safe to handle, and is well defined chemically. In the multilaboratory testing exercise its average recovery was the lowest among the organic compounds examined. Its use as a standard for the TOC suitability test therefore suggests the greatest challenge to oxidation. This presents a prudent choice to the subject of TOC determinations (WQC/

Table 1-19
Average Reduction (%) of Some Volatile Hydrocarbons and Benzene Derivatives during Elimination Tests with EVP Equipment

Model Compounds Tested n = 12	*Distillate with One EVP Unit*	*Distillate with Two EVP Units*
Volatile hydrocarbons		
$CHCl_3$	98.4	99.1
$CHBrCl_2$	99.8	99.7
$CHBr_2Cl$	98.9	98.8
$CHCl_3$	77.4	86.5
Benzene derivatives		
Touene	41.7	85.8
Total	96.0	97.1

Kroneld (1991); Courtesy, *J. Parenteral Science and Technology*

PhRMA, 1996). To attest to the suitability of a TOC instrument, the suitability standard would require being detected to the extent of 100 ±15% by that measuring device.

The recommended standard would apply to the total organic carbon measured as NPOC (non-purgeable oxidizable carbon) for nonpackaged Purified Water and Water for Injection. The setting of TOC standards for containerized pharmaceutical water must await a more extended testing experience over time.

Volatile organics (see page 318). In the differentiation between organic and inorganic carbon, a distinction necessary to the accurate determination of TOC, the presence of purgeable organics must be considered lest some TOC be lost by volatization (Cohen, 1995). The operations and manipulations involved in the TOC analyses are beyond the scope of this writing. However, the subject of volatile TOC merits treatment.

Total organic carbon can consist of some proportion of volatile or purgeable organic compounds. Volatile contaminants such as the lower hydrocarbons, their chlorinated derivatives such as the trihalomethanes, and various benzene compounds can each and all be present in high-purity waters. The chlorinated molecules may derive from the addition of the chlorine intended as a biocide. Other molecules, highly oxidized (such as epoxides, peroxides, and various oxygenated structures) may be formed by the action of ozone. It has been known that the injection of such volatile organics (contained in high-purity water used for pharmaceutical preparations) results in body burdens of long duration. Being lipophilic, they become stored in the fatty tissues of the injected humans, leading to long-term exposures.

Table 1-16 presents a listing of such volatile organics and some of their properties. Kroneld (1991) analyzed a collection of pharmaceutical solutions from hospitals and laboratories for their volatile organic contents. The presence of the trihalomethanes and certain other chlorinated volatile organics was evident, as shown in Table 1-17.

Such purgeable organic compounds might escape analysis by certain of the TOC instruments because of their volatilization and loss under the oxidative conditions characteristic of these instruments. The WQC/PMA survey discloses, however, that only 8 or 9% of the TOC are volatile, and that only 5% would be expected to exceed 20 ppb. It is concluded, therefore, that the influence of

* Kroneld (1991) analyzed the blood samples of patients undergoing hemodialysis. It was found that the volatile organics accumulated in the patients' blood during the 2 to 3 times weekly treatments. Table 1-18 illustrates different methods used to eliminate volatile organics from aqueous solutions. The investigator found most efficacious the use of an airstream flowing countercurrent to the feedwater being cleansed. This method also efficiently removed the fugacious organics, as shown in Table 1-19. The coupling of this "eliminator of volatile pollutants" (EVP) as a pretreatment to water being directed to distillation is advocated. The temperature of the water being treated was at 130 °C under 5-bar pressure (72.5 psig), and the water-to-air ratio was 1.5. Carcinogenic, mutagenic, and teratogenic properties have been imputed to volatile organics in pharmaceutical contexts; as has their interference in cell culture work.

purgeable organic carbon on the TOC determinations of pharmaceutical waters can be ignored.*

Drinking water as feedwater sources. Currently, USP Purified Water must start with water that complies with the EPA's National Primary Drinking Water Regulations (EPA NPDWR). Source water is not specified in the *USP 23* monographs for WFI or its various sterile derivatives. However, *USP 23* in its informational chapter (p. 1984) states, "Drinking water, which is subject to federal EPA regulations and which is delivered by the municipal or other local public system or drawn from a private well or reservoir, is the starting material for most forms of water covered by Pharmacopoeial monographs. Water prepared from other starting materials may have to be processed to meet drinking water standards."

Coliform testing. USP Purified Water had been required to be tested as being free of coliforms. However, it was also specified that the potable water from which the Purified Water is prepared must be free of coliforms. The testing of the prepared Purified Water for coliforms was, therefore, redundant. Cooper (February 1993) emphasize that "the relevance of the coliform test is based upon its function as an indicator of occult mammalian pathogens, either bacterial or virus in origin." Therefore, the only reason to again perform the test for coliforms would be to ensure against the unlikely occurrence of fecal contamination after the potable water was at hand. This requirement was eliminated (*USP XXII*, Ninth Supplement).

It is proposed that all forms of USP water initially utilize source water meeting the quality attribute requirements of the EPA NPDWR, which will be set forth. This source water would be exempt from requirements that it contain additives such as chlorine, provided that quality attributes guarded by these additives are suitably met and maintained.

***Pseudomonas* presence**. The FDA had stated that the presence of *Pseudomonas* in WFI would be cause for its rejection. There was objection to this ruling since these organisms are native to waters; their presence to some small extent could be expected and may be innocuous. Whether WFI containing some *Pseudomonas* is acceptable or not will be decided on a case-by-case basis, by considering the intended use of the product to be formulated. Munson (1993) statc that FDA does not require that no *Pseudomonas* species be present in the water system. Indeed, that species need not be monitored for specifically unless the presence of such organisms represent hazard to the product. The presence of pseudomonads in topicals would be objected to, *Pseudomonas aeruginosa* having been implicated in the infection of abraded skin or wounds. The water system needs to be free only of those organisms that represent potential pathogens in the products involved. (See, however, page 123, Objectionable Organisms.)

Added substances. The USP monograph on Purified Water stipulates that "it contains no added substances." This is interpreted by some as meaning that no chemical or reagents of any kind are to be added. Actually, chemical additives of many sorts are used, whether as flocculating agents, for water softening, to avoid mineral scale, to control microbial growth, or to regulate pH, etc. What is required is simply that the added chemicals should be removed in subsequent processing steps (WQC/PMA, 1993). Monitoring steps should be part of the water purification system to make sure that such removals are effected.

The PW monograph unambiguously states of PW that "It contains no added substances." There are those who believe, however, that chlorine is not a foreign substance in Purified Waters prepared from chlorinated potable water. It is likely that FDA inspectors will disagree.

The USP limitations against chloride ions in PW would seem in themselves to rule against the presence of chlorine, for that substance undergoes reaction with water to form chloride ions, as expressed below.

$$H_2O + Cl_2 \longleftrightarrow H^+ + Cl^- + HOCl \qquad \text{Eq. 1-2}$$

Furthermore, chlorine is an oxidant. It reacts with various substances and becomes reduced, generating chloride ions. The chief objection to the presence of chlorine in PW is its potential degradative action upon the drug product formulated with that water.

Increasingly, ozone is being used in place of chlorine. Its presence could also constitute an added substance were it not for its short half-life. Its destructive

Table 1-20
Maximum Contaminant Levels (MCL) for Drinking Water

Element	*EPA MCL*
Silver	100 ppb
Arsenic	50 ppb
Cadmium	5 ppb
Copper	1,000 ppb
Mercury	2 ppb
Lead	50 ppb
Bismuth	none
Antimony	none
Molybdenum	none
Tin	none

Source: WQC/PMA 1992b. Courtesy of the United States Pharmacopoeia Convention, Inc.

Table 1-21
Summary of National Primary Drinking Water Regulations
(as of July 1990)

Contaminant	*MCLGs*[1,5]	*SMCLs*[1,6]
	(In mg/L unless otherwise noted)	
Microbiological Contaminants		
Coliforms (total)	0	1/100 mL
Giardia lamblia	0	TT[3]
HPC	—	TT[3]
Legionella	0	TT[3]
Virus	0	TT[3]
Turbidity	—	1.5 NTU
Inorganic Contaminants		
Arsenic	—	0.05
Barium	—	1
Cadmium	—	0.010
Chromium	—	0.05
Fluoride	4.0	4.0
Lead	—	0.05
Mercury	—	.002
Nitrate	—	010
Selenium	—	0.01
Silver	—	0.05
Organic Contaminants		
2,4-D	—	0.1
Endrin	—	0.0002
Lindane	—	0.004
Methoxychlor	—	0.1
2,4,5-TP Silvex	—	0.01
Benzene	0	0.005
Carbon tetrachloride	0	0.005
p-Dichlorobenzene	0.075	0.075
1,2-Dichloroethane	0	0.005
1,1-Dichloroethylene	0.007	0.007
1,1,1-Trichloroethane	0.20	0.20
Trichloroethylene	0	0.005
Vinyl chloride	0	0.002
Total trihalomethanes	—	0.10
(Chloroform, bromoform, bromodichloromethane, dibromochloromethane)		
Radionuclides		
Gross alpha particle activity	—	15 pCi/L
Gross beta particle activity	—	4 mrem/yr
Radium 226 and 228 (total)	—	5 pCi/L

MCLG--Maximum Containment Level Goals
SMCLs--Secondary Maximum Containment Levels
Courtesy, *Water Technology* magazine

removal by the action of UV light of 254-nanometer (nm) wavelength would require analytical substantiation. There is some question regarding the reliability of ozone detectors, as they themselves undergo ozone attack. Ozone can be analyzed reliably using wet chemistry (Rice et al., 1986).

Heavy metals. Concern with heavy metals arises from the baleful effects of these elements upon human (or animal) physiology. The USP test for heavy metals, essentially unaltered since its introduction in 1900, measures those elements that produce colored sulfides in slightly acidic solutions. These elements and their Maximum Contamination Levels (MCL) as set by EPA, are shown in Table 1-20 (WQC/PMA, 1992b). The USP stipulates that Purified Water is to be prepared from waters that conform to the EPA standards for potable water. However, the EPA limits exceed in their degree of restriction the test sensitivity of the USP detection, which registers at the parts per million (ppm) level. EPA does require testing for antimony and may come to set limits on that element. It does not currently monitor bismuth, tin, or molybdenum. The EPA heavy-metal regulations are appropriate requirements as well for the potable source water intended for Purified Water and for Water for Injection preparation.

A PMA survey indicates that stainless steels, polytetrafluoroethylene (PTFE), and polyvinylidene fluoride (PVDF), the very materials used in pharmaceutical water systems because of their degrees of inertness to water, do not contribute

Table 1-22
National Secondary Drinking Water Regulations

Turbidity: not more than 1 NTU as a monthly average, or not more than 5 NTU as an average of 2 consecutive days.

NTU is a nephelometric turbidity unit, a measure of the amount of light that is reflected off the water. The turbidity standard applies only to systems using surface water. See Appendix D, Surface Water Treatment Rule, for upcoming changes to the turbidity standard.

Total coliform: For fermentation tube method; not more than 10% of tubes can be positive per month or not more than 3 tubes* positive in more than one sample per month.

For membrane filter method; not more than 1 per 100 mL as a monthly average or not more than 4 per 100 mL* in more than one sample per month.

*These levels trigger a check-sampling requirement.

A result of TNTC (too numerous to count) or CG(confluent growth) may be considered coliform-positive or an invalid sample, in wh'ch case another sample would be required.

Some regulatory agencies calculate a quarterly average instead of a monthly average.

The revised total coliform standard goes into effect on December 31, 1990.

heavy metals to the prepared water. Furthermore, the PMA survey indicated that of 32 plant locations none reported confirmed failures of their Purified Water preparations attributable to heavy-metal contents (WQC/PMA, 1992b). On the basis of these findings, the Water Quality Committee proposed that heavy-metal testing be deleted from the USP bulk pharmaceutical water examinations. However, where heavy metals may be present, the potable water source must periodically be monitored. Lead contamination from pipe and lead fluxes used in piping joints is to be avoided.

Although the routine testing for heavy metals is eliminated, the responsibility for testing, when it is significant and appropriate, falls upon the drug manufacturer.

Aluminum testing. Source waters, particularly potable waters, can be high in their aluminum content, if only as a result of being treated with alum. However, the aluminum is easily removed (see page 47). The WQC/PMA points out that water is not the primary source of aluminum in pharmaceutical products, and that the quantity of aluminum contributed by the bulk waters is less than 5 ppb (parts per billion), a level below that associated with physiological effects (WQC/PMA, 1992c). Packaged pharmaceutical waters contain 5 ppb or less. It appears, therefore, that aluminum testing for the compendial waters is not required.

The large-volume parenterals include peritoneal dialysates. Individuals primarily at risk for aluminum toxicity are patients on hemodialysis or peritoneal

Table 1-23
National Secondary Drinking Water Regulations SMCLs*

Contaminant	*level*
Chloride	250 mg/L
Color	15 color units
Copper	1 mg/L
Corrosivity	non-corrosive
Fluoride	2 mg/L
Foaming agents	0.5 mg/L
Iron	0.3 mg/L
Manganese	0.05 mg/L
Odor	3 threshhold odor number
pH	6.5-8.5 pH units
Sulfate	250 mg/L
Total dissolved solids (TDS)	500 mg/L
Zinc	5 mg/L

*Secondary Maximum Contaminant Levels (SMCLs) are federally nonenforceable; and establish, for contaminants in drinking water, limits that may affect the aesthetic qualities and the public's acceptance of drinking water (e.g., taste and odor).

Courtesy, *U.S. Environmental Protection Agency, EPA, 1990*

dialysis, those on long-term parenterals nutrition, and premature infants. The FDA has recommended a limit of 25 micrograms per liter (µg/L), or 25 ppb of aluminum for large-volume parenterals. Assuming an estimated administration of three liters per day, the aluminum is estimated variously to be from 30 to 80 or from 90 to 100 µg per day. The matter is still under FDA investigation and study (WQC/PMA, 1992c). It had not, at present, been endorsed.

Other Potable Water Impurities. Table 1-21 presents a summary of the National Primary Drinking Water Regulations. Table 1-22 sets forth maximum contaminant levels given under the National Secondary Drinking Water Regulations (NSDWR) for several inorganic and organic contaminants. for several inorganic and organic contaminants. Table 1-23 presents the NSDWR in terms of specific contaminants such as certain metals, and their acceptable maximum levels. The NPDWR differ from the NSDWR in that the Secondary Maximum Contamination Levels (SMCLs) are federally unenforceable. Their levels reflect the water's aesthetic qualities and the public's acceptance thereof. A listing of unregulated contaminants plus surface-water treatment rules and the requirements of the Safe Drinking Water Act, its standards and its reporting procedures are available (EPA, 1990). The concerns are with regard to these potable-water impurities being carried over into compendial waters during their preparation.

Disadvantages of EPA-regulated feedwaters. The USP is an organization whose activity is based on standards. The reliance on EPA-regulated drinking water serves this need. But what if the EPA were to change its standards or even eliminate them, unlikely though it be? There are those who believe the USP should develop its own standards. This would free pharmaceutical houses from the need to perform a multiplicity of tests required by the EPA that are not germane to pharmaceutical usages. As of now, many pharmaceutical manufacturers using well waters feel compelled to perform the entire series of EPA drinking-water tests. Others eliminate the performance of those tests they consider irrelevant. The USP, it is argued, could better define the pertinent tests and secure a more universal adherence thereto. However, if this were done, it would become neccessary again to reinstitute testing for coliforms and heavy metals. The development of a test list by USP would involve a very sizable undertaking.

Large-volume parenterals. Water for Injection is copiously used in the formulation of large-volume parenterals (LVPs). These are preparations intended for the intravenous injection of humans in single doses of 100 mL or more. They are terminally sterilized in single-dose containers, at present exclusively by thermal means. Actually, the term LVPs is meant to include IV infusions, irrigating solutions, peritoneal dialysates, and blood-collecting units containing anticoagulants (Code of Fed. Regs., 21 CFR Part 212, June 1976).

The USP does not use the term "large-volume parenterals." It advisedly says "large-volume intravenous solutions," thereby effectively excluding other uses such as irrigation solutions and peritoneal dialysates (*USP 23*, p. 1650).

Endotoxin level. The WFI endotoxin limits had originally been set at 0.50 EU/mL to be equivalent to the pyrogenic sensitivity of the rabbit test then in use. Although the gel clot limulus amebocyte lysate (LAL) test has a sensitivity of 0.03 EU/mL, the higher (0.5 EU/mL) limit was set to make the substitution of the LAL test for the rabbit test more easily adopted.

However, in the preparation of large-volume parenterals wherein added ingredients are diluted by the WFI, the possibility exists that the added drug components could themselves contribute endotoxin. The standard for the WFI was therefore set lower, at 0.25 EU/mL, so that actual LVPs would not exceed 0.5 EU/mL.

Actually, most WFI as now prepared contains less than 0.001 EU/mL of endotoxin, as measured by more sensitive LAL methods such as kinetic turbidimetry (Gould, 1990). It would be regrettable if the setting of the 0.25 EU/mL standard for WFI served to permit the present level of higher manufacturing quality to slip. The purer water is, in any case, necessary to serve as a standard.

An LVP solution as administered (IV over 1 hour) with its additives (up to six or even eight are used at times) should not result in the patient having to receive more than 5 EU per kilogram (kg) of body weight. At an EU level of 0.50 EU/mL, a 70-kg (154-pound) person could receive more than 7 EU/kg. Human studies show that 5 EU/kg may be too high a limit. A more suitable limit would be 4 EU/kg (Outschoorn, 1990).

References to endotoxin testing are increasingly referred to, more accurately, as bacterial endotoxin testing (BET).

Sterile Water for Injection. Notwithstanding statements made under "Packaging and Storing," Purified Water and Water for Injection are not distributed in containers. They serve as pharmaceutical ingredients, rather than as compendial dosage forms.

According to its *USP 23* monograph (p. 1636), Sterile Water for Injection is Water for Injection sterilized and suitably packaged. It is to be packaged in single-dose containers of not larger than 1 liter. It contains no antimicrobial agent or other added substance, and its endotoxin content is not to exceed 0.25 EU/mL.

The intended purposes of Sterile WFI are set forth in *USP 23* (p. 1984) in the informational text concerning it. Sterile WFI serves as a solvent for solids that must be distributed dry because of their instability in solution form. The Sterile WFI label must state that it is not suitable for intravascular injection without first having been rendered approximately isotonic *USP 23* (p. 1636).

Sterile WFI is a finished drug product, whereas WFI is a drug component. Sterile WFI is WFI rendered sterile by treatment intended specifically to render it sterile. This requirement also pertains to all the other sterile waters listed in the USP water monographs.

Bacteriostatic Water for Injection. As stated by its *USP 23* monograph (p 1636), Bacteriostatic WFI (BWFI) is Sterile WFI containing one or more suitable antimicrobial agents. It may be dispensed as single or multiple doses from containers not exceeding 30 mL in volume. The containers are to be suitably labeled as to the type and proportion of the antimicrobial agent contained, and the label is also to bear the legend "NOT FOR USE IN NEWBORNS."

As set forth in the *USP 23* general information section (p. 1984), Bacteriostatic WFI has the same standards as does Sterile WFI with the exception of its containerization. It is intended essentially for the same purposes.

When the constituted solution is designed for parenteral applications, Sterile WFI must be used. Otherwise, preparations made with the Bacteriostatic Water for Injection are employed. The Bacteriostatic WFI is limited to containers of 30 mL because of its antimicrobial ingredients. However, Sterile WFI, not being safeguarded against invading organisms by an antimicrobial agent, may be containerized only in single-dose packages of no larger than 1 liter. The compatibility of the antimicrobial agent with the drug substance with which the BWFI is to be used is an important consideration, although not detailed within the monograph.

Other sterile waters. The *USP 23* (pp. 1636-1637) also designates Sterile Water for Irrigation and Sterile Water for Inhalation. These types of pharmaceutical waters essentially meet all the standards of Sterile Water for Injection, except that they may be packaged in volumes in excess of 1 liter and must be suitably labeled as to their purpose. A summary of what is expected of Sterile Water for Irrigation

Table 1-24
Sterile Water for Irrigation

- Is WFI-sterilized and suitably packaged
- Single-dose containers may exceed 1 L
- Endotoxin limit 0.25 EU/mL
- Contains no antimicrobial agent or added substance
- Labled ("For Irrigation Only, Not for Injection")
- No particulate standards

Courtesy, Dr. R. Dabbah, USP Convention

and Sterile Water for Inhalation is given in Tables 1-24 and 1-25.

In addition, a new pharmaceutical bulk water classification, Sterile Purified Water, will be created. Its chemical composition will be defined by the characteristics common to that of Purified Water.

Water for washing and rinsing. Washing and rinsing constitute another pharmaceutical water use not involving water as a drug ingredient or dosage form. Its use in pharmaceutical manufacture requires conformation to federal regulations, not to compendial standards.

Potable water is suitable for initial cleaning and rinsing provided its microbial content can be maintained under control. If necessary, the addition of chlorine or the use of heat can be resorted to. Obviously, the use of hot water offers the advantage of better cleaning.

Water for initial cleaning and rinsing bears no regulatory requirements for chemical purity in excess of potable water. It should suffice at least for washing of non-product-contact surfaces, such as floors or walls, in conjunction with soaps or cleaners.

In accordance with the guidance of 21CFR212.224 of the Good Manufacturing Practices proposed (but never finalized) for Large-Volume Parenterals, water used for cleaning or initial rinsing of drug-product-contact surfaces shall:

- Meet the stipulations prescribed in the EPA Standards for drinking water.
- Be subjected to a process such as chlorination for control of the microbial population.
- Contain not more than 50 microorganisms/100 mL.

Purified Water USP or WFI is sometimes used for all phases of cleaning when usage is low or no other pretreatment is available. The most common practice

Table 1-25
Sterile Water for Inhalation

- Prepared by distillation or RO and rendered sterile
- Contains no antimicrobials except where liable to contamination (e.g., humidifiers, long-term usage)
- Single-dose containers
- Endotoxin limit 0.5 EU/mL
- Not for compendial dosage forms
- Labeled ("Not for Parenteral Administration")
- Other specifications similar to USP Purified Water

Courtesy, Dr. R. Dabbah, USP Convention

in the pharmaceutical industry is to use softened or single-pass RO water for prerinse, wash solution, and all postrinses except the final rinse, which is by Purified Water USP for nonsterile products, and WFI for sterile products.

Cooper (1996) advises that equipment washed with USP Purified Water but left wet for extended periods can result in microbial colonization; particularly flexible hoses left in coiled configurations. He suggests disinfection with isopropanol, efficiently applied in spray form.

Microbial levels of WFI and Purified Water. The microbial levels for Water for Injection is set at 10 cfu/100 mL. That for Purified Water is referenced at 100 cfu/mL. In the case of Purified Water the acceptable level will, in each instance, be judged in accordance with the specific application to which the water will be directed.

It should clearly be understood that these stated microbial levels are not intended to be pass/fail limits (*USP 23*, p. 1984). Their purpose is to serve in the establishment and ongoing monitoring of the pharmaceutical water system's trend lines, in conjunction with set alert and action limits.

Water for drug-product cooling. In 1976 the FDA proposed the GMPs for LVPs. Mindful of a then-recent drug recall, it specified microbial limits of 1.0 cfu/100 mL for the drug-product-cooling water. From a practical point of view, concerns about endotoxin were muted. A suitable drug-product-cooling water can be composed of very heavily chlorinated Purified Water. Water for Injection should also serve this purpose. A complete absence of microbes from the water is desired.

Water for bulk chemicals. Regulations are in their rudimentary stage concerning the quality of the water used in the manufacture of bulk pharmaceutical chemicals (BPC) designed ultimately for compounding injectable preparations. The USP stated only that the water used must be of potable water quality. "Drinking water may be used in the preparation of USP drug substances but not in the preparation of dosage forms." (*USP 23*, p. 1984, General Information section). More recently, the FDA Mid-Atlantic Region issued a draft of a "Guide to Inspection of Bulk Pharmaceutical Chemicals" (FDA, March 1991). It stated, "While the USP allows the use of potable or drinking water in the preparation of BPCs, microbial content is of concern. The process water system should be validated. If the final BPC will be used for parenteral products, the potential presence of pyrogens or endotoxins are an additional concern. Routine sampling of the process water and testing for the presence of endotoxins, preferably by the Limulus Amebocyte Lysate (LAL) method, is indicated."

It was noted that the dosage-form manufacturer is "highly dependent upon the BPC producer to provide bulk substances uniform in chemical and physical characteristics." Validation of the process water system is required to demonstrate that it is adequately designed and controlled to produce efficiently water of the required reduced endotoxin levels. This will automatically involve validation of its control microbial content. "End product testing alone is not permitted in the dosage form manufacturing and control process....An end point test for a critical factor such as endotoxin contamination of the bulk substance defeats the quality control procedures employed at the dosage form manufacturer." The FDA inspectors are directed, by this guide, to require justification of the belief that "the process works and works consistently providing adequate control over potential endotoxin development." Since endotoxin normally originates from Gram-negative organisms, this last quotation comes to mean that the microbial validation of the process water system is also required.

Normally, the drug manufacturer, the preparer of the injectable, stipulates the endotoxin level permissible in the bulk pharmaceutical chemical purchased, as from a chemical supplier. The FDA might become involved with the chemical supplier only if the records at the drug preparer indicate problems with the properties of the drug substance. The inspections of product failure or batch rejection records at the pharmaceutical preparer or the customer complaint files usually serve as focal points for an FDA inspectional visit to the bulk pharmaceutical manufacturer. The Mid-Atlantic Region's Guide states, "The inspection of a BPC operation should be the same, whether or not that BPC is referenced as the active ingredient in a pending NDA or ANDA." Overall, the inspection "must determine the bulk substance manufacturer's capability to deliver a product that consistently meets the specifications of the bulk drug substance." Obviously, the bulk pharmaceutical chemical manufacturer will not be permitted to cull good batches from bad. The BPC production must be validated, as also the water process it is part of.

No special compendial water type need be used by the BPC manufacturer; neither Purified Water nor WFI, for instance. However, the process water must be validated as providing the restricted endotoxin and organism counts necessary to the quality of the BPC. Therefore, the preparations of water by the use processes such as of RO, ultrafiltration, and electrodeionization can all serve adequately, provided they are validated with respect to organisms and endotoxins. (See page 520).

Regardless of which procedure is employed to furnish the BPC process water, its storage at elevated temperatures, 65 to 85 °C, would serve to ensure the preservation of its microbiological quality, as would also cold ozonated storage.

The FDA in its "Guide To Inspection Of High Purity Water Systems" (July 1993) says the following about the water concerns connected with bulk pharmaceutical chemical production:

> Currently, the USP, pg. 4, in the General Notices Section, allows

drug substances to be manufactured from Potable Water. It comments that any dosage form must be manufactured from Purified Water, Water For Injection, or one of the forms of Sterile Water. There is some inconsistency in these two statements, since Purified Water has to be used for the granulation of tablets, yet Potable Water can be used for the final purification of the drug substance.

It, the FDA Guide to Inspection of Bulk Pharmaceutical Chemicals, comments on the concern for the quality of the water used for the manufacture of drug substances, particularly those drug substances used in parenteral manufacture. Excessive levels of microbiological and/or endotoxin contamination have been found in drug substances, with the source of contamination being the water used in purification. At this time, Water For Injection does not have to be used in the finishing steps of synthesis/purification of drug substances for parenteral use. However, such water systems used in the final stages of processing of drug substances for parenteral use should be validated to assure minimal endotoxin/ microbiological contamination.

In the bulk drug substance industry, particularly for parenteral grade substances, it is common to see Ultrafiltration (UF) and Reverse Osmosis (RO) systems in use in water systems. While ultrafiltration may not be as efficient at reducing pyrogens, they will reduce the high molecular weight endotoxins that are a contaminant in water systems. As with RO, UF is not absolute, but it will reduce numbers. Additionally, as previously discussed with other cold systems, there is considerable maintenance required to maintain the system.

For the manufacture of drug substances that are not for parenteral use, there is still a microbiological concern, although not to the degree as for parenteral grade drug substances. In some areas of the world, Potable (chlorinated) water may not present a microbiological problem. However, there may be other issues. For example, chlorinated water will generally increase chloride levels. In some areas, process water may be obtained directly from neutral sources.

In one inspection, a manufacturer was obtaining process water from a river located in a farming region. At one point, they had a problem with high levels of pesticides which was (sic) a run-off from farms in the areas. The manufacturing process and analytical methodology was not designed to remove and identify trace pesticide contaminants. Therefore, it would seem that this process water when used in the purification of drug substances would be unacceptable.

Potable Waters Preparation

The USP monograph on Purified Water states that "it is to be prepared from water complying with the regulations of the Federal Environmental Protection Agency with respect to drinking water." Indeed, many pharmaceutical manufacturers prepare their compendial waters from municipally treated water supplies (potable water). It may be profitable, therefore, to consider what is generally involved in producing water of potable quality from raw water sources, and to explore what impact such treatments may have on subsequent high-purity water preparations. The preparation of potable water usually consists of treatment of the source water with an oxidant to remove undesirable tastes and odors (algae, for instance, confer a fishy, musty taste), followed by the clarification of the water by the agglomeration of suspended and colloidal matter, generally by alum treatment. This is succeeded by removal of the flocculated solid particles by deep-bed filtration, usually through sand. A chlorine or other biocide residual is then added, and the pH is adjusted before the water is released for distribution.

Oxidation for taste and odor. Raw source waters in water authority or municipal treatment plants are first treated to destroy objectionable tastes and odors. Treatment with oxidant also reduces the total organism counts to less than 100 cfu/mL, in conformity with EPA goals.* Traditionally, this was, and often still is, achieved by the addition of gaseous chlorine to the water to concentrations of 5 to 10 milligrams per liter (mg/L), or 5 to 10 ppm. The discovery that the organic impurities present in waters were oxidatively modified by chlorine into "potentially" carcinogenic trihalomethanes (THM), such as chloroform, resulted in EPA regulating such contents to a maximum of 0.1 ppm or 100 ppb. This restriction seems likely to be made more severe, to 50 or even 25 ppb of THM. Some water treatment plants substitute other oxidants for chlorine in order to avoid THM formation. Potassium permanganate has found a limited use. Chlorine dioxide has been tried. It seems, however, to give rise to taste and odor problems of its own. Some efforts, at least in research endeavors, utilize hydrogen peroxide, and hydrogen peroxide in combination with ozone. Ozone itself has been applied for this purpose for some 80 years in France. Experimental facilities are being installed in several places, including Fairfax County, Virginia, to study the efficacy of ozone for this application. The chief impediments to the use of ozone are the capital expenditures involved in its on-site generation. More recently, these costs have moderated as a result of advances in the design of ozone generation equipment. By and large, however, chlorine gas is still used as a primary oxidant. Indeed, it has been advocated by some that, to enable the

* This treatment also serves to reduce the heterotrophic organism count and to kill *E. coli* and fecal coliforms. The EPA Maximum Contaminant Level goal is zero organisms. Actually, low hererotrophic counts of some 10 to 20 cfu/mL are hoped for. However, in recognition of the practical realities involved (e.g., sampling), 100 to 500 cfu/mL are accepted for heterotrophic counts. *E. coli* or fecal coliform counts are to be at zero, the presence of these organisms being interpreted as signifying the presence of pathogenic microbes derived from fecal contamination.

continuing use of chlorine, the organic mater should first be removed as much as possible from the raw water by filtration.

The removal of organic matter from the water prior to chlorination not only conserves the use of chlorine and minimizes its costs, but creates less of the objectionable chlorinated by-products, such as the trihalomethanes. This is the practice of several large metropolitan areas, including a large Swiss city that draws its water from the Rhine river, which is overabundant in organic materials.

The oxidation step is also depended upon to convert soluble iron and manganese ions to their insoluble forms. Soluble iron and manganese have no untoward health implications, but their early precipitation by oxidation allows their removal under control of the process; otherwise their deposition could occur haphazardly.

When chlorine is used as the oxidant/biostat, its metered concentration is usually regulated in a looped system utilizing feedback controls. The total amount added can be confirmed gravimetrically as by loss of weight of the chlorine cylinders. *Standard Methods for the Examination of Water and Wastewater* (1989) treats on the methods of analyzing for chlorine.

Alum addition. Removal is then sought of the suspended matter present in the water, as is evident in its turbidity. This includes visible particulates, as well as colloidal bodies too small to be visible to the naked eye. Colloidal removal involves coagulation, flocculation, and precipitation, practices that culminate eventually in a filtration step. The mechanisms of coagulation and flocculation are discussed more fully below, as is also the action of alum in removing colloidal particles. It may not be amiss, however, to anticipate somewhat the subsequent discussion. (See Chapter 6, page 293).

The addition of alum (containing positively charged trivalent ions of aluminum), or of ferric chloride/lime combinations often serves economically to neutralize the mutually repulsive charges that stabilize the common water colloids. As a result of the destabilization of the colloidal suspension, the particles, if large enough, settle out of solution. The process is generally called *coagulation*, and the alum or other inducing agent is called a *coagulant*. The settling-out of the charge-neutralized particles may involve an inordinate amount of time. The process is abetted by the use of flocculants that unite the small particles into larger structures more amenable to settling under the force of gravity. A flocculant bridges the surfaces of separate charge-neutralized particles or their agglomerations (also called *flocs*), building up to a large-size aggregate or floc. Flocculation is promoted by slow mixing; high mixing shears may disrupt flocs. (The proper rate of mixing is determined empirically in jar tests.) (Kemmer, 1988)

The chemistries of iron and particularly of aluminum in solution are complex in the extreme, reflecting the influences of pH and of time-dependent molecular equilibria. Consequently, the coagulation and flocculation phenomena are intricate as well (Bratby, 1980; Kemmer, 1988). They are of interest here, because how the coagulation and flocculation are performed may later on influence the performance of RO filters that encounter these treated waters.

Substances added to water to effect destabilization of the colloidal suspensions are called primary coagulants. Alum (aluminum sulfate) or ferric chloride are the two most commonly used metal coagulants, chiefly on account of their low cost. There is no noteworthy cost difference between them, and the choice is often a matter of personal operator preference. Alum is the coagulant most widely used, perhaps 90% of the time, and usually in concentrations of 20 to 50 ppm. Excess alum is not only wasteful, but may cause reflocculation in conjunction with pH changes, a reversal of the desired effect. The amount of alum required for a given water is determined by jar tests in the laboratory, wherein the flash-mixing of the plant treatment is imitated for 30 to 60 seconds, followed by slow mixing for 20 minutes, followed by a 1-hour settling period. What is sought is a maximum diminution in the water's turbidity.

Polyelectrolytic polymers, called *polymer* in the jargon of the trade, may be added in small ppm quantities to improve the clarification and to reduce the amount of coagulant needed. Because these materials are very expensive as compared to alum, their use is limited.

Polymeric coagulants are usually from 10,000 to 1,000,000 g/moles in molecular weight. They are either polyquaternary amines or polyamines in nature. In the latter case, their charge density will vary with pH. In either case they are cationic in charge. Polymeric flocculants are of high molecular weight, from 1 million to 20 million. The higher the molecular weight, the greater the particle-bridging capacity. Almost all are copolymers of acrylamide or modified polyacrylamide.

Soluble aluminum and reflocculation. Optimum floc formation may be defined differently, depending upon the main objective being sought. It may be gauged by indicators such as the removal of color (usually of humic origins), the removal of turbidity, or the filterability of the water. Optimum floc formation, depending upon the particular water, occurs roughly at pH 5.5 to 6.5 for groundwaters or even higher for others, as measured by the achievement of maximum water clarity with minimum alum addition. However, flocculation can be managed at any pH by the addition of sufficient alum. The precipitative removal from the water of the aluminum ions added as alum occurs optimally at a pH closer to 8. The aluminum does not precipitate as simple aluminum hydroxide but as a polymeric form thereof, whose formation is time-dependent. At a lower pH, despite colloid destabilization and floc formation, the aluminum exists in complex hydrate forms bearing various degrees of ionic charge.

Figure 1-7 depicts the molecular transformations possible for aluminum as a consequence of its pH levels. The more highly positive charged complexes will be increasingly converted to aluminum hydroxide (charge-free hydrated aluminum) as the pH is raised to neutral. This entity is soluble until it forms insoluble polymeric complexes as a function of time through development of coordination compounds. Thus aluminum chloride ($AlCl_3$) is more accurately represented as being Al_2Cl_6, and insoluble aluminum hydroxide may be depicted as being in some hydrated form bearing no ionic charge or only surface charges (Bratby, 1980, Chapter 3).

It is known that partially neutralized Al_2Cl_6 forms polynuclear hydrolyzed species, presumably of kindred structure. As Mangravite (1989) views the situation, the hydrolyzed metal salts (alum) destabilize colloids by charge neutralization, by adsorption through hydroxy ligands, and by enmeshment in precipitated metal hydroxides. At the pH levels where coagulation occurs, the form is $Al(OH_2)_6^{3+}$, a hydrated metal ion (Partridge et al., 1989). Aluminum hydroxide is least soluble at pH 5 to 8 (Figure 1-9). The chemical formula shows $Al(OH)_3$ as without ionic charge, but it does bear surface charges, whether from dissociated hydroxyl groups or by the adsorption of soluble hydrolyzed metal ions.

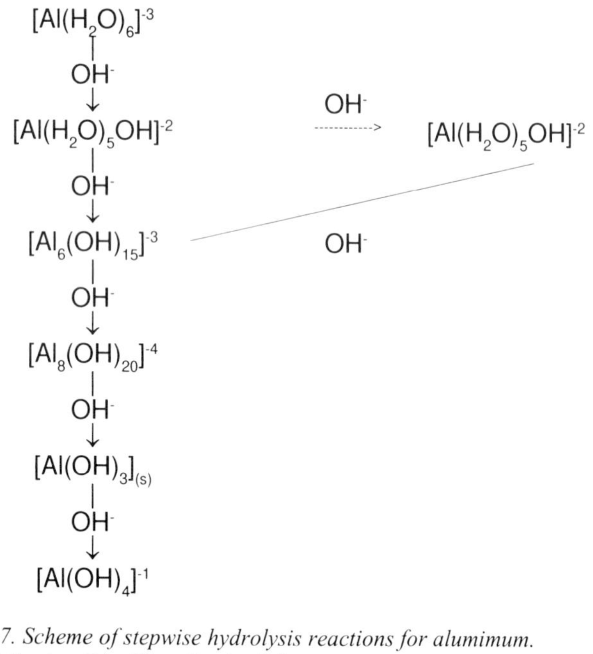

Figure 1-7. Scheme of stepwise hydrolysis reactions for alumimum.
Bratby 1980; Courtesy, Upland Press, Croydon, U.K.

In its more simple, less charged manifestations, aluminum is able to permeate RO membranes to a fair extent. Specifically, between the pH limits of about 6.5 and 8, the aluminum is in the form of heavily hydrated aluminum hydroxide essentially without ionic charges. As a result, it is rejected to only about an 80% extent. As the coordination complexes develop, their increasing size and floc formation will bar their passage through RO filters; their deposits can accumulate to block RO surfaces.

The pH dependence of the aluminum moiety of alum has a very direct influence on subsequent treatments of these waters by RO. Aluminum is an amphoteric element. Below about pH 6, the aluminum is essentially all in the form of trivalent cation, which is rejected by RO. Above about pH 8 the aluminum is largely in the form of aluminate ions, which are also rejected by RO. The minimum rejection of aluminum, then, is largely between pH 6.5 and 8. Within this range, treatment with RO will remove only about 80% of aluminum ions. Where the water is intended for hemodialysis, the 20% that permeates RO membranes is unacceptably high. Therefore, when an alum treatment is used on waters directed to such applications, a deionization following pH adjustment is required in conjunction with reverse osmosis; RO itself will not suffice.

An overdosing of alum is often unavoidable, as the qualities of surface waters can vary considerably over short durations. An operational consideration may on occasion also serve to create aluminum hydroxide floc in the very waters

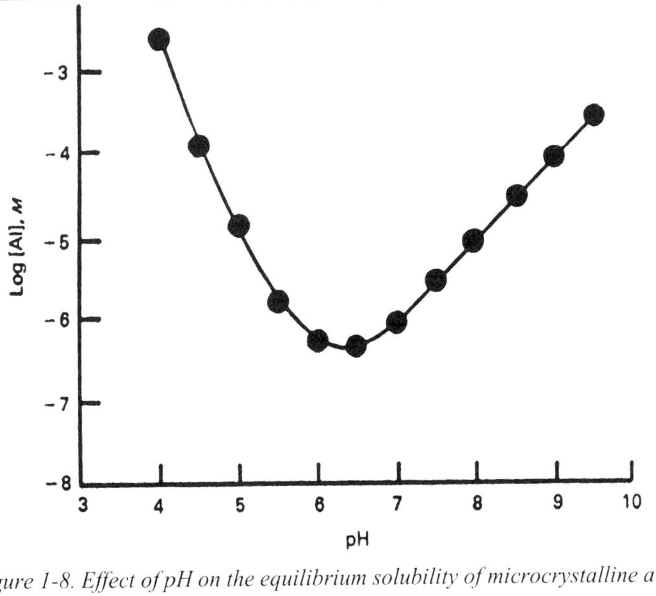

Figure 1-8. Effect of pH on the equilibrium solubility of microcrystalline aluminum hydroxide at 25°C.

released by the water treatment plant. Natural waters may be outside the optimum pH range of floc formation, or at the limits. In Virginia, for example, waters may be at pH 6 or 6.5. To bring these waters to a more neutral pH would require neutralization such as with lime or soda ash. This entails an additional treatment step with its attendant costs. Instead, for optimum floc formation, excess alum can be added to compensate for the deviation from the ideal pH range. The excess aluminum ion will remain in solution in those of its complex molecular manifestations that are appropriate to its pH ambiance (see Figure 1-9), even as the insoluble floc is removed by the subsequent deep-bed filtrations.

It has, however, become an increasing practice to raise the pH of the water, after its deep-bed filtration but just prior to its being released and distributed. Raising the pH value can result in the formation of floc in the distributed waters. This reflocculation need not include aluminum-containing precipitates. The floc formed by adjustments to higher pHs can be precipitates of other ions rendered insoluble by alkalinity. It should be stated, however, that the complexities of aluminum chemistry make possible the formation of aluminum-containing precipitates even at a high pH, despite the amphoteric nature of the element.

Elevated aluminum residuals may increase the turbidity of the water, interfere with its disinfection, and reduce (by depositing upon pipe surfaces) the water-carrying capacity of the distribution system. Additionally, high aluminum intake by humans has possible implications to such neurological disorders as Alzheimer's disease and pre-senile dementia.

In one study, the use of alum at a municipal water treatment plant at a level of 5 mg/L increased the aluminum concentration in the raw water from 10 ± 9 to 49 ± 9 mg/L. Approximately 11% of the added aluminum was released to the distribution system in the treated water (Driscoll et al., 1987).

The effective removal of particulate matter from raw waters was found to minimize the aluminum content of municipally treated waters. The deep-bed filtered water turbidity should best not exceed 0.1 turbidity units (NTU).

In particular, the lime used to make pH adjustments following the deep-bed filtrations was found to be an important source of residual aluminum. It is by no means certain that the pH of the treated waters significantly influences their aluminum concentration (Driscoll et al., 1987).

There exists at present a Secondary Maximum Contaminant Level of 0.05 mg/L for aluminum. Such SMCLs are not federally enforceable. They are advisory in nature, serving as guides, and are usually addressed to aesthetic issues, unlike the Primary Maximum Contaminant Level Goals (MCLGs) that deal with health considerations, such as organism levels. In this case, the matter of concern is the posttreatment generation of turbidity, the very subject of reflocculation.

The deposition of aluminum hydroxide floc on RO membranes can cause severe fouling, as manifest in a sharp drop in the RO permeation rate. Such occurrences are relatively common in the San Francisco area, where high alum concentrations are used. This floc is easily cleaned from the RO membrane by pH adjustment to below 4 or above 8.5. Cellulose-acetate type membranes are not amenable to treatments involving such extremes of pH.

Deep-bed filtration. The majority of the settled particulate is usually separated from the water by the use of a clarifier. However, centrifugal filtration may be used to remove particles down to 20 microns (μm) in size, and devices involving Taylor vortices enjoy increasing application. Clarifiers are employed when the turbidity of the water is greater than 50 ppm. The water bearing the remainder of the particles is put through a deep-bed filter. What is required of the deep-bed filter is that it prevent passage of the suspended matter, that it be capable of accommodating a reasonable volume of suspended material, and that it hold the retained solids so loosely as to be amenable to easy cleansing by backwashing.

Silica sand is the commonly used medium for constructing deep-bed filters (Ogedengbe, 1984). Such beds have nominal porosities of about 10 to 40 μm, with new beds tending to have the lower porosities.

A typical layered deep-bed filter may have, in order moving downward, layers of anthracite or charcoal, then sand, garnet, and a support layer of gravel. This provides three zones within the depth filter wherein particles may filtratively be removed. Such multimedia beds are replacing sand filters. (The subject of deep-bed filters will be discussed more extensively in Chapter 7).

Oil, a particularly noxious impurity, is removed by deposition on the sand granules. It will, however, not be removed by backflushing. Sand beds, for such reasons, require periodic replacement, or washing with detergent solutions.

Chlorination and chloramine formation. Chlorine (1 to 2 ppm) is usually introduced into the water just after it leaves the clarifier but before it enters the filters. This helps to prevent the deep beds from becoming breeding grounds for organisms that would reinfest the water. Polymer is sometimes added to the water at this point to serve as a filter aid, helping to retain fines and other particles smaller than would otherwise be trapped.

Removal or at least diminution of organic material by the clarifier reduces risks of THM formation being caused by the action of the subsequently introduced chlorine.

In any case, the water is retained in a clearwell after the filters for some 30 minutes, during which time it is again treated with 1 to 2 ppm of chlorine. Higher chlorine concentrations are found to impart objectionable tastes. Under this present practice, the EPA limits of 100 ppb of THM are not exceeded. However, more rigorous standards of 50 or 25 ppb of THM seem likely to be mandated. Against that possibility, studies and practices involving chlorine dioxide (ClO_2) or ozone as primary biocide are in place. Chlorine dioxide, while promising, yields chlorates and chlorites to an extent of 1 ppm. At that level there are negative health implications.

The presence of chlorine is terminated after 30 minutes by the introduction of ammonia, which interacts with the chlorine to form chloramines. This cancels out possibilities for further THM production. Each of the three hydrogens of the ammonia molecule can be progressively substituted by a chlorine atom to form primary, secondary, and tertiary chloramine, respectively. The higher the degree of chlorine substitution, the less pleasant is the odor and taste of the chloramine. The formation of the tertiary chloramine is favored by a higher ratio of chlorine to ammonia, as present at the beginning of the ammonia addition.

Indeed, mono- and dichloramines can be removed from water supplies by being oxidatively altered by the action of chlorine intro nitrogen gas, nitrate ion, and volatile trichloramine or nitrogen trichloride. This process, known as breakpoint chlorination, is utilized by certain pharmaceutical processors to remove the chloramines from incoming municipally-treated waters. (See page 316).

Trichloramine is a gas having limited solubility in water and low biocidal properties. Dichloramine is more desirable, being a stronger biocide. A mixture of 1/3 monochloramine and 2/3 dichloramine has both components equally adsorbed by carbon. The presence of the chloramines in water renders it unsuitable for kidney dialysis as these entities cause hemolytic anemia, shortening the life span of the red blood cells by an oxidative degradation of the hemoglobin. The chloramines are removed by carbon adsorption, but at slower rates than is chlorine. Overseas, even with chloramine present, the French and Germans maintain chlorine residues; the Dutch do not.

The EPA regulations require that a disinfectant residual (unspecified) be present in the prepared potable water. The chloramine serves as a secondary disinfectant whose residual presence in the water endows it with bacteriostatic properties. This keeps the bacteria under control while the water is dispersed throughout its distribution network. Even where chlorine conversion to chloramine is practiced, chances exist for chlorine to be present.

Final organism counts in potable water. Regulations for potable water, as controlled by the EPA, have as their focus its suitability as drinking water. No stipulations are made regarding its mineral contents. However, the chief concern is with its microbiological purity.

The regulations regarding the final organism counts permitted in drinking water underwent significant alterations as of December 30, 1990 (*Federal Register* 54(124):27566 June 29, 1989). Confusion on this point may exist because the previous microbial limits were in use for a long time, and their modification is relatively recent.

Bacterial concerns as regards potable water center on the presence or absence of pathogenic organisms. The most likely source of these is fecal contamination.

Testing for possible pathogens would be a very substantial undertaking. It is finessed by analyzing for *Escherichia coli*, whose presence in the water is taken as an indication of recent fecal contamination. Hence, *E. coli* is regarded as an indicator organism. Its presence transcends considerations of its own pathogenicity; it signals the presumed presence of the frank pathogens that accompany it in and from the guts of warm-blooded creatures.

Escherichia coli constitutes a definite and specific type of organism. It is part of a broader group, characterized by a similarity of biological behavior, called the fecal coliforms. Some analysts prefer, for operational reasons, to analyze a water for fecal coliforms rather than for *E. coli*. Not all coliforms are of warm-gut animal origins; therefore not all coliforms imply fecal contamination by their presence. Some coliforms are native to soil, and have ample opportunity thus to be present in surface waters. It is a point of prudence, then, that the new drinking water standards prescribe testing for total coliform organisms. The standards stipulate maximum contaminant level goals (MCLGs) of zero for these organisms and also for *giardia*, viruses, and *Legionella pneumophila*. The zero level for these organisms is considered achievable by the proper application of chlorine, ozone, or other appropriate biocides, in conjunction with floc formation and deep-bed filtration. However, the practical realities governing water analysis are recognized. Thus limitations are inherent, as, for example, in the sampling. The Maximum Contaminant Levels (MCLs) actually achieved may, therefore, register some positive total coliform count.

The final coliform value is rated as being either present or absent, the goal being zero present. No numerical density standard applies. If any coliforms are detected, they are speciated to make sure none is *E. coli* or fecal coliform. (Provisions are made for the repeat of positive results, and for the resolution of conflicting analyses.) The specified organism levels are not regulatory limits; they constitute guidelines. The presence of *E. coli* or of fecal coliform signals that the water purification operation is in need of remediation.

It may be that the choice of total coliforms for the initial testing reflects the ease of performing such analyses. The speciation tests, performed in the event any coliforms are detected, are, at the preference of the analyst, either for *E. coli* or for fecal coliform. Although these organism types are not identical, the presence of either in drinking water is of equal significance. Therefore, testing for either meets the intended purpose.

The regulations had previously stipulated a maximum monthly average of 1 cfu/100 mL for total coliforms. Present specifications are more stringent. No more than 5% of the total monthly samples may register positive for any coliforms. The number of samples mandated per month is set according to the population density served by the water treatment plant. Thus, as Arlington, Virginia, requires 200 samples to be performed per month, only 10 may offer a positive total coliform count before system amelioration becomes necessitated.

It is not uncommon for total organism assays (heterotrophic plate counts) to be performed. These evaluate the microbes generally presumed to derive from the all-pervasive biofilm that coats the insides of pipes and other surfaces that contact the water. (Biofilm and its formation are discussed below). The MCLG for total organisms (as distinct from total coliforms) is zero. The MCL, in recognition of the realities of such testing, is set at 500 cfu/mL. Total heterotrophic plate count numbers in excess of this level have no implications of fecal contamination or the presence of pathogens. The 500-cfu/mL number serves as a working standard. It alerts the water facilities people to appropriate actions, such as flushing the water distribution system or raising the biocidal residue level.

The 500-cfu/mL value was set through the belief that higher levels would interfere with the detection of *E. coli* because the heterotrophic organisms would successfully compete for the growth medium nutrients. Such concerns seem now to have abated. The listing of the 500-cfu/mL value for potable waters in *USP XXII* arises not from the concern for possible suppressing of *E. coli* counts, but rather for the purpose of providing some numerical standard, however arbitrary, for the source water from which compendial waters are to be prepared.

Table 1-21 summarizes the National Primary Drinking Water Regulations for 1990 in terms of their Maximum Contaminant Level Goals (MCLGs), and with regard to Secondary Maximum Contaminant Levels (SMCLs).

Provided that the water source is physically free of fecal contamination, this standard of quality is rather easily attained through the agency of chlorination. The presence of chlorine as a disinfectant in potable water usually endows it with low organism counts.

The *USP 23* contains no monograph on potable water. (See, however, page 17). It relies on the Environmental Protection Agency's definition. There are those who decry this situation, as has been stated, believing that if EPA changes the definition for its own purposes, the USP dependency may conceivably no longer be appropriate. Current USP thinking seeks, however, to avoid the confusion of needless duplication.

Waters reflecting strong regional differences conform to the EPA definition, but they differ sharply in their amenabilities to being purified into compendial waters. A USP definition of a starting water quality could helpfully narrow such differences. Alternatively, the USP could concentrate its efforts on the standards for pharmaceutical water and leave it to the manufacturer to determine how to meet the standards with its starting water quality.

Potable water will most likely not be suitable for the preparation of dosage forms. If not, it has to be processed to make it conform to the compendial monograph standards. What the USP says is, "Drinking water may be used in the preparation of dosage forms, or in the preparation of USP drug substances, but not in the preparation of reagents or test solutions." (*USP 23,* 1995, p. 1984).

Final pH Adjustments

In addition to considerations of floc formation, the pH of the water may influence the corrosion of pipes and conduits distributing the treated water. The concerns are with lead and copper piping whose corrosion would create hazards to health. For this reason, the EPA-stipulated pH tolerance levels of 6.5 to 8.5 have undergone modification to a very narrow range near pH 8. This more alkaline region is seen as being less conducive to metallic corrosion. The adjustment in pH may, however, convert aluminum hydroxide floc to soluble aluminate ion, and may lead to the reflocculation of other materials that are insoluble at alkaline pH levels.

In any case, pH in this regard is really a surrogate measurement; it would be best that lead and/or copper determinations be made directly.

After the deep-bed filtration for floc removal, and the ensurence of a biocidal residue, the pH of the water may be adjusted upward (where pipe corrosion is the concern) by the addition of lime. Attainment of the desired point of alkalinity may be signaled by the precipitating out of calcium carbonate. The deposition of this precipitate as a film upon the inner surfaces of the water-conveying pipes serves to protect them from acidic corrosive attacks.

Particulate Matter in Pharmaceuticals

There is serious anxiety regarding the presence of particles in injectable preparations.

The introduction of particulate matter into the body through the agency of parenteral drugs is normally to be avoided. Such particles are potentially harmful; their introduction, such as by means of parenteral injections, can hardly be considered salubrious. The problem, however, has always been in designating limits beyond which particles may, indeed, be harmless: below or above which size, in what number they may be tolerated, or even in knowing which clinical conditions may predispose patients to greater vulnerability from injected particles.

What is feared is the danger of embolism formation, the direct blockade of blood vessels by injected particles, as well as clot formation resulting from the adherence to the particle by the erythrocytes in the blood (Jonas, 1966; Plumer, 1970). Also, Jonas (1966) indicated the possibilities of antigenic reactions with allergenic responses. Granuloma formation may occur locally as the foreign particle becomes embedded in tissue, a typical inflammatory occurrence.

Some studies have shown encapsulations in the brain, lungs, and elsewhere of particles introduced by injection. The implications of resulting damage to health are clear, but difficult to prove by direct evidence.

Myers (1972) in a study emanating from the Edinburgh Royal Infirmary in Scotland, revealed that a patient undergoing extensive intravenous therapy may have from as low as 100,000 to as high as 20 times that amount of particles larger than 1 µm introduced into the body. Garvan and Gunner (1971) infused IV solutions into rabbits. These IV solutions appeared to be free of particulate matter (none visible to the eye). Yet for every 500 mL infused, 5,000 granulomas were found in the rabbit's lungs. Goddard (1966), in a FDA study, examined more than 300,000 bottles of intravenous solutions supplied to 360 hospitals by six IV solution manufacturers. Visible particles characterized the products of each of the six manufacturers (although not of every bottle, nor of every product). Garvan and Gunner (1971) also discovered that vascular granulomas containing cellulose fibers characterized the lungs of children with a frequency that related to the volume of IV fluid administered, as determined by autopsies. A partial blockage of the central retinal artery by a particle presumably derived from a parenteral infusion has been reported (Jonas, 1966). The condition could have caused blindness in the patient. A granuloma in the brain was found in the case of a patient who had received an intra-arterial saline infusion. The relationship of such untoward occurrences to the receipt of parenteral drug administration seems rather well established.

Particulate Sources

The sources of such particulate material are numerous and varied (Dean, 1985). Glass fragments from the IV solution container bottles; bits and particles of rubber from the closures and liquid-conveying tubing; fibers and particles from filters; carbon fines; deionizing-resin fines; dead bacteria or mycotic spores imperfectly removed by filters; particles worn or abraded from the surfaces of O-rings, pumps, valves, and moving parts in general; imperfectly redissolved lyophilized material; and precipitates formed by drug incompatibilities, may all serve as sources of particulate matter. The consequences of such particulate introduction into the human body may be myocardial damage; injury to the liver, kidneys, lungs, and other organs; and the general peril of embolism formation (Plumer, 1970; Turco, 1981). DeLuca (1983) listed a particularly relevant bibliography.

It is significant that over the many years these standards have been in effect, there has been a lack of adverse reports concerning them.

LVP Particulate Standards

As a consequence of all of the above, the present USP standards for large-volume parenteral solutions stipulate that LVPs may not contain more than 5 particles per milliliter of sizes greater than 25 µm, and not more than 50 particles per milliliter 10 µm in size or larger; "no visible particulates" are permitted.

SVP Particulate Standards

The particulate limits for small-volume parenterals (SVPs) are based on the concept of patient particle loading rather than on existing SVP manufacturing technology. An explanation of this concept may be in order. Consider the particulate standards for large-volume parenterals. On the basis of a 1-liter LVP administration, this translates to a total allowable particle count of 50,000 of 10 μm or larger, and 5,000 of 25 μm or larger. Of significance is that this standard has been in existence for many years and that "these are standards with which patients have been able to live." The limit for the SVPs is, therefore, based on these standards.

The administrations of many SVPs are made by "piggybacking" them onto an LVP infusion. That is, as the LVP is being administered intravenously, intra-arterially, or intrathecally,* the SVP is flowed into it. Very seldom is an LVP, such as of dextrose or saline, given without an SVP additive, or, in fact, many SVP additives. Clearly, there would be no point to limiting the number of particles in LVP solutions if there were no restrictions on the particulate content of the coadministered SVPs. Of course, no one can predict, for any individual patient, how many SVP's will be coadministered. The literature shows, however, that the upper limit seems to be five SVP additives. Therefore, the USP Convention arbitrarily proposed the one-fifth rule. That is, that the total particulate content of any of a listing of frequently administered SVPs be confined in its particulate content to one-fifth the allowable number of particles permitted LVPs on a 1-liter volume basis. Thus, the total maximum quantity of particles to which the patient will be subjected, assuming up to five SVP additives, will not exceed double the amount received from the LVP alone.

It should be noted that the SVP particulate limit is not set on a per-milliliter basis. Regardless of whether the SVP dosage is 1 mL or 99 mL (the upper limiting-volume definition of SVP), the total particle count per dose, of whatever volume, is not to exceed the one-fifth allowed for LVPs. One-fifth of 50,000 of particles 10 μm or larger equals 10,000; one-fifth of 5,000 of particles 25 μm or larger is 1,000 particles. Thus, the smaller doses of SVP can have more particles per milliliter, as far as this particular proposal goes. The concern here is with the cumulative particulate insult to which the patient may be subjected. Not all SVPs are the concern of the particle standards. Of interest are those drugs that are administered intravenously, intra-arterially, or intrathecally.

Drugs whose mode of introduction into the body is subcutaneous or intramuscular are considered of lesser significance. For these, there is more concern with large-volume parenterals solely because of frequency of use. Drugs used in diagnostic settings, such as the radiopharmaceuticals, in cancer treatment, or for episodic (emergency) treatments are not covered by the proposed standards. A list of the drugs to which the proposals do apply has been published by the USP. The list includes SVPs likely to employed in a treatment regimen on a frequent or continual basis.

*Into the subarachnoid space surrounding the spinal cord, as between the fourth and fifth lumbar vertebrae (near the base of the brain).

USP sees this single particulate limit for all SVPs as protecting the interest of the patient while not unduly burdening the drug manufacturers.■

CHAPTER 2

ORGANISMS AND THEIR CONTROL

The need to avoid the presence of microbes in pharmaceutical waters is self-evident. Their presence in injectable formulations could be dangerous in the extreme, and infections can result from the occurrence of organisms even in formulations for oral and topical use. Nor need the organisms necessarily be frank pathogens. Opportunistic microbes pose threats, particularly to debilitated hosts. Thus *Pseudomonas aeruginosa* present in topicals has been implicated in the infection of abraded skin.

Corrosion in connection with organisms and biofilm, particularly in high-temperature waters, has been described (Stoecker and Pope, 1986). The potential of silica deposits can be traced to diatoms. These single-celled plants, whose cell walls are composed almost entirely of silicon dioxides, are a major source of silica. They thrive in warm waters, particularly under the influence of sunlight (EPRI, 1983). Similarly, algae may be plentiful enough to clog cooling-water intakes.

Microbes, both living and dead, are among the sources of organic contaminants. Bacteria will concentrate sodium and potassium ions and heavy metals (Mittelman and Geesey, 1985). Organisms carry a net negative charge; they act as deionization units. They release their concentrated sodium and potassium ions upon their demise, along with organics and mitochondria particles. Yabe et al. (1989) quoted Table 2-1 as revealing the elemental composition of bacteria. Assuming organisms to have a cylindrical shape and dimensions of 1.0 μm by 2.0 μm, a moisture content of 90%, and a specific gravity of 1.0, Yabe et al. (1989) calculated them to contain the number of atoms of the constituting elements as shown in Table 2-2.

Although the concerns of the microelectronics industry regarding the presence of organisms differ from those of pharmaceutical processors, thc methods of microbe detection and assay and the considerations of avoidance and sanitization are the same. It will be instructive to investigate how the microelectronics industry deals with these issues. A similar cross-fertilization of ideas and techniques in the matter of TOC, organic chemical impurities, has already proved beneficial to preparers of pharmaceutical waters.

Motomura and Yabe (1991) isolated 127 species of organisms from semiconductor pure water. Pseudomonads constituted 80% of the population. The remainder were *Acinetobacter, Alcaligenes,* and *Flavobacterium.* The same organisms were found in the source water. These organisms are sterilizable by heat, hydrogen peroxide, and chlorine.

Futatsuki et al. (1991) found that acidic (pH 2 to 3) wastewaters emanating from semiconductor operations are deadly to some Gram-negative bacteria such as *Pseudomonas aeruginosa*, but that filamentous fungi and actinomycetes adapt and multiply. The biofilm that is formed diminishes flowrates. Sanitizations alone do not suffice to restore desired flows, as the interconnected bacterial sheaths themselves require being removed. These investigators found that as extreme acid pH is moderated in the wastewater treatment, the general organisms that are suppressed at low pH become dominant. Spore-forming bacilli can resist pH of 2 and of 12; however, they cannot multiply under those conditions. By contrast, *Nocardia,* filamentous bacteria (actinomycetes) can multiply in pH 2 environments. They are less tolerant of pH 12 conditions, and may thus be managed. Gram-negative organisms are killed completely in a few minutes at pH 2 or 12, as shown in Table 2-3.

As stated earlier, natural waters, perhaps with some very few exceptions, are not sterile. Both Gram-negative and Gram-positive organisms of many species flourish in natural waters, for these normally contain ample nutrients. For example, Adair (1982) said that in the northeastern part of the United States, it is not unusual to find *Pseudomonas* types of microorganisms indigenous to the

Table 2-1
Composition of Bacteria

Element	*Content*
C	50%
O	20%
N	14%
H	8%
P	3%
S	1%
K	1%
Na	1%
Ca	0.5%
Mg	0.5%
Cl	0.5%
Fe	0.2%
Others	-0.3%

Yabe et al. (1989) ;
Courtesy, *Microcontamination*

Table 2-2
Amount of Elements in a Bacteria Cell

Elements	*Weight(g)*	*Atoms*
C	7.9×10^{-14}	3.9×10^{9}
O	3.1×10^{-14}	1.2×10^{9}
N	2.2×10^{-14}	9.5×10^{8}
H	1.3×10^{-14}	7.6×10^{9}
P	4.7×10^{-15}	9.2×10^{7}
S	1.6×10^{-15}	3.0×10^{7}
K	1.6×10^{-15}	2.4×10^{7}
Na	1.6×10^{-15}	4.1×10^{7}
Ca	7.9×10^{-10}	1.2×10^{7}
Mg	7.9×10^{-16}	2.0×10^{7}
Cl	7.9×10^{-16}	1.3×10^{7}
Fe	3.1×10^{-16}	3.4×10^{7}
Others	4.7×10^{-16}	

Calculated - Cell size: 1 μm × 2 μm; S.G. 1.0 Water: 90%
Yabe et al. (1989); Courtesy, *Microcontamination*

water supply. It should be noted, however, that while Gram-negatives find nutritional sources even in extremely pure waters, they are far less indifferent to elevated temperatures. They are killed at temperatures above 60 °C. From the outer membranes of Gram-negatives such as *Pseudomonas* arise the lipopolysaccharides that are the most common causes of pyrogenicity when injected into the blood stream, and that constitute organic matter (TOC).

In water purification contexts, organisms are killed by UV light, chlorine, ozone, heat (as in distillations), and chemicals (as during the regeneration of ion-exchange resins). Largely, however, organisms alive and dead are removed from water sources by filtrations.

Among all the impurities that beset waters and that must be removed in their purification, there is something singular about organisms. Other impurities once removed or diminished in quantity remain so. Organisms reproduce, however, given hospitable circumstances. Their concentrations thus threaten constant renewal and augmentation. Moreover, even when thoroughly removed, they may again reinvade from contact with unsterile air or unsterile surfaces. The effort to control organism levels in water supplies is unending. It would not be too much to say that microbial management is central to the entire water

Table 2-3
The Resistibility of Bacteria against pH 2 and pH 12

	pH 2	*pH 12*
P. vesicularis Gram (-)	X (1 min)	X (1 min)
P. aeruginosa Gram (-)	X (5 min)	X (5 min)
Acinetobacter lwoffii Gram(-)	X (5 min)	X (5 min)
Bacillus sp. Gram(+)	Δ	Δ
Bacillus sp. Gram(+)	0	Δ
Nocardia sp. actinomycetes (filamentous)	@	Δ

x: Killed completely Δ: Decreased
0: Resisted but did not increase @: Multiplied

Futatsuki et al. (1991); Courtesy, Semiconductor Pure Water Conference purification effort.

It is advantageous, however, to reduce the organism densities of feedwaters. Most attempts at removal end in organism density reductions of about 6 logs. Therefore, short of absolute removals, the lower the initial count, the fewer the microbes in the final water.

Gram-Negative Organisms

Organisms can conveniently be divided into two groups, depending upon their retention of a dye after staining and exposure to an eluting solvent. Those organisms that remained dyed are called *Gram-positive*. The microbes that do not retain the stain are called *Gram-negative*. (Christian Gram was the discoverer of the staining method.) Cell wall structure determines whether or not the organism accepts the stain. *Pseudomonads* are Gram-negative.

The majority of aquatic bacteria are Gram-negative, and their presence in waters is noteworthy for at least three reasons. They flourish even in high-purity waters seemingly devoid of nutritional components; this is in distinction to Gram-positive organisms. They are killed at temperatures above 60 °C, and killed rapidly above 80 °C. From their outer membranes they shed endotoxins, a lipopolysaccharidic material that constitutes TOC and is pyrogenic, causing fevers if not more serious debilities when injected into humans. For all of these reasons, control and elimination of these organisms (as well as of all others) is sought in pharmaceutical usages.

Table 2-4
Summary Comparison of UV, Chlorine, Ozone, and Membrane Disinfection

Effect	*UV*	*Ozone*	*Chlorine*	*Membrane*
pH	No	Yes	Yes	No
Temperature	No	Yes	Yes	No
Residual	No	Dependent on pH and temp.	Yes	No
Contact time required	Very short	Medium	Very long	Very short
Operator skill required	Little	High	High	Medium
Equipment maintenance	Little	High	Moderate	Moderate
Dissolved iron interference	Yes	Yes	Yes	No*
Dissolved iron organic (e.g., phenol, humic acid, lignin sulfonates: interference)	Yes	Yes	Yes	No*
Ammonia interference	No	Yes	Yes	No
Water chemistry change	No	Yes	Yes	No
Capital cost	Low	High	Medium	High
Operating cost	Low	High	Medium	High

*Can cause membrane fouling, which will increase operating costs because of increased cleaning requirements.
Cruver, (1990); Courtesy, *Membrane Planning and TechNology Conference*

Effect of heat on Gram-negative organisms. Anderson et al. (1985) measured the effects of heat on pseudomonads, specifically *P. pickettii*, in 0.9% sodium chloride solution. The D value (the time needed to reduce the organism counts by 90%, 10 logs, or tenfold) in minutes at 50 °C (122 °F), was 26.0; at 55 °C (131 °F) was 1.9; and at 60 °C (140 °F) was 0.7. The Z value (the number of degrees in temperature required for the D value to change by a factor of 10) at 60 °C (140 °F) was found to be 6.3 °C (3 °F). It is evident from the above data that pseudomonads, as modeled by *P. pickettii*, are rapidly killed at temperatures above 60 °C (140 °F).

Neither reverse osmosis nor distillation, the two FDA-accepted methods for producing WFI, can be relied on to guarantee the desired product quality independent of a maintenance-free operation. Distillation is favored, not necessarily because of any inherently greater reliability on its part, but because it involves heating the water and producing it at elevated temperatures. As a result, the threat of organisms is eliminated or at least sharply reduced.

As indicated by Husted and Rutkowski (1991) (see Figure 2-1), microbial kill kinetics characteristically obey a time-dependent pattern. Exposure to heat results in organism deaths in exponential fashion in accord with a first-order reaction that increases in rate as a function of temperature. The phenomenon can be described in equation form:

$$kt = \ln(N/N_0)\ t_0 \qquad \text{Eq. 2-1}$$

where N_0 is the percent of viable organisms at t_0, (time zero), N is the percent viable at some later time, t is the time interval between the two measurement points, and k is the thermal death rate constant per unit time for that organism at a given temperature. Plotted, the equation yields a straight line for a given temperature, the slope of which is the thermal death constant. Moist heat is seen to cause organism deaths by denaturation of their enzymatic and structural proteins, and also by nucleic acid damage. The selectivity of their permeable cell membranes is thereby destroyed.

The proposed GMPs for LVPs state that WFI can be stored at 80 °C for as long

Table 2-5
Correlation between LAL Readings and TOC

	Log ng/mL vs. Log cells/mL	*Log ng/mL vs. Log ppm*	*Log cells/mL vs. Log ppm*
Correlation coefficient (r)	0.897	0.605	0.611
Number of samples	113	113	126
Significance	<0.001	<0.001	<0.001

Correlations between endotoxin (ng/mL), cell number (cells/mL), and TOC (ppm) taken from a study of pure water system. Dawson et al. (1988); Courtesy, *Pharmaceutical Engineering* as it meets its desired quality. This type of storage necessitates continuous recirculation of the WFI between its storage tank and its points of use. The 80 °C temperature is that of the WFI taken at the point of its return to the storage tank, presumably when it is at its coldest. This means, of course, that the water in the tank is, if anything, even hotter than the prescribed 80 °C. Water of this temperature is hazardous to handle. In its ultrapurity it is corrosive to many materials, and therefore is known as "hungry water." Maintaining its heat is expensive in terms of energy costs. Pharmaceutical processors have therefore validated WFI systems at lower temperatures. The Upjohn Company reported a WFI system validated at 60 °C, although it was operated at 65 °C to provide a safety margin (Coates et al., 1983).

The interest in a WFI operation centers on elevated temperatures related to the killing of the Gram-negative organisms indigenous to water systems; the pseudomonads are typical. These microbes can find an adequate nutrition even in waters of extremely low nitrogen and carbon content. However, they do not survive temperatures of 60 °C or higher for any extended periods of time, although the contact time required to kill them is longer at 60 °C than at 80 °C. The Gram-negative organisms can survive, however, at 40 °C. By contrast, there are Gram-positive organisms that can live at elevated temperatures. There are thermophilic organisms that can thrive even at 100 °C or above. These are the spores of spore-forming organisms. They can therefore exist even within stills. However, these microbes, unlike the vegetative Gram-negatives do not find adequate nutrition in high-purity water.

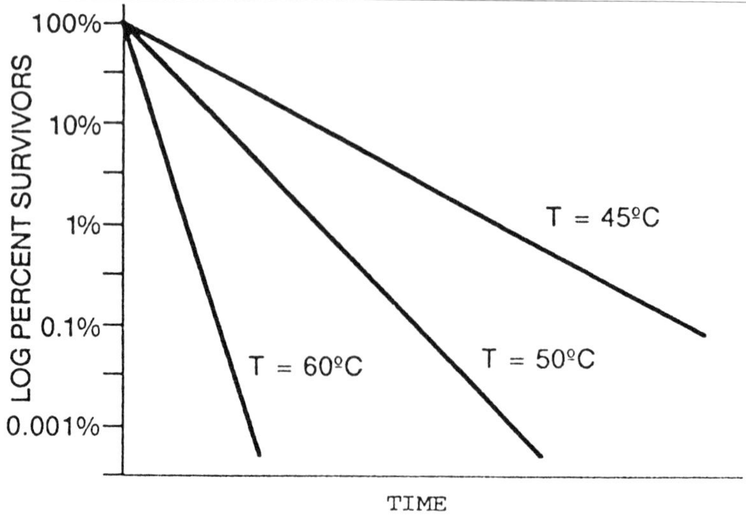

Figure 2-1. Typical kill curve.
Husted and Rutkowski (1992); Courtesy, *UltrapureWater* journal.

Most waterborne organisms are killed at 60 to 80 °C. Most pathogens will not grow above 50 to 60 °C. Moreover, purified waters do not supply them the nutrients they require. Vegetative organisms will not grow above 60 °C, and mesophiles and psychrophiles will not grow above 50 °C. *Legionella pneumophila* is reported as sometimes surviving at 50 to 55 °C. At 80 °C only spores and extreme thermophiles can survive; most thermophiles will not grow above 73 °C.

Distillation is seen as a self-sanitizing process. The use of distillation, when practiced in accord with manufacturer's instructions, therefore produces a WFI free of microbial contamination. Not to operate a still correctly is a violation of the umbrella GMPs regarding equipment and may, in any case, lead to nonsterile water.

Storage of Water

Influence of temperature. Even prior to the issuance in 1976 of the proposed CGMP's for LVP's, the FDA had a strong desire to see WFI stored in a recirculating mode at elevated temperatures, namely, above 80 deg C. Over time, the actual practice often became modified to storage at ambient temperatures with periodic sanitizations at 80 °C for some period of time. Waters stored at room temperatures were initially expected to be dumped to drain after 24 hours. Eventually, these cold non-recirculating waters were permitted to be sanitized by being heated to 80 °C. Their use in the manufacture of injectables was permitted only if the storage and sanitation process was demonstrated to accord wtih the microbiological and endotoxin requirements of WFI. Progressively, other changes came into being. Not all of these gained the approval of FDA investigators.

It should be noted that Noble (1994) concluded from mathematical modelling that dead-legs even of dimensions of lengths only twice the diameter could not be thermally disinfected.

One pharmaceutical company used ambient storage in a 1,500 gallon tank. After the day's water consumption, at a weekly interval, a remaining 250 gallon residual was heated to 85 °C, as a measured by thermometer, and flowed through the points of use for 2 minutes. The FDA disallowed this practice despite a change in the sanitization frequency to a daily operation, and regardless of apparently good microbiological numbers.

At another installation a 10,000 gallon quantity of water is circulated while being heated over a period of an hour or so to 85 °C. It is kept in circulation at that temperature for one hour, and while being permitted to cool to room temperature over a two hour, or so, period of time. While at 85 °C, the water is flushed through the points of use for 15 minutes. This practice, performed weekly, received a recommendation that it be performed daily.

One company circulates a 5,000 gallon quantity of water heated to 85 °C. every day for one hour, plus the time needed to heat and cool the water, with point

Table 2-6
Typical Bacterial Profile of the High-Pressure RO/DI Production Pad

Sample Point	*Analysis Parameter*	*1*	*2*	*3*
Well water	EPI	1.0×10^7	1.5×10^7	7.5×10^6
	LAL	1.92	1.92	0.96
	Live counts	<1	1	3
Multimedia in	EPI	4.6×10^7	4.2×10^7	8.4×10^6
	LAL	0.96	0.96	0.96
	Live counts	<1	<1	<1
Multimedia out (A)	EPI	4.2×10^7	6.2×10^7	4.8×10^6
	LAL	0.96	0.96	0.96
	Live counts	<1	<1	<1
Multimedia out (B)	EPI	2.8×10^7	4.8×10^7	5.2×10^6
	LAL	0.96	0.96	0.96
	Live counts	1	<1	1
Multimedia C	EPI	4.6×10^7	4.8×10^7	6.4×10^6
	LAL	0.96	0.96	0.96
	Live counts	<1	<1	<1
Cartridge filter in	EPI	8.8×10^c	4.2×10^7	6.0×10^6
	LAL	0.96	0.96	0.96
	Live counts	<1	<1	1
Cartridge filter out	EPI	6.4×10^5	8.2×10^5	6.8×10^5
	LAL	0.96	0.96	0.96
	Live counts	<1	<1	<1
RO out (A)	EPI	1.0×10^3	1.0×10^3	1.2×10^3
	LAL	<0.24	<0.24	<0.24
	Live counts	<1	<1	<1
	SEM (0.2 μm)	1,200	1,500	1,800
RO out (B)	EPI	1.8×10^3	1.8×10^3	2.8×10^3
	LAL	<0.24	<0.24	<0.24
	Live counts	12	14	16
	SEM (0.2 μm)	2,200	2,000	3,200
RO out (C)	EPI	1.6×10^3	1.1×10^3	1.8×10^3
	LAL	<0.24	<0.24	<0.24
	Live counts	6	6	10
	SEM (0.2 μm)	1,800	1,500	2,400
RO out (D)	EPI	1.1×10^3	1.0×10^3	1.1×10^3
	LAL	<0.24	<0.24	<0.24
	Live counts	<1	<1	2
	SEM (0.2 μm)	1,500	1,400	1,200
RO out (E)	EPI	1.6×10^3	1.6×10^3	1.6×10^3
	LAL	<0.24	<0.24	<0.24
	Live counts	10	8	18
	SEM (0.2 μm)	2,400	2,600	2,800
RO out (F)	EPI	1.6×10^3	1.7×10^3	2.2×10^3
	LAL	<0.24	<0.24	<0.24
	Live counts	<1	<1	1
	SEM (0.2 μm)	2,200	2,400	2,800

Total RO out	EPI	1.6×10^3	2.2×10^3	2.8×10^3
	LAL	<0.24	<0.24	<0.24
	Live counts	6	6	14
	SEM (0.2 μm)	2,200	2,800	-3,000
Degasifier out	EPI	2.6×10^3	2.8×10^3	4.2×10^3
	LAL	<0.24	<0.24	<0.24
	Live counts	2	4	8
	SEM (0.2 μm)	3,200	3,800	5,500
Carbon purifier out(A)	EPI	1.4×10^3	1.0×10^3	1.0×10^3
	LAL	<0.24	<0.24	<0.24
	Live counts	8	12	12
	SEM (0.2 μm)	2,000	800	1,200
Carbon purifier out (B)	EPI	4.4×10^3	6.4×10^3	8.6×10^3
	LAL	<0.24	<0.24	<0.24
	Live counts	6	18	10
	SEM (0.2 μm)	6,500	8,800	10,800
Carbon purifier out (C)	EPI	5.8×10^3	4.8×10^3	5.0×10^3
	LAL	<0.24	<0.24	<0.24
	Live counts	4	2	6
	SEM (0.2 μm)	8,400	6,500	7,800
Primary MB in	EPI	4.8×10^3	2.8×10^3	2.8×10^3
	LAL	<0.24	<0.24	<0.24
	Live counts	10	14	12
	SEM (0.2μm)	6,800	4,600	5,600
Primary MB out (A)	EPI	1.4×10^3	1.4×10^3	1.4×10^3
	LAL	<0.24	<0.24	<0.24
	Live counts	<1	<1	1
	SEM (0.2 μm)	2,200	2,800	2,600
Primary MB out (B)	EPI	2.4×10^3	2.4×10^3	2.0×10^3
	LAL	<0.24	<0.24	<0.24
	Live counts	<1	<1	<1
	SEM(0.2 μm)	3,200	3,800	2,900
Primary MB out (C)	EPI	1.0×10^3	1.2×10^3	1.1×10^3
	LAL	<0.24	<0.24	<0.24
	Live counts	<1	<1	<1
	SEM (0.2 μm)	1,200	1,600	1,400
Secondary MB out (A)	EPI	8.4×10^3	1.0×10^4	5.6×10^3
	LAL	<0.24	<0.24	<0.24
	Live counts	<1	<1	<1
	SEM (0.2 μm)	10,200	12,800	9,400
Secondary MB out(B)	EPI	1.2×10^3	1.4×10^3	1.8×10^3
	LAL	<0.24	<0.24	<0.24
	Live counts	<1	<1	<1
	SEM (0.2 μm)	1,800	1,600	2,200
Secondary MB out (C)	EPI	1.2×10^3	1.0×10^3	1.0×10^3
	LAL	<0.24	0.24	<0.24
	Live counts	<1	<1	<1
	SEM (0.2 μm)	1,000	1,200	800
Central pad product	EPI	2.0×10^3	2.1×10^2	4.9×10^2
	LAL	<0.24	<0.24	<0.24
	Live counts	1	1	1
	SEM (0.2 μm)	1,500	800	400

Carmody and Martyak (1989); Courtesy, *Microcontamination*

of use flushing for 15 minutes. Yet another drug company utilizes 80 °C sanitizations over a three hour period with 15 minutes point of use flushing. It should be emphasized that many pharmaceutical manufacturers continuously recirculate their 80 °C. WFI without any cooling except when withdrawing a portion for use.

A multinational company utilizes as a standard practice Water for Injection held in tanks at room temperature. The water is circulated daily through heat exchangers sufficient to keep it at 85 °C for 20 minutes. The WFI is then allowed to come to room temperature in the uninsulated tanks. Weekends, the water heating is more rigorously maintained at 85 °C for 2 hours.

A prudent practice would involve the stored water being maintained at 80 °C for about 4 hours weekly. Temperature equilibration for that time period should sufflce as the thermal sanitization for a sizeable stainless steel water storage facility and its contents. The address would be to biofilm as well as to the more easily killed planktonic microbes. Depending upon the water volume, attaining the 80 °C level from room temperature could require 3 or 4 hours, as would also its cooling down. The total operation could take 10 to 12 hours.

Husted (1994) reported that his observations of hot-water systems reveal no evidence of biofilm. To what extent this situation extends to systems that undergo intermittent cooling has not been remarked upon.

Not only is WFI maintained in loops at room temperature, sanitized periodically by being heated to 80 °C for suitable intervals, as directed by validation needs, but it may be stored at lower than room temperatures. This practice is

Table 2-7
The Adsorption of Bacterial Cells to Solid Surfaces Immersed in Very Dilute Organic Solutions

Reversible Adsorption Phase
Mechanism - Balance between double-layer repulsion and van der Waals attraction.
Net Effect - Loosely adherent cells are a finite distance (-2 nm) from adsorbent; cells are easily removed by rinsing.
Influencing Factors - pH, electrolyte concentration, organic carbon concentration, fluid motion.

Irreversible Adsorption Phase
Mechanism - Adhesion due to biologically-mediated adhesions (e.g., polyanionic molecules) or hydrophobicity of cell surface.
Net Effect - Tenaciously adherent cells; biologically-mediated adhesions "bridge" gap between cells and surface; cells can be removed by alteration of adhesions or by harsh physical methods (e.g., brushing or scraping).
Influencing Factors - Time, temperature, surface free energy (γ), critical surface tension (γ_c), interaction parameters (η), free energy of adhesion (ΔF), hydrophobicity.

Mittelman and Geesey, Water Micro Associates; Courtesy, *Biological Fouling of Industrial Water Systems (1987).*

followed in one instance where plasma fractionation makes advisable the maintenance of water temperatures at from 2 to 8 °C to prevent protein denaturation. In another case, the temperature is kept at around 2 °C, largely to discourage organism growths. Over a 10-year period no system contamination has been encountered in either system. In the first example, the loop is sanitized by being heated for 2 hours at 80 °C every Wednesday, followed by a 10-hour heating at that temperature on Saturdays. In the other case, the loop is steamed monthly using steam from a clean-steam generator. In this instance, the use of a heat-exchanger is avoided. In neither case are the refrigeration costs judged to be excessive.

Water for Injection storage at 4 °C is being practiced as a means of discouraging organism growths. At one Danish pharmaceutical company, the WFI is stored at 4 to 7 °C. Periodically, hot-water sanitizations are practiced as needed.

Further modifications to water storage practices derive from the use of ozone. Pharmaceutical waters are reportedly being stored under ozone at room temperature. Several developmental efforts directed to Water for Injection are essaying this storage mode.

Cold-water systems of equivalent capacities entail lower capital costs and operational expenses than heated systems. Purified Water is, therefore, often

Table 2-8
Shear Force on a 1.0-μm-Diameter Section of Pipe Surface as a Function of Velocity (lbf) × (10^{-13})

Normal Pipe Size (Sch. 80-in.)	*Velocity (ft/sec)*						
	0.25	*0.5*	*1.0*	*2.0*	*5.0*	*8.0*	*12.0*
1/2	*	*	*	2.60	13.3	30.1	61.7
1	*	*	0.693	2.28	11.6	26.6	55.5
2	*	0.170	0.575	1.94	10.1	22.3	47.1
3	0.046	0.153	0.524	1.79	8.96	20.9	43.5
4	0.044	0.144	0.500	1.69	8.62	19.4	41.3

as a Function of Velocity (N) × (10^{-13})

Normal Pipe Size (Sch. 80-in.)	*Velocity (ft/sec)*						
	0.25	*0.5*	*1.0*	*2.0*	*5.0*	*8.0*	*12.0*
1/2	*	*	*	11.56	59.16	133.88	274.44
1	*	*	3.08	10.14	51.60	118.31	246.86
2	*	0.76	2.56	8.63	44.92	99.19	209.50
3	0.20	0.68	2.33	7.96	39.85	92.96	193.49
4	0.19	0.64	2.22	7.52	38.34	86.29	183.70

*Flow may or may not be turbulent at these conditions. (English units have been used where appropriate.)
Pittner and Bertler, (1988); Courtesy, ULTRAPURE WATER Expo

produced by such systems, as by the use of ion exchange to demineralize the water. In some cases the Purified Water, although prepared cold, is heated by way of a heat exchanger and is stored at 80 °C (or even higher). This too keeps if free of Gram-negatives (pseudomonads). The heated Purified Water is not necessarily sterile. It may, however unlikely, contain heat-tolerant Gram-positive spores, and is almost certain to have an endotoxin content in excess of 0.25 EU/mL. It will, however, meet the specifications of the Purified Water. In cases where the rate of usage is too great to enable the volume to be adequately and economically handled by the action of a heat exchanger, stored water is periodically heated in a hot-water loop to 80 °C and is maintained at that temperature for 4 hours. This serves to sanitize it. It subsequently cools in the hot-water loop to approximately 50 °C. It may be used as such, or may be blended with Purified Water at room temperature to produce a Purified Water ready for formulation. The proper quality of the product water is assured by microbiological assay.

Pasteurization is increasingly employed to diminish the organism counts of a water. By means of steam-heated stainless steel heat-exchanger plates, the incoming water is elevated in temperature to about 70 °C (158 °F). This serves to sterilize it with regard to vegetative bacteria (some spores survive). This brief heat treatment offers other advantages as well. Reverse osmosis operations perform better at 24 °C (75 °F); degasification of the water is promoted by the heat; and, some believe, adsorption by the carbon beds is enhanced.

The lower the storage temperature of the water, the greater the risk of organism growth. Microbiologists responsible for WFI systems utilizing lower temperatures, either in the water purification or in storage steps, should be aware, possibly from plant bioburden studies, of organisms that can exist at such temperatures. *Stearothermophilus* can thrive at 55 °C. Screening tests for such organisms should be conducted as part of an ongoing validation and maintenance program. To manufacture or store WFI at temperatures below 80 °C requires routine microbiological testing for organisms that can live between those temperatures and 80 °C. Water produced and stored under continuous circulation need not undergo such testing, if stored at 80 °C.

At one Canadian company Purified Water produced at 80 °C is allowed to cool while stored in a 1000 L stainless steel tank. The quantity not consumed within 24 hours is discarded. The tank is sanitized twice weekly with 70% isopropanol delivered through spray balls, and is scrubbed with same. The isopropanol is recirculated overnight. Weekly, the tank is sanitized more aggressively with surfactant and 70% isopropanol. Though there are operational advantages to 60 °C systems, in the event of a shutdown (such as may be required to change a pump or other piece of equipment) these systems will be unable to endure downtimes as extensive as would hotter systems before attaining unacceptably low temperature levels.

Water storage hot versus ozone. Because of its self-sanitizing effect, the historically proven hot water system is preferred by the FDA; ozone-protected systems seem to receive individual scrutinies of a more intense kind. Indeed, one prominent inspector points out, apparently to the disparagement of ozone, that once it is removed its protective influence vanishes. But he approves of systems protected by heat, of which exactly the same can be said. Serious installations are, however, underway in which ozone-protected ambient pharmaceutical waters are stored. In pharmaceutical settings, ozone is injected into the storage tanks. The tank head is sanitized using spray balls.

Ozone costs more than heat, but this disadvantage decreases inversely with the size of the system. Ozone can remove biofilm. Husted (1994) claimed that hot-water systems remain free of biofilm buildup, an important consideration. Ozone is stated to preserve passivation of the stainless steels. This belief, however, remains unassessed in the literature. This beneficial, or at least neutral, effect of ozone on passivation may be advanced on the basis of ozone being an allotrope of oxygen, which is believed to confer passivation in its own right by converting the nickel and chromium metal into the inert oxides. It is these inert oxides that constitute the passivation by protectively cladding the stainless steel surfaces. A contradictory anecdotal account does attribute rouging to the long term use of ozone in at least one particular stainless steel system; but the matter is in dispute. Imperfectly removed iron residuals may have been at fault.

Hot water storage will not provide sterile water; defined as having present fewer than a one-in-a-million probability of live organisms. The elevated temperatures will kill the vegetative microbes, Gram-negative included, but need not necessarily kill Gram-positive spores. Dry steam at 121 °C for 12 minutes is required to kill the most resistant isolates of *Bacillus stearothermophilus* spores. As with all antimicrobials, time and concentration are important factors. In this case, temperature equates with concentration.

With ozone, a concentration of 0.26 mg/L over a 20 minute minimum period would suffice to kill the gram-positive spores; 1.7 minutes at ozone concentrations of 3.5 mg/L. These numbers are based on the 15X relative resistance of spore formers as compared to *E. coli* (Block, 1995). Nebel (1989) showed that ozone residuals in the range of 0.0005 to 0.1 mg/L kill *Bacillus megaterium* spores to a 99% extent in 10 minutes.

The FDA (1993) cited a case where the efficacy of hot-water sanitization was notable:

> It should be pointed out that simply because this is a one-way system, it is not inadequate. With good Standard Operational Procedures, based on validation data, and routine hot flushings of this system, it could be acceptable. A very long system (over 200 yards) with over 50 outlets was found acceptable. This system employed a daily flushing of all outlets with 80 °C water.

In its "Guide to Inspections of High-Purity Water Systems", the FDA (1993) states:

> Because this manufacturer did not have a need for a large amount of water (the total system capacity was about 30 gallons), they attempted to let the system sit for approximately one day. Figure 9 (FDA, 1993) shows that at zero time (at 9 am on 3/10), there were no detectable levels of microorganisms and of endotoxins. After one day, this static non-circulating system was found to be contaminated. The four consecutive one hour samples also illustrate the variability among samples taken from a system. After the last sample at 12 pm was collected, the system was resanitized with 0.5% peroxide solution, flushed, recirculated and resampled. No levels of microbiological contamination were found on daily samples after the system was put back in operation. This is the reason the agency has recommended that non-recirculating water systems be drained daily and water not allowed to sit in the system.

Macroreticulated quaternarized resin effects. An additional means of coping with microbial contaminations of waters was offered by Scruton (1980), who reported on the use of macroreticulated quaternary anion-exchange resins to reduce organism populations. As described below in the section on ion exchange, macroreticulated resin beads are porous. Scruton saw the pores as serving as traps for the retentive demise of microbes. A synergistic effect is offered by the bactericidal properties of the quaternary ammonium groups.

Scruton reported laboratory verification of the resin supplier's claims, namely, that every 6-inch depth of resin bed decreases by one order the number of bacteria remaining in the aqueous medium. Thus, a 36-inch (14-cm) deep bed should remove 99.9999% of the organisms. The laboratory verification was claimed using an 18-inch-long, 1-inch-diameter column challenged by 9×10^6 per mL of *E. coli* for an unspecified total volume or flowrate. An industrial-scale trial was performed using the macroreticulated quaternarized resin as part of a bacterial filter, the other portion of which was a cation-exchange resin included to yield a balanced cation and anion ion exchange. The resin filter canister was 54 inches long and 12.5 inches in diameter and was charged with 2.25 cubic feet of the mixed resins. Its purpose was not to effect ion exchange (previously provided for) but to test the sought-after microbial removal as assayed by total plate counts on 100-mL aliquot volumes of the effluent waters, using the membrane filter technique. The results showed that bacteria appeared only after some weeks of processing consecutive batches of 4,000 liters each.

(Some ambiguity of interpretation on the part of this reviewer is possible. The term *filter* is used both for the mixed-resin canister and for a subsequent 0.22-μm-rated membrane used to retain resin fines. It was not entirely clear to this reviewer whether the testing was done on the effluent before the sterilizing membrane filter, as implied in the tabulated results, or after, as stated in the text. The difference could be very significant.)

In any case, this method of removing organisms, whatever its promise, has received little commercial application.

Filtration. Although not biocidal in its operation, filtration offers a means of controlling the microbial contents of high-purity waters by its removal of particles, both viable and nonviable, from fluid streams. Filters and the filtrative action are discussed below.

Although organism removal by filters can be relied upon, there can be untoward consequences nonetheless. The trapped organisms will live, multiply and die upon the filter. Their multiplication will exacerbate the effects their original numbers would have had. Bacterial endotoxin values will become elevated downstream of the filters, and effluent resistivity levels will fall, a consequence of the inorganic ions released from the dead microbes. TOC values will also increase proportionately.

In an electroplating operation the use of water having 18 megohm-cm resistivity was compromised by the presence of organisms exiting a mixed ion-exchange bed. Their removal was accomplished by means of microporous filters. However, failure periodically to sanitize the filters resulted in a decrease of the water's resistivity.

In such cases the use of ultraviolet light in conjunction with organism-retentive filters will help, but periodic sanitizations of the filters, their frequency defined by LAL and conductivity (resistivity) measurement, are indicated.

An interesting comparison of what is involved in the application of UV light, ozone, chlorine, and membrane filtration in the removal of organisms from their aqueous suspensions was presented by Cruver (1990), given there in Table 2-4. Cruver's conclusion was that "no single method of disinfection is superior in every situation."

Bacterial Endotoxins and their Removal

A component of the Gram-negative organism's cell wall is the principal cause of pyrogenicity induced by the injection of impure aqueous preparations. Called endotoxin, it is a lipopolysaccharide (LPS) that is shed during bacterial cell growth and may be found free, particularly in aqueous environments. (Because Gram-positive organisms do not multiply in high-purity waters, their bacterial pyrogens are of little concern here.) In any case, LPS is found only in Gram-negative cell walls, not in Gram-positive organisms. Endotoxin is quite stable both physically and chemically and is not destroyed by the temperatures used to kill the bacteria themselves. (For endotoxin removal see pages 74, 267, and 580).

The endotoxin unit consists of two parts: a hydrophilic polysaccharide (sugar) chain, and a hydrophobic lipid group. The lipid portion is called lipid A. The polysaccharide chain may vary in its length from one endotoxin unit to another. Therefore, the overall endotoxin unit may be from 3,000 to 25,000 daltons in size. The hydrophobic character of the lipid A moiety predominates to such an extent that the endotoxin molecules aggregate in water, a polar medium. Vesicles and other membranous structures result, depending upon the pH, the ions that are present, and the presence or absence of surfactant. Where divalent ions are present to cross-link individual endotoxin molecules, the molecular weights of the endotoxin aggregates may be in the millions of daltons. In the absence of multivalent ions, the hydrophobic lipid chain ends form micellar aggregates in order to minimize the free energy of the lipid surfaces exposed to water. In this case, the molecular weight of the endotoxin is in the neighborhood of 300,000 daltons. Only in the presence of surfactants that serve to disperse the micelles do endotoxin molecules exhibit their individual molecular weights of about 20,000 daltons (Sweadner et al., 1977).

Pearson (1985) stated, "...from a practical point of view, endotoxin can be considered to have a molecular weight of 10^6 daltons in an aqueous environment in the absence of significant levels of divalent cations and surface-active agents." Thus this is the approximate molecular aggregate most frequently encountered in large-volume parenterals and medical-device rinse solutions. That being the case, endotoxins ought to be filtratively removed from aqueous preparations by ultrafilters having 100,000-dalton cutoffs. The usual practice of employing ultrafilters of 10,000-dalton cutoffs would seem to be needlessly restrictive in the resulting liquid flows where high-purity waters are concerned.

Small quantities of LPS in the blood or spinal fluid, as low as 10^{-9} grams, can cause a series of adverse effects, from fever to shock and death; thus the term *pyrogen* (Gould et al., 1990). The permissible endotoxin contents of pharmaceutical waters has already been remarked upon.

Endotoxin initiates clotting of the blood of the horseshoe crab, *Limulus polyphemus* and/or of certain other marine invertebrates. The Limulus amebocyte lysate (LAL) test based on this activity provides a very sensitive and accurate method of measuring LPS concentrations. Not surprisingly, endotoxin levels may be used to indicate the microbial state of water systems (Novitsky, 1984). See, however, the following paragraphs.

Correlation of endotoxin with organisms. Watson et al. (1977) established that, in samples taken from seawater or laboratory cultures, the concentration of cell-bound LPS correlates with cell counts. These investigators also showed that the growth rate of the laboratory culture could be determined from the rate of increase in LPS. This not-unexpected correlation of bacterial cell counts and LPS has its uses. It is much easier to do LAL assays than to perform microbiological testing. Direct counts may not be sensitive enough to detect low numbers of bacterial cells, and this determination usually requires at least 72 hours to carry out. In high-purity waters, the bacteria are small and few in number because of the dearth of nutrients. They grow very slowly; their doubling time is measured in weeks (Gould et al., 1990). In order to obtain meaningful counts in high-purity water, therefore, the sample volumes must be quite large, possibly hundreds of liters, as has been reported. Plate counts, taken as a measure of "viable" cells, are too insensitive for high-purity waters even where large volumes are used. Finally, there is no known medium capable of supporting the growth of all bacterial types that are adapted to growth in high-purity water. Clearly the LAL test is to be preferred, were it to have an unambiguous relationship to all counts.

It is not possible to state that a given amount of endotoxin represents a certain number of cells. The endotoxin content differs with different organisms, and even with the nutritional state for a given organism. Moreover, endotoxin that is present need not be associated with a bacterial cell. Free endotoxin may have been shed from a cell or may be derived from dead cells.

Similarly, organism numbers hardly represent absolute counts. Direct counting of organisms, as by scanning electron microscopy (SEM) or epifluorescence, yields more reliable numbers than do culture methods, but is seldom used because it is operator-intensive. Epifluorescence and SEM counts agree rather well (Carmody and Martyak, 1989). Direct organism counts may give results from 10 to 1,000 times the numbers obtained from culture methods. This difference is ascribed to limitations of the culture methods. Culture techniques select for those organisms that can grow on the medium they are furnished. No single medium can suit all the organisms in the sample. High nutritional concentrations may actually inhibit the growth of organisms from low nutritional conditions; and the relatively short incubation periods that are practical may mean that the slow growth rates of pure water organisms may not suffice to render them visible for counting. The relationship between LAL values and organism counts is therefore tenuous.

The quantity of endotoxin originating from one microbial cell depends upon the type organism involved. *Escherichia coli* has yielded 50 femtograms per organism, 1 femtogram being equal to 1×10^{-15} grams. Another organism, type unspecified, has produced 15.7 femtograms per cell. A third type of microbe, an unidentified pseudomonad, has given rise to 6.9 femtograms per cell. The cells were counted by epifluorescence (Dawson, 1991).

The detection limit of the LAL method by gel clotting is 0.03 EU/mL. Measured kinetic chromogenically it is 0.005 EU/mL, and by kinetic turbidimetry it is 0.001 EU/mL. Most pharmaceutical water systems measure negative by the gel clot method and are usually at the 0.001-EU/mL level. Assuming 5 femtograms per cell, 20 cells would give 0.1 picograms, equivalent to 0.001 EU. To yield 0.03 EU, 600 cells, a range of 500 to 1,000, would be needed.

Correlation of endotoxins with TOC. It has also seemed logical that in waters essentially prepurified of organic matter, the TOC levels ought to reflect essentially the presence of organisms. If so, TOC would correlate with the LAL readings and could be measured thereby. Table 2-5 shows such a correlation (Dawson et al., 1988). These investigators stated,

> An extensive study of an electronics industry water system demonstrated significant correlations between endotoxin concentration and direct bacterial counts and between endotoxin and TOC measurements. Similar correlations were found in other pure-water systems.
>
> Previously unpublished results of a major water system study show clear and highly significant correlations between endotoxin concentration, epifluorescence direct count and TOC.

Figure 2-1 shows the correlation. A high correlation coefficient requires a range of different values for the parameters being compared. Figure 2-1 shows too great a constancy in each of the parameters for a high correlation to be adduced. The datum point for day eight is an exception, however. It represents the upset of a previously stable condition and overall indicates the sought-for high degree of correlation among the number of bacterial cells, the TOC, and the corresponding LAL values. Whether or not the bacteria are capable of utilizing the TOC that is present ought to determine how strong the correlation (among TOC level, bacteria concentration, and LAL) will be in any given circumstance. Where the TOC serves as a nutrient source, as when it is of biological origin (humic acids), the correlation will be strong. If, however, the organic carbon arises from a chemical or nonbiological source, the correlation may be weaker.

Microbiological Testing

Growth media. A common error in the microbiological examination of Water for Injection is to apply the USP Microbial Limits Tests procedures. These were designed for finished dosage forms assays, and not for the high-purity of WFI. Total counts will be deceptively low for the sparse waterborne organisms grown on these highly nutritional media. Removed from their nutritionally spartan WFI environments, organisms (holds one theory) undergo "catabolic metabolism." They will convert their protein into enzymes in an exaggerated effort at growth in the rich media, and will die in the process, thereby giving rise to counts that are falsely low.

The relatively high nutrient contents of microbiological media preclude growth for many purified water bacteria. Thus, Saleem and Schlitzer (1983) used media containing lower concentrations of nutrient to obtain better growth for such organisms.

Yet it is not enough just to dilute a normal, rich medium to suit it to the microbiological needs of high-purity waters. Corrections, such as for pH and osmotic pressure would also have to be dealt with. Media developed for this purpose should be utilized. One such is known as R2A agar. It is recommended by the EPA for the nutritionally limited environment of (oligotrophic) purified water systems (*APHA Standard Methods*, 1989). It involves a reduced organic carbon content and an increased incubation time at a decreased incubation temperature, namely at 28 °C for 5 to 7 days. A one-half triptocay soy broth is also recommended as a suitable low-metabolite diet. Figure 2-2 shows a scanning electron micrograph of a *Pseudomonas diminuta* culture grown on a minimal saline lactose broth.

Standard Methods (1989) describes the composition of R2A as consisting of 0.5 gram (g) quantities of yeast extract, proteus peptone #3 or polypeptone, casamino acids, glucose, and soluble starch, plus 0.3 g each of dipotassium hydrogen phosphate and sodium pyruvate, plus 0.05 g of magnesium sulfate heptahydrate and 15.0 g of agar. The mixture may be obtained commercially in its dehydrated form and is made up in one liter of distilled water by boiling 18.2 g of the dehydrated form with the water until dissolved. It is sterilized by being steam autoclaved at 121 °C for 15 minutes. The final pH should be 7.2 ± 0.2. The methods and incubation for its use are presented in *Standard Methods*.

Tryptone Glucose Broth, TGB, also mTGE, is used for the growth of some organisms recoverable from high-purity water systems. Its use is suggested for *E. coli* and *Staphylococcus aureus*. However, these are rarely present in pure water systems. The TGB is composed of 6 g of beef extract, 10 g of tryptone, and 2 g of glucose. It is available from, among others, Difco Laboratories, whose manual sets forth the methods of its employment, including incubation at 35 °C for 18 to 24 hours.

Meade and Song (1985) described the use of such media in the semiconductor industry for the recovery of organisms from high-purity waters. Viable cell counts, as distinct from total counts, are obtained using a membrane cassette technique along with appropriate media and incubation times and temperatures. Samples of water issuing from a port are flowed through the membrane positioned within the attached cassette so that the organisms being assayed become retained, to be incubated and counted. Alternatively, samples of water are flowed through a membrane filter held in a funnel in the technique of conventional water microbiology. Meade and Song (1985) utilized Means and Geldreich's (EPA) R2A medium, along with TGB, and also a second minimal, MS-PC, also developed by Means and Geldreich. For generalized recoveries, these investigators employed Mueller Hinton medium.

Reasoner and Geldreich (1985) showed that the R2A agar medium gave counts 5 times as high as plate-count agar (PCA). However, this need not necessarily be true for purified waters. Reasoner and Geldrich also reported that counts after 72 hours at 35 °C were substantially higher than after 48 hours of incubation. After 168 hours of incubation at 30 °C, counts were somewhat higher than after 72 hours.

R2A is widely used, perhaps in part because of the deserved prestige of its formulators. Others report anecdotally that tryptone soy agar (TSA) is found to give higher counts. One comparison made among TSA, R2A, and triptoglucose agar (TGA), a high nutrient, at various incubation times and temperatures concludes that the higher counts reflect the longer incubation times, such as are used with R2A, and the more optimal incubation temperatures. No firm consensus exists on this matter. A common view is that higher counts are not necessarily significant where the data are used to establish trends.

Incubation times and temperatures. There is still controversy regarding optimum incubation times and temperatures, as well as concerning the values of the different sampling methods and recovery techniques. Incubation temperatures in the 35 to 37 °C range may have stemmed from concerns with the growth of pathogens in human systems. This may have no basic bearing on waterborne microbes. The use of R2A medium is generally made at incubation at about 25

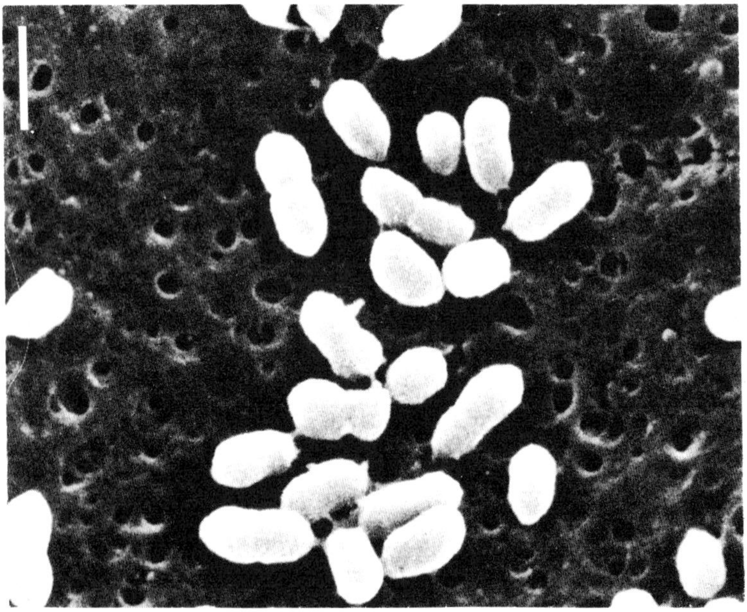

Figure 2-2. SEM of saline lactose broth culture grown for 24 hours at 30 °C. Bar = 1 mm.

Leahy and Sullivan (1978); Courtesy, *Pharmaceutical Technology*

°C for a minimum of 72 hours, and usually for 5 days. The problem is that one does not wish to select for just one portion of the total count. Heterotrophic plate-count agar widely used in general environmental work at 30 °C for 72 hours seems inappropriate for work with high-purity water.

Van Doorne and Neuteboom (1984) reported on some effects of media and incubation temperatures. No differences resulted from using 22 °C or 30 °C. A medium containing 17 g of peptone was shown to be less productive than media containing a lower level of peptone. Five days of incubation was shown to be optimal.

King medium, which contained the same level of peptone as tryptone soy agar but also contained glycerol, was more productive than the tryptone soy agar.

Lilly (1990) referenced a number of investigators, Meade and Song (1985) among them, who found American Society for Testing and Materials (ASTM) incubations at 35 °C for 48 hours inadequate, and productive of misleadingly low organism counts. Lilly advised the use of 20 °C incubations for 96 hours (Figure 2-3). As can be seen, incubations at 35 °C gave far lower counts than those performed at 20 °C. Longer incubation times, as shown in Figure 2-4, were more productive of significantly higher counts.

Cooper (February 1989) stated,

> In *Standard Methods for Examination of Water and Waste Water*, plate-count agar (PCA) and R2A agar are offered as alternatives with the provision that R2A samples are incubated at 35 °C for 5 to 7 days while other media such as PCA are to be incubated for only 48 hours for fresh water samples.

Cooper (February 1996) observes,

> FDA has not yet advised that R2A agar is preferred over Plate Count Agar although articles are been published which demonstrate higher plate counts when R2A agar is employed, using extended incubation and lower temperatares. Whether such higher counts will result from applying these extended conditions to Plate Count Agar is less clear. The debate also revolves about the benefits derived from moderately higher viable counts as opposed to the disadvantages of longer periods required before trends can be detected and appropriate actions taken. If it can be shown that specific undesirable organisms are not detected during the 48-72 hour incubation period at 30-35 °C, then some changes would be in order. To qualify the above definition of an undesirable organism would, of course, depend on the type of product and the process involved in its manufacture.

It would seem that the microbiological assaying of highly purified waters stored at ambient temperatures should require a dilute nutrient, along with incubations at near room temperatures, and for longer terms than 2 or 3 days. Husted (1995) utilizes R2A at one-third concentrations and 1.2% agar at 25 °C for up to seven days. The identity of organisms is more fully revealed. However, this practice is not widespread.

Cooper (February 1989) also said,

> The bottom line in this discussion is simply that if specific quantitative limits for the total aerobic count of process water will prevail, it is obvious that this must be considered within the context of precise microbiological procedures.
>
> The above observations are of considerable importance in pointing out the need for standardized procedures for microbiological analysis of water samples.

Direct counting. The viable count is the most commonly used method of monitoring bacteria. In any situation, the type of medium used as well as the duration and temperature of the incubation select for the organisms that will grow. Unfortunately, the matter becomes increasingly complex where the bacteria being tested for are those present in high-purity water systems. Such water bacteria have slow rates of growth, possibly as an adaptation to low nutrient concentrations. Longer incubation times than the usual 72 hours may be required.

It should be pointed out that the same considerations are involved in the assaying of organisms stressed by exposure to chlorine and UV light. In fact, FDA inspectors may inquire as to how the microbial testing was performed on waters emanating from UV units, to make sure that the organisms attenuated by these treatments were nurtured properly so that their presence could be quantified by enumeration. The fear is that the organisms, attenuated but alive, could be killed by inappropriate growth media and incubations, leading to false negative results in the testing, but could, if left alone, survive to recover and reproduce in the treated water.

Epifluorescence. Direct counting of organisms is performed by collecting them on the surface of a microporous filter and then counting them either by scanning electron microscopy or by utilizing epifluorescence. In this latter technique, the nucleic acids in the bacterial cells are stained with acridine orange. This is a fluorescent dye when viewed under ultraviolet using epifluorescence optics. One is presumably enabled to distinguish bacterial cells from other particles. These cells are considered living cells. Dead cells would lyse; their nucleic acid contents would become dispersed. Actually, dead cells are among those counted.

Clancy and Cimini (1991) utilized a modification of the acridine orange direct-count method (ASTM method D-4455-85) to distinguish between live and dead organisms. The dye stains all organisms, both viable and otherwise. A total organism count of the (stained) microbes is made under the epifluorescence microscope. The organisms are then supplied a yeast extract and nalidixic acid. The yeast extract promotes growth. The nalidixic acid is a deoxyribonucleic acid (DNA) inhibitor. Living bacteria thus treated grow in length but do not undergo cell division. A recount is made of the organisms. The elongated organisms are the viable microbes in the total population of living and dead. The method of conducting the viable count is that of Rollins and Colwell (1986).

Gould (1993) said the following relative to the epifluorescence technique as compared to the bacterial counting methods based on membranes:

> Many bacteria adapted to poor nutrient conditions pass easily through a 0.22-micron sterilizing filter, and they are very difficult to distinguish from the other types of particles with the use of standard light microscopy.
>
> Full appreciation for the numbers of bacteria in low-nutrient environments came only after the development of the acridine orange stain in the 1970s. Compunds like acridine orange bind to nucleic acids in cells. The bound stain fluoresces when viewed with an epifluorescence microscope. The number of bacteria detected in many environments is often three orders of magnitude greater than the number determined by standard plate count methods. Large bacterial populations have since been confirmed using other methods like scanning electron microscopy.

Given that epifluorescence provides a more rapid technique than the plate-count method, why is it not more widely used? The reasons given are various. It is a more expensive technique and it requires the use of a fluorescence microscope, not always available because of its cost. It is more difficult to train operators on its procedures. The acrydine orange stain is carcinogenic, involving questions of safety. Unlike the plate-counting technique, it does not permit the use of organism speciation.

Epifluorescence yields only total counts. The differentiation between viable and dead organisms, claimed to be possible by this technique, is not universally, or even widely, endorsed. Gould (1993) stated that living organisms. containing RNA, exhibit red-orange colorations; dead organisms, because of the presence of DNA, show a green color, also characteristic of organisms present in salt water. Husted (1994) saw the color differences as reflecting the single or double-strandedness of the DNA or ribonucleic acid (RNA) that is present. Confusingly, intermediate colors and blends of color are also present, and offer interferences.

Objections to the obtaining of total counts (the summation of both living and dead organisms) may, however, be wide of the mark. Sessile organisms, those attached to the biofilm, are seen to give rise to the live planktonic, free-floating microbial population. The total count, both living and dead, is perhaps more significant, therefore, to the organism picture than are the more limiting live counts.

The higher counts afforded by epifluorescence are of less importance in situations where trends rather than exact numerical specifications are the consideration. The same holds true for the rapidity of assaying. Rapid organism counting may offer advantages. However, usually trend lines are being plotted, and speed of assaying is then of lesser importance.

Recovery method. Microbiological assays are also performed using microporous membrane filters in a technique known as the *recovery method*. Filtration of the organism suspension collects the microbes on the filter, which is then placed onto nutrient and incubated. The pore-size membrane that is used is 0.45-μm-rated. The retention of organisms by 0.2-μm-rated membrane would likely be greater. However, the recovery of organisms is greater using 0.45-μm-rated filters. It is for this reason that microbiological assays (as of potable or recreational waters) involving the recovery technique utilize 0.45-μm-rated membranes. In the recovery method, the organism suspension is filtered. To repeat, the membrane serves to collect and concentrate the microbes, presumably largely on its surface. The membrane with its positioned organisms is placed within a Petri dish atop a nutritional agar or broth medium, whereupon it is incubated at a proper temperature for an appropriate period of time. This causes the organisms to grow to sizes that (often with the aid of stains) can be detected and counted microscopically (Sladek et al., 1975).

It has been found that 0.2-μm-rated membranes give poorer recoveries than their 0.45-μm-rated counterparts (Bordner, 1987). Presumably, it is rationalized, the larger pores better shelter the surface-retained microbes against fatal desiccations, or else are less restrictive to their being supplied with nutrients being brought to their locations by the capillary action of the pores. Therefore, 0.45-μm-rated membranes, not 0.2-μm-rated membranes, are used in recovery work. This too presumably accounts for the higher recoveries, as of *E. coli* and/or fecal coliform, that are obtained on those surfaces of the asymmetric membranes bearing the larger pores, as used in those water microbiological assays (Presswood and Meltzer, 1980).

The above facts notwithstanding, use is often made of 0.2 μm-rated membranes in recovery work, impelled, no doubt, by a well-intentioned zeal for maximum organism retentions. This practice is furthered by the advocacy of a major membrane manufacturer for the use of his 0.2μm-rated membrane. What should be of interest is that this particular 0.2μm-rated filter would be classified as being 0.46μm-rated on the basis of latex particle retention (Krygier 1986).

Carter et al (1996) in a study of the recovery method confirmed that until the organism loading density exceeds 1 x 10^4 per cm^2 of membrane surface, the 0.45μm-rated filter retains as well as does its 0.2μm-rated counterpart; as previously stated by Bowman et al (1967), and as demonstrated by Leahy and Sullivan (1978). Carter et al found that the 0.45μm-rated filter yielded higher recovery values than the 0.2μm-rated membrane, a confirmation of the Sladek et al (1975) work.

More important, Carter et at (1996) concluded from their studies that the *recovery method* compared favorably in quantitative assay work with the conventional plate count method. This is of real significance in filter validation studies where the recovery method is use to detect organisms that have penetrated the filter undergoing validation. It answers the question of why a 0.45μm-rated referee membrane can be used to detect organisms that may have penetrated the challenged 0.2μm-rated filter.

Sterility testing method. However, 0.45-μm-rated membranes are also stipulated for membrane sterility assays wherein direct counting is not involved (*USP 23*), where the membrane and its retained organisms are immersed in the nutrient broth eventually to give visible evidence of insterility. Clearly, retention is the consideration in this technique, and 0.2-μm-rated membranes ought to be relied on. The use of 0.45-μm-rated membranes for sterility testing was first advocated by Frances Bowman when these filters were the sterilizing filters, the smallest-rated membrane filters available. Subsequently, the 0.22 (0.2) μm-rated filters

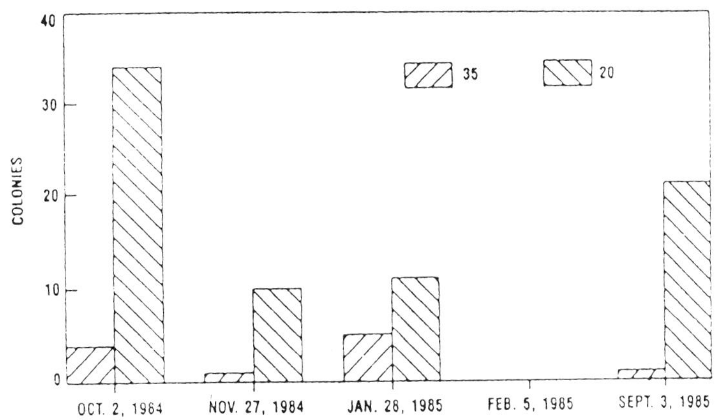

Figure 2-3. Comparative bacteria counts using incubation temperatures of 35 °C and 20 °C.
Lilly (1990); Courtesy, *Microcontamination*

were devised as sterilizing filters (to retain *P. diminuta* ATCC-19146).* However, alteration in the specifications from 0.45-µm-rated to 0.2-µm-rated was never accomplished. It bears reiteration that 0.2-µm-rated membranes ought to be used for sterility assays other than those involving the recovery technique.

It is recognized that the direct-count methods consistently underestimate the bacterial population (Clancy and Cimini, 1991). Heat shock is a technique sometimes used to render culturable bacteria into a dormant stage wherein they are viable but not culturable. In this technique, the organism suspension is heated to 45 °C for 30 minutes. The heat-shock phenomenon is believed to be a thermally controlled genetic mechanism that alters cell metabolism. It has been reported to be effective in the recovery of *Legionella* from potable waters, and in *E. coli* and *Vibrio* recovery from estuarine and marine waters. However, Clancy and Cimini (1991) reported it not to be effective for the organisms (largely pseudomonads) isolated from their high-purity water systems.

Plate count agar. Plate count agar is widely used as an acceptable growth medium in accordance with *Standard Methods* (1989, 17th edition) usage.

Martyak (1988) analyzed for *Pseudomonas* by filtering 100 mL RO/deionized (DI) water samples through a 0.45-µm-rated membrane, which was then incubated on *Pseudomonas* agar or standard plate agar for 24 hours at 28 °C. Direct-count enumeration was made. This procedure is a variant of the ASTM method of analysis. Others have identified *P. aeruginosa, P. cepacia,* and *P. vesicularis* in RO/DI distribution systems.

Indirect methods of assessing microbial numbers and/or identities are by way of fatty acid analyses, by deoxyribose nucleic acid analyses, and through lipopolysaccharide quantitation, as already indicated.

A proper perspective of what has been involved in high-purity water microbiology is given by Gould (1993):

> Full appreciation for the presence of bacteria in water did not come until ways were found to detect them. Failure to grow water bacteria in the laboratory, the inability to trap them on sterilizing filter membranes, and failure to see them under the light microscope had led microbiologists to the conclusion that a pure water environment would be too "stressful" for bacterial growth. But most environments, including pure water, define a medium and a physical state that some kind of bacterium can exploit.
>
> A classic way to enumerate bacteria is to do a plate count, which is to spread a known volume of sample on the surface of a laboratory medium and count the number of visible colonies that develop after

* *Pseudomonas diminuta* has been reclassified to the genus *Prevundimonas*. The genus *Pseudomonas* is used in this writing, however.

> a period of time. A colony arises from one bacterium. The bacterium grows and divides only if it can grow in that specific chemical and physical environment.
>
> Plate counts are often referred to as viable counts that sometimes are equated literally with "living" or "not dead". The assumption of dead cells is a common rationalization for why a direct count under the microscope may indicate far more cells than are indicated by standard plate count methods. Failure to mimic the critical conditions found in the environment in the laboratory does not mean. however, that the cells in the sample were dead. In fact, the majority of bacteria that are growing in pure water may only be grown in pure water; laboratory conditions are simply toxic to bacteria adapted to or selected for growth in high-purity water systems. This leads directly to the phenomenon of viable but non-culturable bacteria. (Dealt with below).

As recent as 1989, Lilly could write,

> A review of the literature reveals that numerous authors have identified point-of-use equipment as being sources of significant wafer contamination due to bacteria. In some manufacturing facilities this problem has been considered so serious that the DI rinse portion of spin/rinse dryers has been shut off.

Lilly pointed out that the use of equipment embodying dead-legs, harboring

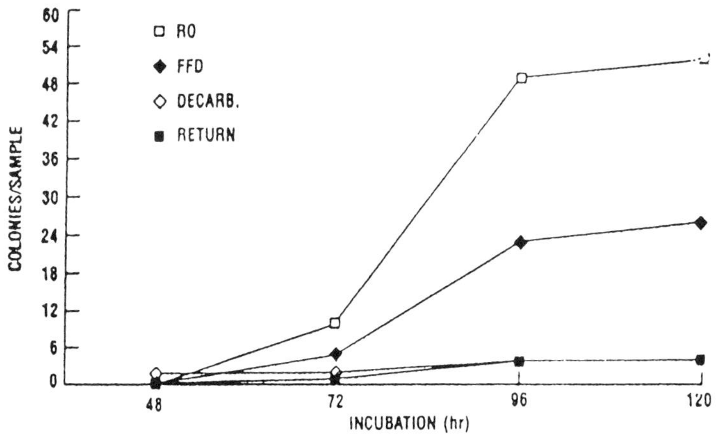

Figure 2-4. Comparative bacteria counts after incubation periods of various lengths.
Lilly, (1990); Courtesy, *Microcontamination*

areas for organisms, is a cause; that too-infrequent sanitization is another; and that the ASTM direct-count method is inappropriate for microbial assays in semiconductor water settings.

Lilly (1989) advocated the use of the epifluorescence technique that permits the direct microscopic counting of organisms stained with acrydine orange. In detailing the epifluorescence method along with the other techniques available for microbiological assays, Mittelman and Geesey (1987, p 279) made plain that the method does not differentiate live cells from dead, nor does it permit the speciation of the organisms. It is, however, a rapid assay procedure with a direct-count enumeration that yields higher counts than are normally obtained from the more conventional methods.

Cooper (Feb. 1996) is, nevertheless, of the opinion that the concerns about nonculturable organisms in monitoring the water for pharmaceutical processing may be overemphasized.

An Application of Microbiological Assays

Carmody and Martyak (1989) described an operational protocol used at IBM's plant in East Fishkill, N.Y., to control bacterial contamination. For this protocol, reliance is placed upon microbiological assays in developing a bacterial profile of the various components of the high-purity water system. This permits proper bacteriostatic contamination controls, and assures the attainment of defect-density and contamination specifications.

Live bacteria are identified using nutrient agar plate counts. A 100-mL sample is passed through a 0.45-μm-rated membrane (recovery technique), which is then placed on heterotrophic *Pseudomonas* agar and incubated at 28 °C for 24 hours. Scanning electron microscopy is used for low-level counting and for total bacterial counts. This includes live, dead, and fragmented organisms. It involves a minimum of 200 liters of sample passed through a 0.2-μm-rated filter. Plate counts and epifluorescence are the other two methods used to secure live bacteria. These are reported in colony-forming units per 100 mL. Total numbers of both viable and dead organisms are reported as numbers per liter. Bacterial endotoxin profiles are used to measure the effectiveness of the microbial control program throughout the system. Such system profiling identifies areas and units involved in bacterial proliferation.

In a separate endeavor, Futatsuki (1991) microbiologically assayed high-purity semiconductor water using M-TGE broth without agar (beef extract, 6.0 g; tryptone, 10.0 g; and dextrose, 2.0 g, in 1,000 mL of high-purity water). Incubation period was 24 hours at 35 °C. A direct-counting method was also used.

Clancy and Cimini (1991) compared, as isolation media for the organisms recovered from a high-purity water system, mTGE, HPC (heterotrophic plate-count media), and R2A, prepared according to manufacturer's directions.

Incubations were performed at 20 °C and at 35 °C for the HPC and mTGE. The R2A samples were incubated at 20 °C. Two different volume samples were assayed for each medium and temperature, namely, 100 mL and 500 mL. The 35 °C incubations showed no differences after 48 hours. All counts were higher after 7 days. Use of mTGE gave the lowest recoveries, too low to reveal differences between 20 °C and 35 °C. When 100-mL water samples were used, recovery was greater using 0.45-μm-rated membranes than with 0.22-μm-rated filters The reverse was true for the 500-mL samples. High-purity-water bacterial recoveries after 7-day incubations at 20 °C were similar for the HPC and R2A media. The data produced from this study do not clearly define advantages to be gained from the use of HPC or R2A. Similarly, the use of 0.22- or 0.45-μm-rated membranes likewise yielded no unambiguous differentiation in recovery numbers.

As stated, the concern with the media is the recovery of oligotrophic microbes. These organisms adapt to survival under low water nutrient conditions, but fail to form colonies under the nutrient-rich circumstances of the usual type of plating conditions. The mTGE medium is an extremely rich extract of beef, tryptone, and dextrose. It is used primarily for standard plate counts on dairy products. The HPC, developed to enumerate the microbial contents of potable water, is composed of peptone, gelation, and glycerol. It is rich in amino acids and in proteins, but not so rich as mTGE.

Typical bacterial profiles obtained by Carmody and Martyak (1989) are partially shown in Table 2-6. What is important is that the microbiological monitoring was done before and after each component in the purification system. This procedure enables trend lines to be drawn. These, in turn, reveal when a particular purification device is in need of refurbishing, as by sanitization or replacement. In the establishing of trend lines, it is not essential that the analyses being depended upon yield the highest possible numbers (although variations in large numbers may be easier to spot). Nor need the relationships between the counts given by different methods require reconciliation. It is enough for trends as a function of time to be made evident and for timely actions to be taken. By this means, the facility reported upon was made dependably to deliver high-purity water of a *consistently* high quality, with fewer than 1 cfu/100 mL of live bacteria, and total counts of less than 35 per liter.

The technique of exercising control over the bacterial contamination of a high-purity water system by way of a rigorous maintenance program based on individual component monitoring is as valid for pharmaceutical and power applications as it is for semiconductor usage.

WQC/PMA Recommendations

WQC/PMA, the Water Quality Committee of the Pharmaceutical Manufacturers Association (now the Pharmaceutical Research and Manufacturers Association,

PhRMA) (1992) has recommended that the pharmaceutical waters be assayed as follows:
Purified Water: Plate-count-agar 1 mL sample Pour plate minimum 48-hour incubation at 30 to35 °C; Water for Injection: plate-count-agar 100 mL sample 0.45 µm-rated filter minimum 48-hour incubation at 30 to 35 °C.

Cooper (Feb. 1993) suggested that a 300-mL sample be used for WFI to give a sufficient count, if any, for the WFI. The FDA likewise would prefer a larger sample for the WFI, its organism population being so low, for a greater accuracy in counting (Munson, 1993). Cooper (Feb. 1993) also prefers that a temperature for incubation be more precisely defined.

The WQC/PMA in its recommendations regarding the microbiological assaying of pharmaceutical waters should serve very helpfully as a guide. However, the responsibility of determining the assay method that is possibly uniquely suitable to a given water rests with the pharmaceutical manufacturer. Different methodologies, nutrients, and incubation times and temperatures may be variously appropriate. Perhaps different media should be tried to see whether different microbial types become disclosed. Perhaps using the same medium for different incubation periods should be explored to see whether the presence of different organisms is made evident. It is ultimately the responsibility of the drug manufacturer to investigate whether different media and different incubation times and temperatures uncover and identify different organisms, and to determine the significances of such findings to the drug product.

The reliance upon preservative formulations to control organism proliferations in non-injectables can be a dangerous and misleading practice. The preservative system developed for the organisms found to be present in a water

Table 2-9
Proportions of *Pseudomonas* Strain EK20 Cells Adhering Reversibly and Irreversibly[a] to a Polysryrene Substration at Different Time Intervals

	% of total bacteria attached	
Time (h)	*Reversibly*	*Irreversibly*
1	*89.5*	*10.5*
2	*70.7*	*29.5*
3	*44.2*	*55.8*
4	*27.3*	*72.7*
5	*22.0*	*78.0*
6	*24.0*	*75.6*
22	*9.4*	*90.6*

a Determined by using 3H-labeled bacterial suspensions in polystyrene petri dishes. After the supernatant was poured off, the washings were retained as the reversibly adhered fraction while the irreversibly adhered fraction remained attached to the substratum.

Marshall (1990) Courtesy ASM News.

system at a given time may not be efficacious should the microflora of that system change to a preservative-resistant variety. The possibilities of such alterations are real and have certainly occurred in the past. Ongoing microbiological investigations and retesting are, therefore, indicated.

Viable but Nonculturable Bacteria

As Colwell (1994) sets forth,

> Viable but non-culturable bacteria have been found to occur in a variety of Gram-negative bacteria, e.g. *Vibrio cholerae* 01 and 0139, *Salmonella spp.*, *Shigella spp.*, *Legionellae*, and *Campylobacter*. Because bacteria in the viable but non-culturable state are reduced in size and frequently in coccoid form, they will pass through 0.45-micron filters and in some cases, 0.2-μm filters. Furthermore, under very low nutrient conditions, the viable but nonculturable state may be predominant. Preparation of water for pharmaceutical and biotechnology applications requires consideration of the presence of bacteria in a nonculturable, dormant stage, especially for the preparation of solutions of injectables or topical reagents for use in the eye or medical therapeutics for burn victims. Water purification systems cannot rely on culturable plate counts for monitoring safety and quality. They must consider the direct count and molecular genetic assay for water safety quality.

Colwell (1994) expatiates upon the situation,

> When bacteria are introduced into a new environment from another, the environmental changes with which they are confronted may include temperature, nutrient concentration, salinity, osmotic pressure, pH, and many others. Bacterial cells dynamically adapt to these shifts in environmental parameters, employing a variety of genotypic and phenotypic mechanism. Bacteria, with the ability to utilize constitutive and inducible enzyme synthesis, can accommodate to growth-limiting nutrients and adjust or rerout metabolic pathways to avoid metabolic and/or structural disruption caused by specific nutrient limitations. Furthermore, they are able to coordinate their rates of synthesis to maintain their cellular structure and function. These adaptive capabilities provide bacterial cells with an extraordinary set of mechanisms by which they are able to respond to their surrounding environment and survive. This is a powerful message for those who prepare water for pharmaceutical and biotechnological applications.

Previously, non-viable cells observed under the microscope were considered dead or vegetative. If these cells could not be grown in the laboratory they were also termed viable cells, *nonviable* cells, *stressed* cells, *moribund* cells, or *injured* cells. Precisely what these particular terms were meant to signify was often obscure. Proof of cell viability was the capability to be cultured in the laboratory on routine bacteriological media. Clearly, such a judgment depended upon the efficiency, limitations, and/or selectivity of the medium employed. Colwell (1994) credits Roszak et al, (1984) with coining the term *viable but non-culturable*. It is meant to designate those bacteria that possess metabolic function but that are not culturable by available means.

Coldwell and Huq (1995) emphasize the unsuitability of plate count methods for the detection of viable but non-culturable organisms. Direct count techniques are required. Operators of pharmaceutical water systems should consider the implications of such organisms.

Small-size bacteria and those with lower metabolic rates have the greatest ability to survive. It has been postulated that morphological changes that result in the "rounding" of cells, or in other size-reduction mechanisms, contribute to cell survival. Such adjustments may attain 15- to 300-fold reductions in size, depending upon the level of nutritional stress (Colwell, 1994).

Gould (1993) states, "When bacteria are introduced with the water source they are in an environment that is relatively rich nutritionally compared to the environment they may end up in further along in the water purification system". Among the survival mechanisms they invoke is minimization of their cell size; thereby maximizing surface-to-volume ratios. "By becoming small round cells or very thin long cells, they minimize the amount of cellular material they need to synthesize" to survive.

The problem often manifests itself as a disparity between direct counts and those that are recovered by the plating or most-probable-number techniques. As Gould (1993) states it , "Plate counts are often referred to as viable counts that sometimes are equated literally with 'living' or 'not dead.' The assumption of dead cells is a common rationalization for why a direct count under the microscope may indicate far more cells than are indicated by standard plate count methods". Therein lies the potential problem! The presence in a pharmaceutical water supply of viable but nonculturable, and hence not detected, bacteria may erroneously lead to the conclusion that the subject water is sterile. This is also the concern regarding the presence of L-form organisms (Thomas et al, 1991). These presumably escape being retained by the 0.45 μm-rated filters commonly utilized in the conventional microbiological recovery method because their defective cell walls render them flexible enough to negotiate the tortuous pore-passageways of the filters (page 235).

The epifluorescence method of microbiological assaying, described on page 80 was developed in response to the limitations of the standard plate count technique. As noted, however, for whatever reasons, the epifluorescence method has thus far gained only limited acceptance. The plate-count technique is still widely used. Indeed, the WQC/PMA recommends that the pour-plate method utilizing plate count agar, in accordance with *Standard Method*'s (1989, 17th edition), be utilized in pharmaceutical water examinations.

Colwell (1994) discusses particular instances whereby difficult-to-grow specific organisms may be cultivated, and provides a rich literature referencing on the subject. She advises direct procedures for ascertaining the organism numbers in water rather than culture techniques. A potential for future study on the subject of bacterial viability is indicated by this author. She writes, in her critique of the epifluorescence technique involving acridine orange stain:

> A more persuasive assay for testing viability is the direct viable count (DVC) developed by Kogure et al (1979) in which active cells are identified by growth, without multiplication, after incubation for 6 hours at 25 °C, in response to addition of yeast extract in the presence of nalidixic acid. Under these conditions active cells carry out protein synthesis in the absence of DNA replication or cell division and produce elongated cells that are easily identified by their size.

Biofilm

A layer of living and dead organisms, their metabolic products, and various organic and inorganic substances trapped within a polymeric matrix of bacterial origin come to characterize virtually all surfaces in contact with water. As will be discussed, the formation of such a glycocalyx over time is the product of many factors. It can, however, develop with rapidity, although different organisms form biofilms at different rates. Marshall (1992) cities evidence, Table 2-9, that tritium-labelled *Pseudomonas* Strain EK-20 begins to form biofilm upon a polystyrene substrate within one hour. It is 75% irreversable at 6 hours, and after 22 hours is 90% so. (It should be noted, however, that the waters Marshall worked with were far more nutritious than the pharmaceutical waters of interest here.)

Biofilms are of interest in the present context because they intermittently shed bits and pieces of their structure into the contacting waters. As self-replicating entities, the shed organisms compromise the microbial integrity of the liquid; inevitably threatening, thereby, the sufficiency of the WFI or Purified Water in contact with the biofilm.

Mittelman (1990) states that virtually all bacteria isolated from purified water systems are Gram-negative rods. The implication of such organisms to the question of "adventitious pathogens" will shortly be explored. The central concern is that even small numbers of such organisms may prove pathogenic to susceptible subjects, and that biofilm may be their point of origin.

Planktonic and Sessile Forms

In the testing of high-purity water, an aliquot sample is assayed. What is being measured is the number of organisms suspended in the aqueous medium. This represents the free-floating or planktonic organism population. Clearly, if an organism (or organisms) were to attach itself to the container wall, it would not flow with the liquid onto the assay membrane's surface. Organisms attached to surfaces are designated by the term *sessile*. Actually, in both environmental and industrial flowing systems the majority of bacteria are attached to surfaces. The ratio of sessile to planktonic organisms (i.e., bacteria per square centimeter to bacteria per milliliter) may exceed 10,000. This may be because the organic matter that serves as nutrient adsorbs to surfaces and is to be found there. Thus, the fraction of sessile organisms tends to increase with decreasing bulk-phase nutrient level (Geesey, 1988). Therefore, in nutrient-limited high-purity water systems, the surface-area-to-volume ratio can be a determinant of the potential for biological contamination (Mittelman, 1985). Biofilm is a surface phenomenon. Therefore, rougher surfaces should exhibit more of it.

Biofilm formation. When surfaces encounter water, they immediately adsorb and become coated by a layer of the trace organics present in all water sources. The adsorption is usually of a hydrophobic nature that results in a diminution of free surface energy. Adsorption phenomena can result from charge-motivated mechanisms as well. The concentration of the organic molecules at the solid-

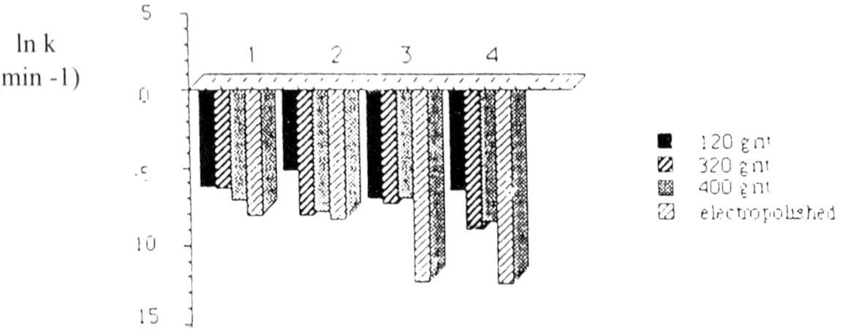

Figure 2-5. Adhesion rate constants of six P. aeruginosa *strains adhering onto a 316-L stainless steel submerged in 0.01-molar phosphate buffered 0.85% saline. A low k-value corresponds with a low adhesion rate onto the stainless steel. Hydrophobic strains: number 1 and 2; hydrophilic strains: number 3 and 4.*
Vanhaeke and Van den Haesevelde, (1991); Courtesy, Interpharm Press

liquid interface is favored because it results in an increase in entropy (Characklis, 1981). Such organic surface adsorption precedes biofilm formation. Cellular adhesion is dependent upon the organic macromolecular film formation. Brownian motion and molecular diffusion (both temperature-dependent), along with flow effects (whether turbulent or laminar), and gravity effects (such as sedimentation and differential settling), all contribute to small-particle (organism) transport in aqueous systems (Hunt, 1982; O'Melia, 1980; Camper et al. 1994). Chemotaxis also plays a role in biofilm formation (Chet et al., 1975; Young and Mitchell, 1972; Young and Mitchell, 1973). Chemotaxis is the movement of organisms in response to a chemical (e.g., nutrient) gradient.

By such mechanisms, organisms first form a reversible phase of attachment to the water-wetted, organic-coated surfaces, and then proceed to establish a permanent or irreversible attachment, as shown in Table 2-7 (Zobell, 1943). One theory of bacterial adhesion to solid substrates holds that the irreversible biofilm formation derives from the action of adhesive extracellular polysaccharides (Costerton et al., 1978). At high bacterial contamination levels and/or at longer contact times, a multilayer of adhering microbial cells is established. Its integrity reflects the bacterial species, the nature of the suspending medium, and the solid surface characteristics. Following this initial phase of organism adherence, a second phase of microcolony formation occurs after several hours of contact. Vanhaecke and Van den Haesevelde (1991) state this to be "due to a remarkable

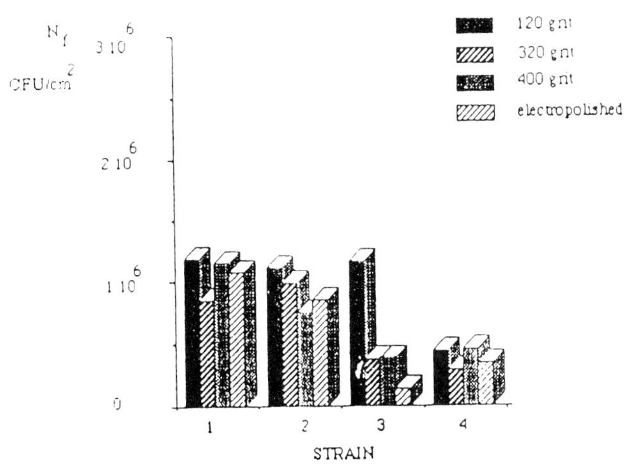

Figure 2-6. Maximum number of adhering bacteria per cm² (N_f values) adhering onto a 316-L stainless steel, after 120 minutes of incubation at room temperature with 2.0 x 10⁷ cfu/mL in 0.01 phosphate-buffered 0.85% saline of P. aeruginosa *cells. Hydrophobic strains: number 1 and 2; hydrophilic strains: number 3 and 4.*
Vanhaeke and Van den Haesevelde, (1991); Courtesy, Interpharm Press

phenotypic plasticity of the bacterial cell." It undergoes an altered metabolic activity upon adhesion. The adhering microbes are completely different with regard to structure and function as compared to freely suspended cells. This difference finds expression in the resistance of adhering cells to chemical agents such as sanitizers.

Surface smoothness. No surfaces have been found that are exempt from biofouling. Surface structure does appear to influence the rate of fouling, but only initially over the first few hours of exposure. In general, smooth surfaces foul at a slower initial rate than do rough ones, but biofilm formation after a period of days is inevitable. Ridgway et al. (1985) cited a well-established film within 16 days. The effect of surfaces has not found consistent experimental expression. Van Loosdrecht et al, (1980) summarize the various relevant findings of different investigators. The qualitative consensus is that surfaces do influence bacterial metabolism. However, evidence for this belief is not conclusive (Van Loosdrecht et al, 1990).

Vanhaecke and Van den Haesevelde (1991), working with stainless steel of

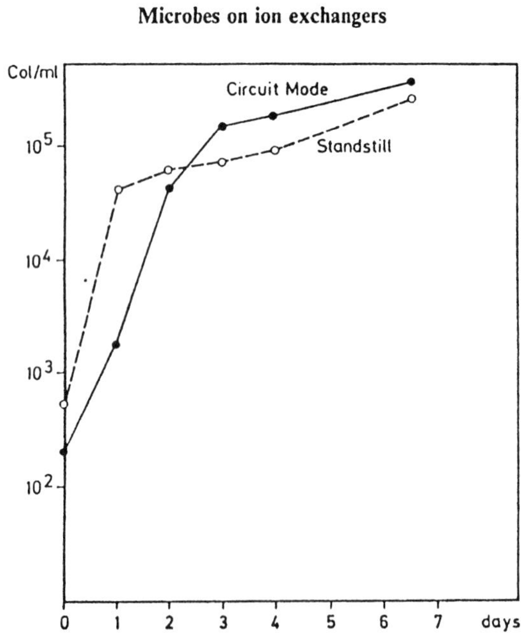

Figure 2-7. Comparison of colony numbers (in colonies per milliliter) in daily random samples from a recirculated (●--●) and from an idly standing (o--o) exchange unit.

Fleming, (1988); Courtesy, Ellis Horwood Ltd., Chichester, U.K.

four different surface roughness, namely, 120, 320, and 400 grit and electropolished 320 grit, found that the differences in bacterial adhesion were minimal when hydrophobic organisms strains were involved. When, however, hydrophilic *P. aeruginosa* types were present, adhesion took place less readily on the smoother surfaces. These investigators concluded that surface roughness has a clear but not exclusive influence on bacterial adhesion kinetics (Figures 2-5 and 2-6). Electropolishing has a minimum influence where hydrophobic strains are involved. In any case, bacterial adhesion to stainless steel occurs nearly instantaneously (Vanhaeke et al., 1990).

The role of surface smoothness in biofilm formation is an especially intriguing one. Costerton and also Geesey stated that surface smoothness does not affect biofilm development (Cooper, July 1987). Nevertheless, these authorities concur that any surface geometry that disrupts laminar water flow will enhance microbial colonization of that surface. Be that as it may, Cooper's wry observation (1984) still bears repeating: "One cannot help but contemplate the effort spent in recent validation programs with the encouragement of 'experts' to assure that inside surfaces were smooth/polished."

Mittelman (1985) stated that "Although surface characteristics do influence biofilm structure, bacterial attachment does not appear to be significantly influenced by construction materials. Smoother surfaces delay the initial build-up of attached bacteria but do not appear to reduce the total number attached."

Surface smoothness should have some influence. Biofilm is a surface phenomenon. The rougher the surface, the more of it. Cracks are in the nature of dead legs. They limit chemical sanitization to a diffusion controlled process.

Effect of water velocity. A similar observation has been made for the influence of flowrates on bacterial attachment. At higher flowrates, a denser, somewhat more tenacious biofilm is formed. As a result, these surfaces often appear to be free from foulants, since they are not slimy to the touch. In closed-loop polishing systems, such as purified-water systems, higher flowrates do result in more frequent filtration and UV (or ozone) contacts, reducing the number of free-floating bacteria and the concentration of nutrients that can contact surfaces. However, higher flowrates will not prevent the attachment of bacteria to pipe surfaces. More work is needed to define the specific role of piping systems design and materials in the biological fouling of high-purity water systems.

Both the structure and induction time for the biofilm formation are influenced by the fluid velocity (McCoy and Costerton, 1982). In high-velocity regimens, the bacteria that accumulate tend to be of a filamentous variety especially suited for attachment by the filaments. Morphological changes in biofilms may partly be due to physiological adaptations to environmental changes. The effects of fluid velocities on biofilms and their formation are still somewhat uncertain. There are, however, no compelling data to affirm that turbulent flows prevent biofilm formation. McCoy et al, (1981) utilized low-flow velocities of 138.5 centimeters per second (cm/sec) and high flow velocities of almost double that amount, 265.4 cm/sec. The low-velocity induction phase, as measured by the frictional resistance to water flow, was 20 hours. The induction phase for the high water velocity was about 65 hours. In each case the occurrence of firmly adherent filamentous bacteria in the biofilm was seen as the cause of the resistance to flow. At the higher velocities the filamentous bacteria became a permanent part of the biofilm only after the surface had acquired great amounts of extracellular material (e.g. polysaccharides). At the lower velocities, considerably less shear presumably permitted filamentous bacteria attachments to grow on cleaner surfaces. The interference with water flows through pipes is ascribed to the presence and growth of such filamentous bacteria.

Regardless of the water velocity, it flows slowest in the layers adjacent to (pipe) surfaces. This favors organism attachments. Bacteria deposit upon the inner surfaces of pipe bends.

Pittner and Bertler (1988) calculated the shear forces that are present under various velocity conditions on 1-µm-diameter sections of five sizes of pipe commonly used in semiconductor pure water distribution systems (Table 2-8). These investigators concluded that in none of the cases are the shear forces strong enough to remove an organism from such a pipe wall. A shear force thousands of times that of the force of gravity would be required because the adhesive force for a 1-µm-diameter particle exceeds the weight of a particle by a factor of 10^6 (Pittner and Bertler, 1988).

Patterson et al. (1991) examined IBM high-purity water with a 18+ megohm-cm resistivity suitable for 4-megabyte dynamic random access memory (DRAM) production (35 bacteria per L), and frequently adequate for 16-megabyte product (8 bacteria per L). They found a marked difference between the results of microbial assays sampled at a pipe-wall tap and those drawn from the center of the water stream. This constituted at least indirect evidence of the existence of biofilm. The removal of a pipe section and the analysis of its coated inner surface confirmed the presence of the biofilm. The presence of the biofilm confounds the generally assumed beliefs that the lack of nutrients and a high Reynolds number keep the pipe walls clean. Indeed, it is noteworthy that numerous Gram-positive isolates were found. These organisms, unlike the Gram-negatives, require significant sources of nutrition.

Patterson et al. (1991) referenced findings that microbial assay methods based on ASTM protocol for standard plate-count methods were not suited to organism detections in high-purity waters. The plating media for viable counts were too rich or selective; the sample volume too small; the incubation time of 24 hours too short; and the incubation temperature of 28 °C too high. Furthermore, the sampling of the bulk water stream failed to assess the presence of biofilm upon the system surfaces. Samples collected from the boundary layer would have yielded cell counts greater than those gathered from the bulk fluid phase. Direct-count methods intended to detect the occurrence of bacterial shedding from the biofilm can only be reliable when the water sampling is large enough so that shedding becomes a uniformly distributed event. That sufficiency in sampling size, both volume and frequency, can become defined only by developing a sampling history leading to a retrospective conclusion.

The situation, then, is that neither smoothness of surface, materials of construction, nor flow velocities long delay the advent of biofilm formation. Costerton (1984) found that organisms form surface biofilm in a number of aquatic systems. The glycocalyx matrix of polysaccharides or of glycoproteins, protected by bacterial slimes, are resistant to biocides..

Recirculation effects. It is firmly and widely believed that organism growth is diminished in flowing (recirculating) waters. As measured by planktonic organism counts per volume of water examined, stagnant waters do yield higher numbers. It does not follow, however, that a continually decreasing count will result from increasing flowrates. Husted et al. (1993) found that flowrates in excess of approximately 3 ft/sec offered no added advantages to organism population diminution.

The cause of the decrease is uncertain in terms of the total number of organisms, both planktonic and sessile. If the oversimplified view is taken that the planktonic count consists of the incoming floater level augmented by a constant release rate from the biofilm, then faster flowrates should show the dilution effects common to diffusion phenomena (such as rates of extraction, for instance). It is also possible that in stationary systems, nutritional or chemotactic gradients between the surface interface and the bulk water diminish and that biofilm attachments become less favored.

If the focus is strictly upon the free-floating population, then the commonly held belief seems true. However, optimal flowrates may be judged using other parameters, such as pumping costs.

In any case, a projection of this phenomenon to recirculation rates optimal for carbon beds or ion-exchange columns cannot safely be made. These each have their own kinetic and equilibria considerations, and these may well be different for each individual installation.

Experimental evidence shows that at least for ion-exchange beds the recirculative flow of water did not yield lower organism counts. Flemming (1988) compared two exchange units characterized by two liters of resin and a flow velocity of 8 meters per hour. One unit was operated in a closed-circuit posture. The other was let stand idle. Bacterial assays were performed daily. As shown in Figure 2-7, recirculation did not prevent, or even diminish organism growth. As Flemming (1988) expressed the findings, "The exchange unit can be considered as being a kind of fermenter operated on a very low level of nutrient.

Growth rates in operating and standing units are very similar, and the low colony numbers of continuously operated units may be due to a dilution effect resulting from the amount of water passed through."

In real systems, recirculations involve multiple passages through units such as ion exchange columns, carbon beds, and filters upon whose surfaces the planktonic organisms may become deposited as biofilm, to their consequent decrease as free-floaters. If recirculated through ultraviolet installations their living numbers would be expected to decrease. Recirculation through heated systems would ensure against cold spots favorable to organisms. As already stated, Reynolds numbers indicative of turbulent flows do not remove biofilm nor significantly retard its formation. There is no reason to believe that microbes in recirculating waters are otherwise inhibited from growing at their normal rates.

Husted's (1995) summation of biofilm formation, and dead leg and velocity effects may be stated as follows: Bacterial nutrients, as also water borne organisms, are distributed rather evenly within a quiescent water volume. (This situation is the one characterizing dead legs). As the velocity of the water is increased to about one foot per second the growth of biofilm increases rapidly. Greater increases in velocity increasingly promote biofilm growth, but not proportionally. The greatest effect of the water velocity upon biofilm growth is between one and three feet per second. Above that range velocity increases are not proportionally influencial. The increased biofilm formation is rationalized as resulting from the organisms migrating to the container walls in a chemotactic response to the nutrients having been deposited thereon by the higher water velocities. The planktonic count decreases in consequence; the sessile population, the biofilm, increases. The nutrients, the organic impurities, tend to migrate out of the water in which they have limited solubility as a result of their cohesive energy densities being substantially different from that of water. They migrate to the water interface, to the tank and pipe walls, where they are adsorbed. The organisms follow in search of food. In static systems there are diffusional impediments to the migration within the stagnant water. Therefore, in static systems the planktonic counts are higher. This hypothesis is given credence by the direct correlation between biofilm build up and nutrient concentration.

The biofilm can be in thicknesses of 20 cells. Such a deposit can exist within the stationary boundary layer proximate to the pipe or tank wall. It remains undislodged regardless of the water velocity and its Reynold's number, contrary to popular belief. The biofilm is highly hydrated. Therefore, higher velocities can compress it. The organisms adapt to new environments. Situated upon surfaces, they may become more hydrophobic than when surrounded by water, a condition that requires hydrophilicity. It may be that the transformation to more hydrophobic forms renders the organisms more resistant to aqueous sanitizing agents.

Dead-leg effect. The examination of waters for the free-floating (planktonic) population of organisms they contained long antedated the current awareness of the biofilm phenomenon. One consequence is that the free-floating microbes and those incorporated into the biofilm, the sessile organisms, are generally considered as if they were unconnected entities, despite the understanding that the free floaters may arise as detachments from the biofilm structure itself. Given this outlook, it is difficult to explain why dead legs should be conducive to organism growth except where heat is involved; turbulence makes for good heat transference. The situation is accepted on a phenomenological basis, part of the belief that stagnant waters encourage bacterial proliferations.

Consider, however, a quiescent pool of water. The organisms resident therein and the organic compounds on which they feed may be roughly idealized as being equally distributed. Flowing of the water would promote contact with and the adsorption or the organic material upon the wall surfaces of the container or pipe. It is Husted's view (1994) that the planktonic organisms, in chemotactic response to their food supply, now adsorbed upon the wall surfaces, migrate thereto to become fixed as biofilm. The overall organism content in the system under consideration need not alter, but the movement of the water serves to decrease the planktonic population, those detected by the microbiological assaying of the water supply.

The subject of dead legs, areas of pipes or containers holding stagnant water, although usually appended to flowing conduits, is discussed in Chapter 11, page 647.

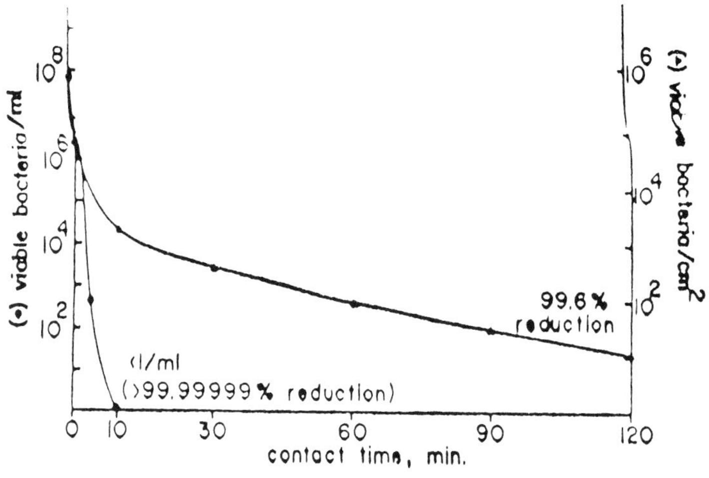

Figure 2-8. Effect of a quaternary ammonium cleaner on sessile and planktonic P. cepacia *populations in purified water.*
Mittelman and Geesey, (1987)

Biofouling of RO membranes. Biological fouling of RO membranes can sharply reduce the cost effectivity of the RO process. The large areas of membrane continuously exposed to feed streams serve to invite such fouling. The result is a diminution in flux and in ion rejection. In RO systems in particular, elevated operating pressures and permeate recoveries promote organism/membrane contact. The tangential flow, while effective in the main, is not completely so. Given sufficient residence time, the bacteria will attach. Clearly the attractive forces involved are more than enough to overcome the fluid shear forces, although in the reversible phase of the adsorption process, gentle rinsing or fluid shear causes bacterial displacement (Zobell, 1943).

Using radioisotopically labeled *Mycobacterium* BT2-4 cells, Ridgway et al. (1984, 1985, 1986) studied biofilm formation on cellulose acetate (CA) RO membranes. The adhesion of the organisms, without the impress of a differential pressure, was surprisingly rapid and showed no log phase. The attachment phenomenon was biphasic; an initial rapid adhesion, straight line with respect to time, was followed by a much slower rate of attachment, also linear with time. In these laboratory studies, the rate of adhesion took place over a 1- to 2-hour period; the slower attachment phase proceeded indefinitely. Typical saturation adsorption kinetics were involved, in keeping with the Langmuir adsorption isotherm equation (Langmuir, 1918). The Langmuir adsorption isotherm bespeaks a monolayer of cells, with no interaction among the adsorbed species, meaning that a higher population in the feedwater would result in a higher fouling rate. This indicates the wisdom of organism level diminution such as by prefiltration. The data also suggested a finite number of adsorption sites on the membrane; once satisfied, no additional adhesion occurred. The number of adsorption sites on the CA membrane studied was about 3.0 x 10^6 per square centimeter (cm^2). Mittelman (1991) questions this latter conclusion stating that an "average" bacterial cell is about 0.51 μm by 1 μm by 1 μm^2 and contains 10^8 μm^2; theoretical space for 2 x 10^8 cells/cm^2.

Table 2-10
Common Physical Methods to Clean Biofouling Deposits from Surfaces

Technique	*Comments*
Flushing	Simplest method; very limited efficacy
Backwashing	Effective for loosely adherent films in tubes, on filters, and in ion-exchange resin beds
Air bumping	Very limited efficacy
Nonabrasive and/or abrasive sponge balls	Extensively used in industry; demonstrated efficacy
Sand scouring	Difficult to control abrasive effects on metal surfaces
Brushing	Expensive; very effective

Courtesy of McCoy, Water Micro Associates (1987); Courtesy, *Biological Fouling of Industrial Water Systems*

Ridgway et al. (1984, 1985) demonstrated that microbial adherence to RO membranes is by hydrophobic adsorption, as illustrated by the strong influence of low concentrations of nonionic surfactant. This is in contrast to the lack of sway by ionic strength or charged-polymer additions.

The nonionic surfactant adsorbs hydrophobically to the organisms and to the adsorptive sites, and serves as a buffer between both entities, preventing their adsorptive interaction. A direct correlation was shown between the relative hydrophobicity of a microbial cell and its adherence to RO membrane surfaces. The ability of nonionic surfactants to disrupt mutual hydrophobic reactions, by masking the hydrophobic ligands and leaving the hydrophilic moiety of the surfactant to interact with the water, justifies the use of such surfactants in the removal of bacterial plaques. Such surfactants are used in many RO cleaning formulas (Adair et al., 1979).

That bacterial attachments may also involve electrostatic interactions is shown by a promotion of adhesion of mycobacteria to cellulose acetate RO membranes caused by certain quaternary ammonium surfactants (Ridgway et al., 1984). This stimulation of adhesion is concentration-dependent, and presumably caused by a differential binding of the surfactant to the organism cell and to the membrane. The effect of the quaternary compound was also to inactivate the organisms. At low surfactant concentrations the quaternary attaches to the organism, imparting a strong cationic charge to it. This enhanced charge interacts more strongly with the more electronegative RO membrane surface. The greatest degree of mycobacterial adhesion is to polyamide RO membranes. These contain anionic carboxylic acid and sulfonic acid groups. The less strongly charged CA membranes show adhesions reduced by five or tenfold. Colonization of cellulose acetate RO surfaces by microbes is quite rapid: 3×10^5 cfu/cm^2 being evident after only 3 days (Ridgway et al., 1984).

Interestingly, the continuous addition of 10 mg/L of monochloramine to the feedwater completely inactivated the fouling bacteria without interfering with their adhesion and subsequent attachment to the membrane surface. The implication is that such attachments are physicochemical in nature, rather than being a result of such metabolic processes as exopolymer-mediated bridging of the electrical double layer.

The developed biofilm consists of predominately rod-shaped bacteria embedded within a glycocalyx matrix. Glycoproteins and heteropolysaccharides constitute an extracellular slime that may be quite extensive. This glycocalyx has a large capacity for hydration, endowing the biofilm with a gelatinous, slippery surface. Increased packing densities for the biofilm contribute to flux declines. These could result from higher stream velocities. The glycocalyx concentrates nutrients and tends, therefore, to elevate metabolic activities and organism growth. It is for this reason that the sessile organisms outgrow their planktonic counterparts (Paerl, 1985). The glycocalyx serves to protect its constituting microbes. Once a surface film is established, the incorporated organisms are resistant even to a free chlorine residual of several ppm (LeChevallier et al., 1984; Ridgway and Olson, 1982; Seyfried and Fraser, 1980).

Patterson et al. (1991) concluded that the majority of microbes observed in the bulk phase of high-purity water systems with a resistivity of 18+ megohm-cm are derived directly from biofilm associated with the system surfaces.

The picture that emerges is that the sessile biofilm deposition serves as a reservoir to replenish, from time to time, the relatively few planktonic organisms that float free in the high-purity water. The organisms differ only in their location. However, there is evidence that the very attachment of an organism to a surface may involve the triggering of a defense mechanism not available to the free-floating microbe. Thus, LeChevallier et al. (1988) showed, for example, that *Klebsiella pneumoniae* attached to glass slides increased their resistance to chlorine by a factor of 150.

Results from an as yet unpublished study concerned the effect of low oxygen levels upon an established biofilm and upon its influence over the growth rates of new biofilm colonizations. Oxygen being a nutrient essential to the growth of aerobic and facultative anaerobic microorganisms, some inhibitory effect was

Table 2-11
Effect of Sanitization on 24-hour Culture of *L. monocytogenes* Attached to Surfaces (cfu/cm²)

Sanitizer (10 Min Exposure)	*Etched Stainless Steel*	*Polyester*	*Polyester/ Polyurethane*
Control	4×10^4	3×10^4	5×10^4
Chlorine	2×10^3	2×10^4	4×10^4
Iodophor	5×10^2	2×10^3	1×10^4
Acid anionic[a]	< 20	< 20	4×10^4
A.O.C.A[b]	< 20	< 20	1×10^2
Fatty acid[c]	< 20	5×10^2	3×10^3
Peracetic acid	< 20	< 20	2×10^3
Mixed halogen	< 20	2×10^3	5×10^2
Neutral QAC	< 20	5×10^2	2×10^3
Acid QAC	< 20	5×10^2	8×10^2
ClO_2	< 20	< 20	9×10^3
ClO_2 + Acid QAC	< 20	< 20	5×10^2
180 °F (29 °C) Water	< 20	< 20	< 20

[a]Acid, anionic, K-SAN
[b]Acidic octenyl succinic anhydride, Divosan x-tend
[c]Fatty acid, Mandate
Courtesy of Krysinski, Brown and Marchisello; Courtesy *Journal of Food Protection*

expected. Studies were made at an oxygen level of less than 50 ppb of oxygen. Preliminary findings were that no long-term effects were evident. An immediate reduction of total bacteria over 24 hours was followed by a resurgence over a 6-day period to original colonization levels.

Reverse osmosis membrane biofouling results in a gradual decline in flux, in a corresponding increase in the transmembrane pressure, and in an increase of membrane permeability to ions. In the practical sense, this translates into reductions in RO process efficiency, coupled with greatly increased maintenance and operating costs, and loss of the RO rejection function. Decrepitude of the RO membrane may result from concentration polarization enhancement within the biofilm layer itself, as well as from the production of enzymes and other metabolites capable of hydrolyzing and otherwise degrading the RO membrane. Numerous cases have been reported of the biodegradation of cellulose acetate. No hard evidence exists to show such alterations to be enzymatic. They may be the result of pH situations in areas directly beneath the organisms, the consequences of acidic or alkaline metabolites.

Filters with their extensive porosities present large surface areas for biofilm formation, as the organisms have a predilection for surface growth. In the case of RO and ultrafiltration membranes, as stated, this results in blockage of the pores leading to the consequences of diminishing effective filtration area. In the case of microporous membranes, it may eventuate also as a passage of the microbes through the filter over time. This phenomenon, known as grow-through, is discussed subsequently in the section on filters. The point being made

Table 2-11
Effect of Cleaners on 24-hour Culture of *L. monocytogenes* Attached to Surfaces (cfu/cm²)

Cleaner (10 min exposure)	*Etched Stainless Steel*	*Polyester/ Polyurethane*
Control	3×10^4	5×10^4
Chlorinated alkaline detergent (1.6%)	*< 20*	1×10^4
Chlorinated alkaline detergent (10%)	*< 20*	9×10^3
Alkaline detergent (1.6%)	*< 20*	6×10^3
Alkaline detergent (10%)	*< 20*	2×10^3
Alkaline peroxide (3%) + phase transfer agent	*< 20*	5×10^2
Enzyme blend	*< 20*	5×10^3
Detergent blend + ClO_2	*< 20*	2×10^3
Anionic detergent (1.6%)	*< 20*	1×10^3

Courtesy of Krysinski, Brown and Marchisello; Courtesy *Journal of Food Protection* here is that grow-through may be concomitant to biofilm formation.

Except for the most exposed bacteria (those not shielded by the biofilm glycocalyx), sanitizing agents meant to control microbial growth by bactericidal action have little effect. The actions of sanitizers, ozone possibly excepted, work principally against planktonic organisms in their vegetative state. Nevertheless, their periodic use leads to a control of the organism levels. The practice of system sanitization should be a routine part of high-purity water manufacture. (See Chapter 9).

Biofilm removal. Given the ubiquity and persistence of biofilm, there is great interest in how to remove it. There is no unanimity regarding how this can be done, nor indeed that it can be done. Sanitization techniques are seen to operate primarily against planktonic organisms, those that break loose from the biofilm itself. The sessile population, variously estimated as being 1,000 to 10,000 times as numerous as the floaters, may be reduced in the outer layers of the film but remain viable in the deeper regions protected by the glycocalyx and may remain free to assert themselves over time.

Figure 2-8 from Mittelman and Geesey (1987) shows a quaternary ammonium compound to be very effective against planktonic organisms but relatively ineffective against the biofilm. Mittelman (1991) advised that, contrary to some common beliefs, hydrogen peroxide has the same type of limitations. It is effective against free-floating organisms, but far less so against those ensconced in biofilm. The cleansing effect of ozone against established scale and biofilm in cooling tower contexts (Merrill and Drago, 1980) leads to the belief that ozone can disrupt and remove biofilm. Anecdotal confirmation is forthcoming from semiconductor sources. Mittelman (1991) believed, however, that ozone effectiveness against biofilm, because the low solubility of ozone in water limits its available concentrations, necessitates its continuing usage or frequent reuse following early and effective applications. Given the equivocations regarding the effectiveness of aggressive reagents such as ozone against biofilm, it is curious that a composition of 10% sodium chloride and 5% sodium hydroxide is said to be a proven remedy to remove biofilm. Presumably, the action of caustic in disrupting proteinaceous matter is seen as the underlying action. The salt-lye formulation is advocated specifically for the removal of organic matter from anion-exchange resins.

Some claims to "lifting the biofilm" from surfaces are made in the literature without any supportive data being offered. One such statement is made on behalf of sodium percarbonate.

Costerton and Geesey (1979) stated that pulse chlorination has been relatively effective in killing adherent bacteria and effecting their removal by causing a sloughing of the bacterial matrix. Freezing also destroys the organisms in the glycocalyx. This can be done while keeping the system fluid through use of ethylene glycol. Sanitizations by ozone or other agencies may promote the release of bacterial endotoxins. These should be tested for.

McCoy (1987) lists in Table 2-10 the relative effectiveness of various physical methods in removing biofilm from surfaces. A common observation following such treatments is the increase in rate of biofilm regrowth. Flushing, the simplest method, has a very limited effectiveness. However, rapid rates of water flow over surfaces, as also the practice of recirculation, are viewed as compressing the biofilm and possibly minimizing by this densification the release of planktonic organisms (other than those loose organisms that are easily and early-on removed). Backwashing is effective for loosely adhered biofilm on filters or in deep beds. Sand blasting is difficult to control and may be too abrasive. Brushing is very effective, although expensive.

In consequence of mechanical or hydraulic cleaning being required to remove biofilm from tank surfaces, Youngberg (1985) advocated installation of a high-pressure tank-cleaning nozzle at the top of storage tanks.

Traditional concentrations of disinfectants at normal contact times will destroy planktonic but not sessile organisms of a given type. Suspended *P. aeruginosa* cells were killed within 8 hours by 50 mg/mL of tobramycin. However, even at 1,000 mg/mL, a 12-hour contact did not sufficiently destroy the cells of the biofilm on a urinary catheter material (Nickel et al., 1985). Sanitation by aldehydes (10% for 48 hours), or chlorine (10 mg/L for 24 hours) of contaminated surfaces was shown by Exner et al. (1987) not to be effective on

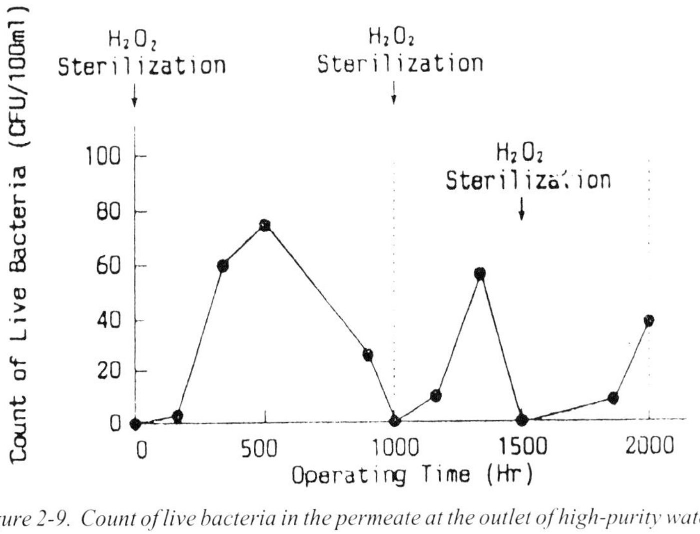

Figure 2-9. Count of live bacteria in the permeate at the outlet of high-purity water line that was sterilized intermittently with H_2O_2.
Matsuo (1991) Courtesy; *Tenth Annual Semiconductor Pure Water Conference*

the biofilm, nor were hydrogen peroxide or peracids. Only mechanical removal of the biofilm seemed to avail. However, Mittelman (1991) stated that 50 ppm of sodium hypochlorite at room temperature for 2 hours at below pH 7 is effective.

One impressive study demonstrating biofilm removal and a technique for ascertaining same derives from the food industry (Krysinski et al. 1992). It involved the removal of biofilms of *Listeria monocytogenes*, an organism whose biofilm poses risks in food processing because this pathogen is widespread and grows under refrigerated conditions.

Coupons of stainless steel, and of various polymeric belting used sterile trypticase soy broth containing glucose. The coupons were 1 by 1 cm. square in size. Assays of the organisms present in the biofilm were made by their abrasive removal over a 2-minute period through the use of vortexing with sterile microscopic glass beads 90 to 120 μm in diameter. The organisms thus removed were enumerated by plating serial dilutions to brain heart infusion agar; plates were incubated at 35 °C for 24 hours. A comparison of the quantity of biofilm grown upon the coupons with that present after particular sanitizing and cleaning treatments led conclusions regarding the biofilm-removal efficacy of such treatments. Some 20% of the bacterial cells were found to undergo cellular damage, rendering them unculturable. However, the abrasive biofilm dislodging technique was shown to lead to highly producible results (Frank and Kaffi 1990).

Krysinski et al. (1992) found that complete biofilm removal and/or inactivation was realized in many cases when the coupon surface was cleaned prior to undergoing sanitization; cleaning must precede sanitization in order to remove and inactivate the organisms.

These investigators found polyester/polyurethane surfaces particularly difficult to clean, more so than the polyesters they examined. Stainless steel was

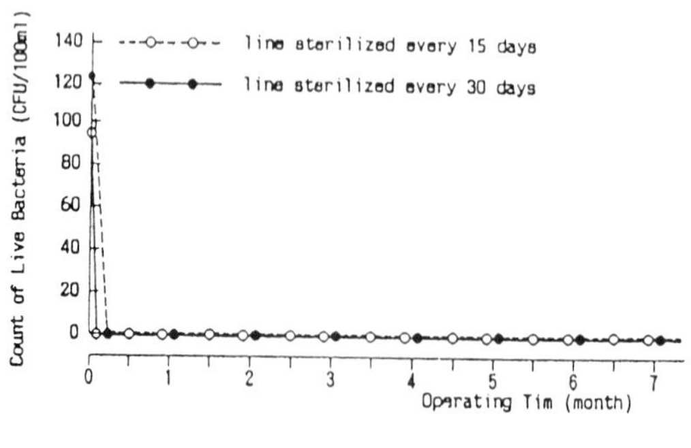

Figure 2-10. Count of live bacteria in the permeate at the outlet of high-purity water line that was sterilized intermittently with hot water.
Matsuo (1991) Courtesy; *Tenth Annual Semiconductor Pure Water Conference*

found to be the easiest material to clean of those they tested. The resistance of adherent cells to sanitizers was influenced by the surfaces upon which the biofilm became established.

Krysinski et al. (1992) detailed by way of scanning electron microscopy the relative effects of various commercial sanitizers and cleaners upon their *L. monocytogenes* biofilms. Table 2-11 shows the effects of various sanitizers; Table 2-12 illustrates the influences of various cleaning agents.

Sanitization

Sanitization, as of membranes, is often considered a part of membrane or system cleaning; more than just a killing of organisms, it should also be a removal of the biofilm itself, where possible. Reverse osmosis membrane cleaning is treated in Chapter 9.

Sanitization is not an absolute phenomenon. It is a partial removal of organisms. Depending on the system, a sanitization operation should reduce the organism population by some 90%, and should completely eliminate *Salmonella* and *E. coli*. With regard to pharmaceutical practices, 80 to 90 °C water is often used to effect intermittent sanitization, particularly of filter systems. With regard to sanitizers for non-food-contact surfaces, the EPA stated that the organism reduction should be at least 99.9% (EPA, 1982, p 55).

As stated, control and elimination of organisms from water purification systems is the paramount challenge of the entire operations of these systems. Once the seemingly inevitable biofouling films become established upon the various surfaces within the purification system (including the surfaces of the purification system and of RO and other membranes), their removal becomes problematical. Organism control through the practice of sanitization serves largely to eliminate the planktonic or free-floating bacterial population; the sessile or surface attached organisms in their much larger numbers (possibly 10,000 times the counts of the planktonic), remain largely protected by the glycocalyx and bacterial exfoliations that constitute the attached biofilm. Thus periodic sanitization is necessitated, as the periodic breakaway of organisms from the biofilm causes recontamination of the water stream.

Sanitizations must be directed to the sessile population, as shown by Figure 2-8. The practice must be repeated at a frequency to prevent new biofilm formation.

Sessile organisms, those incorporated into the biofilm matrix, have an enhanced resistance to sanitizers and antimicrobial agents. This has been documented for medical prosthetic devices (Anwar et al. 1990), in aquatic contexts (Le Chavallier et al. 1988), and upon biofilm deposited upon glass and stainless steel (Frank and Kaffi 1990, Shin-Ho-Lee and Frank 1991), and upon polypropylene and rubber (Mafu et al 1990).

The subject of sanitization has been dealt with extensively; nevertheless, ambiguities and at least some confusion exist. According to Mittelman (1986), chlorine in concentrations of 50 to 100 mg/L over contact times of 1 to 2 hours is effective in killing the organisms and inducing the sloughing of the bacterial matrix. Husted (1994) reports the absence of biofilm from water systems maintained at 80 °C.

Table 2-13 presents a list of agents, their dosages, and their contact times as usually recommended for use in water distribution systems (Mittelman, 1987). This investigation lists the relative effectiveness of certain of these reagents on a milligram-per-liter basis as being in the following decreasing order: ozone, sodium hypochlorite, iodine, quaternary ammonium compounds, hydrogen peroxide, formaldehyde or glutaraldehyde, ionic surfactants, and nonionic surfactants (Mittelman, 1986). What is of note is that sodium hypochlorite is more effective than hydrogen peroxide. The contrary is often assumed from the widespread use of hydrogen peroxide. Often this reagent is used because its ultimate decomposition into innocuous oxygen and water makes less threatening its imperfect rinsing from the water system. Sodium hypochlorite is not perceived to possess this advantage. Moreover, its application is limited by the poor stability of its concentrated solutions. Table 2-14 lists the definition of terms related to the action of chemical sanitizing agents as given by Mittelman (1985).

Sodium hypochlorite. As noted, chlorine, usually delivered as a gas to the water, forms hypochlorous acid:

$$Cl_2 + H_2O \longrightarrow HOCl + H^+ + Cl^- \qquad \text{Eq 2-2}$$

Actually, most water supplies are sufficiently buffered by their ingredients not to show a pH reduction caused by chlorine addition. The hypochlorous acid that is formed undergoes partial dissociation, however, into hypochlorite ions.

$$HOCl \longrightarrow H^+ + OCl^- \qquad \text{Eq 2-3}$$

The hypochlorite ion is significantly less biocidal than the undissociated hypochlorous acid (Haas and Karra, 1984; White, 1985; Wheeler, 1978).

The pK_a at 25 °C for hypochlorous acid, the point where it exists half in its undissociated and half in its dissociated forms, is at 7.4. Therefore, at the alkaline pH of sodium hypochlorite, above the pK_a of 7.4, there is less free hypochlorous acid. The available chlorine is in a less effective form. By contrast, the pK_a of hypobromous acid (HOBr) is at 8.8. This signifies that hypobromous acid would be more effective at the high pHs of its sodium salt, pHs of 7 to 10, than is hypochlorous acid. Unfortunately, the higher costs of sodium hypobromite are a deterrent to its use. The significance of the pK_a has received ample applicational confirmation (Beckwith and Moser, 1933; Conley and Puzig, 1987; Sergent, 1986).

One semiconductor high-purity water manufacturer uses a 5% to 10% equal-volume mixture of 30% hydrogen peroxide and sodium hypochlorite for 2 to 4 hours of contact time during a 24-hour sanitization operation once every week. Stainless steels are reported to be impervious to the action of 10 ppm of sodium hypochlorite solutions over contact times of 30 minutes at pH 6, as distinct from the stabilized pH 12 characteristics of Chlorox. Usually, however, sodium hypochlorite seems to be used in concentrations as high as 0.1% to 0.5%. One gallon of bleach per 1,000 gallons of water is a much-used formula. The use of sodium hypochlorite may require the neutralization of its residuals using sodium bisulfite or sulfite before release to municipal drains. Cellulose diacetate RO modules are said to endure treatments of 30-minute duration with chlorine concentrations not exceeding 10 mg/L. However, thin-film composite RO membranes composed of polyamide are ordinarily ruined by exposures to almost

Table 2-13
Methods for Monitoring Residual Levels of Treatment Chemicals

Biocide *	*Dosage Level (mg/L)*	*Contact Time (hours)*
Chlorine	50-100	1-2
Ozone	10-50	<1
Chlorine dioxide	50-100	1-2
Hydrogen peroxide	10%(v/v)	2-3
Iodine	100-200	1-2
Quaternary ammonium compounds	300-1,000	2-3
Formaldehyde	1%-2%(v/v)	2-3
Anionic and nonionic surface-active agents	300-500	3-4

Chemical	*Analytical Method(s)*	*Analytical Sensitivity (mg/L)*
Chlorine	1. Free total chlorine iodometric (colorimetric)	0.1
	2. Free/total chlorine amperometric	0.05
(Chloride)	1. Ion chromatography	-0.00005
Ozone	1. Ozone iodometric (colorimetric)	-0.03
Chlorine dioxide	1. Iodometric (colorimetric)	0.05
	2. Amperometric	0.03
Hydrogen peroxide	1. Permanganate reduction:0.10	
Quaternary ammonium compounds	1. Sulfonphthalein dye tablets/papers	-0.5
	2. Sublation	-0.3
Formaldehyde	1. Hydrazone derivatization (HPLC)	0.05
Anionic and nonionic surface-active agents	1. Sublation	-0.5
	2. Methylene-blue-substances (MBAS)	0.02

HPLC--high-pressure liwuid chromatography

*Typical biocide dosage levels. Levels reflect concentrations of active ingredients. Ozone levels were at 1 to 2 mg/L residual. Manufacturers should always be contacted concerning recommended dosages and applications.

Mittelman (1985); Courtesy, *Microcontamination*

any bactericidal concentrations of sodium hypochlorite. It is true that certain of these RO membranes are said to tolerate 0.1 ppm of sodium hypochlorite. Such concentrations may not sufficiently sanitize, however.

Martyak (1988) achieved specifications of fewer than 1 cfu/100 mL for RO-treated waters with the aid of continuously injected sodium hypochlorite to maintain 5.0 ppm of concentration levels. The hypochlorous acid that resulted was readily destructive of viable bacteria. Ion-exchange units were sterilized using 0.5% solutions of formaldehyde.

The bulk sodium hypochlorite solution commercially available could vary in concentration from 13% to 21%, and could degrade because of heat and light effects to 8% of concentration within 7 days at 24 °C (75 °F). To avoid dilution problems, an on-line titration/controller and daily analyses were used. Residual

TABLE 2-14
Definition of Terms Related to the Application of Chemical Agents

Term	*Definition*	*Applications*
Antibiotic	A substance produced by certain microorganisms that, in dilute solutions, can kill or prevent the growth of microorganisms.	Treatment/prevention of disease in humans, animals, and plants; animal feeds.
Antiseptic	A disinfecting agent applied to living tissues (see definition of *disinfectant*).	Treatment/prevention of infections in humans and animals.
Bactericide	An agent that kills bacteria, both disease-causing and non-disease-causing. Spores and nonbacterial microorganisms (e.g., algae, fungi, and viruses) are not necessarily killed.	Industrial water systems, equipment cleaning, dairy and food operations, treatment of infections in humans and animals, surgical scrubs.
Bacteriostat	An agent that prevents the growth of bacteria and their spores. These organisms are not necessarily killed by a bacteriostat.	Equipment cleaning, chemical-processing fluids, metal-cutting fluids.
Biocide	An agent that kills all living organisms and their spores. Since spores are the most resistant of all life forms, a biocide may properly be defined as a sterilizing agent.	Industrial and potable water systems; recreational and reservoir waters; secondary oil-recovery operations; cooling towers; treatment of infections in humans, animals, and plants.
Biostat	Similar to a bacteriostat but prevents the growth of all living organisms.	Equipment cleaning, chemical-processing fluids, metal-cutting fluids, recreational and reservoir waters.
Disinfectant	An agent that kills living organisms that are capable of producing disease or infection. Non-disease-causing microorganisms are therefore not necessarily killed. A disinfectant is often defined in terms of the application for which it is intended. Disinfectants are also required to act within a relatively short period of time, generally 10 minutes. Application of disinfectants is by definition restricted to inanimate objects.	Equipment and institutional cleaning, dairy and food operations.

analyses were relied upon.

Others pointedly avoid sodium hypochlorite, sodium ions being one of the worst contaminants in the electronics industry.

Hydrogen peroxide. Hydrogen peroxide is widely used in solution strengths varying from 3% to 10% over contact times of up to 12 hours prior to having its residues removed by flushing. For instance, 2-hour contacts weekly of a solution of 2 liters of 30% hydrogen peroxide diluted with 15 liters of filtered water are used. The actual concentrations and contact times require being determined experimentally. They depend upon, among other things, the organism load and the amount of oxidizable organic matter that is present. A large amount of the latter would be wasteful of the peroxide. The maximum use temperature is about 25 °C. Dump sinks are cleaned with 10% hydrogen peroxide by volume for 30 minutes, followed by scrubbing. Industrial grades of hydrogen peroxide contain heavy metals. Reagent-grade hydrogen peroxide contains 1 ppm of zinc and 0.5 ppm of iron. Interestingly, combinations of hydrogen peroxide and ammonium hydroxide have been stated to destroy organisms partly because the ammonia, it is said, renders surfaces hydrophobic. (Experimental evidence was not furnished.)

A very common surface cleanser is composed of 0.25% to 0.5% hydrogen peroxide in a 1% solution of sodium hydroxide. (Actually, 2% of a 50% caustic soda solution is used). The pH of this mixture is 14. High pH, where it can be

TABLE 2-14 Cont.

Term	*Definition*	*Applications*
Germicide	Similar to an antiseptic but kills all disease-causing microorganisms. As with a disinfectant, non-disease-causing microorganisms are not necessarily killed.	Equipment cleaning, dairy and food operations, industrial and potable water systems, recreational and reservoir waters, treatment/prevention of infections in humans and animals, surgical scrubs.
Microbicide	Similar to biocide but does not necessarily kill macroscopic organisms.	Same as biocide.
Preservative	An agent that prevents the deterioration of materials. Usually associated with the prevention of biological deterioration.	RO membranes, DI resins, food products, pharmaceuticals and medical devices.
Sanitizer	An agent that results in the reduction of bacterial number to public health limits. Application of sanitizers is by definition restricted to cleaning operations (inanimate objects).	Food and dairy processing operations, institutional cleaning.
Sporicide	Agent that destroys microbial spores. By definition, a sterilizing agent.	Surgical instruments, medical devices, and other inanimate objects.

Mittelman, (1985); Courtesy, *Microcontamination*

endured, is an effective remover of proteinaceous and organic matter. In the wine industry, a very common cleaning solution used is a mixture of anionic surfactant in caustic to remove organic foulants.

Hydrogen peroxide is commonly used in conjunction with sodium hydroxide at high pH. Sodium hypochlorite, on the other hand, is used at pH below 7.4 in order to achieve the maximum biocidal benefits of undissociated hypochlorous acid.

Hydrogen peroxide in 10% concentrations is used to cleanse organic matter from ultrafilters. Some users recommend more dilute solutions of 100 to 200 ppm of H_2O_2, motivated, perhaps, by the expense of the reagent. An advantage of hydrogen peroxide is its half-life of about 7 hours, and its decomposition into harmless molecules. A 30% solution placed into water on Friday will have decomposed on Monday, particularly under the influence of UV light. Thin-film composite membranes can sustain 0.1% of hydrogen peroxide; CA membranes, 2%. Time/concentration equivalents for hydrogen peroxide are said to be 3% for 1-hour contact, 10% for 10 minutes, and 1% for 48 hours. The 0.1% H_2O_2 strength is not very effective.

Hydrogen peroxide is increasingly favored over sodium hypochlorite because the ultimate decomposition of its residues leads to oxygen and water. It should be noted, however, that the oxidative action of hydrogen peroxide on organic molecules can produce such ionizable entities as carboxylic acids and various long-lived free radical intermediates before it achieves its ultimate potential, if ever, of converting them to carbon dioxide and water. The same may be said for ozone.

Ozone. Slowly but steadily, ozone use increases in the water purification picture. Efforts have been made to utilize ozone for the total removal of biofilm from the surfaces of semiconductor pure water systems. Anecdotal accounts say such efforts (unidentified) have been successful, but at the cost of initially loosening a flood of particulate matter, presumably derived from the biofilm, disintegrating under the action of the ozone. As the conventional wisdom has it, therefore, the water system should be treated early, hopefully to prevent substantial biofilm formation; and frequently, to make more easy its removal and less burdensome its decomposition. Best of all would be the maintenance of an ozone residual to prevent biofilm formation.

Ozone has less of an electrical potential, namely, 1.77 volts. It is, however, very effective in doses of 0.2 to 0.4 ppm. In several semiconductor installations, the ozonization sanitizations are performed on a weekly schedule.

A growing use of ozone is being made in sanitization. A problem associated with its use is the need to replace the sensors in the ozone detectors with some frequency. Maintenance is required, and the calibration of the ozone detectors is a weak point. At least one topical drug manufacturer maintains 5 ppm of ozone in his Purified Water storage tank. Ozone is discussed in Chapter 3, "Ozone and its Applications."

Hot water. Matsuo (1991) flowed highly purified water through a 100-meter-long pipe at a linear velocity of 0.5 m/sec (1.5 feet per second). As the two graphs of Figures 2-9 and 2-10 disclose, he found that the sanitization effects of intermittent treatments with 90 °C water during a 7-month period were more lasting by far than intermittent sanitizations with (undisclosed) concentrations of hydrogen peroxide. The bacterial counts in the feedwaters were 10 to 200 cfu/mL. The hot-water treatments were performed in two ways; sanitizations at 15-day intervals, and at 30-day intervals. No organisms were observed during the test period. After sanitizations with the hydrogen peroxide, the organism counts remained at zero for 5 to 6 days. The numbers then mounted. It is possible that the 90 °C water, in addition to killing organisms, may also have disrupted (or removed) the biofilm, possibly by differential thermal expansion between the biofilm and surface. The hydrogen peroxide in its sanitization action may, however, have caused only a killing of organisms in the outermost accessible layers of biofilm.

Obviously, the heat component of hot water systems performs a self-sanitizing function. It is not surprising, therefore, that heat is used in some water systems primarily as a sanitizer; the water is otherwise intended to be retained at ambient temperatures. There is perhaps a subtle difference here from systems involving alternations of hot and cold wherein a balance is sought in terms of heat cost minimizations.

Some drug companies recirculate their systems overnight at 80 °C. For example, at a New England pharmaceutical company, the water exiting mixed

Table 2-15
Biocide Efficacy Results

Exposure Time	*Minncare (1%)*	*Formaldehyde (2%)*	*Sodium Hypochlorite (0.001%)*	*Hydrogen Peroxide (0.2%)*	*Hydrogen Peroxide (5%)*	*Hydrogen Peroxide (10%)*
0 minutes	2.3×10^6	2.3×10^6	2.1×10^6	2.2×10^6	2.1×10^6	2.0×10^6
15 minutes	1.1×10^6	2.3×10^6	2.2×10^6	2.3×10^6	2.0×10^6	2.0×10^6
30 minutes	3.0×10^6	2.1×10^6	1.1×10^6	2.3×10^6	2.0×10^6	2.0×10^5
60 minutes	<10	2.0×10^6	4.0×10^4	2.0×10^6	1.0×10^5	<10
2 hours	<10	1.5×10^5	1.0×10^4	2.0×10^6	<10	<10
4 hours	<10	1.2×10^5	1.0×10^3	1.5×10^6	<10	<10
6 hours	<10	1.0×10^3	<10	1.0×10^6	<10	<10
12 hours	<10	<10	<10	1.0×10^3	<10	<10
24 hours	<10	<10	<10	<10	<10	<10
D values	6 min.	113 min.	69 min.	250 min.	22 min.	11 min.
6D	36 min.	678 min.	414 min.	1,500 min.	132 min.	66 min.

Maltais and Stern (1990); Courtesy, Ultrapure Water Expo '89-West beds is pumped through a heat exchanger operating at 180 to 190 °F (82 to 88 °C). It then is filtered through a 0.45-µm-rated membrane filter, passed through a UV installation, and then passed through a 0.2-µm-rated membrane filter to a loop bearing point-of-use (POU) final filters before rejoining the line before the pump, but just after (omitting) the mixed beds. In the morning each POU is flushed for 2 minutes, and the hot water is dumped, to be replaced by cold water from the makeup loop.

In another instance, the water is heated to 85 °C and is then permitted to circulate overnight as it cools, eventually to a use temperature of 35 °C.

The distinction between hot-water sanitization and alternate hot and cold balancing during storage is more evident in the semiconductor industry where systems are run cold, and where heat is used explicitly for its sanitizing effect. Otherwise in electronics, chemical sanitization is used.

It seems worthwhile to emphasize that system sanitization need not rely upon chemical agents. Thus, it has been reported that 90 °C water was more effective over longer durations than was hydrogen peroxide (Matsuo, 1991), detailed on page 113). More recently, Yagi et al. (1992) successfully practiced hot-water sanitizations at 80 °C over a 2 hour period every 15 days. These practices could be a trend in the making, freeing sanitizing operations from chemical intrusions. This would constitute a significant achievement.

Peracetic acid. There seems to be widespread agreement that peracetic acid is an effective biocide safe to use even with polyamide membrane structures. Table 2-15 from Maltais and Stern (1990) compares the relative biocidal efficiencies of formaldehyde, sodium hypochlorite, hydrogen peroxide, and a commercially available proprietary mixture of hydrogen peroxide and peracetic acid against *Bacillus Subtilis* var *niger* (ATOC 9372) spores using, not comparable concentration, but concentrations normally recommended for cleaning RO membranes and water systems. The results show that the 6 D values, these generally accepted as representing the times required for disinfection, were substantially lower than for the other biocides: 36 minutes for 1% polyacrylic acid (PAA) as compared with 678 minutes for 2% formaldehyde, 414 minutes for 0.001% sodium hypochlorite (stronger concentrations would be ruinous for polyamide RO membrane), and 66 minutes for 10% hydrogen peroxide.

Flemming (1984), in a review of peracetic acid, stated that, unlike the case for formaldehyde or hydrogen peroxide, no organism resistant to peracetic acid has been found. Of major importance is that the bacterial spores are killed as well, albeit by higher concentrations of PAA. Additionally, viruses and bacteriophages are also very sensitive to its influences. Lange (1969) reported that 0.1% PAA solutions drastically reduced pyrogen concentrations within 30 minutes, presumably because of the acid sensitivity of lipopolysaccharides.

Unlike its commercial mixtures with hydrogen peroxide, peracetic acid seems largely unaffected in its effectivity by temperature. The range of minus 40 to plus 37 °C has little influence on its bactericidal effects. Disinfection is normally not possible at these lower temperature extremes. Although more prone to dissociation by alkali, it performs equally at every pH (Mücke, 1977). Interestingly, water hardness reduces the effectiveness of PAA, as is also said to be the case for other disinfectants. Peracetic acid can be enhanced by the presence of alcohols such as ethanol, isopropanol, and n-propanol; and by hydrogen peroxide. PAA can be neutralized by reducing agents such as thiosulfate and, as stated, it can be destroyed by being dissociated by the action of alkali, sodium hydroxide. Of advantage to the use of peracetic acid is that its oxidative action leaves no residue of it other than acetic acid and water.

In one application, peracetic acid was used in concentrations of 50 to 100 ppm at a contact time of 1 hour. (A 1% concentration was judged an overkill, although others use 1% and even 4% to sanitize a CA/RO). The peracetic acid can be purchased commercially in stabilized form containing also hydrogen peroxide from Minntec, Echo Laboratories (Nenkel), and FMC.

Steam-in-place. Preeminent in the sanitization of pharmaceutical processing systems is the use of steam. Perhaps this practice can gainfully be extended to pharmaceutical water purification systems as well. Steam-in-place is a valuable concept that is of particular usefulness in pharmaceutical process sanitizations (Berman et al., 1986; Kovary et al., 1983).

Steam, usually superheated above 125 °C to provide margin for cooling, is permitted to flow through the system whose sanitization is being sought. The air occupying the equipment provides an impediment to penetration by the steam. Unlike a steam autoclave, the system cannot usually be evacuated of air by the use of vacuum. Instead, (numerous) vents and bleed valves are provided through which the advancing steam is allowed to displace the air. These vents are so positioned as to encourage the escape of the entrapped air. Bleed valves are particularly placed at the ends of dead-legs, if any.

Bleed points should be positioned at each low point in the system and at the terminus of each leg, particularly at loci furthest from the steam supply, to facilitate steam flow and penetration (Agalloco, 1990a). Air bleeding can be managed using a constant orifice or a thermostatic trap. It is more prudent to be wasteful of steam, if necessary, to insure the removal of air and the consequent avoidance of cold spots. Therefore, system design should encourage a greater number and larger bleeds (Agalloco, 1990a and 1990b).

Displacement of the occupying air by the invading steam will subject all the equipment in the system to the heating engendered by the superheated system. This, in short, is the very principle of the steam-in-place sanitization. (Individual units not amenable to direct contact with steam can be bypassed by way of appropriate valves and piping, but will, in consequence, remain unsanitized.) In the process of transferring its heat, the steam will lose temperature and itself undergo condensation into water. Such condensation will continue to take place until the entire system attains a temperature of at least 100 °C. Due to their complexity, the units composing the water purification systems are seldom, if ever, lagged or jacketed to retain heat. Therefore, the amount of steam condensing into water in such systems would be considerable (Berman et al., 1986; Kovary et al. 1983).

It is mandatory that the condensed steam, now liquid water, be removed from the system. As water at atmospheric pressure, it will not attain temperatures higher than 100 °C. Its presence will, therefore, militate against the attainment of the 125 °C level required for steam sanitization. Removal of condensate is achieved by way of drains set out at the various low points of the system. Lines set so as to slope to these low points would be an advantage.

Condensate drains may consist of a steam trap, regulating ball valve, or globe valve (Agalloco, 1990a and 1990b).

No actual water purification systems now known to be in use rely upon steam-in-place sanitization. Such is often advocated for certain of the purification units, such as the carbon beds. More extensive adaptation of sanitization by steam-in-place to water purifications may be a useful technique to consider and to adopt where possible.

Cleaning and sanitizing of RO membranes. The cleaning of RO membranes will be treated in greater detail in Chapter 9, page 537. It may be helpful, however, to reference the subject here.

Reverse osmosis devices utilizing polyamide membranes, including the most widely used thin-film composites, are susceptible to degradation by oxidizing agents, especially to chlorine and hypochlorite. Low concentrations may be endured for some period of time, but they are usually too weak to have much effect as sanitizers. Hydrogen peroxide or hydrogen peroxide/peracetic acid mixtures may not be used in strengths exceeding 0.2% and at temperatures above 25 °C (77 °F). If hydrogen peroxide is used, heavy-metal ions should not be present lest they catalyze the destruction of the membrane by the peroxide.

McAfee et al. (1990) sanitized their polyamide (PA) RO unit using weekly treatments of 20 mg/L of aqueous potassium dimethyldithiocarbamate for 1 hour. The RO unit was cleaned only yearly, using solution of 10% EDTA (ethylene diamine tetraacetic acid), a chelating agent, and 1% caustic soda. The removal of silica, would it appear necessary, would be essayed using an alkaline wash followed by an acidic ammonium difluoride solution.

Because of their susceptibility to oxidizing agents, polyamide membranes are sometimes sanitized with formaldehyde. However, because of its toxicity, formaldehyde is no longer recommended. Its homologue, the less volatile glutaraldehyde, is replacing it. Formaldehyde is also implicated in the formation of an insoluble white powder, its linear polymer, paraformaldehyde. When used, it is at concentrations of from 0.5% to 3%, usually at the higher concentration over a 3-hour contact time. It is not restrained from permeating CA RO. Glutaraldehyde is used in somewhat lower concentrations, namely, 0.5% to 2%. Unlike its lower-molecular-weight homologue, it is reported not to permeate cellulose acetate RO membranes. When formaldehyde is used, it should not be employed on new membranes lest it cause a serious loss in flux. In any event, its use will cause a one-time 10% flux loss. The effect of glutaraldehyde remains unreported. The use of iodine, of quaternary amines, or of phenols causes flux loss and is, therefore, not recommended. However, Pohland and Bettinger (1981) have said that PA RO film can tolerate iodine. The control of algae can be managed by the use of 0.1 to 0.5 ppm of copper sulfate (Petersen, FilmTec Corp).

In these circumstances, Zoccolante recommends 0.2% peracetic acid to be used in weekly applications for the sanitization of polyamide RO units.

Iodine is used as a sanitizing agent with CA RO. At a southwestern pharmaceutical installation, chlorinated city water is first softened and is then treated with activated carbon to remove the chlorine. Iodine is then added to the water, which then permeates a CA RO. It is then subjected to steam degasification. The steam is filtered through a stainless steel metal filter that is changed yearly. The water then enters a 10,000-gallon storage tank where the iodine concentration is maintained by means of an iodine monitor. A circulation loop includes a mixed bed that is regenerated every 3 to 4 days. The iodine is removed by strongly-basic anion exchange. The water feeds a Stillmas 6-effect still. The distilled water is held in a 800-liter tank, to be dumped after 8 hours.

Continuous versus Intermittent Feeds

As with all chemical reactions, the kinetic characteristics that determine the extents to which sanitizations take place are products of reactant concentrations and time, albeit modified by relevant factors such as temperature.

Thus, a single dose of ozone, for example, may suffice to destroy oxidatively within a given time a set concentration of organisms or TOC that is present. If not, a larger dose may be administered within the same time frame, or the smaller dose may be repeated intermittently over longer durations to accomplish the same goal. Alternatively, smaller ozone concentrations may be applied continuously; to achieve the objective somewhat more slowly, but also to serve prophylactically against the impurities newly added over the time. A continuous ozone feed may well be required where the organism or TOC concentration is not fixed but is augmented over time. However managed in terms of time, whether intermittent or continuous, the ozone concentration being supplied requires being matched with the organism or TOC density, and with the kinetics of the oxidation/reduction reaction that is taking place.

Microbiological Specifications for Compendial Waters

In summary, it can be stated that there is wide agreement among the FDA, USP, and WQC/PDA that the microbiological specifications for Purified Water be at no more than 100 cfu/mL. This is so stated in *USP 23*. It is recommended that the microbiological assay method entail using plate count agar and the pour plate technique on 1-mL samples. Incubation is to be at 30 to 35 °C for from 48 to 72 hours.

The use of R2A as growth medium requires longer induction periods, but no advantage is seen to be gained thereby, although this is often disputed.

Water for Injection is to contain no more than 10 cfu/100 mL. The assay is to be performed on 100 mL samples using the membrane technique (0.45 µm-rated) with the plate-count agar and incubations at 30 to 35 °C for from 48 to 72 hours. Given the relative freedom from organism content, samples smaller than 100 mL would likely not provide sufficient organisms for reliable counting. By the same token, assaying samples of Purified Water larger than 1 mL could be expected to provide overwhelming numbers of organisms, too large for accurate counting. The basic reference is the *Standard Methods for Examination for Water and Wastewater*.

These microbiological criteria are set forth in the USP Informational Chapter; they are not monography specifications. They are, therefore, to serve as action points, to signal when measures are to be taken to bring the performance of the water system into conformity with its intended operations. Cooper (Feb 1993), as usual, succinctly defines the situation:

> It is important that this distinction be maintained. If microbiological criteria were monography specifications, it would indicate that the product prepared from this water would not meet USP quality and could result in regulatory enforcement actions. This becomes particularly onerous since the microbiological results are not recorded until several days after the lot of product has been formulated. Perhaps at some time in the future when rapid microbiological methods such as epifluorescence are widely accepted and the water is prepared on a batch basis, it could be feasible to consider monograph specifications.

Inevitably, there will be those who, perhaps seeking the simplicity and security of precisely defined numbers, will see organism levels as constituting FDA acceptance/rejection criteria. That such an interpretation is incorrect is explicitly stated by Munson (1993) of the FDA:

> Failure to meet these action limits does not mean automatic rejection of products. As the definition indicates, action limits are points which signal a drift from normal operating conditions and which

require action on the part of the firm. When these limits are exceeded you should conduct an investigation designed to determine why the action limit is being exceeded. Then identify and implement the corrective action needed to restore the system to normal operation. You should also recheck products made prior to the corrective action to determine if the contamination has affected the quality of the product. You should increase your sampling rate for a period after the corrective action is implemented to insure that the system has returned to a state of control. This also does not mean that if you get a count of 110 CFU per mL for your Purified Water that you must shut down the system during the investigation.

Because microbial test results are already two to five days old you should not wait for two consecutive samples to exceed the action limit before you perform an investigation. This is when control charts or trend analysis can be a very useful tool. If the organism(s) isolated do not represent a potential problem and the historical profile of the system indicates that his single result is unusual and not part of an upward trend, then the follow-up action may simply consist of resampling or stepping up the rate of sampling for a short period so that a more accurate determination of whether the system is truly out of control or not can be made. The important thing is that you document what follow-up action you took and that the problem was corrected. No documentation means no follow-up action and no correction.

FDA Statements Concerning Microbial Limits

The FDA "Guide to Inspection of High Purity Water Systems" (July 1993) states the following as regards the microbial limits of pharmaceutical waters:

Water For Injection systems. Regarding microbiological results, for Water For Injection, it is expected that they be essentially sterile. Since sampling frequently is performed in non-sterile areas and is not truly aseptic, occasional low level counts due to sampling errors may occur. Agency policy, is that less than 10 cfu/100mL is an acceptable action limit. None of the limits for water are pass/fail limits. All limits are action limits. When action limits are exceeded, correct the problem and assess the impact of the microbial contamination on products manufactured with the water and document the results of their investigation. With regard to sample size, 100-300 mL is preferred when sampling Water for Injection systems. Sample volumes less than 100 mL are unacceptable.

The real concern in WFI is endotoxins. Because WFI can pass the

LAL endotoxin test and still fail the above microbial action limit, it is important to monitor WFI systems for both endotoxins and microorganisms.

Purified Water Systems. For purified water systems, microbiological specifications are not as clear. *USP XXII* specifications, that it complies with federal Environmental Protection Agency regulations for drinking water, are attempts by some to establish meaningful microbiological specifications for purified water. The [Cosmetics Toiletries and Fragrance Association] CTFA proposed a specification of not more than 500 organisms per ml. The USP 23 has an action guideline of not greater than 100 organisms per mL. Although microbiological specifications have been discussed, none (other than EPA standards) have been established. Agency policy is that any action limit over 100 cfu/mL for a purified water system is unacceptable.

The purpose of establishing any action limit or level is to assure that the water system is under control. Any action limit established will depend upon the overall purified water system and further processing of the finished product and its use. For example, purified water used to manufacture drug products by cold processing should be free of objectionable organisms. We have defined "objectionable organisms" as any organisms that can cause infections when the drug product is used as directed or any organism capable of growth in the drug product. As pointed out in the Guide to Inspections of Microbiological Pharmaceutical Quality Control Laboratories, the specific contaminant, rather than the number is generally more significant.

Organisms exist in a water system either as free floating in the water or attached to the walls of the pipes and tanks. When they are attached to the walls they are known as biofilm, which continuously slough of organisms. Thus, contamination is not uniformly distributed in a system and the sample may not be representative of the type and level of contamination. A count of 10 cfu/mL in one sample and 100 or even 1000 cfu/mL in a subsequent sample would not be unrealistic.

Thus, in establishing the level of contamination allowed in a high purity water system used in the manufacture of a non-sterile product requires an understanding of the use of the product, the formulation (preservative system) and manufacturing process. For example, antacids, which do not have an effective preservative system, require

> an action limit below the 100 cfu/mL maximum.
>
> The USP gives some guidance in their monograph on Microbiological Attributes of Non-Sterile Products. It points out that, "The significance of microorganisms in non-sterile pharmaceutical products should be evaluated in terms of the use of the product, the nature of the product, and the potential harm to the user." Thus, not just the indicator organisms listed in some of the specific monographs present problems. It is up to each manufacturer to evaluate their product, the way it is manufactured, and establish an acceptable action level of contamination, not to exceed the maximum, for the water system, based on the highest risk product manufactured with the water.

Munson (1993) in "FDA Views on Pharmaceutical Water" adds the following:

> We consider 10 colony forming units per 100 mL to be the appropriate total microbial count action limit for Water for Injection and 100 colony forming units per mL for purified water. If you manufacture products that are susceptible to microbial growth, such as antacids, the action limit for your water system may have to be lower to reduce the potential for growth in the product. The action limit for any water system should be determined by the product with the highest risk of microbial growth.
>
> In addition to the total microbial count action limit for purified water, the type of microorganism(s) present must also be considered. The microorganism(s) present should not be capable of growth in the product nor should it (they) represent a potential health hazard when the product is used as directed. I would like to state that FDA does not require that no Pseudomonas species be present in the water system. You also do not have to specifically monitor for Pseudomonas species, unless they represent a potential hazard to your products. We do not require that water systems be free of certain organisms unless those microorganisms represent potential pathogens in the products involved. For example, we would object to the presence of pseudomonads in a water system used in the production of topical products which could be applied to abraded skins or wounds.

With regard to the microbiological assay procedure proper to compendial water examination, the FDA (Munson 1993) observes the following:

> The major problem we find when reviewing the laboratory controls

> for purified water systems is that scientifically sound and appropriate microbiological test procedures are not being used. There has been such debate over the correct microbial test procedure to be used. The Pharmaceutical Manufacturers Association is recommending to USP that for Purified Water, a pour plate method using a sample size of 1 mL and Plate Count Agar, incubated for 48 hours at 30-35 °C be used as a general water method. For Water for Injection the proposal is to use a membrane filtration method using a sample size of 100 mL and Plate Count Agar, incubated for 48 hours at 30-35 °C. FDA does not have any significant problems with these proposals except that the sample size for water for injection should be 250 to 300 mL to obtain a more accurate determination of the microbial count. We also know that these methods are not the only methods that can be used and they may not work for all water systems across the country. It is simply a starting point. If you use this method and still have product failures, then you will still have to develop a method appropriate for your water system.

Additionally, to emphasize FDA views on USP published statements concerning the microbial quality of compendial water, Munson (1993) says as follows:

> The USP does have an information chapter on pharmaceutical waters which does suggest microbial action limits. We do not consider the action limits in the USP informational chapter to be standards nor do they serve as the GMP requirements for appropriate specifications.

In an aside Munson (1993) cautions, "Typically, conductivity meters are used on water systems to monitor chemical quality and have no meaning regarding microbiological quality.

Microbial Control Levels

The purpose of designating microbiological limits is to serve as a benchmark. The setting of precise limits for Purified Water is difficult given the different uses to which this type water is applied. Thus, to manufacture a nasal solution by cold processing, the water should best be sterile. By contrast, the preparation of a topical which would subsequently receive high temperature treatment could accommodate a much higher bacterial load.

The organisms most commonly encountered are potentially pathogenic Gram negative bacilli. In an independent study, 6 of 14 microbiological contaminants of cosmetics found in process waters were pseudomonads. Dunnigan (1970) offers the opinion that the presence of Gram negative organisms in topical preparations poses a moderate threat to health. The well known contamination of Povidone Iodine by *P. Cepacia* was a cause of hospital infections (Berkelman et at 1984).

In its unedited draft on *"Microbiological Attributes of Pharmaceutical Ingredients and Excipients, Drug Substances and Non-Sterile Dosage Forms"* the USP in its Open Conference on Microbiological Compendial Issues (1996) has proposed microbial limits for non-sterile dosage forms based upon the route of administration. For inhalants, the organisms of concern are *E. coli, P. fluorescens, and Salmonella* species; for (1) vaginal applications, *E. coli, Staphylococcus aureus, P. Aeruginosa*, and *Candida albicans*; for (2) nasal/otic/rectal/topical, *E. coli, Staphylococcus aureus, P. Aeruginosa*, and only for the nasal form, salmonella species; for (3) oral-liquid and (4) oral-solid with synthetic ingredients or excipients, (5) oral-solids with natural ingredient or excipients, E. Coil and salmonella species.

The corresponding total aerobic microbial counts permitted in cfu/g or mL for each administrative route are <10, <100, <100, <100, <1000, <3000; the respective permitted yeast and mold counts are <2, <2, <10, <10, <100, <300.

Table 2-16.
Assignment of Microbial Limit Tests for Non-sterile Finished Dosage Forms, by Route of Administration

Route of Administration	*Total Aerobic Microbial Count (CFU/g or mL)*	*Yeast and Mold Count (CFU/g or mL)*	*Absence of Specified Microorganisms*
Inhalants	≤10	≤2	Escherichia coil, Pseudomonas fluorescens, Salmonella species
Vaginal	≤100	≤2	Escherichia coil, Staphylococcus aureus, Pseudomonas aeruginosa, Candida albicans
Nasal/Otic/Rectal/Topical	≤100	≤10	Escherichia coli, Staphylococcus aureus, Pseudomonas aeruginosa, Salmonella* species
Oral-Liquid	≤100	≤10	Escherichia coli, Salmonella species
Oral-Solid, with synthetic ingredients/excipients	≤1,000	≤100	Escherichia coli, Salmonella species
Oral-Solid, with natural ingredients/excipients	≤3,000	≤300	Escherichia coli, Salmonella species

Only for nasal dosage forms.
Courtesy: USP Convention Inc.

(See Table 2-16).

Objectionable Organisms

The USP not only stipulates the maximum action limites for Purified Water but specifies as well that it not contain objectionable organisms. It is obvious that frank pathogens should be precluded. If present in the water used to compound drugs, they may come to be present in the drugs themselves. Fortunately, very few types of organisms grow on drugs, given the presence of solvents, the limitations posed by pH, and by heat. The total counts of Gram-positives and of Gram-negatives usually serve to describe the microbiological quality of the finished drug form.

The significance of organisms in non-sterile drugs requires being evaluated with regard to the product application, the nature of the preparation, and the potential hazard to the user. Gram-negative microbes, such as *Pseudomonas sp.* while rarely pathogenic, are considered opportunistic pathogens. Under certain conditions proper for them, they may prove pathogenic. Almost all organisms are potentially pathogenic, depending, upon other things, on the health and robustness of the subject exposed to the drugs. Usually, pharmaceutical houses require low counts and a complete absence of pathogens; but realistically this comes to mean opportunistic pathogens as well. This prohibition is applied to the compounding Purified Water as well.

It is unreasonable to expect Water for Injection and Purified Water to be free of pseudomonads whose natural habitat is water. Therefore, one settles for low counts. If, for instance, the total cfu/mL count includes some 50 cfu pseudomonads, the water system is considered to require amelioration. If, however, the count is about 10 cfu, the preservative system is expected to handle that level. Unfortunately, preservative systems have their own limitations, and, increasingly, pseudomonads are identified with pathogenic situations. The undesirability of *P. aeruginosa* in topicals has been referred to; *P. cepacia* has been known to infect Povidone Iodine; and P. fluorescence has been implicated in encephalitis.

A complete freedom from pseudomonads would be ideal. However, even if sterile Purified Water could be prepared, its storage under normal conditions would expose it to organisms shed from the biofilm. Clearly, the elimination of biofilm is required. Storage of the prepared Purified Water within elevated temperature (80 °C) systems, or its storage under ozone is called for. At least each of two multinational pharmaceutical manufacturers, each with plants in both Canada and the U.S. do just that. The Canadian plants store the Purified Water at 80 °C; the U.S. plants, under ozone. In effect, these drug processors use sterile bulk Purified Water; freeing themselves from the problem of objectionable organisms, opportunistic pathogens, as defined by the health of some unknown user, and exempting themselves, thereby, from untoward liabilities.■

CHAPTER 3

OZONE AND ITS APPLICATIONS

The application of ozone to high-purity process waters shows an inexorable, if slow, advance. Whatever problems are associated with its use, it offers real advantages over chlorine as a disinfectant in that the removal of its residuals need not depend upon the use of carbon beds with their usual pyrogenic accompaniments, but is effected by exposure to 254-nm UV light. Its presence in stored waters may offer an alternative to storage at elevated temperatures (80°C). Moreover, being a strong oxidant, it offers promise in pyrogenic lipopolysaccharides destruction. Additionally, ozone has a higher lethality coefficient than chlorine against most organisms and readily destroys viruses, which is a matter of interest in work with cell lines and in sewage water reclamation. The use of ozone as a bactericide or bacteriostat has found application over a period of about 80 years, particularly in France and in areas under French influence.

The organisms whose presence and proliferation cause the biofouling that is the concern in various water applications can be considered organic molecular systems that, for their viability, depend on the specifics of their protoplasmic arrangements. Disruption of these exact molecular dispositions, as can occur during chemical oxidative degradations, can inactivate and/or kill these organisms. The nonviable residues may also interfere with the utilization of the water. Some of these may be removed by filtration, distillation, and other treatment procedures, but also by chemical oxidation. One purpose of UV radiation, and/or of ozone, and/or either of these techniques with synergistic or catalytic reagents such as hydrogen peroxide, is to effect such disinfection and/or oxidative degradations leading to the destruction and removal of organic matter.

Free Radicals

The actions of ozone and/or UV radiation often are through the agency of free radicals, produced by or from the incorporation of these two treatment processes. The covalent bond connecting two atoms consists of the mutual sharing by these atoms of two bonding electrons. This valence bond may break in one of two ways. In one process, one of the atoms may acquire both bonding electrons, leaving the other with none. This type of bond cleavage gives rise to ions. The electron being the seat of negative electricity, that atom now possessing more than its original share of electrons is negatively charged; it is an anion. The other atom, deprived of its normal complement of electrons, is positively charged as a result. It is the cation. There is in the water purification community a familiarity with the reactions and interactions common to ions; but there is generally less understanding of free-radical processes.

The covalent bond may also rupture, leaving each of the two constituent atoms with one of the bonding electrons. These atoms are thus now free radicals, which require combinations with other free radicals to form stable molecules. Alternatively, a free radical may form a labile linkage with a molecule it encounters to abstract an atom and a bonding electron. This action stabilizes the free radical in the form of a complete molecule; in the process, however, a new free radical is formed from what had been a stable molecule before it lost its abstracted atom-cum-electron.

A series of repetitions of free-radical attacks upon molecules to form new free radicals, which then attack other molecules to coproduce more free radicals, and so on, is common in free-radical chemistry. The oxidative degradation of organic compounds is a case in point. The result is a free-radical chain. The production of the free radicals is called the initiation step. It leads to and is succeeded by the propagation step. Eventually, the free-radical chain terminates, by combination of free radicals, in what is appropriately called the termination step. Free radicals are uncharged electrically.

Free radicals have half-life durations whose lengths are inverse expressions of their stabilities. Thus, the more structurally unstable a free radical (i.e., the more avid its need to participate in new covalent bonding), the greater its interaction with a broader spectrum of molecules, and the shorter, therefore, its half-life. Less aggressive free radicals endure longer, being less prone to react with their neighboring molecules.

Free radicals satisfy their need to form covalent bonds by joining one another, each contributing its lone electron to the new covalent bond. Such dimer formation is, however, the hallmark of less reactive (more highly stabilized) free radicals. The more aggressive species will rupture, for example, a carbon/hydrogen bond, by abstracting the hydrogen atom with its bonding electron. This reaction will satisfy the need of the free radical to form a stable (new) covalent bond, but will leave the abstracted carbon atom as a free radical. The newly created free radical may stabilize in a number of ways, depending upon its own reactivity. It may dimerize to create carbon-carbon branching; it may abstract a hydrogen and one bonding electron from less stable carbon/hydrogen bonds; or it may combine with oxygen to form oxygenated structures when oxygen is present. Oxygenated structures may also be formed when peroxidic or hydroperoxidic structures undergo fission into free radicals; or when hydroxyl free radicals stabilize by terminating free-radical chains. Free radicals may also cleave carbon-carbon linkages. Such cleavages become easier when oxygenated groups are present on neighboring carbons within carbon/carbon chains, such as those that constitute organic matter.

In the proliferation of a free-radical attack upon an organic compound, both chain scission and branching occur; the latter, from a free radical joining to the free-radical site upon an inner carbon of another chain. Overall, the oxidative degradation of a long-chain organic compound (such as a linear polyethylene) transforms it into shorter, stubby, multibranched molecules.

Alterations in the mechanical properties of the modified molecules result, as do changes in their electrical polarity. Polypropylene easily suffers abstraction of its tertiary hydrogens. Its free-radical degradation produces a brittle material that generates solid particles. Other organics or polymerics may fare differently, according to their molecular structures.

Hydrogen abstraction from carbon atoms, as well as carbon-carbon bond cleavage to create free-radical chains, can be initiated by the hydroxyl free radicals caused by the action of the ozone upon water:

$$O_3 + H_2O \longrightarrow O_2 + 2\cdot OH \qquad \text{Eq. 3-1}$$

Hydroxyl free radicals are generated by ozone in water in a several-step reaction (Baumann and Stucki, 1988). They can also be promoted by the energy inherent in UV light, following hydroperoxide (ROOH) formation by oxygen catalyzed by UV. Thus, the oxidation by way of peroxide formation is catalyzed by UV and near-UV light (Shelton, 1978):

Table 3-1
Relative Oxidation Power of Various Oxidizing Species

Species	*Oxidation Potential (Volts)*	*Relative Oxidation (Power*)*
Fluorine	3.06	2.25
Hydroxyl free radical	2.80	2.05
Atomic oxygen	2.42	1.78
Ozone	2.07	1.52
Hydrogen peroxide	1.77	1.30
Perhydroxyl free radical	1.70	1.25
Hypochlorous acid	1.49	1.10
Chlorine	1.36	1.00

*Based on chlorine as reference (= 1.00)

Table 3-2
Lethality Coefficients for Ozone at pH 7 and 10-15 °C

Organism	*A*	C_{99}*:10**
Escherichia coli	4,600	0.0010
Streptococcus faecalis	3,000	0.0015
Mycobacterium tuberculosis	1,000	0.0500
Poliovirus	460	0.0100
Bacillus megaterium (spores)	150	0.1000
Endamoeba histolytica	50	0.0300

*C_{99}:10 = concentration in mg/L for 99% destruction in 10 minutes.

Mittelman and Geesey (1987); Courtesy, Water Micro Associates

$$R\text{-}H + O_3 \xrightarrow{UV} R\text{-}OO\text{-}H \qquad \text{Eq. 3-2}$$
$$ROOH \longrightarrow RO\cdot + \cdot OH$$
$$2ROOH \longrightarrow RO\cdot + ROO\cdot + H_2O$$

It is these initiation reactions that are the basis for the use of UV and/or ozone and/or hydrogen peroxide for the destructive removal of organic compounds from water.

The introduction of oxygenated groups into the organic molecule speeds its destruction. Guillet (1978) stated that although hydroperoxide is the main carrier of the photooxidative chain, it is the buildup of ketonic and aldehydic groups that contribute to direct photolysis by their absorption of the UV. It is the absorption of the light energy that contributes to the breakdown of the organic molecule even at low degrees of oxidation.

Not surprisingly, ketonic and aldehydic compounds are encountered when organic materials present in waters are oxidized (Glaze et al., 1989). Such compounds are the precursors of the carboxylic acids whose presence is often noted when ozone or UV treatments are utilized. The further free-radical oxidation of carboxylic acids involves abstraction of the hydrogen atoms alpha to the carboxylic acid group. This reaction results in the release of carbon dioxide. Eventually, then, most organic substances can be degraded oxidatively to carbon dioxide and water. Carbon dioxide is, however, the final product of the oxidative free-radical chain. It may be more practical and less expensive to remove the altered organic material when it is in its carboxylic acid stage, by means of ion exchange.

Table 3-1 (Mittleman and Geesey, 1987) presents a comparison of different oxidants and their oxidizing potentials. It is seen that ozone is a very powerful oxidizing agent, the most powerful readily available for water treatment. By the same token, the hydroxyl free radical is seen to be even more powerful as an oxidizing agent.

Properties of Ozone

Ordinary molecular oxygen consists of two atoms of oxygen in peaceful chemical union. Normally quite stable, molecular oxygen can be decomposed, through the agency of UV radiation or by the application of high electrical energy, into two reactive oxygen atoms or free radicals. In aqueous solutions, the interaction of atomic oxygen with water molecules may give rise to two hydroxyl free radicals:

$$O\cdot + H\text{-}O\text{-}H \longrightarrow (HO\cdot) + (\cdot OH) \qquad \text{Eq. 3-3}$$

Ozone is an allotrope of oxygen consisting of three oxygen atoms. It is relatively unstable. Liquid ozone (100% pure) is readily exploded. Gaseous compositions containing ozone/oxygen mixtures in excess of 20% of ozone constitute potentially explosive mixtures. In the commercial generation of ozone from air or from oxygen, however, concentrations above 10% ozone are difficult to prepare. At such concentrations, gaseous compositions containing ozone have not been reported to be explosive. The decomposition product of gaseous ozone is oxygen. Certain catalysts, as well as organic matter with which ozone can react, facilitate its decomposition to elemental oxygen.

Gaseous ozone is only sparingly soluble in water, in general about 13 times as soluble as oxygen. Its specific solubility is dictated by Henry's Law, which relates solubility of a partially soluble gas in a liquid to its partial pressure above that liquid. Different liquid media have different Henry's Law constants.

The rates of chemical reactions with ozone usually bear some relationship to reagent concentration, as well as to temperature, pH, and the chemical nature of the oxidizable solutes and inorganic impurities. Therefore, efforts sometimes are made to combine the action of ozone with UV radiation or/and hydrogen peroxide so that the more reactive hydroxyl free radicals may be produced in high concentrations.

Half-Life of Ozone

The half-life of ozone in once-distilled water is about 25 minutes at 20 °C. In the presence of impurities with which it can react, however, its half-life is considerably less.

The ready destruction of ozone can be beneficial. Ultraviolet radiation of 254-nm wavelength converts it into oxygen and hydroxyl free radicals. This can be accomplished conveniently in a recirculating loop, with the water being released upon signal from an ozone detector.

The rate of ozone decomposition in water is pH-dependent. At pH 8, typical of many drinking water supplies, ozone has a half-life of much less than 25 minutes. Its decomposition rate, initiated by hydroxyl ions, increases with pH

Table 3-3
Specific Lethality Coefficients at 5°C

Agent	*Enteric Bacteria*	*Amoebic Cysts*	*Viruses*	*Spores*
Ozone (O_3)	500	0.5	5	2
HOCl as Cl_2	20	0.05	1.0 up	0.05
OCl^- as Cl_2	0.2	0.0005	<0.02	<0.0005
NH_2Cl as Cl_2	0.1	0.02	0.005	0.001

Morris (1975)

(Glaze et al., 1987a, Glaze 1987b).

The short half- life of ozone in solution is sometimes mentioned as if it were a shortcoming of that reagent. That is not so. The half-life brevity is an index of ozone's powerful oxidative reactivity with other molecules. In the process the ozone is consumed, generating the hydroxyl free radicals that, in turn, alter and destroy the molecules being oxidized. In this chemical transformation the specific molecular arrangements that are oxidized also become altered. When these "molecular arrangements" are in the form of organisms, the chemical alteration leads to their demise. This is the essence of sanitization not only by ozone but also by other oxidizing agents.

The oxidizing chemistry is by way of a free-radical chain reaction involving initiation, propagation, and termination steps (See page 126). These oxidative chains are initiated by ozone molecules reacting to produce hydroxyl free adicals, often abetted by ultraviolet light and/or hydrogen peroxide. This reaction is rapid and leads to the prompt disappearance of the ozone. Hence its short half-life. But the ozone has done its job. The generated hydroxyl free radicals carry on the destruction of the organisms (or of TOC in general) in the propagation step of the oxidative chain reaction, after the ozone molecule is gone. The brief half- life of ozone, therefore, is not a shortcoming of that reagent. On the contrary, it directly reflects the useful aggressivity of ozone; its ready transformation into free radicals, the very characteristic that renders it a desirable sanitizing agent.

Comparisons with Chlorine

The control of microbial growths has been managed by the use of numerous disinfectants or sterilants. Each has been shown to have its merits and limitations. Inevitably, ozone comes to be compared with chlorine for this type of application. The relatively quite short half-life of ozone in water means that significant concentrations of dissolved residual ozone probably will not endure over the reach of an extensive water distribution system. The microorganism population, controlled to that point, will begin to flourish again.

Long-lived chlorine would not be so fugitive as ozone. Chlorine is, relatively, a stable compound, and hence is not described by any half-life characteristic. Once chlorine has served its useful purpose, however, it and many of its by-products can be more difficult to remove. Adsorption by activated carbon or reaction with bisulfite (reducing) solutions are the usual means, and each has its complications. Also, chlorine may convert many organic substances into trihalomethanes and other halogenated derivatives. Some of these have been identified with carcinogenicity.

Because it can be removed easily, as by UV destruction, ozone finds applications in-line. Chlorine and other chemicals requiring more complicated removals cannot be so employed. In pharmaceutical contexts ozone is used in-line. In biotech applications it is more often confined to storage tanks.

Multiple feed points can reinforce the ozone concentration throughout the zone of operations (though cost efficiency then becomes a practical consideration). The short half-life of ozone means that upon discharge, treated waters are less likely to be toxic to aquatic life. Indeed, the decomposition serves to increase the dissolved oxygen level of the water being treated. This is usually desirable; however, increased corrosion also may result.

Action upon Microorganisms

It is cited that ozone kills *E. coli* bacteria 3,125 times faster than the same molar concentration of chlorine as measured by a lethality coefficient, A, which has the dimensions of both oxidant contact time and oxidant dosage level (Nebel and Nebel, 1984):

$$A = \text{In } 100/C_{t^{99}} \qquad \text{Eq. 3-4}$$

where C is the residual oxidant concentration (in mg/L) and t^{99} is the time in minutes required to kill 99% of the organisms (Morris, 1975). The comparison of the effects of 0.1-mg/L doses of ozone and chlorine against 60,000-cfu levels of *E. coli* showed that 99% destructions required 2,570 minutes for chlorine against 0.8 minutes for ozone. The ratio is 3.125 to 1, as stated. In this case, the action of ozone may be so rapid that contact times pose no problems, assuming that efficient transfer of ozone to the aqueous phase has been effected.

Table 3-4
Concentration-Time Data for 99% Inactivation of *Giardia* Cysts with Ozone at pH 7

	Giardia lamblia			*Giardia muris*		
Temperature °C	*C mg/L*	*t' min*	*C-t' mg-min/L*	*C mg/L*	*t' min*	*C-t' mg-min/L*
25	0.15	0.97	0.15	0.18	1.3	0.24
	0.082	1.9	0.16	0.10	2.2	0.22
	0.034	5.5	0.19	0.080	3.4	0.27
				0.034	8.2	0.28
			0.17*			0.25*
5	0.48	0.95	0.46	0.70	2.5	1.8
	0.20	3.2	0.64	0.40	5.0	2.0
	0.11	5.0	0.55	0.31	6.4	2.0
				0.21	9.6	2.0
			0.55*			1.9*

* Average C-t' value at given temperature

Wickramanayake et al. (1985); Courtesy, American Water Works Assoc.

When ozone is added to water using an efficiently operated in-line static mixer, bacteria are killed within seconds (Nebel et al., 1973). Chlorine requires diffusion through the cell walls of the organisms in order to degrade enzymes. Ozone lyses the cell walls directly. In disinfection applications, ozone is more powerful than chlorine by factors of from 5 to 1,000, depending upon the form in which the chlorine is dispensed, and upon the organisms being disinfected. Chlorine as hypochlorous acid, the gas dissolved in water with pH at or below 7.4, is the most effective form of chlorine; chloramine is the least; and hypochlorite ion (present at pH above 7.4) is of intermediate germicidal activity.

Table 3-2 illustrates the action of ozone against certain organisms. Table 3-3 compares the bactericidal efficiency of ozone to that of other chlorine disinfectants (Morris, 1975). The ozone residual levels represented range from 0.0005 to 0.5 mg/L (Nebel and Nebel, 1984).

The presence of viruses in waters is of considerable current concern. Enteroviruses and viruses of infectious hepatitis can exist for long periods, even in well-maintained potable water distribution systems. Ozone is far more effective than UV radiation or chlorine in inactivating such viruses. For example, complete inactivation of polio-type viruses was effected within 30 seconds using a dissolved ozone residual of less than 0.5 mg/L (Majumdar et al., 1974, and Glassman 1974).

French public health officials (Coin et al., 1967a, 1967b) specify ozone concentrations of 0.4 mg/L maintained over a minimum contact period of 4 minutes, to guarantee a 99.9% inactivation of Poliovirus Types I, II, and III.

Pseudomonas, Staphylococcus, Candida, Penicillium, Proteus, Clostridium, Schistosoma, Salmonella, Shigella, Vibrio cholera, and *Endamoebic* cysts are readily destroyed by ozone in their aqueous suspensions. Sterilization is a very rapid first-order reaction. Vegetative bacteria at concentrations of 10^6 to 10^7/mL are totally destroyed at ozone concentrations of 0.01 to 1.0 mg/L within 5 minutes. *Escherichia coli, Streptococcus,* and *Bacillus* attain zero levels at ozone concentrations of less than 0.2 mg/L within 30 seconds. Bacterial spores are 10 to 15 times more resistant. *Bacillus* and *Clostridium* spores at levels of 10^7/mL require higher ozone doses and contact times to reach sterilization. Ozone concentrations of 0.2 to 0.5 mg/L and contact times of 10 minutes are recommended for water sterilization where large bacterial spore populations are involved. Viruses are extremely susceptible to ozone. Residual ozone concentrations of 0.1 to 0.8 mg/L and contact times of less than 30 seconds suffice for polio, encephalomyocarditis, coxsackie, enterovirus, vasicular stomatitis, GDVII, rhabdovirus, and herpes viruses (Gurley, 1985).

In France, where ozone treatment is used widely for primary disinfection of potable water supplies, the residual ozone level is maintained at 0.4 mg/L for 8 to 12 minutes. Such a level is sufficient to inactivate in excess of 99% *of Giardia* cysts, even at low temperatures.

Wickramanayake et al. (1985) showed that the contact times required to inactivate two logs of *Giardia lamblia* cysts with 0.15 mg/L of residual ozone at pH 7 are 1 and 4 minutes at 25 and 5 °C, respectively. Cysts of *G. muris* are 1.5 and 3.5 times more resistant to ozone at 25 and 5 °C, respectively. Table 3-4 shows concentration time relationships for 99% inactivation of *Giardia* cysts.

Ozone Generation

Nearly all large-scale commercial ozone generators employ the corona discharge principle. Properly dried air, or oxygen itself, is passed between a high-voltage electrode and a ground electrode separated by a dielectric material (Figure 3-1). Considerable electrical energy is required for the ozone-producing electrical discharge field to be formed. A minimal energy expenditure requires the use of dry air (maximum dew point of minus 60 °C). Using dried air, usually 1% to 2% of ozone is produced in the air. When dry oxygen is used, double that concentration of ozone is obtained for the same amount of electrical energy applied to the generator. In excess of 80% of the applied energy is converted to heat that, if not rapidly removed, causes the produced ozone to decompose, particularly above 35 °C (95 °F). Proper cooling of the ozone generator is crucial to maintaining consistent ozone yields.

Air can be used to generate the ozone but, consisting of 80% nitrogen, it gives rise to unwanted oxides of nitrogen. The nitrogenic oxide content can be minimized, however, if dry air is used.

In pharmaceutical contexts, nitrogen oxides that are generated will, along with carbon dioxide, give the water a pH lower than that permitted. For these uses, ozone generated from oxygen is required. This is conveniently prepared by means of a swing generator. Air under pressure is exposed to molecular sieves in a tower. The nitrogen, carbon dioxide, and even oxides of sulfur (should these be present) are preferentially adsorbed. The oxygen passes through to become

Table 3-5
Chemical Costs vs. Blowdown Water and Sewage Costs in San Francisco Area

Tower Size (tons)	*Cycles of Conc.*	*Chemical Costs ($/yr)*	*Water & Sewage Costs ($/yr*
4,000	8.5	6,000	19,200
1,600	3.2	6,100	13,000
1,200	3.6	13,300	18,000
700	3.5	5,400	7,300
500	3.0	5,200	9,300

Pryor and Bukay (1990); Courtesy, *Ultrapure Water* journal

exposed to the corona discharge. Following the pressure release, the nitrogen desorbs from the molecular sieve, to be swept away by an oxygen stream. During this tower renewal, a twin tower is operated. Alternation of the towers furnishes a steady feed stream enriched to 90% to 95% oxygen.

Ozone generator design alternatives as well as considerations of using oxygen rather than air were discussed by Rice and Bollyky (1981).

A more convenient, though expensive, method for preparing ozone uses its generation from water by way of electrolysis (the Membrel method). This method introduces fewer by-products and less oxygen into the water. Since the ozone is generated in water, the problem of introducing it into the water is obviated. During its electrolysis, water decomposes at the anode to yield ozone and oxygen. Hydrogen forms at the cathode. The anodic reactions are as follows:

$$3H_2O \text{ ---->} O_3 + 6H^+ + 6e^- \qquad \text{Eq. 3-5}$$

The theoretical potential of the reaction, E_o=1.51 V. Oxygen is simultaneously formed at the anode:

$$2H_2O \text{ ---->} O_2 + 4H^+ + 4e^- \qquad \text{Eq. 3-6}$$
$$E_o = 1.23V.$$

The production of ozone is favored by the use of an anode having a high oxygen overpotential, at least 1 volt above 1.23. Lead (IV) oxide, the anode material used industrially in this ozone production process, encourages the catalytic formation of ozone.

Ozone (mixed with oxygen) is generated directly in the water by commercial devices of this design. The water used should be demineralized, or softened at the very least. Its conductivity should be lower than 20 microsiemens μS/cm (about 10 ppm). Hydrogen gas formed at the cathode is released into the atmosphere. The water electrolysis occurs at a potential of 3 to 5 volts, with an applied current density of 0.5 to 2 amperes per cm^2. The ozone production can be controlled by variation of the current density. Concentrated ozone solutions of greater than 100 mg/L can be obtained by operating the cell under pressure (Stucki et al., 1985). Regardless of its advantages in more easily introducing the ozone into the water, the electrolysis method of ozone production is not commonly perceived as suitable for enabling slugs of higher ozone concentration to be generated. For this, it is held, the corona discharge method is required.

In the corona discharge method of generating ozone, some unconverted oxygen is present. Less, but some oxygen is also present when ozone is generated electrolytically. This oxygen content may be objectionable in semiconductor usage where silicon oxide formation may be influenced thereby. MABOS, a method for generating oxygen-free ozone and applying it intermittently to cooling towers, may be useful in such applications.

Developed by a Japanese team (Nakayama et al., 1980), MABOS is a unique system that generates ozone from pure oxygen, then adsorbs the ozone onto silica gel. This allows the oxygen to be rerouted back to the ozone generator without recleaning or redrying. When ozone must be added to the water, it is simply desorbed from the silica by heating the gel and drawing the gas into the water by suction.

Several major advantages result from this system. First, generating ozone from pure oxygen allows smaller generators to be used than would be required

Table 3-6
Ozone Exposure Test: Pressure Decay-Data for High Ozone Concentration (500-1,200 ppb)

Filter	*Media/Support*	*Cumulative Ozone (ppm-hours)*	*Starting Pressure (psig)*	*Pressure Drop (psig)*
A	PTFE/PTFE	0	15	1.5
		5	15	1.4
		12	15	1.4
		30	15	1.4
		45	15	1.4
		100	15	1.4
B	PVDF/polypropylene	0	50	2.1
	(2-layer)	0	50	2.1
		12	50	2.1
		30	50	2.2
		65	50	2.2
		100	50	2.1
C	PVDF/polyester	0	50	2.0
	(1-layer)	5	50	1.3
		12	50	1.4
		30	50	1.4
		45	50	25.0
D	Nylon/polyester	0	30	0.4
	co-casted zeta	5	30	0.2
		12	30	0.6
		30	30	20.0
E	Nylon/polyester	0	30	2.2
	(coated zeta)	5	30	3.5
		12	30	15.0
F	Polysulfone/polypropylene	0	30	1.0
		5	30	1.3
		12	30	1.0
		30	30	30.0
G	PVDF/polysulfone	0	25	1.1
	(ultrafilter)	5	25	0.7
		12	25	0.7
		30	25	0.7
		65	25	0.7
		100	25	0.7

Pate (1990); Courtesy, *Ultrapure Water* journal

using air; thus capital costs are lower. Second, the oxygen gas exiting the adsorption columns can be recycled to produce ozone. Thus only minimal amounts of oxygen actually are consumed. Finally, when ozone is desorbed and added to the water, only ozone is added to the cooling water. No oxygen is added other than that which is formed as the solubilized ozone decomposes.

The original description of the MABOS system (Nakayama et al., 1980) pointed its application to freshwater cooling towers. A later description (Nakayama et al., 1985) showed its use for seawater cooling-water circuits. The system applies high concentrations of ozone to the cooling water once each day for 5 to 10 minutes. This prevents algae and slimes from attaching to the condenser tube walls.

A German modification of the MABOS concept (Joel, 1987) is called SORBOZON. Following the two silica-gel ozone adsorbers is an "ozone surge tank" into which ozone desorbed from the two adsorbers is collected. From this surge tank, ozone can be fed continuously to the contacting system.

Except in the Membrel electrolysis method, whatever gases emerge from an ozone generator are fed directly into the water. Thus a lot of oxygen is added to the water. Off-gassing is a consequence for both the oxygen and ozone. Usually the gaseous stream is fed into water storage tanks. Provisions are therefore made for vent decomposers wherein off-gassing ozone is destroyed by conversion to oxygen through the agency of UV light of 254 nm.

Unfortunately, its strong oxidizing powers lead ozone to degrade elastomeric O-rings, seals, and gaskets that come in contact with it. Elastomers based upon butyl rubbers and ethylene-propylene rubbers (EPR) are primarily susceptible, probably because of their content of molecular branching and unsaturated bonding. Specialty rubbers designed for oxidative resistance, such as the Vitons, may be more immune to attack. In the electronics industry, where an ozone residual in component rinsewater is sometimes used to destroy organic impurities, the use of fluorinated elastomers such as Kalrez and Vitons (both from E.I. duPont, Wilmington, Del.) is necessitated. The more usual elastomers can be used in Teflon-encapsulated form, chiefly in contexts where static rather than dynamic stressing of the elastomer is involved. Few organic materials, whatever their form—filters, gaskets, pipes, or containers—are impervious to the ravages of ozone. The effects of 0.5 ppm of ozone on ion-exchange resins is said to be devastating.

Yarnell et al. (1989) studied the effects of 0.1-ppm concentrations of ozone on mixed-bed resins. Oxidative degradations ensued, but at what could be considered acceptable levels of risk for up to 200 hours.

The materials that come in contact with ozone require being selected for that purpose. Polyvinylchloride (PVC) is not immune to attack by ozone. Polytetrafluoroethylene (PTFE) and polyvinylidene fluoride (PVDF) can be used with ozone. Stainless steels, which are pitted by chlorine, resist ozone.

Therefore, ozone will not damage stainless steel stills and will be removed in the distillation process.

Operational Considerations

The ozone generated for biofouling control can be effective only to the extent that

Table 3-7
Ozone Exposure Test: TOC and Resistivity Rinse-up Data for High Ozone Concentration (600-1,200 ppb) after Approximately 1 Day of Rinse-up at 2 gpm/10 °C.

Filter	*Media/Support*	*Cumulative Ozone (ppm-hours)*	*Rinse Time, hours at (3 gpm/10" Cart)*	*Δ TOC (ppb)*	*Δ Resistivity (Mohms-cm)*
A	PTFE/PTFE	0	10	0.0	0.0
		5	24	0.2	0.0
		12	24	0.2	0.0
		30	24	0.2	0.0
		65	35	0.1	0.0
		100	35	0.1	0.0
B	PVDF/polypropylene (2-layer)	0	5	0.7	0.0
		5	20	0.7	0.7
		12	20	3.0	1.0
		30	21	8.0	2.5
		65	22	12.1	3.1
		100	24	15.4	3.1
C	PVDF/polyester (1-layer)	0	7	0.4	0.0
		5	33	1.0	0.7
		12	33	2.0	2.0
		30	21	5.2	7.9
		65	21	5.8	10.6
D	Nylon/polyester co-casted zeta	0	7	1.3	0.2
		5	26	2.9	0.6
		12	26	7.7	1.1
		30	34	10.2	4.4
E	Nylon/polyester (coated zeta)	0	9	6.5	0.0
		5	28	2.2	0.4
		12	26	11.1	1.5
F	Polysulfone/polypropylene	0	20	0.0	0.0
		5	24	5.9	2.7
		12	37	6.0	2.4
		30	23	22.7	4.2
G	PVDF/polysulfone (ultrafilter)	0	23	0.0	0.1
		5	23	0.0	0.3
		12	23	0.0	0.3
		30	2.2	0.9	0.9
		65	24	2.8	0.9
		100	24	2.8	0.9

Pate (1990); Courtesy, *Ultrapure Water* journal

it dissolves in the conveying water. In accordance with Henry's Law, ozone concentration varies directly with its partial pressure, and inversely with temperature. Therefore, it is recommended that the generated ozone be injected into the water stream after the circulation pump and before any heat exchanger.

Ozone introduction into solutions is best done by employing an Otto-type aspirator/injector that sprays the water into the ozone chamber. This device has a high power requirement, however, which confines its use to smaller systems. In general, there are two types of ozone injectors or mixers. The first, intended for fast reactions, is mass-transfer limited; the second, for slow reactions, is rate-reaction limited. Either countercurrent or co-current flows are used. The in-line mixers can be a grouping of helices that form cavities leading to vortices. The flow through these is, however, limited to about 4 to 7 feet per second (Nebel et al., 1973). The faster the flow, the smaller the bubbles and thus the more rapid their solution. Porous stone baffles can also be used to break the ozone stream into smaller bubbles. Diffusion tanks of such construction can service flows of 450 gallons per minute.

Electrolytic generation of ozone results in the formed ozone being rapidly dissolved in water. However, the small quantity of ozone-containing water involved must be dispersed throughout the water being treated. Static mixers are used for this purpose.

The first quantities of ozone introduced are consumed by reaction with the organics that are present. Only after these excessive initial requirements of ozone been assuaged can maintenance of a proper ozone residual level relative to the biocidal action be made. Also, some quantity of ozone must be expected to be lost by decomposition.

Further addition to a concentration of 0.04 to 2 ppm provides an ozone residue level discouraging to organism growth. Systems based on such residual concentration have been used successfully on a continual three-shift basis, 7 days per week, for extended periods of time. Ozone serves admirably as a sterilant for water systems. However, its low water solubility slows its destruction of the biofilm glycocalix. Therefore, its continuous application is advocated for this purpose. Ozone is also used in intermittent operations. In one such, the use-cycle is of a 2-hour duration for every 4-hour interval.

Because the ozone requires time to be dissolved and to act, generators supplying 1 ppm of ozone are used, even though only tenths of a ppm are required. Not all the generated ozone gets dissolved and used. The gas stream exits from the generator at 10 to 15 psig. This suffices to introduce it into storage tanks, the common practice in pharmaceuticals. If it must be introduced into a pressurized system, say at 80 psig, it is first dissolved in a small quantity of water that is then discharged by a pump.

Ozone Generation by UV Radiation

Ozone also can be generated in oxygen or air by UV radiation itself, although only in relatively low concentrations per unit time. This is insufficient to treat large volumes of water economically. Thus, more than 44 kilowatts (kW) are required to generate 1 kg of ozone from dried air under high gas flowrates (Nebel, 1981) by UV, compared with 12 to 17 KW by corona discharge.

The oxidative effects of UV radiation on aqueous solutions are often ascribed to the presence of ozone. The more likely occurrence is the generation by the UV radiation of hydroxyl free radicals in solution. Ozone probably is not involved, except to provide some of the feed source of the hydroxyl free radicals.

Table 3-8
Ozone Exposure Test: Pressure, Decay Data for Low Ozone Concentration (40-60 ppb)

Filter Media/Support	*Cumulative Ozone (ppm-hours)*	*Starting Pressure (psig)*	*Pressure Drop (psig)*
A PTFE/PTFE	0.0	15	1.5
	1.2	15	1.4
	4.0	15	1.4
	7.5	15	1.4
	10.0	15	1.4
B PVDF/polypropylene (2-layer)	0.0	50	3.2
	1.2	50	2.3
	4.0	50	1.9
	7.5	50	1.9
	10.0	50	3.0
C PVDF/polyester (1-layer)	0.0	50	0.5
	1.2	50	1.0
	4.0	50	21.0
D Nylon/polyester co-casted zeta	0.0	30	0.7
	1.2	30	0.6
	4.0	30	1.6
E Nylon/polyester (coated zeta)	0.0	30	0.8
	1.2	30	0.9
	4.0	30	30.0
F Polysulfone/polypropylene	0.0	30	1.0
	1.2	30	30.0
G PVDF/polysulfone (ultrafilter)	0.0	25	1.1
	1.2	25	0.8
	4.0	25	0.6
	7.5	25	0.6
	10.0	25	0.6

Pate (1990); Courtesy, *Ultrapure Water* journal

Being so strong an oxidant, whether by its own direct action or through the agency of generating free hydroxyl radicals, ozone can be used to destroy organic materials of various molecular compositions. It is this capability that commends ozone for use in physically removing organisms as well as their pyrogenic products, along with all manner of organic extractables that constitute TOC. Ozone champions enthuse that it can convert organics to carbon dioxide and water (Nebel and Nebel, 1984; Francis, 1987). But, as already discussed, such a total transformation is difficult, and possibly impractical to achieve (Francis, 1987). Reliance can, however, be placed on attaining so definite a degree of oxidative alteration of the organic molecule or system as to neutralize its viability (organisms) or physiological effect (pyrogens). The statement that ozone leaves no residues is therefore only partly true. It leaves no trace of its own molecular existence, but the altered organic may still exist, albeit in less objectionable form, often to be removed as a carboxylic acid derivative by ion-exchange reaction. The transformation to carbon dioxide is catalyzed by titanium dioxide.

Ozone Usage

Performing ozone analyses for off-line batch or grab samples poses no special problems. It is somewhat more difficult to measure ozone in real time in systems. The calibration monitors are of somewhat uncertain reliability; the detectors, being exposed constantly to an aggressive ambience, suffer in dependability. Indeed, ozone detectors lag behind the rest of ozone technology. Therefore, all the in-line meters are backed up by wet chemistry.

That ozone concentrations are not measurable with the greatest accuracy provides room for uncertainties. How can one be certain, for instance, concerning the possible effects of 1 ppb of ozone on monoclonal antibodies? Undoubtedly, however, much of the uncertainty derives from the novelty of ozone applications rather than from demonstrated concerns.

In semiconductor contexts, there are also problems associated with ozone use. Low conductivities are among the steadfast goals of this application. Yet in ozone's oxidation of organic compounds, carbon dioxide is released and ionizable carboxylic acids are produced. These elevate the conductivity values of the water being purified. Obviously, the carboxylic acids, carbon dioxide (where such is produced), and other ionic by-products of the TOC oxidation require appropriate removal. This gives pause, in some cases, to the use of ozone.

Removal of Ozone

Ultraviolet radiation of 254-nm wavelength (the germicidal frequency) destroys ozone in water in seconds, converting it into oxygen (Nebel and Nebel, 1984). Stated in quantitative terms, 90,000 microrads/cm^2/sec of UV light energy are required to eliminate quantitatively 1 ppm of ozone. Higher concentrations require higher energy levels for their destruction. Such higher energy levels for low-level concentrations may accomplish the ozone destruction in fractions of a second. There is a strong advantage to the destructive removal of ozone by UV; no reagents having been added, no residues need be removed.

Ozone can also be destroyed by adsorption and/or reaction with wet granulated activated carbon; catalytically by contact with manganese dioxide; and by chemical reductions, as by thiosulfate. Ozone dissolved in water stored in tanks is destroyed when vented through manganese dioxide catalyzed tank vents. It is decomposed into oxygen.

The 254-nm UV irradiation of waters containing ozone is the device used to

Table 3-9
Ozone Exposure Test: TOC and Resistivity Rinse-up Data for Low Ozone Concentration (40-60 ppb) after Approximately 1 Day of Rinse-up at 2 gpm/10 °C.

Filter Media/Support	*Cumulative Ozone (ppm-hours)*	*Rinse Time, hours at (3gpm/10" Cart)*	*Δ TOC (ppb)*	*Δ Resistivity (Mohms-cm)*
A PTFE/PTFE	0.0	10	0.0	0.0
	1.3	30	0.0	0.0
	4.0	30	0.0	0.0
	7.5	33	0.0	0.0
	10.0	6	0.0	0.0
B PVDF/polypropylene	0.0	8	0.7	0.0
(2-layer)	1.3	22	0.4	0.5
	4.0	23	0.6	0.6
	7.5	27	2.4	0.7
	10.0	23	2.8	0.7
C PVDF/polyester	0.0	7	0.4	0.0
(1-layer)	1.2	22	0.6	0.3
	4.0	22	0.0	0.6
D Nylon/polyester	0.0	7	1.3	0.2
co-casted zeta	1.2	21	2.1	0.3
	4.0	21	5.4	0.6
E Nylon/polyester	0.0	9	6.5	0.0
(coated zeta)	1.2	21	0.6	0.0
	4.0	20	1.6	0.1
F Polysulfone/polypropylene	0.0	20	0.0	0.0
	1.2	23	1.6	0.3
G PVDF/polysulfone	0.0	23	0.0	0.0
(ultrafilter)	1.2	21	0.0	0.3
	4.0	20	0.0	0.3
	7.5	20	0.0	0.3
	10.0	19	0.2	0.2

Pate (1990); Courtesy, *Ultrapure Water* journal

free them of its residuals.

It has been recommended that deozonation by UV light, in order to provide an ample dosage, be done on water moving at flowrates that are 40% of those employed when UV light is used for germicidal effects. Thus, if the flowrate through a UV device is set at 60 gpm to achieve germicidal destruction, then a slower flowrate of 24 gpm should be used for deozonation. This flowrate recommendation was established for ozone concentrations of parts per million. The more recent use of sub-ppm levels of ozone for germicidal purposes finds complete ozone destruction by UV to be attained even at full germicidal flowrates. Where prudence is required, the oversized UV dosages forthcoming from lower flowrates may be relied upon.

In an ultraconservative approach to the removal of ozone from processed waters, one eastern pharmaceutical manufacturer employs two ozone-destruct units in series. The ozone monitor is not quite relied upon in its signalling of zero ozone content. The compatibility of the processed water with the product is monitored very carefully by product stability studies.

Rice (1987) outlines an ozone utilization scheme as follows:

↗Destroy exhaust gas
Gas preparation ---> Ozone generator ---> Contactor
↑
↘Utilize the ozone
Power generation

Ozone in Microbiological Control

Gurley (1985) believed that available ozone generation and water-ozone contactor equipment make ozone a cost-competitive sterilization technique for the phar-

Table 3-10
Filter Description for Ozone Exposure Testing

Filter	*Media*	*Support*	*μm Rating*	*Type*
A	PTFE	PTFE	0.1	Cartridge
B	PVDF (2-layer)	Polypropylene	0.1	Cartridge
C	PVDF	Polyester	0.1	Cartridge
D	Nylon (co-casted zeta)	Polyester	0.1	Cartridge
E	Nylon (coated zeta)	Polyester	0.2	Cartridge
F	Polysulfone	Polypropylene	0.1	Cartridge
G	PVDF (ultrafilter)	Polysulfone	0.03	Rej. flow

Pate (1990), ULTRAPURE WATER journal

maceuticals industry, especially as regards parenterals. Ozone can be used gainfully in the preparation of sterile process water; for the terminal sterilization of aqueous drug formulations without organic components; and in the sterilization of glass and certain plastic containers, notably polyvinylchloride.

Empty glass bottles have been sterilized using ozone-containing air at concentrations of about 30 ppm of compressed gas. Control bottles inoculated with 10^3 cfu of yeasts, molds, spores, and vegetative cells were sterilized by the end of an 18-second period. The ozone-containing air was removed by sweeping with sterile air (Torricelli, 1959). Schneider and Rump (1983) used ozone-containing rinse solutions to sterilize glass containers. Control bottles contained 10^4 cfu of yeasts and bacterial cells. Ozone doses of 2.5 to 3.0 mg/L rendered them sterile upon rinsing.

Pyrogenic material is destroyed rapidly by ozone. Glass and PVC containers are simultaneously sterilized and depyrogenated by ozone (Nebel and Nebel, 1984; Matsaoka et al., 1982).

Ozone usage in microbiological control generally assumes one of two types of arrangements. In the first, ozone is applied continuously in distribution with removal at points of use (POU). In the second, it is applied intermittently, usually for extended periods daily, to provide sanitization of distribution systems during nonproduction periods. Continuous distribution with removal at the POU by the

Table 3-11
Filter Inlet and Outlet Ozone Concentration Data

Filter	*Media/Support*	*Inlet Ozone Concentration, ppb*	*Outlet Ozone Concentration, ppb*
A	PTFE/PTFE	52 500	52 500
B	PVDF/polypropylene 2-layer)	46 931	42 416
C	PVDF/polyester 1-layer)	47 842	7 468
D	Nylon/polyester co-casted zeta)	50 904	16 0
E	Nylon/polyester (coated zeta)	52 1,114	0 0
F	Polysulfone/polypropylene	52 832	0 21
G	PVDF/polysulfone (ultrafilter)	52 832	21 343

Pate 1990; Courtesy, *Ultrapure Water* journal

action of 254-nm UV sterilizers is designed for long runs of distribution piping that culminate in relatively few points of use.

The cost of UV-sterilizers to destroy the ozone precludes large numbers of POU stations. At the POU, the activation of the UV can be interlocked with a fill valve to the tank and with an ozone monitor on the effluent to assure that all ozone has been destroyed before the water enters the compounding tank. A typical continuous ozone system is shown in Figure 3-2. All water purification, either by membrane systems or demineralization or a combination of both, occurs prior to the pure water storage tank. Ozone is applied to the storage tank continuously and remains in distribution at levels that typically range from 0.1 to 2 ppm.

In-line UV sterilizers are employed at use points in the system. These in-line UV sterilizers are turned on when water is drawn at a use point. This design is practical where there are minimal use points and where these use points typically draw infrequently, as in batch operations. The principle advantage of this design is that the storage and distribution system is continually in the presence of ozone.

The continuous application design requires careful attention to operation, and should include automatic controls to assure that ozonated water will not be produced at the use points. Since this may be difficult to control in some facilities, a more common design involves the intermittent application of ozone to the distribution system. A system of this type is shown in Figure 3-3. In this system, as in the previous system, all demineralization of water takes place prior to the storage tank. Ozone is still applied continuously to the storage tank by either the corona-discharge process or the Membrel process. An in-line UV sterilizer at the tank outlet to the distribution system removes ozone continuously during compounding hours.

When water is no longer required for production, as during off shifts, the in-line UV sterilizer is turned off. This allows ozone to pass to the distribution for several hours daily. The UV sterilizer is turned on prior to the beginning of production in the morning, and ozone is immediately removed from the water that passes to the distribution system. As soon as all of the water that was ozonated and in the distribution piping is displaced, the distribution system is ozone-free.

Table 3-12
Inactivation of *E. coli* Using Ozone and Peroxone

Test Number	*Peroxide/Ozone Applied Dosages, mg/L*	E.Coli/*100 mL*		*Percent Removal*
		Influent	*Effluent*	
1001	0/1.2	5.4×10^7	33	99.99994
1002	0/4.0	4.8×10^7	0	>99.9999998
1003	0.48/1.4	8.1×10^7	68	99.99992
1004	1.9/4.0	6.3×10^7	22	99.999996

Where extremely high purity of water is required, as in some biotechnology applications, it may be a necessity to have purification equipment (such as mixed-bed demineralizers and ultrafilters) in the distributing system. These designs preclude the continuous application of ozone to the distribution system. Systems of this type operate similarly to the previously described storage tank, which is normally placed downstream of makeup equipment and upstream of high purity polishing equipment. An in-line UV sterilizer at the tank outlet prior to distribution removes ozone during production hours. During nonproduction hours, the UV sterilizer is turned off; and equipment such as demineralizers and ultrafilters, which would be harmed by ozone, are bypassed during sanitization of the distribution system. Figure 3-4 illustrates a design of this type with conventional ozone generation. Figure 3-5 illustrates a design of this type with Membrel ozone generation.

All of the systems previously described used the storage tank in the system as an ozone contact chamber. Contact time plays a major role in the effectiveness of ozone for bacterial control. Some system designs preclude the use of the storage tank for ozone application. In these system designs, ozone is produced and injected at some point in the distribution system and after brief contact (10 to 30 seconds), the ozone is removed by UV light. Ozone applied even at this low contact time can prove effective. Generally these systems will produce low bacterial counts, but these counts may not be as low as in other systems where ozone is applied for several hours daily. In all cases, for ozone to be most effective, the distribution system must be hit with appropriate ozone levels for several hours on at least a weekly basis. A short-contact ozone system of this type is shown in Figure 3-6.

Ozone-generating equipment has a wide range of costs, depending upon the production method involved. In many cases, the ancillary equipment required (such as stainless steel tanks and piping, ozone monitors, and Teflon gaskets) will cost more than the ozone-generating equipment.

Table 3-13
Ozone and Hydrogen Peroxide Residuals

	Oxidant Dosages, mgL		*Pilot Plant Effluent Oxidant Residuals, mg/L*	
Test Number	*Hydrogen Peroxide*	*Ozone*	*Hydrogen Peroxide*	*Ozone*
1001	0	1.2	0.01	<0.01
1002	0	4.0	0.01	<0.01
1003	0.48	1.4	0.05	<0.01
1004	1.9	4.0	0.12	<0.01

McGuire and Davis, (1988); Courtesy, *Water Engineering and Management*

A 1-pound-per-day conventional ozone unit would be required to apply 1.0 ppm of ozone to an 80-gpm water stream. Although 1.0 ppm is applied, the actual dissolved ozone level is in the range of 0.2 to 0.5 ppm. A complete ozone package consisting of the ozone generator, oxygen enrichment unit, two dissolved ozone monitors, one ambient ozone monitor, and one catalytic vent decomposer would cost in the range of $35,000. An oxygen analyzer can be added to the ozone generator for about $5,000. A high-concentration ozone monitor can be added to the generator outlet for about $6,000.

A Membrel system to ozonate the same 80-gpm stream with equal effectiveness would be sized to produce ozone at about 0.15 ppm. A package including the Membrel unit and two dissolved ozone monitors would cost about $58,000.

At higher flowrates the cost goes up. At 300 gpm, the cost of the conventional ozone package would be about $80,000, while the Membrel system would be about $140,000.

That ozone is so effective against individual organisms does not signify as speedy an action against microbes ensconced within and protected by biofilm. For this reason, ozonated water systems may be under microbiological control but by no means be sterile. The ozone content may become expended against planktonic microbes, and in the oxidation of organic matter. It is, indeed, for this reason that ozone system sizing depends upon the organic level (TOC) in the water as well as upon the microbial density. There may, in any instance, not be enough ozone or reaction time to destroy totally the glycocalyx as well as the free-floating organisms and organic molecules. New colonies may thus from time to time be able to break loose from the biofilm. However, the higher the ozone concentration and the longer its residence time within the system, the lower will be the prevailing organism count. In any case, the use of ozone, particularly in a continual mode, should give water systems that are controlled to very low organism levels. Ozone is credited with the destruction of biofilm.

The use of ozone to disintegrate established biofilms will result in the generation and release of particles from the disrupted glycocalyx. Where this is objectionable, as in semiconductor usage, intermittent applications of ozone might not be suitable. To the extent that reformation of new biofilm between ozone applications is possible, cyclical particle releases would result. To avoid this occurrence, a continuous presence of ozone is required to prevent biofilm reformation once it has been removed. Concentrations down to 0.1 ppm ought to suffice, provided the bioburden is not excessive. Where it is unusually high, proportionately greater ozone concentrations would, of course, be needed.

The use of ozone in concentrations of 0.1 to 2 ppm for the control of microorganisms is far more widespread in the pharmaceutical industry than is apparent from accounts published in the literature. One such report dealt with the preparation of USP Purified Water. The feedwater passed through the system, which was made up of a 10-μm-rated depth-type filter followed by a carbon bed;

this was succeeded by a 7-μm-rated depth filter and UV light installation. The water was then demineralized by a three-bed ion-exchange arrangement of cation, anion, and another cation exchanger. The effluent water passed through a UV sterilization into a 4,000-gallon tank into which ozone was fed. Water from the tank was used for tablet, liquid, and ointment preparation after being freed of its ozone content by passage through a UV light unit. The ozone was made from oxygen prepared by a swing generator using air. It employed twin molecular-sieve towers equipped with a low-oxygen alarm to signal possible dysfunctions.

Ozone is efficacious against endotoxin, particularly at higher dosages or over longer contact times. Ozone, and more pertinently the hydroxyl radicals generated by ozone with or without hydrogen peroxide or UV light catalysis, do oxidatively degrade organic molecules. Lipopolysaccharide molecules are no exception. To be sure, the oxidized entity would still exist, probably in smaller, altered molecular dispositions. However, its pyrogenic properties may well be destroyed. Continuous versus intermittent use is discussed on page 117.

Ozone and TOC

An example of how ozone decomposes TOC is demonstrated by its action in

Table 3-14
Generation of Hydroxyl Free Radicals in Ozone

Theoretical Amounts of Oxidants and UV Required for Formation of Hydroxyl Radical in Ozone/Peroxide/UV Systems

	Moles of Oxidant Consumed per Mole of OH Formed		
System	O_3	*UV*[a]	H_2O_2
Ozone/hydroxide ion[b]	1.5	---	---
Ozone/UV	1.5	0.5	(0.5)[c]
Ozone/hydrogen peroxide[b]	1.0	---	0.5
Hydrogen peroxide/UV	---	0.5	0.5

Theoretical Formation of Hydroxyl Radicals from Photolysis of Ozone and Hydrogen Peroxide

Molecule	*Molar Absorbtivity 254 ($M^{-1}cm^{-1}$)*	*OH Radicals Formed*[d] *Stoichiometry*	*per Incident Photon*
H_2O_2	20	$H_2O_2 \longrightarrow 2(OH)$	0.09
O_3	3,300	$3(O_3) \longrightarrow 2(OH)$	2.00

[a]Moles of photons (Einsteins) required for each mole of OH formed.
[b]Assumes that superoxide formed in the primary step yields one OH radical per O_2^-, which may not be the case in certain waters.
[c]Hydrogen peroxide formed *in situ* .
[d]Assumes 10-cm path length; quantum yield as predicted from stoichiometry; $[O_3]$ and $[H_2O_2]$ at 1×10^{-4}M.
Glaze et al., (1987-B); Courtesy, *Ozone Science and Engineering*

cooling tower maintenance. The conditions surrounding cooling towers (i.e., microbial contamination, organic nutrients, and temperatures conducive to organism replication) all act to encourage problems such as microbial water fouling and the luxuriant growth of algae.

Biofouling of heat exchangers, often manifested by slime formation on the inside of condenser tubes, results in reduction of heat-transfer efficiency, in corrosion of metal, and in diminution of water flowrates. In large electric power plants, biofouling results in large, recurring economic losses to the power industry.

Various chemical additives have been employed to minimize and/or prevent biofouling, chlorine being chief among these additives. Ozone also has been used to achieve this goal, and studies often have shown it to be technologically superior. Sugam and Guera (1981) conducted a comparative study at an electrical utility power-generating station on a polluted, brackish water. Chlorine was found to be more effective on a weight basis, but ozone could be used at a level less injurious to the indigenous aquatic species. This advantage could be heightened by intermittent use of ozone as the biocide. Advantages accrue to ozone from its scale-inhibiting action in addition to its biocidal effects (Merrill and Drago, 1980).

Studies have been made of the current use of ozone in cooling-water towers of air-conditioning systems at four locations in California (Merrill and Drago, 1980). In physical appearance, the ozone-treated towers generally were good, scaling and biological growth being limited to the outer edges, in areas alternatively wetting and drying. The waters generally were clean, but sometimes colored. The ozone dose was estimated at a maximum of about 0.03 mg/L, based on circulating water flow. No heat transference problems were evident.

Biofouling was judged to be controlled by the ozone. The heat exchange surfaces were not observed directly, but the waters appeared clear; their plate counts were relatively low at 7,000 to 54,000 colonies/mL; the cooling towers were comparatively clean; and the air conditioners operated well.

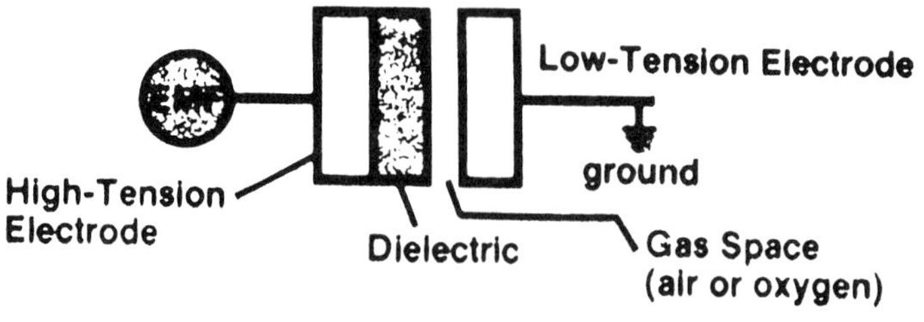

Figure 3-1. Diagram of ozone generator based on corona discharge principle.
Meltzer and Rice *(1987);* Courtesy, Water Micro Associates

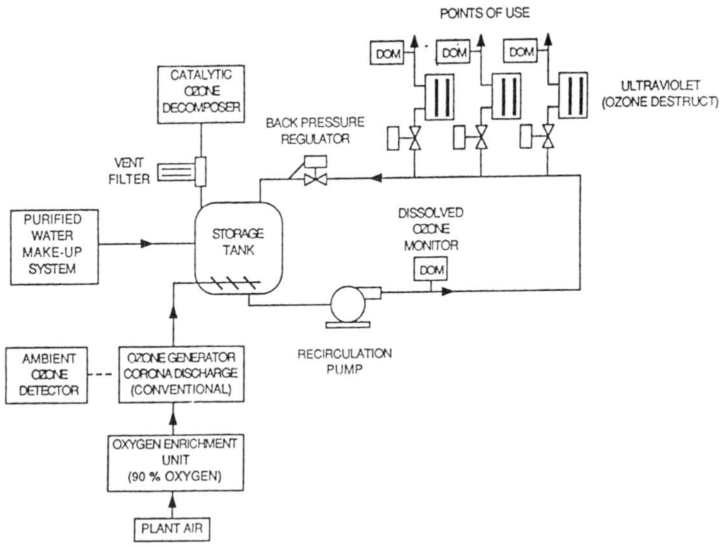

Figure 3-2. Conventional ozone production with point-of-use UV ozone destruction.

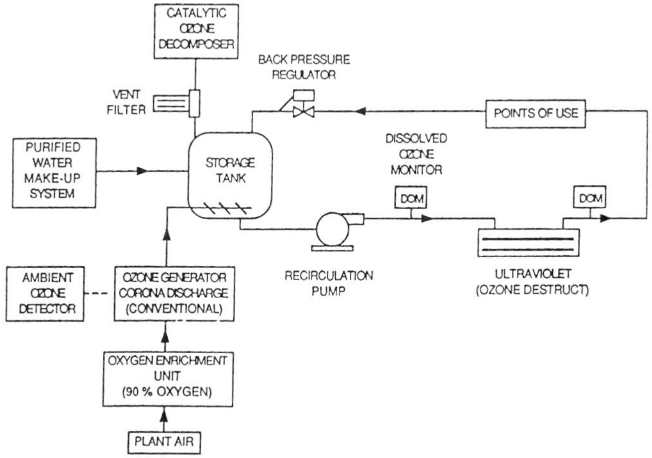

Figure 3-3. Conventional ozone production with central UV ozone destruction.
Courtesy, Continental Penfield Water Systems

An installation in Alhambra, Cal., consisted of a high-frequency ozone generator, including an air predrying unit, of 90 grams per hour ozone generation capacity. Eight months after installation the operation remained flawless. It provided ozone for a model 372-102 Marley cooling tower, servicing condenser water for 1,236 tons of air conditioning. The water was clear and odor-free. Its average usage declined from 2,300 gallons per day (gpd) to 900 gpd. The condenser pressure underwent a corresponding reduction of 2 pounds. Inspection of the condenser showed it to be sludge-free, with only a slight scale formation. Old scale continued to disintegrate for periodic removal. The ozonation system was operated on a 20-minute off/on cycle. Plans were to prolong the off stage to 30 minutes. The tower, an automatic operation, was inspected daily. Originally, the operation was planned for 8 hours a day; it actually operated for only 3 hours. A 65% cost savings was projected, attributed by Stopka (1981) to the 2% (by weight) concentration of ozone in the air generated, coupled with a highly efficient ozone contactor.

An installation in Los Angeles based on the same type of 90 g/h ozone generator utilizes two independent ozone contactors, each supplying a 2-inch in-line static mixer contactor. The basins of each of two 750-ton cooling towers are supplied separately with water that is ozonized, and is received from an 8-inch main under pressure. Algae and scale disintegrated after 8 days of ozone treatment. The scale, as removed, deposits on the bottom of the basin for eventual removal. The water, previously dirty and yellow in color, now is crystal clear. There has been no need to add water treatment chemicals, and hence no need to remove their accumulation by any blowdown. The planned treatment cycle was decreased by 50%. The ozonized cooling waters are clear and odorless.

Cooling towers are engineered so that the cascading water droplets exchange their unwanted heat with an upward cooling draft of air. Roughly 72 cubic feet of air are swept through every gallon of water every minute. The water contains the ozone, the air does not. Therefore, the air current serves to strip the water of its ozone content. Additionally, the forced-air draft introduces new populations of organisms into the aqueous system. A substantial decline in ozone content marks the descending waters. This becomes progressive as the remaining ozone encounters and reacts with the organisms harbored within the cooling tower fill. As a result, the cooling-tower sump contains water with the lowest concentration of ozone in the system. Assessment of the sufficiency of ozone residual concentrations should be made at this very point. The sump itself is not static. It recirculates at 1- to 2-minute intervals.

Generally, 5 to 10 minutes of contact time are desired for total control of organisms in circulating water when residual ozone levels of 0.4 mg/L are involved. If even as low an ozone residual as 0.02 mg/L continuously bathes the cooling-tower fill and sump, organism control should be satisfactory, provided a prolonged, nearly infinite contact time is allowed in the cooling tower.

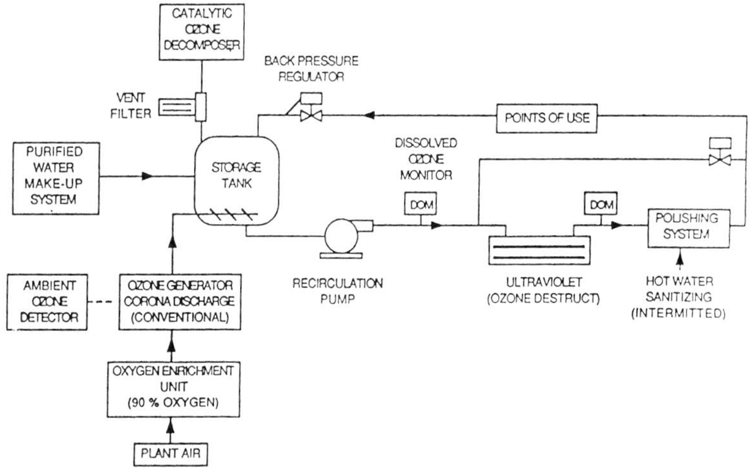

Figure 3-4. Conventional ozone production with central UV ozone destruction and polishing system.

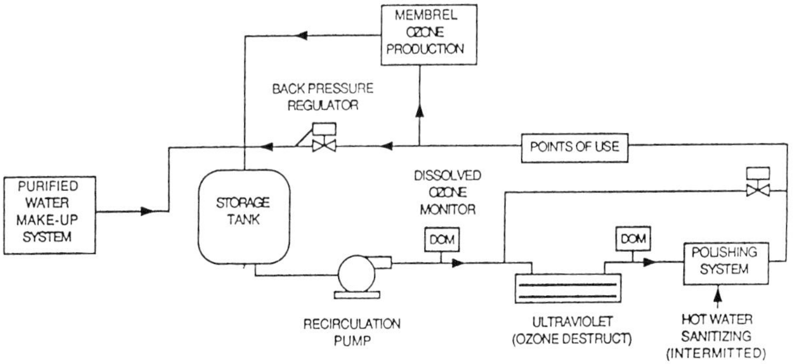

Figure 3-5. Membrel ozone production with central UV ozone destruction and polishing system.

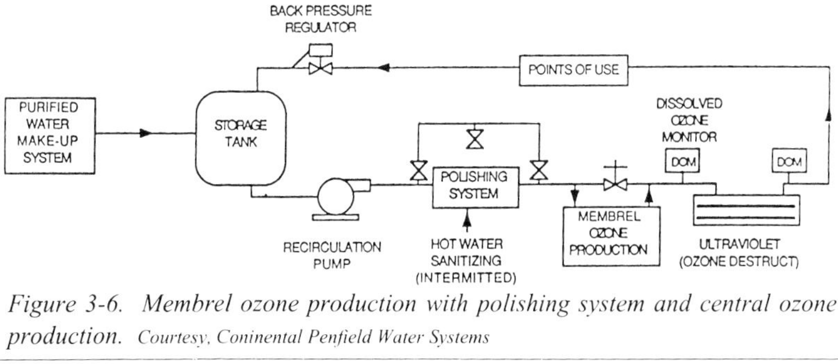

Figure 3-6. Membrel ozone production with polishing system and central ozone production. Courtesy, Coninental Penfield Water Systems

However, to attain even so low an ozone residual concentration, a 0.4 mg/L residual level must be present in the circulating waters. At these residual ozone concentrations, the microbes suspended in the circulating waters are "completely" eliminated within 1 to 2 minutes. Those adhering to the tower-fill surfaces or resident within the tower sump are held to a bacteriostatic condition by the prolonged exposures to lower ozone concentrations there present. Either way, ozone is useful in achieving the biofouling control necessary for cooling tower operations.

Pryor and Bukay (1990) stated that the ozonation of cooling tower waters can reduce the blowdown volume requirements of such installations by 90%. *Blowdown water* refers to the water that is discharged from cooling towers in order to prevent the excessive buildup of mineral salts that occurs as a result of evaporation of water. Pryor and Bukay termed the blowdown water one of the industry's largest sources of wasted water. They advocated the use of ozone in cooling-tower applications to control scale formation, corrosion, and microbiological growth. Table 3-5 and Figure 3-7 project the attendant water and costs savings that are possible.

There are those who believe that the economic benefits of ozone in such contexts are exaggerated (Puckorius, 1990). No one disputes, however, the devastating effects of ozone on microbiological growth.

Effect of Ozone on Filters

The aggressiveness of ozone and its free-radical progeny upon organic materials holds also for the polymeric materials of which filters are composed. Yet it is the high amount of surface areas that these very filters offer for biofilm formation, and their purposes as microorganism collectors, that put them often in need of sanitization, as by ozone. The molecular features that dispose the various commercially available membrane filters to succumb to or to resist oxidative attacks have been detailed (Meltzer, 1989). These features include such susceptible linkages as allylic and tertiary carbon-hydrogen bonds, and such impervious linkages as the carbon/fluorine bonds. It is the high resistivities of the latter that particularly suit filters composed of PTFE and PVDF for contact with ozone. Such filter compositions can be costly, however. It is thus possible that filters of less resistant natures may offer a sufficiently long service to be cost-effective. All-PTFE (Teflon, duPont trademark for PTFE) filters are available in the marketplace (Lukaszewicz et al., 1986).

Pate (1990, 1991) compared the performances of seven different commercially available membranes in their responses to ozone. The microporous filters tested were an all-PTFE construction, a 2-layer PVDF with polypropylene support, a 1-layer PVDF with polyester support, a nylon membrane co-cast with charge modifiers and with polyester support, and a polysulfone membrane with polypropylene support. Additionally, an ultrafilter, a PVDF membrane utilizing a polysulfone support, was tested.

As shown in Tables 3-6 to 3-9, each filter was tested at two different ozone concentrations, at a low concentration of between 40 and 60 ppb and a high one of between 500 and 1,200 ppb. Exposures to ozone are customarily expressed as cumulative ozone exposure, E, wherein E (ppm-hours) equals the product of ozone ppm and hours of exposure. In this relationship, the ppm concentration and the exposure duration are of equal influence. For example, sanitizations of final filters in a deionization (DI) arrangement using 200 ppb (0.2 ppm) over an

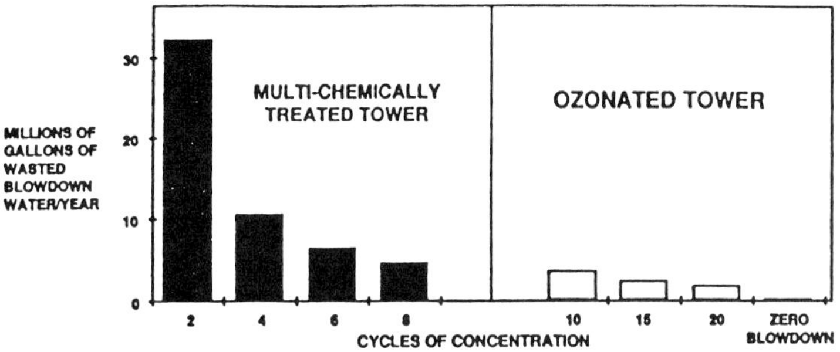

Figure 3-7. The amount of water typically wasted in a 2,400-ton cooling system operated at 85% of its capacity. Ozonation allows operation at high cycles of concentration, thus greatly reducing water waste.
Pryor and Bukay (1990); Courtesy, *Ultrapure Water* journal

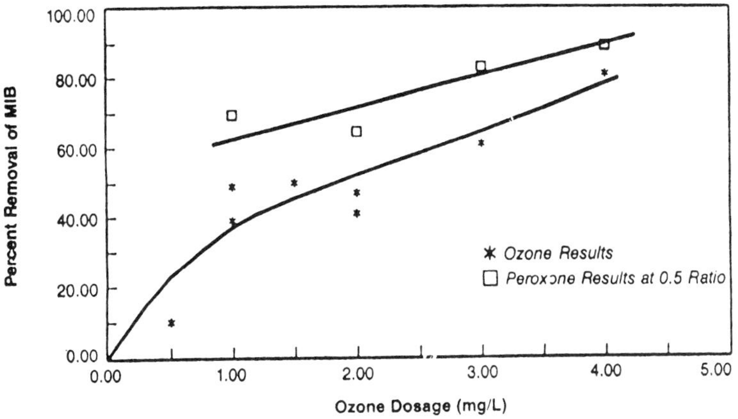

Figure 3-8. Methylisoborneol oxidation in bench-scale tests.
McGuire and Davis, (1988); Courtesy, *Water Engineering and Management*

exposure time of 2 hours, repeated quarterly over a 2-year period, would give an E value of 3.2 ppm-hours. The study of Pate (1990) investigated the following assumption:

$$0.05 \text{ ppm} \times 20 \text{ hours} = 1.0 \text{ ppm-hr} \qquad \text{Eq. 3-7}$$

is equivalent to

$$0.5 \text{ ppm} \times 2 \text{ hours} = 1.0 \text{ ppm hr.} \qquad \text{Eq. 3-8}$$

It was found that equivalence was *not* the case. Failure of the filters was judged by their failure to maintain their integrity or to rinse up, as measured by TOC and resistivity, after the ozone exposure. Long-term, low-level exposures were found to be more deleterious than high-level, short-term exposures. Pate (1990) suggests, therefore that a better expression of E ppm-hours for ozone exposures would be forthcoming from the relationship :

$$E = C_{ppm} \times T^2 \text{ hours.} \qquad \text{Eq. 3-9}$$

As shown in Tables 3-10 and 3-11, the ozone concentration was recorded going into and out of each filter. Decreases in the ozone concentrations were presumably caused by reaction with the filter. What was sought was a low consumption of ozone by the filter during an exposure to 100 ppm-hours of ozone, a level typical of the range of 1 to 100 ppm-hours that a filter might experience over its useful service life. This level would encompass initial and periodic sanitizations. Filters were expected to maintain their integrity over this exposure, and to rinse up rapidly to acceptable TOC and resistivity levels. The ozone consumption did not necessarily need to reflect upon the integrity of the membrane layer, however. It could be caused by reaction with the support layers that, while contributory to adsorptive particle retentions, are used more to optimize the filter's flow patterns than to effect particle removals. Thus, had a PTFE/polypropylene filter been tested, the PTFE would not have been affected by the ozone and would not diminish its concentration. The filter would retain its overall integrity. The polypropylene separation layer, however, would have been involved in reaction with ozone, with concomitant generation of TOC and conductivity. By the same token, an imagined filter made of polypropylene membrane separated by a diffuse PTFE separation layer would also consume ozone and generate TOC and conductivity. However, the damage or destruction of the microporous filter would compromise its retentive function, as attested to by the loss of filter integrity. The maintenance of filter integrity under ozone attack is the key point to the particle-retention function. The generation of TOC and conductivity is not without practical importance, however.

Pate (1990) found the all-PTFE cartridge filter to be the best, the most resistant to ozone. He believed, however, that its cost would normally be prohibitive for DI water applications. The PVDF filters also maintained their integrity. (The

PVDF data showed some aberrations. Such are always possible, however, when a single, individual filter is evaluated as representative of the entire class of filters.)

The situation ideally requires a statistically significant number of samples of each type. The exigencies of such testing, regrettably, render the implementation impractical. Pate concluded that the charge-modified nylon filters showed "respectable ozone resistance" that could sustain periodic periods of ozone sterilization to a total of 1.2 ppm-hours. This should be of interest; the ultimate in resistance to ozone may or may not be required in particular situations. The concept of cost effectiveness may be a useful one. The polysulfone filter, alone among all those evaluated, did not demonstrate a sufficient resistance to ozone; it was not acceptable even at less than 1-ppm-hour doses.

The evaluation of filter resistance to ozone as reported by Pate (1990) accords with earlier findings by Zahka and Smith (1988). These investigators found that a PTFE membrane on polyfluoroallomer (PFA) stacked disks, as judged by integrity testing, alone proved to be completely resistant to ozone, at an exposure of 30 hours at 1 ppm concentration. This was not surprising, given the totality of carbon/fluorine substituent bonding on the carbon/carbon polymer backbone of PTFE; the total lack of carbon/hydrogen linkages whatever; and the very high degree of fluorination for the PFA that makes up the heat-tractable fluorocarbon portion of the total filter combination. Zahka and Smith (1989) also demonstrated that PVDF membrane also withstands ozone well. The filter maintained its integrity after 20 hours at 1 ppm of exposure. To be sure, the hydrophilic coating that was grafted to the PVDF membrane to render it wettable by water was removed by oxidative degradation. The inherent PVDF filter maintained its integrity, however, and remained wetted by water. This experience agrees with the successful mediation by hydrophilic surface treatments in the wetting of hydrophobic surfaces by water. The surfaces will remain wetted, unless allowed to dry out, despite the eventual removal of the wetting agent.

Pate (1990) found that the ultrafilter combination of PVDF membrane and polysulfone separation layers preserved its integrity through a full 100-ppm-hour exposure, and showed a satisfactory ozone resistance as measured by acceptable rinse-ups even after 10 ppm-hours of exposure. Zahka and Vakhshoori (1990) came to the same conclusion after exposing the PVDF/polysulfone ultrafilter to 6,000 ppm-hours of ozone (3 ppm for a total of 200 hours). The filter integrity remained unchanged, as did also its colloidal-silica retention.

Scanning electron micrography examination of the PVDF membrane surface revealed no structural changes. However, Fourier transform infrared (FTIR) was revelatory at 1,700-nm wavelength of carboxyl group formation, an index of oxidative alteration. Some effects were also evident at 2,800 nm. Conceivably, the changes detected by FTIR may ultimately impinge upon life-controlling events. They found no expression, however, in the filter properties of interest to

600 ppm-hour ozone applications. What is significant, however, is that these findings give substantiation to the claims of Pate et al. (1990) that high-intensity UV light has degrading effects upon PVDF piping.

Effect of Ozone on Ion-Exchange Resins

Yarnell et al. (1989) investigated the effects of ozone concentrations of 0.10 and 0.02 ppm upon mixed-bed ion-exchange resins. It was found that the effects were cumulative with time and involved steadily increasing TOC generation and progressively decreasing effluent resistivity. The observed resin degradations varied inversely with the cross-link density of the resin, being especially marked for the cation-exchange resins. It is known that oxidative free-radical attack on organic polymer will result, among other reactions, in scission of the polymer chains. Higher cross-link densities, by providing alternative linkages that maintain the long-chain configurations, help to maintain the integrity of the polymer structure against its fragmentation. The decrease in resistivity derives from a loss of the ion-exchange functional groups to attack by the free radicals initiated by the ozone, and from the ionic compounds (chiefly carboxylic acids) generated by such attack. The increase in TOC mirrors the organic entities formed by the ozone (hydroxyl free radical) degradation of the long-chain polymer molecules. Strong correlation exists between increase in TOC and the decrease in resistivity, an indication that the TOC is ionic (carboxylic acids) in nature.

It was found that macroreticular resins (which are inherently more highly cross-linked) better resisted ozone than did the gel type. Yarnell et al. (1989) found that routine property tests, such as those to evaluate the moisture-holding, weight, and volume capacities of ion-exchange resins, were inadequate in assessing deterioration in the resin performance, although moisture-holding capacity is ordinarily useful in gauging oxidative damage to resin. Kinetic performance as measured by mass-transfer tests showed no impairment for sodium, but did substantially for sulfate. These investigators concluded that the degradation caused by ozone preferentially attacks the cation resin component; that the resulting degradation fouls the anion resin component, impairing its kinetic performance; and that it is this impairment that is responsible for the increased TOC throw and the decreased effluent resistivity.

Combinations of Ozone, UV, and Hydrogen Peroxide

As explained, the oxidative destruction of TOC under free-radical attack, such as is forthcoming from ozone, UV light, and oxidizers such as hydrogen peroxide, results (among other effects) in the cleavage of carbon/carbon bonds. As a result, complex organic molecules become fragmented, ultimately into derivatives of methane, the archetype of one-carbon compounds. When chlorine is the oxidizer, progressively halogenated methanes are the reaction products.

This is the origin of the trihalomethanes, the THMs. Due to the stability of the carbon/chlorine bond, the THMs and their higher homologs, unlike methane and its homologs such as ethane, are difficult to degrade to carbon dioxide, even by the action of ozone.

Glaze and Kang (1988) found in laboratory experiments, however, that trichloroethylene (TCE) and tetrachloroethylene underwent ozone attack when accelerated by hydrogen peroxide. This was attributed to the generation of hydroxyl free radicals. High levels of bicarbonate served to significantly reduce the efficiency of the reaction. Prior water softening would seem to be indicated. At up to H_2O_2/O_3 ratios of 0.5 to 0.7 weight-to-weight (w/w), the oxidation is accelerated about 2 or 3 times for TCE and 2 to 6 times for perchloroethylene (PCE) (where a carbon/carbon bond is available for attack). Higher hydrogen peroxide concentrations are not more effective, being mass-transfer limited; higher ozone dosage rates may be. Bicarbonate and carbonate ions interfere with the process because of their free-radical scavenging propensities. The utility of ozone/hydrogen peroxide combinations to reduce the TOC contents of softened waters is seen as being justified.

Aieta et al. (1988) successfully extended Glaze and Kang's laboratory studies to pilot plant evaluations. The results indicated the optimum ratio of hydrogen peroxide to ozone to be 0.4 and 0.5 by weight. The constancy of the rate of TCE and PCE oxidation was dependent upon the constancy of the mass-transfer rate of the ozone from the gas phase to the liquid phase. The rate of oxidation by ozone/hydrogen peroxide was almost instantaneous. According to Aieta and his colleagues, a cost analysis of the process indicated it to be competitive with more conventional technologies. The actual process economics would, however, be strongly dependent upon the specific water quality being dealt with.

McGuire and Davis (1988) stated that the combined use of hydrogen peroxide and ozone promised to be effective against microorganisms and against disinfection by-products, such as the THMs, at half the cost of ozone itself. Figure 3-8 shows the superiority of Peroxone, as McGuire and Davis termed the combination of hydrogen peroxide and ozone, compared with ozone alone against 2-methylisoborneol (MIB), a difficult-to-oxidize organic compound. These findings were confirmed in pilot plant studies. These investigators found the ratio of hydrogen peroxide to ozone to be optimal at 0.5 to 1.0, presumably by weight. Table 3-12 indicates the more salubrious effects of Peroxone against *E. coli*; Table 3-13 demonstrates the desired freedom from reagent residuals that attended these treatments.

A review article by Glaze et al. (1987) covered the potentiation of the destruction of organic compounds by ozone combined with hydrogen peroxide, UV radiation, or both. Glaze and his associates referred to such systems as "advanced oxidation processes."

It is worth noting that among such processes were included other hydroxyl free-radical initiators such as certain metals and metal oxides. It is interesting that certain commercial TOC analyzers utilized combinations of titanium dioxide and UV light to degrade organic molecules (TOC) into measurable carbon dioxide. Glaze and his coworkers discussed the mechanisms of these processes.

In very pure water, hydroxyl free radicals whose proximate presence may be owed to either UV radiation or to hydrogen peroxide (or certain other causes) react with ozone to form additional free radicals. From such a single initiation step, then, results a propagation chain involving hundreds of ozone molecules. It is for this reason that ozone can have a short half-life in distilled water presumably free of TOC. The chain may be broken (terminated) by the presence of organic matter, bicarbonate or carbonate ions, or other entities that interact with the hydroxyl free radical, and also by dimerization of any other radical/radical coupling reaction. The rate constants for hydroxyl free-radical reactions are extremely large, meaning that the reactions are very fast. It is these hydroxyl free radicals that are made increasingly available from the ozone by UV or H_2O_2 that serve oxidatively to transform the TOC, subject of course to the action of other free-radical "traps" such as bicarbonate/carbonate ions that may competitively preempt the hydroxyl free radical's attack.

Ozone in water reacts with UV radiant energy to produce hydrogen peroxide:

$$O_3 + \eta u + H_2O \text{ ----> } H_2O_2 \qquad \text{Eq. 3-10}$$

It would appear, then, that the reaction path between an organic molecule and a hydroxyl free radical would be the same whether the free radical was generated from the ozone by UV radiation, or directly by hydrogen peroxide. This is so except where the organic molecule is itself absorptive of UV light. In such cases, direct photolysis may contribute importantly to the decomposition of the organic molecule. In effect, for certain organic molecules, the molecular alterations are results of simultaneous photolysis and oxidation processes when ozone and UV are used in combination. (Zeff et al., 1988).

Baumann and Stuki (1988) performed laboratory experiments, utilizing electrolytically generated ozone and 185-nm UV radiation to accomplish, in aqueous solutions, the removal of such organic compounds as isopropanol, acetone, methanol, and trichloroethylene (all solvents being used in semiconductor operations), and of humic acid. Isopropanol and acetone showed high removal rates. Trichloroethylene also exhibited a high removal rate, despite the relative stability of its carbon/chlorine bonds, probably because ozone itself directly attacks double bonds, whereas TOC otherwise is degraded by the hydroxyl free radicals generated by ozone from water. Methanol and humic acid were more resistant. All the test compounds in concentrations of 0.77 ppm were efficiently converted to carboxylic acids, which can be removed by ion-exchange resins. Baumann and Stuki (1989) concluded from their rates-of-removal studies that the optimum ozone concentration for such UV-potentiated TOC destructions is in the region of 2 to 10 mg of ozone per L of water, and that total ozone dosages in the order of 1 to 100 grams per cubic meter would be involved, depending upon the TOC content of the water. The ozone-generating capacity needed for TOC destruction when abetted by UV is several magnitudes larger than that needed for disinfection.

Glaze et al. (1987) compared the reaction rates at pH 2 of dichloroethylene and trichloroethylene with ozone and with ozone abetted by UV light:

	Ozone	Ozone + UV
Dichloroethylene	4.3	25
Trichloroethylene	17	130

Glaze et al. (1987) saw the ozone-UV light combination as a product of free hydroxyl radicals by way of hydrogen peroxide formation from water. The UV boosts the energy level of some organic compounds, promoting their destruction by the ozone.

Hydrogen peroxide itself photolyzes under the influences of UV radiation to yield hydroxyl free radicals:

$$H_2O_2 + \eta v = 2\ OH^{\cdot} \qquad \text{Eq. 3-11}$$

The stoichiometric yield of these free radicals is greater than from the photolysis of ozone. However, ozone has a higher molar extinction coefficient than does H_2O_2. Therefore, in practice, the photolytic generation by UV of hydroxyl free radicals is greater than from hydrogen peroxide, which has an exceptionally low molar extinction coefficient; this is shown in Table 3-14. Glaze et al. (1987) concluded that, of the advanced oxidation processes, the combination of ozone and hydrogen peroxide is best suited for adoption to water purification plants and should be relatively cost-effective. These investigators expected, on the other hand, that ozone/UV systems may be difficult to adopt on a large scale but may be useful for smaller installations, especially when the organic materials involved are strong absorbers of UV radiation.

The hydrogen peroxide/UV combination is being offered as skid-mounted equipment by at least one company. In one application designed for the removal of trichloroethylene from groundwaters, it was said to be more effective and economical than TCE removals based on granular-activated carbon adsorptions (Hagar et al., 1988).

Depyrogenation of Water

Lee et al. (1991) investigated the kinetics of the reaction of bacterial endotoxin and ozone as catalyzed by UV radiation. They found the rate of destruction to be first order, following a nonlinear phase. The initial phase of some 1 to 3 minutes duration varied from a rapid rate to one that evinced a plateau. Bacteria levels in feedwaters are variable, and the organisms are killed by ozone within the first 3 minutes. Endotoxin released from these sources probably accounted for the initial variations. The effects of temperature were not explored. The endotoxin concentrations were measured by way of the LAL technique (see page 75) using a Kinetic Turbidimetric Analyzer. The levels of endotoxin used in the study were much higher than would be expected in practice. Normally, the initial level could be expected to be about 0.5 to 5 EU/mL. The solutions studied consisted of deionized water to which endotoxin was added. The initial endotoxin concentrations varied from 0.843 to 238 EU/mL in strength. Except for one test, a 4 to 5 log reduction in endotoxin was attained within 30 minutes. The D value of between 6 and 10 minutes was obtained on endotoxin concentrations as high as 100 EU/mL. The spread in the D value may reflect the uninvestigated effect of temperature. Regrettably, neither the ozone concentration (continuously bubbled into the test solution) nor the UV dosage (furnished by six lamps of unspecified provenance) were quantified. Lee et al. (1991) by this investigation would seem to have demonstrated that DI-treated waters can rapidly and efficiently be simultaneously rendered sterile and free of endotoxin (to detectable limits) by use of the oxidizing action of ozone catalyzed by UV radiation.

Destruction of TOC

Hango et al. (1981) utilized ozone in combination with hydrogen peroxide in the reclamation of recycled semiconductor rinsewater. The removal of organic compounds, largely isopropanol and acetone, was sought. At pH 7.5 and using a weight ratio of 5:1 ozone to hydrogen peroxide, TOC levels of 18 mg/L were completely removed in 60 minutes. The ratio of ozone to TOC was 14:1. Neither ozone by itself, nor with UV radiation, was as cost-effective. The use of 1.7 pounds of ozone plus 0.42 pounds of H_2O_2 per 1,000 gallons was estimated at 1981 prices to cost 83 cents per 1,000 gallons.

Francis (1987) preferred the combination of UV radiation and ozone for the removal of TOC. Ultraviolet radiation by itself does not occasion the total oxidation of organic materials. Also, its organism kill rate, particularly of spores, is less. Ozone itself reacts more slowly with organics than does the hydroxyl free radical, and is less effective against the carboxylic acids that are some of the standard intermediates produced during the oxidation of organic compounds. Ozone transformed into hydroxyl free radicals by combination with UV radiation of 254-nm wavelength was the course favored by Francis.

The oxidative aggressivity of these reactive entities is depended upon to destroy TOC. The combination of ozone and UV offers another advantage in addition to the conversion of ozone into a more aggressive oxidizer. The solubility of ozone in water is relatively low (about 13 times higher than oxygen, depending upon temperature and concentration of ozone in the gas phase applied), and its transference from the gas phase into the water phase reflects, at any partial pressure, its concentration gradient between gas and water. The ozone-decomposing action of the UV light serves to enhance the gas-to-liquid mass transfer of the ozone by converting it to hydroxyl free radicals in the water.

Water was circulated through an ozone/UV reactor at a flowrate of 240 L/h. A steady-state TOC level of 100 μg/L was reduced to under 20 μg/L. Series or parallel arrangements of such reactors could be used to achieve lower TOC levels at fixed flowrates, or to obtain such TOC values at higher flowrates. This technique lends itself to the recovery of rinsewater, its customary application in the semiconductor industry, but also to the primary preparation of low TOC water. In either case, reliance usually is placed upon DI resins for the removal of the carboxylic acids that are generated oxidatively. The introduction of ozone or hydroxyl radicals into DI beds can result in the degradation of the resins with concomitant generation of new TOC.

An interesting application of the synergistic oxidative effects of a combination of ozone and UV was made by Governal and Shadman (1992) for the removal of particles of humic acids and lipopolysaccharides as measured by particle counting. Monitoring was made of particles in the size range 0.05 to 0.2 μm. The TOC, resistivity, temperature, flowrate, and pressure were also monitored. The effects of 30 ppb of ozone alone, of 185 nm of UV alone, and of the combinations of both over time periods up to 30 minutes were measured against humic acid concentrations of 4 ppb and of 40 ppb, as well as against 20 ppb and 4 ppb of polysaccharides. The results indicated a disappearance of the TOC-particles as occasioned especially by the simultaneous application of the ultraviolet light and the ozone. It is hypothesized that the TOC particle removals resulted from an oxidative fragmentation of the larger particles, resulting in a shift of the particle-size distribution, accompanied by a simultaneous solubilization of the smaller particles.

It will be recalled that for the ozone to function effectively as a sterilant, a residual concentration must remain in the water system until its removal becomes mandated. Francis (1987) achieved this objective by the use of multiple ozone injection points. This ensured a maximum hydroxyl free-radical concentration.

On the other hand, Glaze et al. (1987) quantified the quenching effect of alkalinity (concentration of bicarbonate/carbonate ions) on hydroxyl free-radical oxidations. The higher the alkalinity, the less efficient is the radical oxidative mechanistic route, because of the destruction of the free radicals by the alkalinity-causing ions.

Safety Issues with Respect to Ozone

Because ozone is one of the most powerful oxidizing agents known to mankind (see Table 3-1), it should be considered to be a hazardous material, one that should be handled carefully and with understanding. In practice, well-designed ozonation systems incorporate subsystems for the destruction of excess ozone that may be present after the ozone contact chamber. Such subsystems insure that no ozone will leak into the ambient atmosphere during normal operations.

Hazardous though ozone is, it has been handled successfully and routinely in water plants for 80 years, and has been used for some 4 decades by segments of the U.S. chemical industry. There are, however, those to whom ozone usage is novel; some are hesitant regarding its use, equating their own unfamiliarity with actual risk. Avallone (1987) references one pharmaceutical installation at which "because of potential problems with employee safety ozone was removed from the water prior to placing it in their recirculating system." Unanswered are the questions as to whether the concerns were not exaggerated and whether they could not have been satisfactorily addressed. Perhaps a more realistic assessment of the hazards involving ozone usage derives from its long-term routine use.

If leaks develop in the ozonation system, the smell of ozone will become apparent. Most people can detect about 0.01 ppm in the air. This is well within the general comfort level. Symptoms experienced with concentrations of 0.1 to 1 ppm are headaches, irritation and burning of the eyes, and dryness of the throat. The action level of 0.1 ppm of the ozone monitored in the ambient air is the level that the Occupational Safety and Health Administration (OSHA) has adopted as its Maximum Exposure level, for exposure of workers to ozone, on a time-weighted average over an 8-hour working day, 5 days per week.

To provide for accidental discharges of ozone, however, it is customary to install an ambient air ozone monitor at an appropriate point or points in the equipment room(s). These monitors usually are set to signal, as a minimum, an alarm at an ozone level of 0.1 ppm. Additionally, such monitors can be connected to exhaust fans, as well as to break the flow of electrical energy to the ozone generator itself. Once electricity ceases to be provided to the ozone generator, the generation of ozone ceases immediately. Exhaust fans rapidly remove any leaked ozone from the room, preventing large quantities of ozone from accumulating.

As is the case with the commercial use of many hazardous materials, understanding the properties and potential hazards associated with ozone and with UV radiation is fundamental to the design and operation of the appropriate equipment.

Summary of Ozone Application

Rice (1987) summarizes the application areas for ozone in water treatments as consisting of the oxidation of iron, manganese and arsenic; the oxidative destruction of TOC in waters to prevent the fouling of ion-exchange, reverse osmosis, and activated carbon units; and the maintenance of organism-free waters. These different functions, depending upon the water volumes handled in the installation, can be optimized by the use of multistage ozonation arrangements. Thus, a groundwater containing TOC will be filtered after ozonation, and the treated water will be stored. A single ozone system can be used; the first stage will be employed for the TOC oxidation, the second to supply a residual ozone content to the storage tank. Interestingly, it is reported that the substitution of ozone for heat in a water-storage application showed no indications of rouging even after one year of service.

Rice (1987) described an "oxidation-reduction potential" meter for monitoring the potential of water, to be used to determine the amount of ozone necessary to maintain the water organism-free in the storage tank. Such meters can be set to call for ozone when the potential of free water drops below 700 mV, and to cease its being supplied when the potential level reaches 840 mV. Such voltage levels, at least in the case of waters treated with chlorine, were quoted by Rice (Carlson et al., 1968) as having a kill capability for *E. coli* equivalent to 0.2 mg/L (or higher) of free chlorine. Such control devices would be most useful in the multistage ozone operations based on a single ozone-generating system.

Analysis for Ozone

Oxidation of iodide ion by ozone releases elemental iodine, that, in turn, in the presence of starch produces a deep blue color that is titratable by standardized sodium thiosulfate solution (iodimetric method). This is a very convenient method for measuring dissolved ozone concentrations. This method is not specific for ozone alone, however. Other materials capable of oxidizing iodide ion to iodine may interfere (e.g., organic peroxides, hypochlorite ion, chlorine dioxide, hydrogen peroxide). Actually, the iodide ion method measures the total oxidant level in solution. It has been widely employed for several decades for ozone analysis, however, for its convenience. Nevertheless, its use no longer is recommended (Gordon and Pacey, 1986).

Ultraviolet absorption is selective for ozone at 253.7 nm, in the liquid or gaseous phases. Single- or double-beam spectrophotometers may be used; the more expensive double-beam instrument more conveniently compares the water to be treated with that containing ozone. Otherwise, blank determinations must be made to correct for background effects.

The primary limitation of UV absorption spectroscopy is the current lack of agreement as to the value of the molar extinction coefficient to be employed. Thus, the accuracy of this method can vary by about 30% in either direction, depending upon which value of the molar extinction coefficient is taken (Gordon and Pacey, 1986).

An amperometric method based on the electrochemical conversion of ozone to oxygen also is in use in many ozonation facilities to measure levels of dissolved ozone. The electrical current required to effect the conversion is measured, and is proportional to the dissolved ozone concentration. The sensitivity of this method is good. Its chief limitations are the potential fouling of the electrodes by organic contaminants, scale-forming entities, or sulfides present in the waters; and the fact that calibrations are based on the iodimetric method.

A newer method involves the use of a membrane in conjunction with the amperometric electrode methodology. Dissolved ozone diffuses through a membrane to the electrode, where decomposition to oxygen occurs. Electrode fouling is minimized by the membrane. Interference from other oxidizing agents is minimal (Rice et al., 1986). Decolorization of indigo disulfonate solutions by ozone is the basis for the determination of ozone. This method is subject to fewer interferences than any of the earlier procedures.

Ozone rapidly and stoichiometrically decolorizes indigo trisulfonate in an acidic solution. The decrease in absorbance at 600 nm is linear with ozone residual. This test was reported to be accurate levels as low as 10 ppb (Bader and Hoigné, 1982), and is the basis of the most accepted wet-chemistry analysis for ozone. It involves a change in the absorbance of 600-nm light. Basically, a colored solution adsorbs light in linear relationship to its concentration. It becomes decolorized by the action of ozone, and the change in light absorption reflects the ozone concentration. Further discussion of all analytical methods for determining ozone in gaseous or water phases can be found in work by Rice et al. (1986).

Summary of Ozone Applicational Considerations

The oxidative aggressivity merits it to the dependable killing in low concentrations of microbial life, and to the destruction of TOC at room temperatures. Ozone kills bacteria about 1,000 times faster than chlorine, and is lethal as well to viruses and cysts. It has the advantages of being low in applicational and maintenance costs.

However, its chemical aggressivity neccessitates its use with inert and expensive materials of construction, such as PTFE, PVDF, and stainless steels. Its use requires careful management in that it poses risks to safety. These can, however, be accomodated.

The use of ozone can prevent biofilm formation. It can also remove old biofilm glycocalyx over time. It can readily and reliably be removed from water systems by the irradiative action of 254 nm ultraviolet light.■

CHAPTER 4

ULTRAVIOLET RADIATION AND ITS APPLICATION

It has been known (Schenk, 1981) for a century that the ultraviolet wavelengths present in sunlight have germicidal effects. The practical utility of UV radiation for the control of organisms followed the devising of the mercury vapor lamp. This form of radiant energy induces photochemical reactions involving biomolecules in microorganisms. The resulting molecular alterations inhibit the growth of the microorganisms, and in higher doses will kill them.

The UV light spectrum is broad enough to include wavelengths of unequal effects upon organisms. Even for efficacious wavelengths, the influence of the UV radiation may differ. Also, the devices designed to discharge UV light are not all alike in the radiant energy they generate. Moreover, the UV emanations are susceptible to absorption by the molecules of the organism-suspending medium, and their germicidal influence may become attenuated by the time they reach the microbe. That UV radiation is of practical utility in controlling most organisms is beyond challenge. The devising of effective UV systems requires careful engineering, however; more than a UV radiation source is needed. Finally, removal of the UV-killed microbes may be required (as by filtration) whenever the presence of particles is undesired, or when their catabolic products may manifest total organic carbon levels or pyrogenic lipopolysaccharides. In addition to its biocidal properties, ultraviolet lights may catalyze the destruction of TOC, and the decomposition of ozone.

Generation of Ultraviolet Radiation

The subject of UV generation is complex. Those interested in its extensive details are directed to Meyer and Seitz (1949).

The most common method of generating UV radiation is by discharge lamps. Typically, a glass or quartz tube contains an inert gas plus a metal, usually mercury. Electrodes, located at each end of the tube, may be cold or preheated. In either case, an ignition voltage is required to begin the discharge. The minimum value of the voltage is dependent upon the length of the tubes (i.e., the distance between the electrodes), and upon the contents and internal pressure of the tube; and may range from 20 to several thousand volts. Preheated electrodes, which are promotive of ions, electrons, and electron carriers, require lower ignition voltages. If the lamp-burning voltage is less than half that of the line voltage, then the lamp can be started easily by means of ballast and starter. Otherwise a stray-field transformer is needed.

Lamps based on mercury/argon mixtures exhibit the highest efficiencies (Meltzer and Rice, 1987); are the easiest to handle; and are the best performing (Dobiasch, 1986). Mercury lamps generally used are designated as high or low pressure. The partial pressure within the discharge tube will depend upon the lowest temperature along the tube, a cool spot. Typically, the pressure may range from 0.025 pascals (Pa) at 0 °C, to 0.8 Pa at 40 °C, 10^5 Pa (atmospheric pressure) at 360 °C, and to Pa values above 10^7 at temperatures above 800 °C. The mercury vapor pressure will be from 0.001 to 0.1 (atm Hg) in the low temperature regions, and from 0.1 to 10 atm Hg in the high regions.

Ultraviolet Wavelengths

During discharge, particularly at low pressures, mercury atoms in their excited states radiate mainly at wavelengths of 184.9 nm, the resonance line; and 253.7 nm, the intercombination line. This results in a large generation of the short UV lines (Dobiasch, 1986). The efficiency of this type of generation may be above 60%, depending largely upon the current density and the tube cross section. Whether the 185-nm line can penetrate the bulb depends upon its material of construction. Quartz permits the passage of lower wavelengths.

Increasing the pressure within the tube (i.e., the density) promotes collisions of mercury molecules. These tend to decrease the incidence of excited states, with concomitant increase in energetically lower-lying states (i.e., the longer wavelengths become stronger). At typical medium pressures of 10^5 Pa, about 2% of the input power is radiated at 254 nm, and about 10% at wavelengths below 300 nm. At higher pressures, the radiations below 260 nm become absorbed, and the longer wavelengths broaden into a continuum.

Special lamp constructions, not yet used in organism control applications, can amplify given wavelengths: Cadmium enhances emanations of below 270 nm; while adding iron, nickel, or cobalt increases those between 280 and 450 nm.

Visible light is at wave lengths above 400. Ultraviolet radiation can, for practical reasons, be divided into four sections: UV-A between 400 and 315 nm, UV-B between 315 and 280 nm, UV-C covering from about 280 to 200 nm, and vacuum-UV, below 200 nm. The last is strongly absorbed by air. The UV-C is used primarily to destroy organisms. The 253.7-nm line emitted by low-pressure mercury discharge lamps can inactivate microorganisms such as protozoa, bacteria, molds, yeasts, viruses, fungi, and algae. It is not so effective against cysts such as are assumed by most forms of *Giardia*. It is this type of lamp that is used primarily in the UV disinfection of water. The broadband emanations of medium-pressured mercury lamps are also suitable for UV germicidal applications. DNA strongly absorbs 254 nm UV light.

Germicidal Ultraviolet Spectra

The germicidal effectiveness of UV radiation is dependent upon its wavelength. Different organisms show slightly different sensitivities to various parts of the UV spectrum. However, an average sensitivity can be characterized. Figure 4-1 presents the germicidal action curve, roughly Gaussian, wherein relative germicidal effectiveness is plotted against wavelength. The action maximum is at about 265 nm. The 253.7-nm line, about 0.85 times as effective, corresponds to a conversion of 35% of the input power. Table 4-1 illustrates the relative germicidal effectiveness of various UV wavelengths (Meulemans, 1986).

Disinfection action is dependent not only upon the UV emission spectrum, but also upon the radiation intensity, the duration of the organism exposure, the sensitivity of the organism involved, and the UV transmission of the medium that suspends the organisms. Clear air offers little impediment to transmission. However, water, even if it appears clear, may contain certain dissolved molecular species or suspended particles that would absorb the radiation and attenuate its germicidal effects. Optically clear solutions of humic acids; of certain hydrocarbons, sugars, and colored materials in solution; and of iron and/or manganese salts have such adsorptive effects (Gelzhäuser, 1986). Therefore, prior to UV disinfection, suspended particulate matter should be removed, and the iron and manganese concentrations should be reduced to below 1 and 2 mg/L, respec-

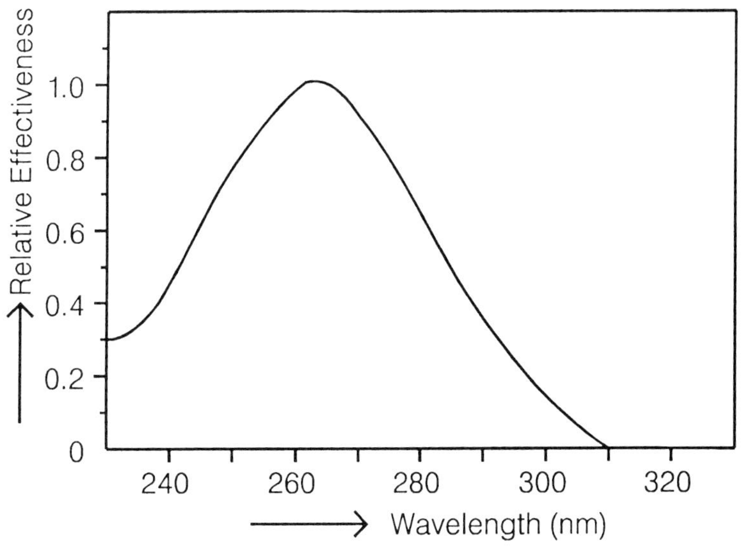

Figure 4-1. Germicidal action curve in the UV region of the energy spectrum.
Meulemans, (1986); Courtesy, International Ozone Association

tively.

Fouling of the UV tube also causes interference. Thus, the quartz tube that protects the UV lamp should be cleaned at least each time the UV bulb is replaced. In applications in which slimes are built up, such as in fish hatchery waters, the tubes are fitted with automatic wipers, which help to maintain the constancy of UV transmission.

Ultraviolet Dosage

Ultraviolet devices are rated by their capacities to treat water at specific flowrates. Actually, the UV dosage is the real consideration. It is the product of radiation intensity and the exposure time, and is expressed as microwatts-seconds per square centimeter (μWs/cm^2). Restated, it is a quantity of energy (the irradiance in the case of UV radiation) in watts/m^2 multiplied by time in seconds, and symbolized as joules per square meter (J/m$^{2)}$. It is dosage that defines the effectiveness of the UV radiation, not the watt input or radiated output of the UV lamps.

The area figure derives from the surface of the lamp wherein the UV is being generated. The time/dose dependency is usually based upon a 10-second dosage. The dwell time in the reactor is specified by the UV lamp manufacturer. As stated, organism elimination by UV radiation is a matter of log reductions; it is not a matter of absolute organism kills. Most reactors are designed for 6-log reductions of organisms. The effective UV dose is tied to the percentage of the energy transmitted by the lamp. At 16,000 μm/mW^2 it is 99%; at 63,000 m/cm^2 it is 77%. Ultraviolet lamp life is normally from 500 to 8,000 hours. Lamps deteriorate as a result of solarization (crystallization), or from becoming fouled.

Ellner and Ellner (1986) devised a biological method for measuring the actual dosages delivered by UV devices. A standard curve is constructed by plotting test bacterium survivors against graded UV radiation doses. Water seeded with the test organism is treated in the device. By reference to the standard curve, the effluent cultured for survivors reveals the actual delivered dose.

There is no possibility of overdosage in terms of negative effects, except in relation to economic considerations of overdesign. No minimum UV dosage standard has been established by the beverage industry. Some use 50 mJ/cm^2. Most firms specify a dosage level of 30,000 mW/cm^2 EOL (end of lamp life), which is equivalent to 50,000 to 60,000 mW/cm^2 new life dosage. In high-purity water treatment, 100 mJ/cm^2 is used (but not universally) as a minimum dosage standard. In the treatment of potable waters, a minimum of 25 microjoules per square meter (mJ/cm$^{2)}$ had long been held to be both effective and economical. However, the National Sanitation Foundation (NSF, 1989) has recently published a new standard (Number 55). A virus reduction of 3 to 4 log against a poliovirus and rotavirus challenge and a bacteriological reduction of greater than 6 log against a challenge of a coliform, *E. coli,* may be accomplished by a UV dosage of 30,000 mW/cm^2. A 5-log reduction of poliovirus takes place at 40,000 mW/cm^2. Therefore, a minimum dosage of 38,000 mW/cm^2 is set as a fail-safe end point to achieve a 4-log virus reduction. It should be remembered, however, that the "set point" level is 40% to 50% of the new life or day-one dosage level.

The radiation output of a UV lamp depends upon the life span of the device. This is not constant, and may also vary from lamp to lamp. Guarantees of stipulated service levels differ from 500 to 8,000 hours. Beyond this duration, the performance of the lamp is undependable, and the lamp should be replaced. Some UV units are equipped with light-emitting diodes (LED) that indicate when the UV lamp has burned out.

At the end of lamp life, the dosage level is typically 30,000 μW/sec/cm^2 (Veloz, 1991). Most waterborne organisms are destroyed by dosages below 15,000 μW/sec/cm^2.

The radiation exposure time is a function of the water flow velocity and the geometry of the radiation chamber. The organisms suspended in the conveying fluid must reside in the radiation zone long enough to absorb a minimum lethal dose. If the suspending medium has too rapid a velocity though the chamber, the minimum dosage may not be achieved. The flow pattern is of importance as well. Film reactors are available to minimize the thickness of the flow channel.

The basic design of a UV unit involves a treatment chamber within which are the UV lamps housed within quartz sleeves or jackets. The sleeves are transparent to UV radiation and act as temperature buffers to optimize the temperature effect by insulating the UV lamp against water temperature. Ultraviolet absorption by water varies with temperature (Figure 4-2). The purity of the water is a factor also. The UV absorption effect by water is affected by whatever molecules are in solution, and by the water molecules themselves.

Random flow is promoted

Table 4-1
S(l) as a Function of the Wavelength

Wavelength *n m*	*Relative Germicidal Effectiveness*
210	0.02
215	0.06
220	0.12
225	0.18
230	0.26
235	0.36
240	0.47
245	0.61
250	0.75
255	0.88
260	0.97
265	1.00
270	0.93
275	0.83
280	0.72
285	0.58
290	0.45
295	0.31
300	0.18
305	0.10
310	0.05
315	0

Meulemans (1986); Courtesy, International Ozone Assoc.

by the turbulence created by baffles. This minimizes the distance from the UV source that an organism could maintain in a radiation chamber, were it to be suspended in a laminar flow layer farthest from the UV tube.

Useful observations regarding the design and performance of single-lamp low-pressure mercury arc UV devices were offered by Powitz and Hunter (1985). It is such lamps that are traditionally used in water disinfection treatments. For water disinfection, such units are suitable for treating flowrates of 10 gpm (0.038 m^3/m) or less. Greater flows necessitate the use of additional lamps. Flows exceeding 100 gpm (0.38m^3/m) generally utilize an array of several multilamp reactors in parallel. Inherent design limitations cause UV lamp manufacturers to overcompensate by using extra lamps in multilamp arrangements.

The operating characteristics of low-pressure mercury arc lamps result in the use of either of two lamp designs, the offset or the annular types. The offset designs utilize a central water-carrying tube surrounded by the UV lamps. The central tube may be constructed of quartz, glass, or PTFE polymer (DuPont's trademark for which is Teflon). Quartz is very completely penetrable by UV; the Teflon only to a 40% extent. A virtue of the offset design is the ease of lamp replacement, and the better control of lamp temperature. It relies upon reflectors to capture and redirect much of the UV light output. Polished aluminum reflectors serve very well. However, they oxidize under UV light. Meyers (1987) reports that aluminum coated with magnesium fluoride will reflect 80% of the UV light. It is cheaper to use stainless steel reflectors. One listing states them to be only 3% reflective of UV light; however, Veloz (1991) holds that value to be low. Westinghouse lists polished nickel as reflecting 60% to 65%. Stainless steel should have similar reflective values. Electropolished stainless steel reflects 75% of UV light. To compensate for the lost light, additional lamps, space for these lamps, and the electrical costs for their operation become involved.

The disadvantages of lost light are absent from the annular UV lamp design. In this configuration, the UV lamps are shielded in a quartz sleeve within the reaction vessel. This arrangement has the advantage of being more space and energy-efficient. Powitz and Hunter (1985) referenced several investigators as demonstrating that most such commercially available reactors are not of an optimally efficient design. Largely, they suffer from inefficient flow patterns that, coupled with uneven UV radiation levels, may permit organisms to escape receiving lethal UV doses.

Powitz and Hunter (1985) described the design of a superior type of UV lamp that had been evaluated by several investigators, and was reported on favorably. This design involved reconfigured electrodes. The lamp can be inserted in the water main perpendicular to the path of the water flow, thereby making possible optimal or plug flows through the reactor. The design features lower vapor pressure and increased current density. As a result, UV light is emitted by the entire cross section of the lamp. In one comparison it was found to consume 25 times the electrical energy, but generated over 200 times the germicidal light. Field tests of this type UV lamp revealed 2-log organism reductions at flowrates of 880 gpm (3.3 m^3/m) using waters having absorption coefficients of about 0.07/cm. Serially disposed multiple units would yield higher disinfection levels, or allow more elevated flowrates.

With one exception, all U.S. UV equipment manufacturers use low-pressure UV lamps in various multilamp configurations. A typical low-pressure UV lamp is 36 inches long, produces an intensity of 120 $\mu w/cm^2$ per second at 254 nm, at a distance of 1 meter. The lamp is rated at 39 watts of power consumption; combined with power supply, its consumption is increased to about 65 watts. All of the emissions vary between 220 nm and 290 nm, with 90% of them at 254 nm.

To reduce TOC, the 185-nm UV lamps are used to induce the production of hydroxyl free radicals. The 185-nm UV lamps are manufactured with a special quartz envelope that allows 5% of the total emissions to be at 185 nm, with the balance up in the 220-nm to 290-nm range (Veloz, 1988). The 185-nm lamps give about as much 254-nm radiation as the 254-nm lamps.

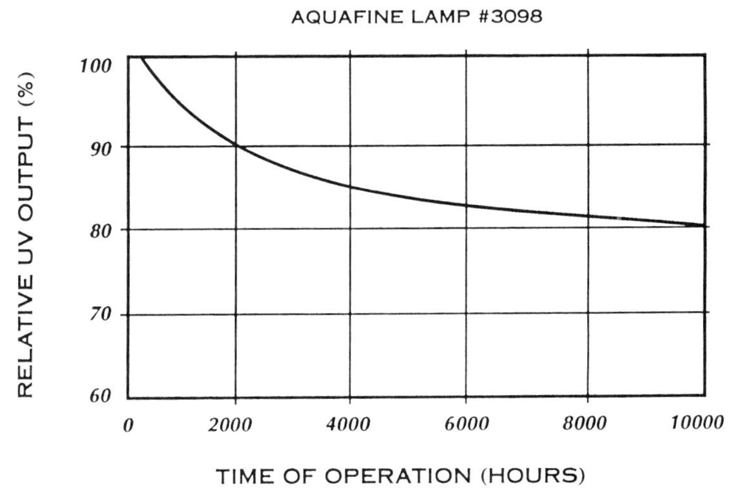

- Relative UV lamp intensity: 253.7 nm
- UV lamp after 100 hours burn-in
- Standard UV equipment

Figure 4-2. Relative UV intensity vs. water temperature.
Courtesy, Aquafine Corp.

Monitoring of Ultraviolet Devices

The automation of a UV system so that it operates efficiently and effectively without supervision was detailed by Zinnbauer (1985). He dealt also with the installation of wall-mounted UV sensors and intensity monitors; and he cautioned that the UV absorbency of the water being treated must be measured, since suspensions and particular components may diminish the radiated energy available for germicidal purposes.

In a treatment of ultraviolet lamp design, Powitz and Hunter (1985) referenced work by Tobin et al. (1983), who reported that not all UV light monitors accurately measure UV light intensities. Powitz and Hunter (1985) discussed the shortcomings of various UV light arrangements, and offered an improved version.

In order to be effective in its degradative actions, whether bactericidal or other, the destructive energy of electromagnetic emanations must be adsorbed by the molecules of the host substance. The UV adsorption ability of a material is described by its adsorption coefficient. This value is characteristic for different materials. Within the host molecule or organism, the optical energy is transformed into disruptive heat.

In accordance with the Bouger-Lambert-Beer law, when a parallel beam of such electromagnetic radiation passes through successive layers of a nondiffusing adsorbing medium, the degree of penetration falls off exponentially with thickness. If, therefore, one wishes to irradiate a volume of water by means of such a UV lamp in order to effect sterilization, the water layer about the lamp will require as thin a dimension as possible. The water should be as free of extraneous UV light-adsorbing molecular species as possible, and it must flow sufficiently slowly to assure adequate residence time of the organism in the radiation zone, so that sufficient photons of the effective wavelength may be adsorbed. The effective depths of penetration are not very large, and are particularly apt to be rendered even smaller in waters that are turbid, or even in clear waters that contain UV-absorbing molecules such as sugars. The effective dosage is a function of time and intensity. There is a trade-off between ray intensity and exposure time.

In all of this, the intensity of the UV light issuing from the lamp is of interest. Indeed, the lamp must be made of quartz or Vicar, adsorptive to the necessary wavelength of energy. In actual usage, the light intensity generated by the lamp is found to deteriorate with time. There is also variability among lamps. It would seem necessary, therefore, for UV lamps to be characterized by minimum threshold emission values, and for some history to be available regarding the likelihood of their required replacement (e.g., their maximum number of operating hours or life expectancy). Figure 4-3 shows how the relative UV output varies with the UV lamp life.

In defining the extent of transmission by a given solution, the measurement is made at 254-nm wavelength; and the depth of water, whether 10 or 100 nm, is stipulated.

Mode of Action of Ultraviolet Radiation

Chemical disinfectants initially attack the outside surfaces of organisms. Hence, considerable contact time may be required. However, UV radiation penetrates the organism carapace, being absorbed by DNA, RNA (ribonucleic acid), and enzyme molecules. Achieving the required dose within an organism depends upon the morphology of the organism. Gram-positive bacteria, having thicker outer membranes, are more difficult to destroy than the Gram-negatives. Spores with their thicker capsules are more resistant than are vegetative cells. Organism types differ in their resistance to UV radiation. Environment and the states of growth and nutrition may contribute. Thus, in water, about 30 J/m^2 of UV radiation is required to kill *E. coli* bacteria to an extent of about 90%. Lower doses are needed to kill organisms in air (Gelzhäuser, 1986).

Microbes exposed to UV radiation are not all killed or inactivated at once; a constant fraction of the living number dies in each increment of time (Harm, 1980). The survival ratio, that fraction of the initial number surviving at any given time, can be approximated by an exponential function of the product of the radiation intensity and the exposure time. Plots of this ratio are straight lines on

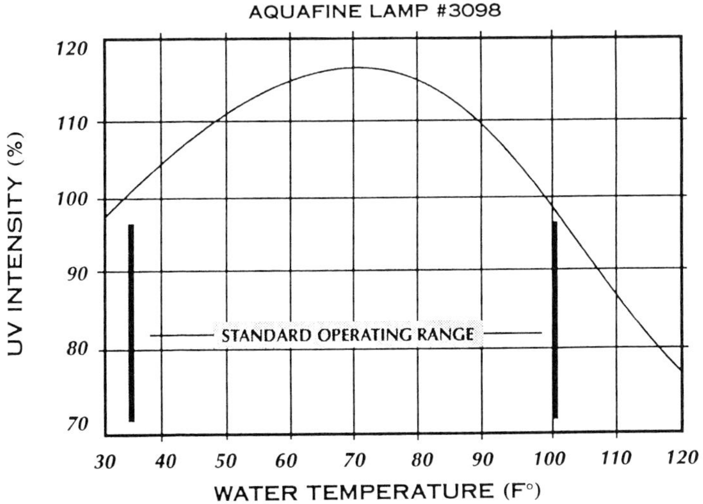

- Relative UV lamp intensity: 253.7 nm
- UV lamp after 100 hours burn-in
- Standard UV equipment

Figure 4-3. Relative UV output vs. lamp life.
Courtesy, Aquafine Corp.

semilog paper. This means that to decrease the survival ratio from 0.1 to 0.01 (i.e., one order of magnitude), double the dose of UV radiation is required. If a survival ratio of 0.00001 is needed, the dose corresponding to the survival ratio of 0.1 must be increased fivefold. Table 4-2 lists the 0.1 survival dosages for a number of organisms.

Ultrasonic effects promote a more efficient UV germicidal action, possibly by promoting the separation of individual organisms from one another and/or from sheltering particulate matter, thus exposing them more fully. A Westinghouse Electric report, Table 4-3, lists a number of organisms and the UV energy levels required to destroy them.

Influencing Factors

Certain commercial designations need to be set clear. Ultraviolet lamps with double intensities do not necessarily mean double dosages, unless the flow capacity is identical. One UV generator designed for treating 100-gpm volumes and having twice the intensity of a unit intended for 50 gpm of water flow does not yield double the dosage of that smaller generator. All else being equal, the dosages could be the same.

The UV unit should be sized for the proper flowrate. Often customers buy UV units 3 and 4 times the size needed, seeking performance insurance in a massive UV dose. However, if a flowrate of 30 gpm is to be used in a device normally intended for a 100-gpm flow, the internal baffling of the unit must be altered to provide the requisite turbulent, swirling flows. Otherwise, quantities of water may flow through the unit at a distance of 1 to 2 inches from the lamps. This is too distant to receive the desired time/intensity dosage of UV that was intended, as UV radiation undergoes rapid attenuation with distance. It may well be that anecdotal accounts of UV unreliability stem from considerations of this sort. Even water temperature seems to influence the relative UV intensity. (See Figure 4-2.) However, the data may reflect the water purity.

Meyers (1987) reports an instance in which a UV lamp rated at a flowrate of 20 gpm effected a maximum TOC reduction at 0.2 to 0.4 gpm from 300 ppb to less than 5 ppb at a single pass through the light. At lower or higher rates of flow the results were not so good. Lower rates may have entailed laminar flows that placed some TOC molecules too far from the lamps. Higher flowrates, while supplying the turbulence required for adequate proximity to the UV lights, might not have permitted a residence time sufficient for proper UV dosages. Since not all TOC molecules exhibit the same susceptibility to UV light, different waters may well exhibit different flowrate requirements when TOC destruction is the goal. The easier susceptibility of microorganisms to UV irradiation may mask individual differences regarding flow-pattern needs. Flowrates for UV installations are rated for sterilization effects, not for TOC removal.

Ultraviolet Intensity Meters

It is very possible for the UV sterilizer to lose intensity through a clouding of the quartz sleeves, as by silt or by particulate matter from the incoming water. Also, the UV lamps may fail, as from bad ballast resistors, yielding low voltages and thus low intensities. The glass envelope may itself undergo structural changes, called *solarization*, that may cause wavelength changes. Therefore, all UV devices should be equipped with intensity monitors, but most are not. At least some FDA inspectors are insisting upon in-line UV intensity meters.

Ultraviolet bulbs require an annual changeout. There are 8,760 hours per year, except in leap years. The lamps are usually rated for about 8,000 hours of operation. They lose intensity continuously, however, and after 8,000 hours have lost about 30%. To provide a safety margin, they normally are rated by most of the UV manufacturers at a few hundred percent of what is required for the effective kill of the most common microorganisms.

The calibration of UV intensity does have some uncertainties. It is presently done largely by relative comparisons. Initially, the UV lamps have a very high intensity. After 1 or 2 days of operation, the intensity decreases to a level from which it continues to decay at a more constant, gradual rate. In accordance with

Table 4-2
Approximate Dose Values for 1 Survival Ratio of 0.1 DE Various Microorganisms at 253.7 nm

Bacteria	*Dose*	*Bacteria*	*Dose*
Bacillus anthracis	45	*Pseudomonas aeruginosa*	55
B. megatherium (veg)	11	*P. fluorescens*	35
B. megatherium (spores)	27	*Salmonella enteritidis*	40
B. parathyphosus	32	*S.typhosa*-Typhoid fever	22
B. subtilus	70	*S. paratyphi*-Enteric fever	32
(spores)	120	*S.typhimurium*	80
Micrococcus luteus	197	*Sarcina lutea*	197
Serratia marcescens	24	*Serratia marcescens*	24
Clostridium tetani	130	*Shigela dysenteriae*	
Corynebact. diphtheriae	34	dysentry form	22
Eberthela typhosa	21	*Shigela flexneri*	
Escherichia coli	30	dysentery form	17
Leptospira Sp-		*Shigela paradysenteriae*	17
infectious jaundice	32	*Spirillum rubrum*	44
Micrococcus candidus	61	*Staphylococcus albus*	18
Micrococcus piltonencis	81	*Staphylococcus aureus*	26
Micrococcus sphaeroides	100	*Streptococcus hemolyticus*	22
Mycobacterium tuberculosis	62	*Streptococcus lactis*	62
Neisseria catarrhalis	44	*Streptococcus viridans*	20
Phytomonas tumefaciens	44	*Mycobacterium tuberculi*	100
Proteus vulgaris	26	*Virbio comma* cholera	34

Meulemans (1986); Courtesy, International Ozone Association

the UV manufacturer's manuals, the intensity level after the 1- or 2-day period of time is set as being 100%; the initial very high intensity is ignored. Further UV lamp deteriorations are compared to the 100% level.

Instruments are being developed that will read UV intensity directly in lumens. Their costs may be some 4 times that of the present intensity meters (which run about $800) that register in relative intensity readings. Direct-light intensity meters will be useful to calibrate the relative-reading meters.

Effect on organisms. It is not enough to speak of percentage reductions in colony-forming organism concentrations. If the raw water contained 10^6 cfu in a specific volume, then a 99.99% reduction would mean that 10^2 cfu still are present in the water volume, a very high number. In designing a UV treatment unit, the number of permissible surviving organisms should be stipulated as well. The treatment system then can be designed not to yield populations in excess of this number.

Table 4-3
Ultraviolet Energy Required for Destruction of Various Organisms

Bacteria	*μW-s/cm²*
Bacillus anthracis	8,700
Clostridium tetani	22,000
Corynebacterium diphtheria	6,500
Eberthella typhosa	4,100
Escherichia coli	6,600
Leptospira	6,000
Micrococcus sphaeroides	15,400
Mycobacterium tuberculosis	10,000
Neisseria catarrhalis	8,500
Phytomonas tumefaciens	8,500
Proteus vulgaris	6,600
Pseudomonas aeruginosa	10,500
Salmonella typhosa	4,100
Sarcina lutea	26,400
Serratia marcescens	6,160
Shigella dysenteriae	4,200
Spirillum rubrum	6,160
Staphylococcus albus	5,720
Streptococcus hemolyticus	5,500
Streptococcus lactis	8,800
Vibrio cholerae	6,500

Mold Spores	*μW-s/cm²*
Aspergillus flavus	99,000
Mucor racemosus	35,200
Oospora lactis	11,000
Penicillium expensum	22,000
Penicillium roqueforti	26,400
Protozoa	
Chlorella vulgaris (algae)	22,000
Nematode eggs	92,000
Paramecium	200,000
Virus	
Bacteriophage (*E. coli*)	6,600
Influenza	6,600
Poliovirus	6,000
Virus of infectious hepatitis	8,000
Yeast	
Baker's yeast	8,800
Brewer's yeast	6,600
Common yeast cake	13,200

Abshire et al., (1983); Courtesy, *J. Parenteral Science and Technology*

Antopol and Ellner (1979) reported that *Legionella pneumophila,* the causative agent of Legionnaires' disease that has been found in cooling towers of air conditioners, is inactivated by UV light. Approximately 380 $\mu W/cm^2$ killed 50%; 920 $\mu W/cm^2$, 90%; 1,840 $\mu W/cm^2$, 99%; and 2,760 $\mu W/cm^2$ killed 99.9% of the test population of microorganisms. The UV dosages required to produce 90% inhibition of *E. coli, Salmonella typhi, Serratia marcescens,* and *Pseudomonas aeruginosa* are 2,110, 2,140, 2,200, and 5,500 $\mu W/cm^2$, respectively (Rice et al., 1986).

Muraca et al. (1990) made a study of the eradication of *Legionella pneumophila* from hospital water systems, comparing the use of UV radiation with other

Table 4-4
UV Resistance Data— Alcon's Dose Results Compared to Literature References

	UV Doses (ergs/mm²)		
Organism[a]	*Alcon*	*Literature*	*Author(s)*
Micrococcus radiodurans ATCC 13939	14,400-57,600[b]	16,000 (99.999%)[Fc]	Bowling, Setlow
Micrococcus luteus ATCC 9341	2,400-3,600	3,000 (99.0%)	Rubbo, Gardner
Escherichia coli ATCC 23224	120-80	462 (99.999%)	Greenberg, Karrer
Bacillus cereus ATCC 11778	1,200-1,800	No reference found	
Bacillus subtilis NCTC 2479	Not tested	40,000 (99.99%)	Rubbo, Gardner
Bacillus subtilis (niger)ATCC 9372	57,600-72,000	No reference found	
Bacillus pumilus[d] BMT-18	36,000-72,000	No reference found	
Bacillus stearothermo philus ATCC 7950	14,400-28,000	No reference found	
Saccharomyces cerevisieae DJ-52875	2,000-3,600	68,000 (99.99%)	Rubbo, Gardner

[a] Particular strains listed are those studied at Alcon. All *Bacillus* strainse were spores. Strains not listed by authors in the literature.
[b] 10^6 Organisms — dose range or "survival-kill window" (i.e., some kill vs. all kill) exposed to a UV intensity of 400 $\mu W/cm^2$ for various periods of time.
[c] Represents % kill of 10^7 organisms per mL in water.
[d] Isolated from Alcon Manufacturing area.

Abshire et al., (1983); Courtesy, *J. Parenteral Science and Technology* modalities such as chlorine, ozone, instantaneous steam-heating, hot-water heat and flush, and metal ionization. The various methods were discussed for their advantages, disadvantages, and costs.

Ultraviolet Sterilization in the Pharmaceutical Industry

Abshire (1986) investigated three different types of UV lamps in a study aimed at evaluating UV radiation as a sterilant for the pharmaceuticals industry. He found the method applicable. *Bacillus pumilus* in its spore form, being relatively resistant, served as a microbiological indicator for the validation of the UV irradiative process.

Abshire et al. (1983) also utilized spores of *Bacillus pumilus* as a biological indicator in the UV sterilization of translucent polyethylene bottles. At a population level of 10^6, 90% of the spores were consistently destroyed in 2 minutes (i.e., D value) using minimal doses of 360,000 ergs/mm^2 per 30 minutes. No spores survived a 10-minute exposure. A minimal dose of 252,000 ergs/mm^2 per 30 minutes gave a D-value of 4 minutes. After 21 minutes, there were no surviving spores from a 10^6 population in the 2-mL aqueous test suspension.

Table 4-4 lists the organisms tested by Abshire and details their UV resistances in terms of the UV doses in ergs/mm^2. The measured doses compare with those listed in the literature.

Table 4-5 from Abshire et al. gives a classification of organism resistance to UV irradiation in terms of the dosage required. Table 4-6 presents the authors' findings relative to the decimal reduction times of selected organism strains following exposure to a UV intensity of only 100 UV/cm^2. The use of 100 /cm^2 intensities rather than 1,000 UV/cm^2 was made in order to allow more accurate

Table 4-5
Resistance Date for Bacterial Isolates

UV Resistance Category	*UV Dose*[a]	*Isolates*[b] *Bacterial*
Extremely sensitive	<1,000 ergs/mm^2	19% (26/137)[c]
Sensitive	1,000-5,000 ergs/mm^2	46% (63/137)
Resistant	5,000-50,000 ergs/mm^2	34% (47/137)
Extremely resistant	>50,000 ergs/mm^2	<1%[d] (1/137)

[a] UV dose obtained using UV intensity of 400 μW/cm^2 for various exposure times.
[b] Included vegetative cells and spores at a level of 104 to 105 organisms per inoculum spotted on the surfaces of agar plates (102 strains were environmental isolates and 35 strains were bioburden isolates).
[c] Number of strains surviving dose range/total number of strains tested.
[d] *B. pumilus* BMT-18 spores were the most resistant bacterial isolate tested.

Abshire et al. (1983)

calculation of the D-values. Survival times were only on the order of seconds at the higher doses. *Micrococcus radiodurans* ATCC 13939 was the most resistant of the vegetative forms studied. *Candida albicans* ATGCC 10231 also was resistant. The other organisms studied, including those of specific interest in ophthalmology drug manufacture, were sensitive to UV irradiation, most of the D-values being between 1 and 2 minutes under static conditions.

There is no intention in this writing of endorsing any commercial products. However, Abshire's observations (1986) on certain of these are repeated. The Sterilamp Model 782L-30 (Westinghouse Electric Corporation, Bloomfield, NJ) is a low-pressure mercury lamp. These emit about 95% of their light in the 254-nm region, near the peak of germicidal effectiveness. The lamp can discharge

Table 4-6
Resistance Data on Selected Organisms Exposed to 100-mW/cm² UV Intensity

		D-Value[a]	
Organism	*Test #1*	*Test #2*	*Test #3*
Micrococcus radiodurans ATCC 13939	33.25 (0.974)[b]	32.99 (0.988)	33.06 (0.981)
Staphylococcus aureus ATCC 6528	0.90 (0.988)	0.97 (0.986)	0.92 (0.986)
Streptococcus faecium ATCC 10541	2.00 (0.988)	1.97 (0.986)	2.02 (0.988)
Candida albicans ATCC 10231	7.31 (0.993)	7.51 (0.995)	7.55 (0.989)
Escherichia coli ATCC 8739	1.36 (0.983)	1.38 (0.989)	1.33 (0.998)
Pseudomonas aeruginosa ATCC 9027	0.63 (0.992)	0.57 (0.994)	0.60 (0.987)
P. diminuta ATCC 19146	1.23 (0.984)	1.27 (0.981)	1.20 (0.983)
P. diminuta ATCC 11568	1.94 (0.992)	2.02 (0.990)	1.97 (0.993)
P. maltophilia ATCC 13637	1.14 (0.978)	1.17 (0.981)	1.19 (0.985)
P. cepacia ATCC 25416	0.96 (0.988)	0.95 (0.982)	1.00 (0.987)
P. putrefaciens ATCC 8071	1.48 (0.990)	1.41 (0.987)	1.44 (0.988)

[a] UV dose obtained using UV intensity of 400 mW/cm2 for various exposure times.

Abshire et al. (1983)

UV radiation with an intensity of 10,000 μW/cm^2 at its surface.

A high-intensity lamp able to transmit UV radiation through a quartz window with an intensity of 100,000 μW/cm^2 and more is forthcoming from Brown, Boveri & Company, Ltd. (BBC) of Baden, Switzerland.

According to Hanselka, the common combination of UV irradiation followed by use of a sterilizing-grade filter is so sufficiently effective in eliminating organisms as to significantly reduce the need for sanitizations.

FDA Inspector Comments on Ultraviolet

Avallone (1985) and Farina emphasized that water, to be treated effectively by UV light units, must have a high degree of clarity. Additionally, they state that the quartz tube envelope within which the UV is generated must be regularly cleaned so that its output does not become attenuated and interfered with. This should be a regular maintenance activity for which a schedule should be established and adhered to, and regarding which records should be kept. As noted, the UV lamps deteriorate with age. The lamps solarize over time; they will turn tan in color after about 1 year's use. The sufficiency of their intensity outputs requires periodic, scheduled, monitored, and recorded measurement by way of an intensity meter. When so indicated, lamps should be replaced. The monitoring of UV radiation is done by measuring UV light adsorption. Validation of the UV operation will require establishing the frequency of UV lamp replacement and documented proof of the sufficiency of a lamp's intensity as a function of time. In-line intensity meters have been required by some FDA inspectors.

Interestingly, as referenced by Collentro (1986), Carson and Petersen (1975),

Table 4-7
UV Dose* Required for Microbial Kill

Organism Types	*90%*	*99.99%*
Gram-negative fermenters *Coliforms, Salmonella, Serratia marcescens*	2-8	8-32
Gram-negative nonfermenters *Pseudomonas*	6	24
Gram-positive rods (spores) *Bacillus, Clostridium*	4-7(9-12)	16-28(36-48)
Gram-positive cocci *Micrococcus*	6-23	24-92
Fungi Mildew, pigmented water molds	30-300	120-1200

*μW/cm^2 at 254 nm
Courtesy, J.M. Martin, Pall Corp.

reported that *Pseudomonas cepacia* can undergo a photoreactivation of UV-damaged cells, resulting in their regrowth to higher levels than were present in the feedwater. Although this was subsequently disputed by Abshire and Dunton (1981), its possibilities are intriguing in their implication.

Ultraviolet Radiation and TOC Removal

The generation of hydroxyl free radicals by the interaction of UV light and/or ozone and/or hydrogen peroxide addressed to the oxidative destruction of TOC has been discussed. However, UV radiation by itself has also been utilized for this purpose, based upon its lysing of water to produce hydroxyl free radicals. (See also Chapter 6 on "Trihalomethane Removal".

Organic material in semiconductor rinse waters creates unwanted "haze" in silicon chips. Additionally, it serves as nourishment for the organisms whose proliferation results in biofouling.

The photon energy emitted by UV radiation is, according to Plank's equation, inversely proportional to the wavelength of the radiation. Thus, the shorter UV rays are better suited to the oxidation of organic matter. The destruction of organisms by UV radiation generally relies on wavelengths close to 254 nm. The 185-nm radiations, being shorter, consequently are more powerful. It is this wavelength that, in conjunction with catalysts such as titanium dioxide or in combi-

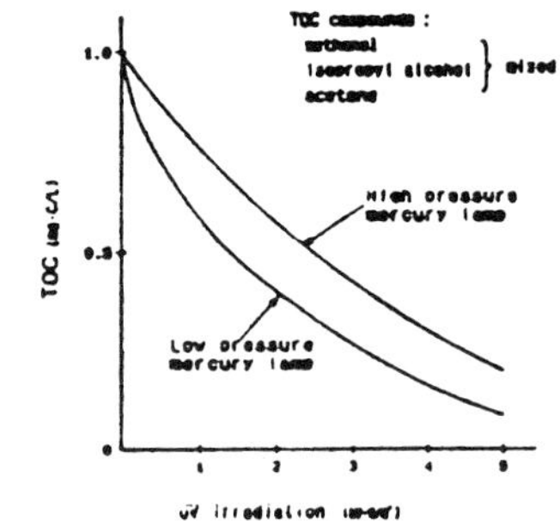

TOC reduction low- vs. 1-gm-pressure mercury.

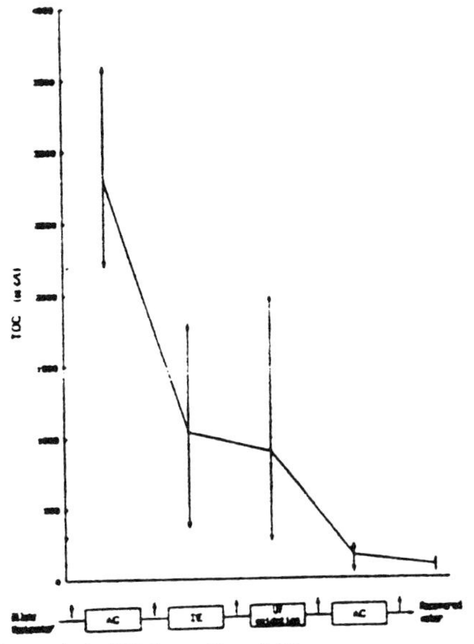

Figure 4-4. TOC profile of dilute wastewater.
Kosaka et al. (1988); Courtesy, *Ultrapure Water* journal.

nation with persulfate, is used commonly to degrade oxidatively the organic matter, or TOC, present in high-purity waters. Indeed, such conversion of organic entities into carbon dioxide is the basis upon which some TOC-analysis instruments function.

Poirier and Kantor (1987) established that TOC removal efficiencies from semiconductor rinse waters are a function of the flowrate of water through the UV treatment apparatus. As expected, the lowest flowrate produced the largest reduction in TOC levels. Even a single pass sufficed to reduce TOC levels from 100 mg/L to 5 μg/L. Unfortunately, designing a 185-nm UV system to remove 98% of the TOC in a single-pass mode presently would require sizing the system an order of magnitude larger than conventional systems.

Immediate practicality is evidenced by a multipass UV system. The polishing loop consists of 185-nm radiation applied upstream of the deionizing resin polishing beds and storage tank. This removes carboxylic acids generated by the UV-caused oxidation of some of the organics. The storage tank is so sized that its volume level does not fall below 50%. Consequently, the full organic burden brought to the UV lights by the primary deionized water is diluted by the recirculating water from the storage tank, and the UV installation is not overburdened. Poirier and Kantor (1987) reported that their system stabilized to TOC levels of under 10 mg/L after a 3-week operation, and ultimately, after 3 months, to less than 5 mg/L.

Irradiation by UV is used widely to recover spent high-purity water in integrated circuit manufacture, and also in pharmaceutical process waters. Many of these applications are proprietary, and are largely kept confidential. Kosaka et al. (1988) detailed one such semiconductor usage, utilizing the greater efficiency of a low-pressure lamp over a high-pressure lamp for the destruction of TOC. Extension of this practice has been made from the wastewater recovery line to the primary production of high-purity water. The low-pressure UV lamps

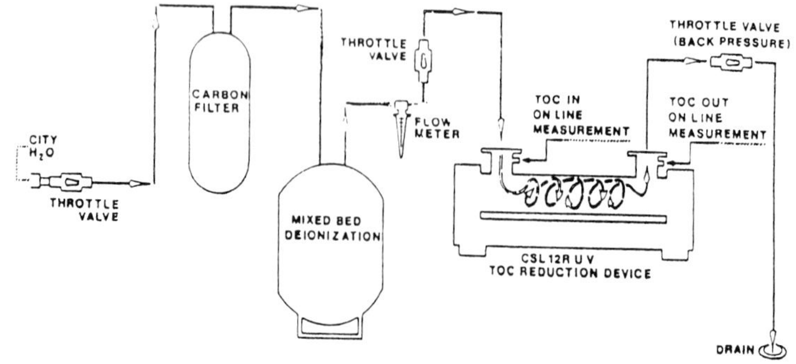

Figure 4-5. Plumbing flow schematic - UV TOC reduction evaluation equipment.
Veloz (1988); Courtesy, Aquafine Corp.

used each had capacities of 670 watts. Employment of a 1-kilowatt lamp simplified the power source facilities and, by minimizing the number of lamps used, diminished the equipment costs. Figure 4-4 shows the TOC profile of a wastewater obtained by such UV treatment. The efficacy of UV irradiation in the removal of TOC is clearly indicated.

Tyldesley et al. (1988) utilized a 2.5-kw arc tube with a quartz sleeve housed in a stainless steel reactor to photooxidize TOC by UV radiation of 185 nm. It was found that water exiting an anion-exchange bed had its TOC and haloform concentrations reduced by about 50% to 60% by an exposure of 6,000 mW/cm. The water effluent from a cation-exchange bed showed much less decrease in its TOC and haloform contents, but absorbed much more of the energy. The greater effect on the TOC emanating from the anion exchanger was ascribed to the greater availability of UV light, less of it having been absorbed by other ingredients in the water. Although concentrations and time details were not

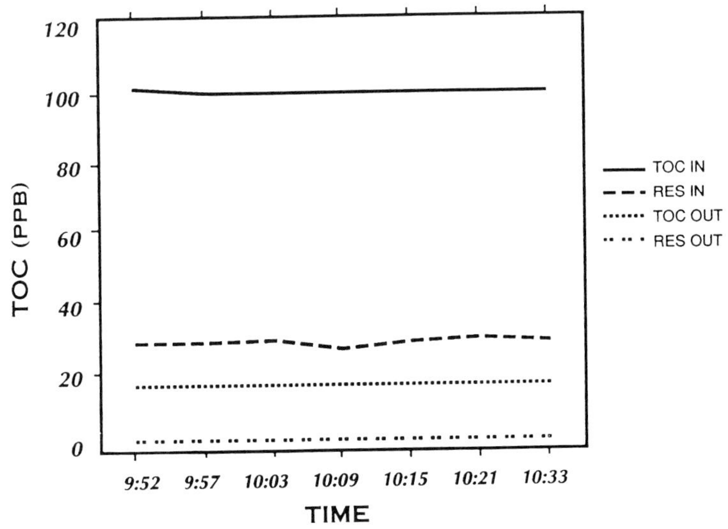

	TIME	TOC IN	RES IN	TOC OUT	RES OUT
1	9:52	101	16.7	26.6	1.6
2	9:57	100	16.7	26.8	1.6
3	10:03	100	16.6	27.4	1.6
4	10:09	100	16.7	24.5	1.5
5	10:15	100	16.7	25.8	1.5
6	10:21	100	16.8	27.8	1.7
7	10:33	100	16.8	27.4	1.7

Average Percent Reduction: 73.4%

Figure 4-6. CSL-12R TOC in-line test (horizontal 4 gpm).
Courtesy , Aquafine Corp.

disclosed, Tyldesley et al. (1988) stated that hydrogen peroxide added to the UV treatment caused an improvement in the effluent water quality, as did also a prolongation of the contact time.

A recirculating loop was constructed of a reservoir, pump, UV reactor, and a mixed-bed resin unit. Water of 280-µg/kg of TOC was circulated. After 75 minutes the TOC was reduced to 240 µg/kg by adsorption in the mixed bed. Application of the UV light decreased the TOC value to below 50 µg/kg within 15 minutes.

Chu and Houskova (1985) found an increase in the levels of inorganic anions, and a corresponding decrease in resistivity in water exposed to UV radiation. The source was chlorinated organics, the irradiative degradation of which ruptured the carbon/chlorine bond to create chloride ions.

Yabe et al. (1989) in Table 4-8 list the relative bonding energies of various organic linkages, and predict the possibilities of their being dissociated by 185-nm UV irradiation (See "Removal of THMs," in Chapter 6).

An intracompany report from a UV device manufacturer (Aquafine Corp.)

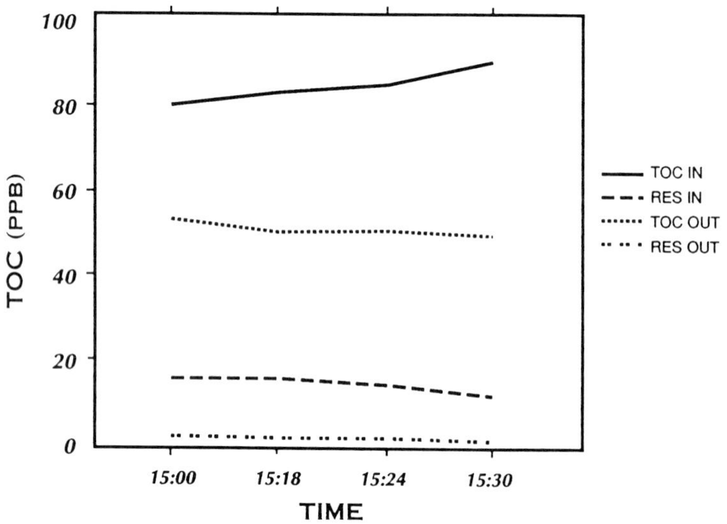

	TIME	TOC IN	RES IN	TOC OUT	RES OUT
1	15:00	81.4	17.2	51.9	2.4
2	15:18	84.3	17.5	49.3	2.2
3	15.24	85.9	16.5	50.8	2.2
4	15:30	90.7	12.7	49.5	2.0

Average Percent Reduction: 41.3%

Figure 4-7. CSL-12R TOC in-line test (horizontal 6 gpm).
Courtesy, Aquafine Corp.

detailed the effects on TOC destruction by an otherwise typical low-pressure UV lamp modified for the purpose of investigating the influences of various design configurations (Veloz, 1988) (Figure 4-5). As would be expected, TOC was reduced by 185 nm of ultraviolet (actually 5% 185 nm, with the balance in the range of 220 to 290 nm; 254 nm), in direct proportion to the applied dosage levels. On the other hand, "pure" 254-nm emissions did not significantly reduce the TOC levels. Interestingly, vertically mounted UV lamps were less efficient than horizontally mounted lamps; and the performance of the vertical posture was not improved by cross-flow. Also, as might have been expected, thin-film lamps became less efficient above flows of 8 gpm (30 liters per minute), as the residence time and dosage diminished with increased water velocity. The influence of water velocities is shown in Figure 4-6, wherein TOC and resistivity levels for influent and effluent waters are shown as a function of flowrate, namely 4 gpm (15 Lpm); in Figure 4-7 of 6 gpm (22.5 Lpm); and in Figure 4-8 of 8 gpm.

Ammerer (1989) reported on the use of 185-nm UV light catalyzed by

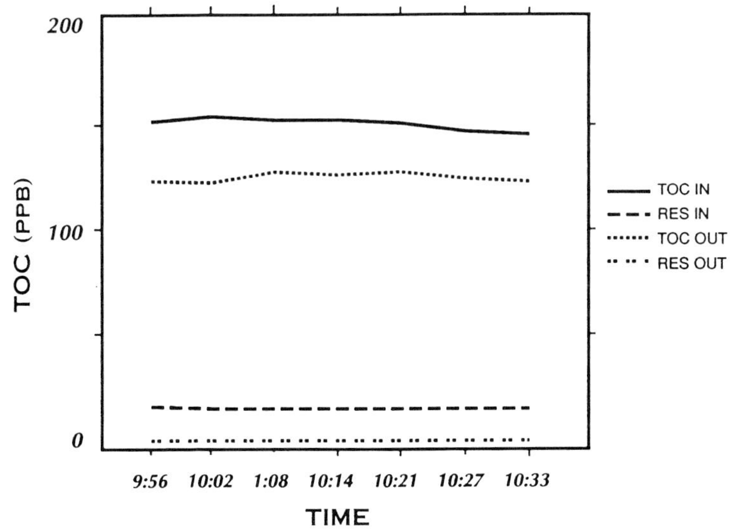

	TIME	TOC IN	RES IN	TOC OUT	RES OUT
1	9:56	152	16.0	120	2.7
2	10:02	153	15.7	118	2.4
3	10:08	153	15.7	122	2.5
4	10:14	152	15.7	121	2.6
5	10:21	152	15.8	121	2.6
6	10:27	148	15.9	117	2.6
7	1:33	144	16.0	116	2.8

Average Percent Reduction: 20.8%

Figure 4-8. CSL-12R TOC in-line test (horizontal 8 gpm).
Courtesy, Aquafine Corp.

titanium dioxide to destroy the TOC extractables emanating from ion-exchange resins. This was done in an off-line water loop dedicated to the purpose. The organic matter extracted by the recirculating water flowed through the UV contact chamber to become photooxidized, and hence removable substances such as as carbon dioxide and carboxylic acids. Multiple UV contact chambers were arranged in series to promote sufficient UV dosage and, therefore, TOC reduction efficiency. It was advocated, reasonably, that the use of this off-line treatment, for which a patent was applied, will shorten the on-line flushing of ion-exchange resins to acceptable TOC levels.

Wiegler and Anderson (1990) found the removal of THMs by adsorption onto activated carbon to be unsatisfactory because of early breakthroughs. The use of UV irradiation reduces the overall THM concentration. However, the chloroform portion of THM is left unaffected. A desired goal of 15 ppb maximum can be attained by use of 185-nm UV lamps, provided the THM concentration does not exceed 100 to 110 ppb. These investigators concluded that the UV destruction of THM (except for the chloroform portion) can be an acceptable procedure until the THM water feed concentration exceeds 150 ppb.

The photolytic UV lamp should be preceded by an RO unit in order to remove as much as possible of UV-absorbing substances. It should be followed by the mixed-bed polishers, which will remove the ion-containing molecules, the carboxylic acids, created by the UV action.

Ozone Destruction

As stated earlier, 254-nm UV radiation dosage levels of 90,000 μW/sec/cm^2 catalyze the destruction of dissolved ozone at 1 ppm concentrations to below detectable levels. Higher ozone concentrations require higher UV dosages. 90,000 microrads/cm^2/sec of UV light energy are required per 1 ppm ozone.

Ultraviolet Safety Concerns

Ultraviolet radiation is hazardous in the because it can damage the human cornea. Consequently, UV-producing bulbs normally are contained in housings that prevent UV radiation from exiting the equipment. Many UV systems additionally are designed so that whenever the housing to the UV bulb is opened inadvertently during operation, the electrical supply to the equipment is broken, thus eliminating the possibility of accidental exposure to UV radiation.

An Example of Ultraviolet Treatment in Pharmaceuticals

In one case, following deionization by way of DI resin beds, the water is filtered through a sintered stainless steel cartridge of 2-μm nominal rating, which is cleaned weekly by reverse flushing, and whose purpose is to retain resin particles. The water then enters an oversized UV facility. Its capacity is rated at 120 gpm (450 Lpm); its use load is, however, only 40 gpm (150 Lpm). The

UV bulbs are equipped with intensity meters and wipers. Daily inspections have yet to reveal the presence of slime.

The treated water has a somewhat lower resistivity, possibly caused by ozone or by some transient ionization produced by the UV. The water entering the system shows a resistivity of 16 to 18 megohm-cm. If the light is switched off, however, the exiting water again exhibits the 16- to 18-megohm-cm value. This effect, in any case, is ephemeral and manifests no untoward consequences, and

Table 4-8
Dissociation Energies for Interatomic Bonds in Organic Substances

Bond	*Dissociation Energy*	*Maximum Wavelength for Dissociation*	*Possibility of Dissociation with184.9-nm UV(154kcal)*
C-C	82.6	346.1	Yes
C=C	145.8	196.1	Yes
C=C	199.6	143.2	No
C-Cl	81.0	353.0	Yes
C-F	116.0	246.5	Yes
C-H	98.7	289.7	Yes
C-N	72.8	392.7	Yes
C=N	147.0	194.5	Yes
C≡N	212.6	134.5	No
C-O	85.5	334.4	Yes
C=O (aldehydes)	176.0	162.4	No
C=O (ketones)	179.0	159.7	No
C-S	65.0	439.9	Yes
C-S	166.0	172.2	No
H-H	104.2	274.4	Yes
N-N	52.0	549.8	Yes
N=N	60.0	476.5	Yes
N≡N	226.0	126.6	No
N-N (NH)	85.0	336.4	Yes
N-N (NH_3)	102.2	280.3	Yes
N-O	48.0	595.6	Yes
N-O	162.0	176.5	No
O-O (O_2)	119.1	240.1	Yes
-O-O-	47.0	608.3	Yes
O-H (water)	117.5	243.3	Yes
S-H	83.0	344.5	Yes
S-N	115.2	248.6	Yes
S-O	119.0	240.3	Yes

Yabe et al. (1989)

of their pore-size distributions, which, in turn, are consequences of the technologies of their manufacture (Lukaszewicz et al., 1981). Membrane filters are thin, with relatively narrow pore-size distributions. If chosen with the correct pore-size rating for an application, their use tends toward particle removal by a sieving action. Depth-type filters, usually mats of fibers, much thicker in their construction, have broader pore-size distributions. Their pore architecture promotes the removal of particles by adsorptive sequestrations. Both depth-type and membrane filters will be discussed in this chapter.

Depth-Type Composite Filters

Depth-type filters, usually used as prefilters, are most often constructed of nonwoven mats of long fibers of such materials as polypropylene, glass, metals, and (before the interdiction of its use on account of its carcinogenicity), of asbestos. These mats are constructed by the random deposition of the individual fibers whose permanence of positioning is sought through gluing, melting, entanglements, or other forms of fixing. The pores of such filter constructions are the interstices among the fibers. As shown in Figure 5-1, the random deposition of the fibers during construction of the filter mat results in a broad pore-size distribution. That is, whatever the mean pore-size, there is a broad difference on either side representing larger and smaller pore sizes. The retention implications of this phenomenon will shortly be considered. Suffice it to say for

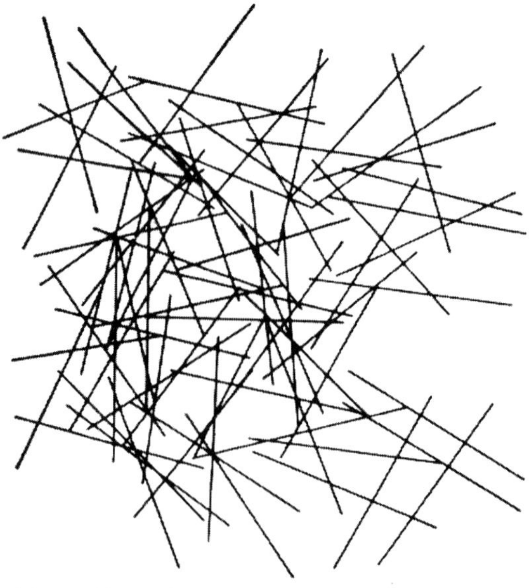

Figure 5-1. Modeling a fibrous filter by a system of lines drawn at random.
Davies (1973); Courtesy, Academic Press.

the present that the adsorptive capture of particles rather than sieve retention is a feature of this type of filter.

Composed of fibers and/or of other discrete particles, these filters are properly regarded as being fiber-releasing. This property is not necessarily eliminated by liquid flushing. Therefore, at least in the case of injectables, their use must be followed by a final membrane filter among whose purposes is the capture of fibers generated by the migration of the medium from the depth-type filter.

Sand beds (multimedia beds), carbon beds, and even ion-exchange columns, all composed of layers or depths of discrete particles, are also depth-type filters, albeit of a nonstructured variety. Consequently, they do exhibit the phenomenon of media (properly, medium) migration. That is to say, under the impetus of the velocity of their permeating fluids they carry bits and pieces of their bed constructions downstream. For this reason, structured depth-type filters, usually of polypropylene or cellulosic fibers, are employed downstream of deep beds to restrain the passage of such particles. Membrane filters with their narrower pore-size distributions would be even more retentive.

Usually being of finer pore sizes, however, these membrane filters are more restrictive of flow. Higher applied differential pressures are required for them to produce a given rate of fluid flow. Moreover, they are usually much more expensive than depth-type filters. Membrane filters are used downstream of deep-bed filters; and particularly are used after ion-exchange beds in pharmaceutical water preparation when the concern is the retention of *Pseudomonas cepacia* (and other organisms) released from ion-exchange beds (Michels, 1981).

Solution-Cast Membranes

Most ultrafilters, nanofilters, RO membranes, and the familiar microporous membrane filters of commerce are prepared from cast solutions of polymeric substances. By a process known as phase inversion or reverse-phase casting, usually involving an exchange of a nonsolvent for a solvent, the polymeric material emerges as a porous membrane. Depending upon the particulars involved in the casting process, the pores may be made to have different size dimensions, and the membranes themselves may even be anisotropic: that is, the pore sizes characterizing one surface may be substantially different from those at the other.

Genesis of Porosity

In the polymeric bulk state, the polymeric chain segments bear a spatial relationship to one another that reflects the balancing of the attractive and repulsive forces present in all matter. Out of this dynamic equilibrium of forces arise the void spaces, some 10 and 100 times smaller than the dimensions of the artificial pores of microporous membranes.

Certain materials, given the opportunity, will develop the orderly, relatively closely packed and dense arrangements of crystallinity. Other polymer chains and segments will maintain the less fixed geometric orders common to an amorphous state. Whatever the polymeric segmental relationship, however, there are distinct spacings involved among the chain segments of all polymers.

The chief determinant of this special relationship is temperature. Generally, the size of the spaces increases with temperature. Higher thermal energies increase the conformational entropy; greater repulsive forces prevail against the attractive forces.

When permitted to develop and equilibrate at a given temperature, a polymeric material, whether in thin-film form or in some other more substantial dimension, will possess those internal intersegmental spacings characteristic of its bulk properties at that temperature. These dimensions, of course, may differ from one substance to another, but will be on the order of 3 to perhaps 10 angstroms in size.

Accordingly, when a polymeric film is deposited in melt form, or as a casting in solution form, its constituting molecules (or more properly the intersegmental sections of its long molecular chains) are spaced from one another by the disruptive influence of thermal energy or by the space-intruding interferences of solvent molecules. As the polymeric disruption is minimized by cooling of the melt or by solvent molecule removal (as by evaporation), the polymeric segments are enabled to approach one another more closely and the intersegmental spaces decrease in size. At room temperature, however, or when all the solvent has been removed, intersegmental spaces still exist. Their finite dimensions express an equilibrium position defined by the mutual attractive-repulsive forces that operate among the constituting atoms and molecules of the polymeric mass. In essence, then, even "solid" polymeric films contain definite spaces because every atom, constituting any form of matter, including solids, is surrounded by such spaces.

It is these intersegmental spaces at angstrom levels that permit the use of solid polymeric films as sieve or screen filters in certain separation contexts, including reverse osmosis applications.

Intersegmental Space Dimensions

The intersegmental spacings depend on the molecular structure of the material. Where the architectural regularity is great, the atoms or molecular segments can approach one another more closely; a denser material results. Indeed, the regularity may be of such a high order that the spatially defined patterns characteristic of crystals may result. Such crystalline regions have high densities. Their intersegmental spaces are small. Such substances serve well, therefore, as barrier films.

Within the fixed atomic arrangements of the crystalline state there is atomic movement, as indeed there is for all atoms above the absolute zero temperature. The vigor of this atomic movement is not enough, however, to disrupt the crystal bonding, which is strong. This is in accordance with the inverse square law governing the influence of such forces, because it need operate only over the short spaces prevalent within the crystals. Thus metallic structures such as aluminum foils are crystalline. The atoms approach one another closely because they are small. Hence, the bonding is strong and predisposes the small, regular atoms to the close packing of the crystalline state. Thus thin films (foils) of metal provide the best packaging barriers against moisture and air passage.

The polyethylenes are semicrystalline polymers, the high-density variety more so than the low-density polymer. In the high-density material, the molecular chains are long and essentially unbranched, permitting close approaches. Low-density polyethylene has shorter chains with more extensive branching. The more frequent chain ends of the lower-molecular-weight chains are more disruptive of close packing, and the chain branches act as spatial buffers or fenders to keep main-chain segments from approaching one another as closely as they do in the case of the straight-chain, high-density polyethylene molecules. The result is a less dense polyethylene whose intersegmental spaces are large enough to permit the passage of small molecules, and to permit their filtrative differentiation from larger molecules. Permeation of such films will also most strongly reflect the solubility of the permeating molecular species in the film.

Cellulose is also a semicrystalline material. Its technology of handling and fabrication determines the extent to which its latent crystallinity will assert itself. In applications where greater permeabilities are desired in regenerated cellulose films, the handling is such that the result is the random packing of the amorphous state rather than the patterning of crystalline regions. Thus, the resulting membrane permits not only the permeation by small gas molecules, as in a membrane heart/lung machine, but also of larger molecules in the liquid phase, as in an artificial kidney device.

The artificial kidney membranes, based on the conventional Cupraphane (regenerated cellulose) and cellulosic tubular forms, also offer openings reflective of the bulk state of the polymer. The technology of their membrane formation may, however, be manipulated to minimize the densifying effects of crystallinity that make for smaller pores. The resulting regenerated cellulose membrane has a porosity, enhanced somewhat by plasticization, that permits practical rates of permeation by molecules as large as substances such as urea, water, and salts; but that is still too tight to permit the passage of serum albumin, the smallest of the blood proteins.

The Phase-Inversion Process

Casting solutions intended for microporous membranes manufacture contain, usually, not only polymer in solution, but also a quantity of high-boiling (low-volatile) nonsolvent. The resulting solution consists, then, of polymer molecules dispersed in a single homogeneous liquid phase. As solvent (a lower-boiling substance) evaporates and the volume of solution diminishes, the polymer segments progressively come closer to one another. However, achievement of their potentially ultimate degree of propinquity is prevented by the action of the nonsolvent, for the point is reached where the composition of the remaining solution, modified from the original by loss of solvent, is too rich in nonsolvent to support further the solubility of both the nonsolvent and the polymer. As described by Kesting (1971), phase inversion occurs at this point with the appearance of two heterogeneous liquid phases—one rich in polymer and solvent, the other in nonsolvent. With further evaporation of solvent, coalescence of the polymer-rich droplets into a wet gel distorts their spherical shapes into polyhedra (Maier and Scheuermann, 1960). (A similar point, for particular casting solutions, may be reached by temperature manipulations, temperature triggered, rather than by evaporation of solvent.)

In a somewhat oversimplified sequence, droplets of nonsolvent separate within the solvent/polymer solution, and the polymer begins to condense out of solution. The polymer then concentrates at the phase interfaces as it comes out of solution, thus leading to the formation of small droplets of nonsolvent surrounded by a swollen polymer shell. As further solvent evaporation (or temperature lowering) takes place, more and more polymer comes out of solution and a thickening of the polymer shell occurs. The polymer-in-solution phase disappears and the polymer-surrounded droplets come into contact with each other, forming clusters that consolidate and distort into closed polyhedral cells filled with residual nonsolvent. Finally, the edges of the closed polyhedral cells accumulate polymer at the expense of the polyhedral cell walls, thereby leading to the thinning of such cell walls and their eventual rupture. An interconnecting, porous polymeric continuum is the result.

With the rupture and disappearance of the cell walls, the interconnecting pores are created, permitting the removal, by washing or evaporation, of the remaining solvent and nonsolvent. The additional solvent removal, however, does not permit further significant spatial adjustments by the polymer segments. Such movements are frustrated by the high viscosity of the wet-gel state.

The attainment of phase inversion need not involve nonsolvent pore formers. Solution of the polymer can be managed by the use of cosolvents, systems wherein two (or more) liquids, neither of them alone a solvent for the polymer, in combination do serve to dissolve it. Evaporative loss of one of the liquids upsets the system solvent properties and causes phase inversion.

Solution of polymer, as well as its precipitation from solution (the phase inversion) can both be managed also by temperature manipulations rather than by solvent evaporation (Hiatt et al., 1984).

Asymmetric or Anisotropic Morphology

Evaporation of solvent from the casting solution leads eventually to phase inversion and formation of the wet-gel form of the microporous membrane. In evaporation of the solvent, two different diffusion mechanisms are involved: diffusion of the liquid-phase solvent from the interior of the casting to its surface, and diffusion from the casting surface into the surrounding air. Hence, the evaporation is affected by the temperature of the casting solution, and also by the air velocity over the surrounding air, by the ambient relative humidity, and by the air velocity over the casting surface.

If the evaporation of solvent from the casting surface into the air is greater than the rate of solvent diffusion from the interior of the cast film to the surface, the result will be *skinning*, the formation of a dense layer on the surface of the cast film. The evaporation of the solvent without adequate replacement by liquid diffusion from the film interior causes the surface of the liquid casting to represent "bad" solvent conditions; polymer precipitation results. The high rate of this process does not permit the formation of droplets of the nonsolvent phase, or at best permits the formation only of very small droplets. The result is that the surface skin can have a high degree of impermeability. However, this dense surface skin will moderate the solvent evaporation in the liquid layers below it. In these layers, therefore, coacervation will occur, and the bulk of the casting will be microporous.

The Loeb-Sourirajan (1962) RO cellulose diacetate membrane devised for water desalination is of such a morphology. Such structures are called asymmetric, because their opposite surfaces differ in their pore-size characteristics. The advantages of such a structure is that the dense metering layer performs the desired discriminating function, while its thin dimension serves only minimally to impede bulk liquid permeations. This condition is facilitated by the relatively open structure of the remainder of the film, whose existence serves solely as a mechanical support for the dense, functional skin.

It is of course possible to moderate the degree of skin density. Also, by the proper manipulation of operating conditions, it is possible to construct microporous membranes that are without skins, but that are characterized by a gradient of pore sizes from one side to the other, and to control these variations to different extents, as desired. Such filters are also asymmetric and are commonly called such. Kesting (1971) suggests, however, that the term *asymmetric* be reserved for skinned structures, and that the appellation *anisotropic* be employed for the nonskinned, pore-size gradient types. Less often, the term *anisomorphic* is used interchangeably with *anisotropic*, and even with *asymmetric*.

Reverse Osmosis Membranes and Asymmetry

It so happens that certain polymers, the cellulose diacetates and a class of polyamides among them, have intersegmental spaces large enough to permit the passage of water molecules, but too small to accommodate the chloride ion in its hydrated form. These polymerics, when arranged in the form of thin films or hollow fibers, desalinate aqueous salt solutions. Under pressure, water permeates the intersegmental spaces and exits on the other side of the polymeric membrane. The hydrated chloride ions are too large to pass through the available spaces. The oppositely charged sodium ions, or other cations, remain behind to maintain electrical neutrality. The result is a polymeric "solid" filter that separates ions from their aqueous solvent. The process is also referred to as hyperfiltration, and RO membranes are, therefore, also called hyperfilters.

While influenced by salt concentration and certain operational manipulations, the interdiction to ionic passage by RO membranes is rather complete, at least with regard to ordinary desalination usage for potable water production. It is compromised to some degree, however, presumably by the flaws that for such membranes seem the inevitable result of their manufacturing process (Carter, 1976)*.

The flux—the rate of water permeation per square area per unit of time—is rather small. To optimize this rate to practical levels, the polymeric barrier is fashioned into membrane compositions wherein the discriminating polymeric film is only some 100 angstroms thick. After the casting formula is deposited on a suitable casting surface, the evaporation of the solvent, moderated by reduced temperature, is allowed to take place for a specified brief time. Solvent evaporation of course occurs preferentially from the top surface of the casting, that surface interfacing with the surrounding atmosphere. As a result, the dense film structure with its salt-rejecting properties forms on this top surface. The interval permitted for evaporation is so brief, however, that the film formed is very thin. Further evaporation and film development are interrupted by soaking the casting in water, whereupon the remaining thickness of the casting is converted into a porous mass. The finished RO membrane has a dense layer thick enough for rejections, but thin enough to minimize the impediment to water passage. The thicker underlayer of the membrane serves essentially to give structural support to the dense functional layer. It is too open to limit the water flux (Loeb and Sourirajan, 1962). In the technology of asymmetric membrane formation, the density of the skin can be varied to a certain extent, within the bounds of the bulk property, to give tighter structures or more open membranes.

There are other methods for enhancing RO filter flux properties. Alternatively, the polymeric film is laid up in spiral-wound jelly-roll arrangements to optimize flux by increasing the surface-area-to-volume ratio. This increases

* It is not that RO or ultrafiltration membranes lack the manufacturing accomplishments common to microporous membranes. Rather, it is that the discriminating dense layer is so thin that its perfection is easily marred by small flaws, perhaps caused in the casting solutions by dust particles that have no significance in microporous membranes where the operative film thickness is so much greater.

membrane surface/solution contacts. The polymer film can also be disposed as hollow fibers in order to maximize the flux through surface aggrandizement. Hollow fibers may be spun with the rejecting skin layer either on their insides or their outsides, as desired. The cylindrical form is inherently strong mechanically, and can therefore withstand a considerable pressure differential. (See Chapter 9, "Reverse Osmosis, Ultrafiltration, and Electrically Driven Demineralizations", for further discussion of the different modes whereby RO filters with their limited fluxes are arranged into devices with enhanced permeation rates.)

Ultrafiltration Membranes

The chain segments of a polymer molecule have a tendency to associate with each other. As the temperature drops, this tendency increases. It may result in a great degree of order among the molecules within given regions of the polymer. Such order in the arrangement of the polymeric chains confers a crystal-like structure to local regions, in some cases up to 1,000 angstroms in size. The ultimate degree of intersegmental contact that is potentially possible during the formation of a solid polymeric film is not necessarily automatically realized, however. There is a relaxation phenomenon, a time factor, associated with the adjustment of the polymer segments to one another. When the temperature is reduced, the rate of segmental movement is also much reduced, so that the chains and their segments may become locked into less ordered arrays. It is a competition between the driving forces striving for order, which increases with lowered temperature; and the speed with which this order can be accomplished, which is reduced with lowered temperature. The transitional structure, or morphology, can be locked into a metastable state simply by the rapidity of the transition.

Time is a factor, as is the maintenance (usually by careful temperature control) of that degree of polymer fluidity (or viscosity) necessary to segmental movement as the melt temperature cools, or the solvent is removed. Thus, if in the preparation of an RO membrane the process is hurried, the resulting film will feature larger intersegmental spaces. In the too-hurried process, a high level of viscosity is so rapidly attained as to prevent closer segmental togetherness. For all these reasons, the bulk polymer state may, in practice, be represented by some span of intersegmental distances. Thus, a given polymer may be prepared in film form to possess larger or smaller intersegmental distances. None of these configurational possibilities is considered an artificiality, although strictly speaking, only one configuration represents the bulk polymer in its most thermodynamically stable state.

Chains that are well aligned and highly ordered are crystalline; have lower solubility for foreign molecules; and, as the chains are tightly packed, inhibit diffusion. Hence the permeability is low. On the other hand, randomly oriented chains and their fragments are amorphous, entertain the inclusion of solvent molecules, and do not present diffusional restraints. Hence the permeability is high.

By the preparative manipulations of the polymer casting formulas it is thus possible to manufacture a spectrum of "solid" polymeric membranes characterized by differing intersegmental space dimensions. It is these more open film forms that are used in the practices of ultrafiltration. These differences in spacings translate to cutoff values, usually defined in terms of the ability of the ultrafilter to retain protein molecules of different sizes as related to molecular weights. The shape of the protein molecules also exerts its influence.

The implication of the cutoff ratings of the ultrafilters is that they retain larger molecules while permitting the passage of smaller ones. They would seem suitable, therefore, for the separation of different sizes of protein molecules. Achieving the separation of proteins by the use of ultrafiltration is far from simple, however. A suitably devised ultrafilter may permit the passage of serum albumin, and may be capable of retaining globulin. Yet it may not smoothly permit their separation from a solution of both, because of the associative hydrogen bonding among protein molecules (Van Oss and Bronson, 1970).

Ultrafilters made of cellulose diacetate, as distinct from RO membranes composed of that polymer, would not be capable of ion rejection because of their larger intersegmental spacings. They would, however, offer higher flux rates, and ought to be reassuringly retentive with regard to organisms. In actual practice, UF membranes, like RO filters, seem not always to retain organisms with requisite dependability. Use has been made of ultrafilters in pharmaceutical applications, however, not for enhanced particle retention, but largely for the removal of bacterial endotoxins and for separations utilizing their cutoff propensities.

The very tightness of the RO membrane that results in salt retention also necessitates the application of higher pressures to achieve meaningful flux. This must be paid for in larger pumps and larger pumping costs, in sturdier vessels and pipe construction, and in more expensive equipment requirements all around, but particularly in slower throughput rates. The more open structure of ultrafilters endows them with larger water fluxes. Their operation is therefore less costly than that of RO, in that less pressure need be applied and accommodated. On the other hand, ultrafiltration units are generally more costly to clean. It is worth noting that filtration, like all operational practices, has its economic component.

Nanofilters

The same preparative manipulation (a less-than-complete attainment of the closest positioning of one polymeric segment to another) that permits the making of ultrafilters also allows the formulation of more open RO membranes. Being more open, they require lower differential pressures to achieve practical flowrates. They are less retentive, however. They do not restrain the passage of monovalent ions (in their hydrated forms), but do hold back the larger divalent ions made even larger by their envelopes of hydration. The resulting "open ROs" are used in water-softening contexts to remove calcium, magnesium, and the other alkaline earth elements from aqueous solutions while avoiding the problems (pollution) of salt-regenerating systems. These filter structures are also called nanofilters. The process is also often referred to as membrane softening. Nanofilters also serve to reject organics that are too large to permeate their pores, described by some manufacturers as being retentive of molecular-weight entities of 300 to 1,000.

The application of these low-rejection RO membranes to municipal water softening avoids the use of sodium ion exchange, a process in which calcium, magnesium, and other hard-water elements are removed; but in which sodium ions, often contraindicated for health reason are substituted. The use of nanofilters adds no ions to the water. Indeed, they accomplish sufficient desalting to permit waters to meet the health standards in certain states. Also, these filters are tight enough to remove (from waters being rendered potable) at least some of the organic molecules that serve as precursors for trihalomethane formation under oxidative attack by chlorine. Nanofilters have been applied to the removal of nitrates, lead, radium, and arsenic. As is common to all RO operations, the disposal of their reject concentrate poses a problem.

The RO membranes are tighter than the nanofilters, which are tighter than the ultrafilters; and both are tighter than the 0.2-μm-rated membranes that are used as sterilizing filters. It is thus often believed that RO and UF filters must also be sterilizing filters. For whatever reasons, this is not so, at least not consistently enough to make them dependable for organism retentions.

These membrane filters are used over long periods of time. This provides opportunities for biofouling to occur. Additionally, their tighter structures accumulate polarization layers of substances such as debris, salts, and proteins, depending upon the application. To ensure their proper functioning, these filters require much attention: sanitization, cleaning, proper prefiltration, and periodic replacement. Users sometimes slight these requirements. In time, these filters can degrade, from whatever causes. The signal for their replacement is usually the detection of their dysfunction.

Tangential Flow versus Dead-End Flow

In the conventional filtration mode, the liquid flow is perpendicular to the filter surface; and the particulate burden filtered from the fluid permeating the filter inevitably becomes deposited on or within it. Filter blocking and/or clogging is the unavoidable consequence. To offset the undesirable effects of the accumulative particle deposition, prefilters are utilized, especially with heavily laden liquids. The prefilter serves to intercept a portion of the particulate load, and to that extent ameliorates the amount of blockage and/or clogging that would otherwise occur. However, it may not always be suitable to use prefilters. Consider a filtrative separation where the desired product is the particulate material. The use of prefilters would render its recovery more difficult. Even where the product is the liquid, the more extensive the prefilter/final filter system, the greater the volume of liquid retained within it. There are, therefore, instances where the conventional dead-ended filtration mode is substituted for by tangential flow filtration.

In tangential flow arrangements, the liquid permeating the filter still deposits its particulate matter on the filter surface, but the liquid on the upstream side of the filter is circulated tangential to or across that filter surface in a manner that serves to sweep the surface clean of deposited particles (Figure 5-2). To be sure, some finite amount of deposition usually does remain. A progressive buildup is avoided, however, as is its interferences with the filtration. To achieve a sweeping action, the liquid encounters the filter surface at one edge and exits in its recirculation path at the opposite edge. Meanwhile, a portion permeates the filter and becomes free of its particulate content. That the point of entry of the liquid is situated at one edge or another of the filter module does not constitute tangential flow. Rather it is that the liquid stream on the upside of the filter is recirculated, an action that results in a liquid sweep of that upper surface, that is the essence of the crossflow or tangential flow principle.

Tangential flow is particularly suited to the use of RO and UF membranes, for these are so tight as to avidly trap particulate matter at rates of accumulation that would render the service life of a dead-end filter impractical in its brevity. The cleansing sweep of the tangential flow serves, however, to limit particle polarization upon the membrane and to prolong its service life to acceptable durations.

Anisotropic Membranes

Every filter is composed of pores represented by some spread or distribution of pore sizes. For most membranes, these various pores of whatever sizes are presumed to be equally scattered throughout any given section or area of filter. There exist membranes, however, wherein there has been purposefully achieved a segregation of pore sizes from one side of the filter to the other. These are called

Table 5-1
Percent Retention of 0.198-μm Latex Particles by Various 0.2-μm-Rated Membranes Using Turbidity Measurements

Filter Type	*In Water*	*In 0.05% Triton X-100*
Polycarbonate	100.0	100.0
Asymmetric polysulfone	100.0	100.0
Polyvinylidene fluoride	74.8	19.2
Nylon 66	82.1	1.0
Cellulose esters	89.4	25.1

Tolliver and Schroeder (1983); Courtesy, *Microcontamination anisotropic*, *anisomorphic*, or more commonly *asymmetric* membranes (Figure 5-3). Where the pores are essentially the same from side to side, the filter is termed *isomorphic*, *isotropic*, or *isometric*.

Processing or industrial applications are those in which relatively large quantities of liquids are involved. As a result, there is the need for an adequacy of the particle retention that is the purpose of the filtrative exercise, along with an expeditious passage of the liquid through the filter. Processing costs must be considered, and time means money. Anisotropic filters permit faster flow rates.

In the case of isotropic membranes, there is trade-off between particle retention and rates of flow. This is shown in Figure 5-4. The pore size pictured on the left is the only proper one of the three shown. The one on the right fails in its retention purposes. The pore depicted in the center, while retentive, unduly restricts the rate of liquid flow. In the isotropic morphology, the more one strives for surety of retention by reducing the pore size, the more one compromises the rate of flow.

In the case of the anisotropic filter that is not so. The pore geometry, to oversimplify somewhat, is funnel-shaped. The restricted area serves to effect the necessary particle retentions. However, the broader spaces of the upper portions

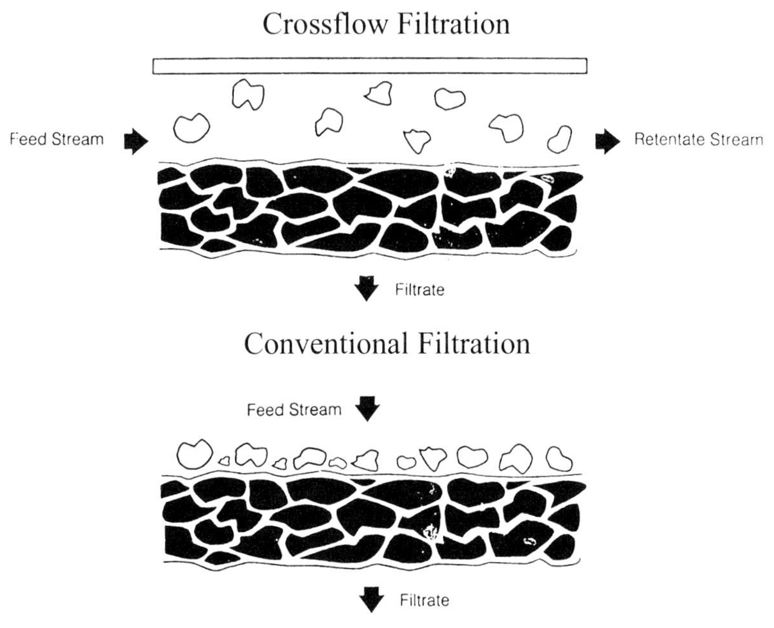

Figure 5-2. Crossflow filtration feed stream.
Gabler (1987); Courtesy, Marcel Dekker, Inc.

of the funnel-shaped pore so little restrict liquid flow that for an equal-pore-size-rated anisotropic membrane, the liquid flow can be 4 times that of the isomorphic filter (Kesting et al., 1981). Therefore, it is possible to tighten the filter rating at the expense of some of the flow advantage and to obtain greater surety of retention along with better flowrates than those shown by comparable isomorphic membranes.

Wallhäusser (1983a) reported similarly advantaged flows resulting from the use of 0.1-μm-rated asymmetric membranes in comparison with conventional isometric 0.1-μm-rated filters.

The result of using anisotropic morphology to obtain surety of particle retention was shown in work by Tolliver and Schroeder (1983) (Table 5-1). The 0.2-μm-rated asymmetric filter alone among its competitive reverse-phase-type membranes was shown to retain completely 0.198-μm-size latex spheres (Simonetti et al., 1986).

The track-etch 0.2-μm membrane also completely retains 0.198-μm latex particles. However, its pore-size distribution is narrower: Only 10% of its pores are smaller than the 0.2-μm. Filtrations such as are encountered in real-life situations involve polydispersant particle challenges. For such removals, the broader pore-size distributions of the reverse-phase anisotropic membranes are superior. (See Table 5-2.)

Badenhop et al. (1970) demonstrated on a laboratory scale the advantage of processing proteinaceous solutions through asymmetric membranes. Kesting et al. (1981) were first to produce asymmetric membranes dedicated to the processing industries. The asymmetry of the Kesting membrane was 10 to 1 (i.e., the pores on one side were 10 times the size of those on the other). The degree of anisotropy can be determined by a comparison of scanning electron micrographs of the two membrane surfaces. Another determination is by an ink test

Table 5-2
Retention of Various Size Latex Particles for 0.2-μm-Rated Membranes

Latex Particle Size (μm)	*0.091*	*0.198*	*0.305*	*0.460*
Membrane Type			*Percent Retention*	
Asymmetric polysulfone	54.3	100	100	100
Charge-modified nylon	10.5	100	100	100
Polycarbonate (track-etched)	6.3	100	100	100
Polyvinylidene fluoride	23.4	19.2	84.5	100
Cellulose esters	17.7	25.1	48.6	100
Nylon 66	1.0	1.0	1.0	100

All solutions 0.04% latex in 0.05% Triton X-100.
Wrasidlo et al. (1983); Courtesy, Parenteral Drug Association

wherein an inked area on the side featuring the larger pores is seen to produce a much larger area marked out on the opposite side characterized by the smaller pores, presumably in proportion to the degree of asymmetry.

Wrasidlo and Mysels (1984) described a membrane defined by an asymmetry of 100 to 1. An asymmetric polysulfone membrane has a degree of asymmetry of 50 to 1. At present not enough work has been done to learn what degrees of

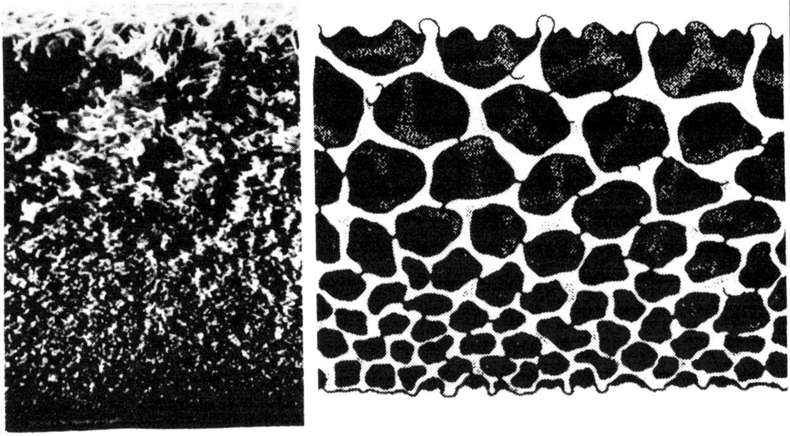

Figure 5-3. Actual micrograph and idealized representation of anisomorphic membrane filter.
Meltzer (1986); Courtesy, *Ultrapure Water* journal

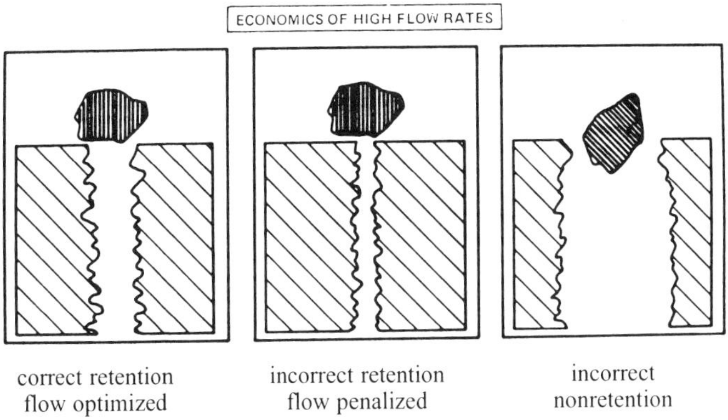

Figure 5-4. Correct pore sizing for desired retention of particulates and avoidance of unnecessary flow restrictions.
Meltzer (1987a); Courtesy, Marcel Dekker, Inc.

asymmetry, if any, are optimum for which applications. As with RO and UF membranes, damage to a discriminating dense layer is more critical than it is to any one side of an isometric membrane. To that extent, asymmetric filters are more prone to flaws than are the conventional types. The greater the degree of asymmetry, the more critical the effect of the flaw. There is a subtlety here. That a flaw in the filter becomes more critical when present does not necessarily mean that the filter is more easily damaged; only that the result produces greater unwanted effects. In any case, once the membrane has been assembled into cartridge form it is shielded from harmful handling. The integrity of the filter cartridge can be assessed by any of the conventional integrity tests (e.g., bubble point, diffusive airflow, pressure-hold, or in the case of hydrophobic filters, water intrusion test). (See page 249).

Anysotropic Bubble-Point Values

Figures 5-5 and 5-6 show the sharp bubble point that is given by membranes of very narrow pore-size distributions (Pall and Kirnbauer, 1978). Filters with broader distributions present a less acute transition before onset of the bubble point. In the case of asymmetric filters, the diffusive airflow through the thinned liquid layers within the anisotropic pores so masks the intrinsic bubble-point values as to give apparent bubble points whose low values would, in isotropic membranes, represent integrity failure readings.

Because of this phenomenon, asymmetric membranes have sometimes found only a qualified acceptance in the marketplace. The manufacturers of asymmetric filters have addressed the problem by using double layers. The upstream layer with the larger pores facing the liquid flow offers the advantages of asymmetry. The downstream layer has its smaller pores facing upstream so that the funnel-shaped pores are not thinned of their liquid content during the integrity testing.

The result of this double layer is a "normal," but indistinct bubble point acceptable to users. A sacrifice in the flowrates is involved in the use of repetitive filters. However, this is acceptable in the case of asymmetric membranes because of the margin of added flowrate advantage they offer. Repetitive filters serve also to ensure particle retentions.

As with all microporous membranes, the bubble-point and diffusive airflow values that denote integral filters are derived from correlations with organism retention experiences. Such anisotropic membranes are retentive of *Pseudomonas diminuta* at a level of 1×10^7 organisms per square centimeter of membrane surface. (Kesting et al., 1981; Wrasidlo and Hofmann, 1982; Wrasidlo and Mysels, 1984). (See page 260).

Charge-Modified Membranes

There are on the market microporous nylon membranes that have been modified chemically so that they bear the positive ions of quaternary amine groups. These

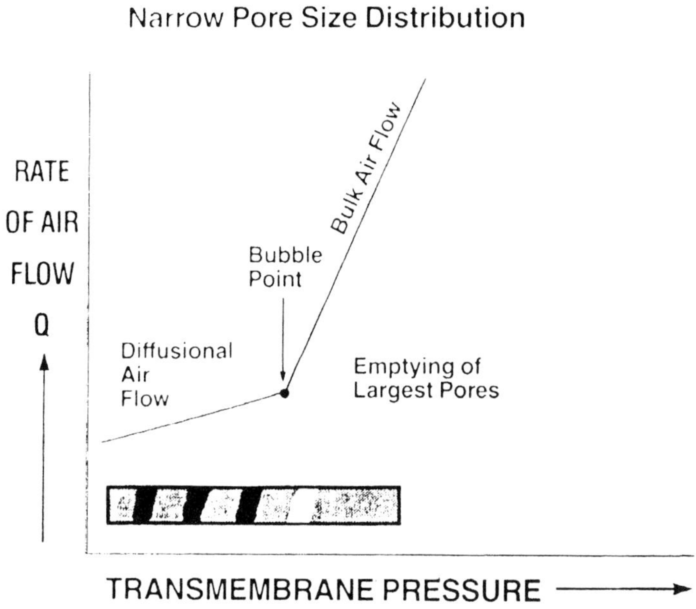

Figure 5-5. Airflow through wetted filters: narrow pore-size distribution.

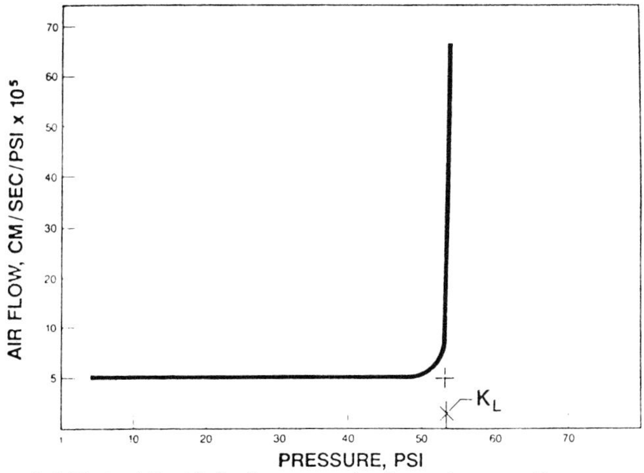

Figure 5-6. Typical liquid displacement plot for an intact uniform pore membrane (Nylon 66).

Pall and Kirnbauer (1978); Courtesy, Univ. of Tennessee

ionic sites, at pH levels conducive to their development, are characterized by positive charges. In consequence, they attract and retain negatively charged entities, such as most particles, and the bacterial endotoxins.

Charge-modified polyvinylidene fluoride membranes are also available. Parekh et al. (1993) measured the efficiency of a charge-modified PVDF membrane of a proprietary composition by assessing its ability to remove colloidal silica particles reputedly spherical and of 0.02-μm diameter size in concentrations of 5 ppm and 50 ppm.

Charge-modified filters are very efficacious at removing the colloidal material often present in waters being prepared for electronic rinsing. Such filters are widely used, as are also charge-modified depth filters, for the removal of pyrogenic lipopolysaccharides (as from the fermentation products of antibiotic productions). They are very effective (Hou and Zaniewski, 1990).

The limitation of these filters is that they operate on a stoichiometric basis. That is, one positive charge site is essentially saturated, and hence neutralized, by one negative particle. There is a finite capacity to these membranes. Once exhausted, they no longer function as charged filters. When ordinary microporous membranes become nonoperative by the accumulation of retained solids, they signal the exhaustion of their capacities by the fact that higher applied differential pressures are required to maintain given rates of liquid flow through them. There is in the degree of elevation of the differential pressure an index to the remainder of the useful life of the filter. This is not the case, however, for the charge-modified filters. Here, the consumption of the positive charges is not marked by a change in pressure. There is no outward signal given regarding the demise of this filter function.

As a result it becomes necessary, as by a pre-use titration, or by the use of two-in-series charge-modified filters (Fig. 5-8, to establish just how much of a given preparation can be treated by such a filter. The validation of such a filter for such an application must rest heavily upon the analysis of the end product to ascertain that it has, in effect, been correctly handled filtratively.

Parks (1967) has shown that the zero or isoelectric point charge of composite surfaces is the weighted average of the individual zero-point charges of the constituents (Fiore and Babineau, 1979). Thus, the adsorption of charge-neutralizing entities onto the filter serves to diminish its remaining charge value. Raistrick (1982) states, therefore, that such charge-modified filters may have only limited utilities where complex fluids such as wines, beers, and whiskeys are involved. The same holds true for protein solutions. Raistrick shows that such filters exhibit high removal efficiencies toward latex particles suspended in aqueous acetate buffer, but show only low efficiencies vis-a-vis such particles suspended in potable liquids. Likewise, yeast cells are removed from buffered aqueous suspensions by zeta-positive filters, but may fail to be removed in the presence of anionic molecules. The sulfate anions, such as those of dextran sulfate or chondroitin sulfate, adsorb to the positively charged sites to cause a reversal of the charge sign on the membrane surface, there being two negative charges to each sulfate ion adsorbed onto a positive-charged site. The resulting negatively charged filters fail to adsorb yeast.

Raistrick's observations confirm findings that the adsorption of negatively-charged particles may shift the surface charge of positively charged filters. This may inhibit further retention of negatively charged particles, leading to particle breakthrough. Furthermore, particle unloading has been observed at this point. Similarly, it is indicated (Rossitto, 1983) that a charge-modified filter medium that is effective in removing a given species of particle from one solution medium may not be effective in its removal of the same particles from a second or different liquid composition. This is a consequence of charged particles of different species competing for the same adsorptive surface. Raistrick's finding relative to latex particle retention from potable liquids, mentioned above, is a case in point.

Charge-modified prefilters are characterized by a maximum pressure value above which they may not function properly because of the possibilities of desorption (unloading) and filter medium migration. The filter efficiency may actually decrease as the applied pressure increases. Therefore, when used with heavily loaded liquids, they should be preceded by prefilters. Otherwise, their maximum allowable pressure levels may become exceeded by high loadings of particulates (whether trapped electrokinetically or by sieve retention), necessitating replacement. Excessive pressure surges must, therefore, also be guarded against. Also, moderation of flowrates may be required to optimize colloid and endotoxin removal. The adequacy of fluid/filter contact time is an issue.

The particle size may influence the capture mechanism whereby charge-modified filters perform. Hou et al. (1980) neutralized the electrokinetic effectivity of such filters by operating at high pH. It was found that particles larger than approximately 1 μm were retained nonetheless. Smaller particles, however, though retained at pH levels where positive charges were operative, did escape capture at the high pH. It was concluded that the larger particles were captured by sieve retention when electrokinetic influences were absent, but that particles too small to be thus retained required charge interactions for their arrest.

Bacterial Endotoxin and Organism Removal by Charge-Modified Filters

Charge-modified filters are widely used in antibiotic manufacture to remove pyrogenic endotoxin. It is an application whose success is widely attested to. Yet the operation requires care because charge-modified filters do have finite capacities, can have their charge sites preempted by competitive adsorption, and can even have their charge polarities reversed by such adsorptions. It is essential that characterizations of both the solution and the filter be performed in a validation exercise to ensure that the conditions favorable to a proper application of these useful filters do indeed obtain.

Carazzone et al. (1985) showed that charge-modified nylon membranes removed bacterial endotoxins from solutions with an efficiency that depended upon the composition of the liquid. The endotoxins used were extracted from *Escherichia coli* 055:B5. The removed bacterial endotoxins were firmly adsorbed. They were not released during continuation of the filtration process. However, the charged nylon filters exhibited a finite adsorption capacity. The bacterial endotoxins removal efficiency decreased with the successive aliquots being filtered. In the case of deionized water containing bacterial endotoxins concentrations comparable to 12 nanograms of *E. coli* endotoxin, the adsorptive removal can be complete (depending upon the filter). With 5% glucose solutions, bacterial endotoxins removal was not interfered with. However, 0.9% sodium chloride solution containing the same bacterial endotoxins concentrations was not depyrogenated to any extent by these charge-modified nylon membranes. Similarly, the presence of 2% peptone solutions at either pH 3.8 or 8.3 inhibited the removal of endotoxin from solutions by the charged nylon filters.

Using 1-liter aliquots of *Serratia marcescens* suspensions containing 1×10^7 cfu/mL, filtered through 47 millimeter (mm) disk filters (15.9 cm^2 effective filtration area) at 6 to 10 psig (0.4 to 0.7 bar), Carazzone et al. (1985) found that organism retention was decidedly higher for positively charge-modified nylon

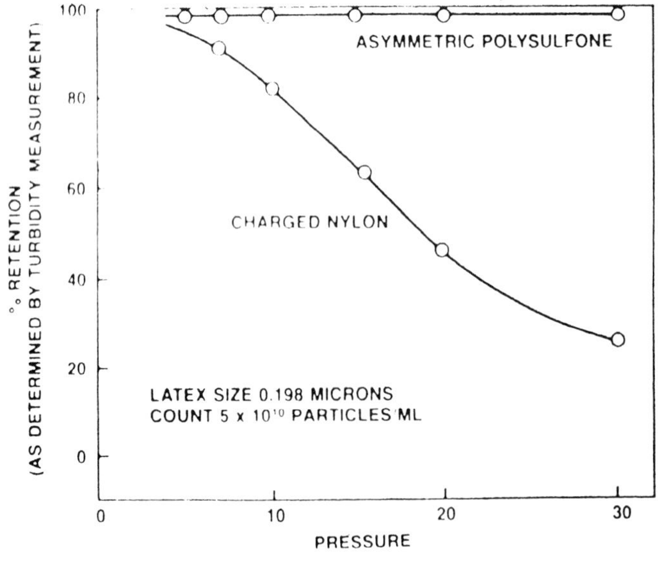

Figure 5-7. Retention by charge-modified membranes.
Pall and Kirnbauer (1978).

filters than it was for conventional mixed esters of cellulose membranes of equal pore-size ratings. Moreover, as in the case of endotoxin removal, the presence of electrolyte or of peptone almost totally reduced the efficiency of organism removal by the charge-modified membranes. The protein was seen as competing with the *Serratia marcescens* for the adsorptive sites and as successfully preempting them. (Van Doorne 1993).

There is another limitation to charge-modified filters, useful as they are. The filter efficiency is dependent upon the fluid flow velocity (Figure 5-7). At lower rates of flow there is enough time for the particles to encounter the charge-modified (quaternary amine) sites, and to become adsorptively arrested. The rates of flow can be so high, however, that the charged sites become swamped by the high number of particles confronting them per unit of time. The result is a decrease in the efficiency of these filters. By the same token, the filter efficiency can vary inversely with the particle density level.

Despite their limitations, as has been said, charge-modified filters find dependable application in bacterial endotoxin removal in pharmaceutical filtrations (Blanden et al., 1991), and for colloid removal in semiconductor rinsewater preparation, often in the polishing loops. As stated on page 579, charge-modified filters are used as prefilters for distillation operations to remove, or reduce to acceptable levels, the bacterial endotoxins that may be present in the still feeds.

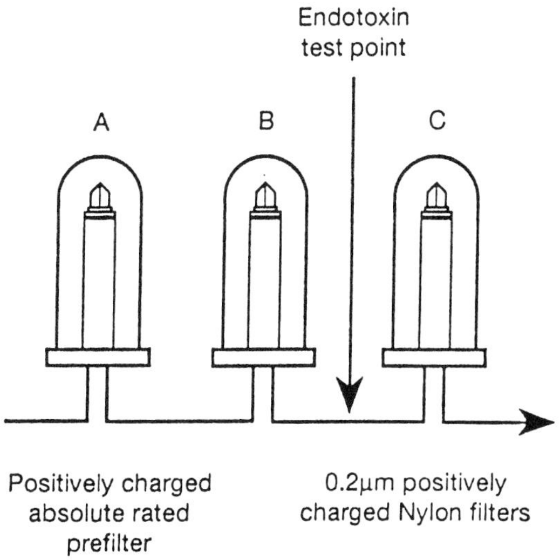

Figure 5-8. Filter arrangement.
Wickert (1993), Courtesy, *Pharmaceutical Engineering.*

Because the eventual saturation of the positive-charge sites by the filter-retained endotoxin does not overtly signal filter disfunction for such further removals, it becomes necessary to ensure that additional lipopolysaccharide does not escape capture. Wickert (1993) discusses how this can be done. An arrangement is made of two charge-modified filters in series, separated by a testing part, as shown in Figure 5-8. When assaying, as by LAL testing, indicates an exhaustion of the upstream filter, that filter is discarded. It is replaced by the downstream filter, which in turn is substituted for by a new charge-modified filter. In this manner, by timely testing, the second charge-modified filter in the series ensures the capture of whatever lipopolysaccharide may have permeated the first filter. Such filter removal is practiced as often as is necessary during the purification process.

Martin (1995) illustrated that at least one particular charge-modified nylon membrane showned no detectable effect of temperature upon the removal capacity for endotoxin from *E. coli* within the range of 4 to greater than 60 °C. The endotoxin removal capacity remained unimpaired as well by pH changes of 4 to 10. Only below pH 3 did the binding capacity becomne weaker, the result of approaching the 1.8 to 2.0 isoelectric point of the endotoxin (Figure 5-9). Increasing flow rate, as expected, did cause a decline in adsorptive endotoxin removal. The charge-modified membrane examined exhibited an endotoxin breakthrough level of 0.125 EU/mL at flowrates of 6 L/min. However, substantial bacterial endotoxin removal took place even at flowrates of 10 L/min.

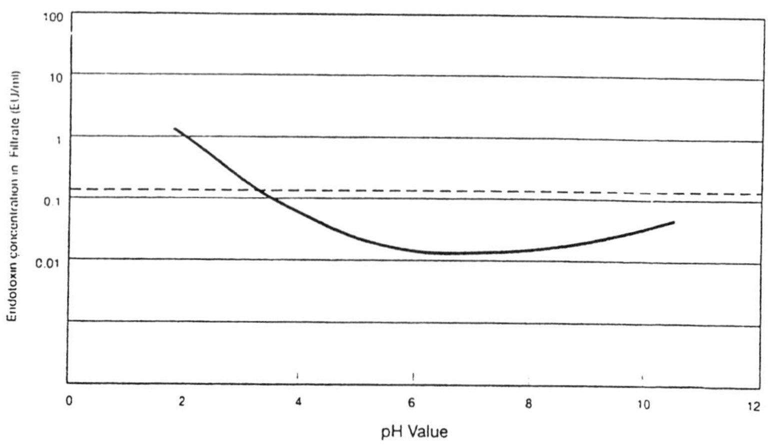

Figure 5-9. Effect of pH on purified (LP5) endotoxin removal capacity of Pall 0.2-µm-rated (NFZ grade) N_{66} Posidyne filters.

(Figure 5-10). The suitability of such charge-modified filters for the removal and reduction of the endotoxin contents of water is demonstrated thereby.

Track-Etch Membranes

Track-etch membranes are unique in their pore geometrics. For their manufacture, thin polymeric films are bombarded by high-energy particles. The polymer is damaged along the bombardment track so that exposure to a caustic solution results in a pore being etched through the polymer film. The resulting pore is of a straight-through columnar shape whose diameter is a function of the etching line. This pore shape is distinct among filters and can be precisely measured under the scanning electron microscope. Although the manufacturers dispute this, it is generally held that in an effort to produce a high density of pores (that is, a large total porosity or pore volume) there is caused an overlapping of pore paths. Double or even multiple hits produce occasional larger pores. Of unpredictable occurrence, they compromise the dependability of retention of the track-etch membranes (see Figure 5-11). (Alkan and Groves 1978, Pall 1975, Wallhäusser 1977, and Stamm 1971).

Several manufacturers furnish filters of this type. Utilized are 1-mil (thousandth of an inch thickness) films of polycarbonate or of Mylar (a DuPont polyester) that have been bombarded by high-energy particles from a nuclear reactor. A process of French origin employs high-energy krypton ions to effect the same result (albeit, it is claimed, a somewhat higher total porosity). The total porosity of about 15% is generally not sufficient to give a filter of high flux. However, the thinness of the membrane enables cartridges to contain enough effective surface area to impart adequate flowrates to these filter devices.

Traditionally, track-etch filters have not been amenable to integrity testing, which has precluded their use in critical pharmaceutical processing. Recently, there have been promising improvements in this regard.

Alone among all the microporous membranes

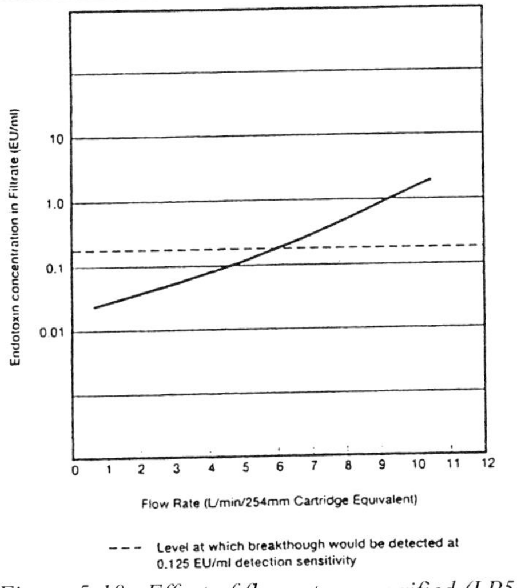

Figure 5-10. Effect of flowrate on purified (LP5) endotoxin removal capacity of Pall 0.2-µm-rated (NFZ grade) N_{66} Posidyne filters.

of commerce, the track-etch filters have pores whose dimensions can be measured directly and unambiguously, albeit under a scanning electron microscope. They may have the narrowest pore-size distribution of all membranes. This property is generally regarded as better ensuring the retention of particles larger than the filter's pore-size rating. However, by the same token, it is lacking in the surety of retention for smaller particles.

The unique straight-through columnar pores offer less wall surface for adsorptive particle arrests than do the more conventional microporous membranes with their particle-trapping tortuous passageways. However, the track-etch filters are successfully used in electronic rinsewater applications. Possibly because they are manufactured from preformed polymeric film, these are clean filters. Newly installed, they rinse up to acceptable resistivity levels using minimum flush volumes at least partly because of thin, straight columnar pores that predispose them to free drainage. In at least one study, filters of this type were found to shed very little when used in rinsewater contexts (Meltzer, 1987f).

Stretched PTFE Membranes

Polytetrafluoroethylene (PTFE) polymer is best known by the DuPont trademark name Teflon. Aside from its carbon-carbon backbone linkages, it consists essentially solely of carbon-to-fluorine bonds. These are very stable chemically. The polymer is thus chemically inert to an exceptional degree. This suits the microporous membranes made of it for use with aggressive solvents. The polymer is hydrophobic, difficult to become wetted by water. This makes its microporous filters advantageous to use as air filters, given the relative ease with which water, accidentally condensed or intruded therein, can be expelled.

Microporous PTFE membranes can be manufactured from extruded films of PTFE by a stretching process. The resulting structure, as seen under a scanning electron microscope, consists of slits among separated strands of PTFE that are periodically bound together at nodules (Figure 5-12). The pore sizes of these microporous PTFE membranes become defined by the degree of stretch to which the PTFE film is subjected. It should be noted, however, that their pore shapes and ratings are different from those of conventional microporous filters, and that this may have unusual implications for particle and organism retentions.

PTFE filters are widely used in pharmaceuticals as sterilizing vent filters because of their hydrophobicity; and as filters for aggressive solvents, as in antibiotic manufacture, because of their chemical imperviousness. Their chemical inertness also suits them for the filtration of very reactive reagents and oxidants in semiconductor applications. Because of their resistivity to ozone (Meltzer, 1989), it has been advocated that they may be used for the filtration of water containing ozone, with the filters rendered hydrophilic by the mediation of an aqueous alcoholic prerinse. The alcohol (TOC) is then to be gotten rid of by aqueous flushing. The high cost of PTFE or "all-Teflon" filters tends their use

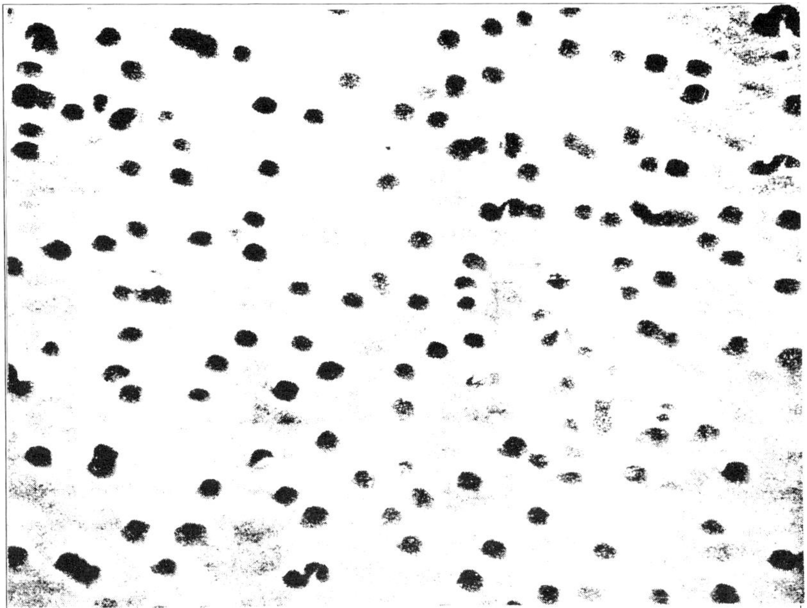

Figure 5-11. Track-etch polycarbonate membrane; overlapping pores.
Meltzer (1987b); Courtesy, Nuclepore Corp.

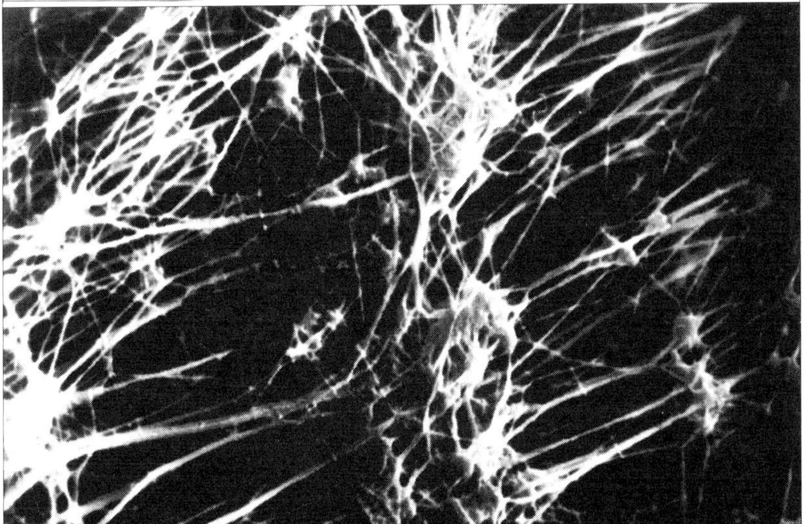

Figure 5-12. Microporous PTFE membrane seen under a scanning electron microscope.
Meltzer (1987b); Courtesy, W.L. Gore and Associates, Inc.

A third procedure involves disconnecting the vent-filter housing from the tank and steaming each component separately. This is done where large tanks are involved, and where the volume of steam exceeds the capacity of the vent filter. Aseptic connection is then made.

It is also possible to steam the tank and its connected vent filter individually using bypass techniques.

Because steam passage through the vent filters, as well as the airflow, can be in either direction, the filters must be so constructed as to withstand a full and adequate pressure in either direction of flow. A robust construction is required. The level of the pressure resistance of which the filter is capable should clearly be stipulated by the filter manufacturer.

Liquid can intrude into the vent filters by splashing, or by the overfilling of tanks, as when level controls fail. Condensate may also form from the vapors of heated solutions. For these reasons it is prudent to mount the vent filter at the highest point of the tank.

Cole (1977) pointed out that after steam flow to the tank has ceased, internal cooling and simultaneous steam condensation occur within the tank. The cooling causes the normal thermal contraction in the volume of the air that is present—a diminution of about one-half to one-third the volume. However, the steam volume decreases most dramatically during its condensation to liquid water. The change of state for the water molecules from gas to liquid at 100 °C, as roughly calculated from the ideal gas law, $PV = nRT$, where the gas constant, $R = 0.08$ liter-atm/deg mol, shows that approximately 32 L of steam contract in volume to 18 mL of water. A vacuum results. If the tank is not strong enough to withstand the negative pressure, it will collapse unless air enters the tank readily enough through the vent filters to eliminate the vacuum, whether partial or otherwise. Figure 5-29 from Cole (1977) permits the approximation of the airflow in cubic feet per minute required per square foot of vessel surface to compensate for the steam condensation, provided one knows the temperature difference between the steam and the ambient air, the thickness of the vessel's insulation, and its location (indoors or out). Such knowledge permits sizing the vent filter to accommodate the needed inward rush of air to prevent tank collapse.

Sizing of Vent Filters

It is generally not a problem to size a vent filter for the amount and rate of air passage required by the liquid addition to or drainage from a storage tank. The service air required by antibiotic fermentors is another matter. Hundreds of standard cubic feet per minute of air may be required. An antibiotic installation in Italy utilizes a special housing containing 105 ten-inch (24.9-cm) cartridges in parallel to furnish the needed filtered air at low pressure drops.

Where vent filters on tanks are concerned, the critical sizing operation involves the inflow of air into a tank, occasioned by its cooling down after being steam sterilized. An insufficient flow, caused by too rapid a cooling, could cause collapse of the tank. The rate of cooling is influenced by factors such as the tank dimensions, its wall thickness, whether or not it is insulated, and the ambient temperature. To size vent filters for such applications requires the services of an experienced professional. Conway (1984) presented a study of vent sizing/tank-cooling considerations.

Given the costly damage of a tank collapse, the use of rupture disks seems proper and prudent. Such a disk can be equipped with a sensor wire so that its rupture would simultaneously signal an alarm. To avoid the costly occurrence of tank collapse, most vent filters are generously oversized.

Exhaust gases emanating from fermentations and being vented may be at temperatures of 80 or 85 °C. They usually contain aerosolized vapors. To minimize their watery content, demisters are used, then coalescers (usually composed of knitted metal yarn meshes). On occasion, cyclone separators and catch tanks are used to remove entrained water. These devices are followed by the membrane filters intended to prevent the passage of organisms to the outside environment. The membrane filters should be capable of withstanding oxidations at 85 °C.

Definitions

Usage has given a strong identity to certain terms and definitions. Thus, *depth-type filters*, *nominal ratings*, and *prefilters* all have a similar context. *Final filters*, *surface retention*, and *absolute ratings* have a commonality, but one that is different from the first group.

Depth-type filters. Because of the technology of their manufacture, these filters are characterized by a broad pore-size distribution. Therefore, many particles find pores large enough to enter, and penetrate into the depth of the filter before being retained, often by adsorptive particle arrests. Because the vast internal surfaces of the depth filter are used to trap particles, these filters have high particle-holding capacities.

Nominal ratings. While depth-type filters can be rated by an ability to retain a certain high percentage of some arbitrarily selected particles, the broad pore-size distribution renders it unlikely that 100% of that particle will be retained. Furthermore, the retention rating is heavily dependent upon the type of particle, its particle-size distribution, the particle load, the polarity of the suspending liquid, its viscosity, its temperature, and above all, the differential pressure. The rating assigned is, therefore, of very limited significance, if any, and is referred to as *nominal*.

Prefiltration. The lack of precise numerical definition to prefilter ratings is not a result of technical neglect or inability to cope. Depth-type filters are largely utilized as prefilters, instruments whose purpose it is to spare the final filter by the removal of some inexact portion of the particulate burden. The service life of the final filter is prolonged by sacrificing the prefilter. How much of the particulate load is best removed by the prefilter has to be determined in each case by actual trial and error. What is sought is the longest service life possible for the combination of prefilter/final filter. The prefilter can remove too much of the burden, thereby unduly shortening its own life. Or it can remove too little, thus abbreviating the life of the final filter. Prefilter ratings can do little to help predict the outcome. Hence nominal ratings, however unenlightening, serve well enough.

From the foregoing the identity among the terms *depth-type filters*, *prefilters*, and *nominal ratings* becomes evident.

Final filters. Final filters are used to remove, to reliable extents, the objectionable viable and nonviable particulate matter from pharmaceutical preparations. The narrow pore-size distributions of membrane filters suit them for this purpose, as attested to by ample experience. Filtration sterilizations are a particularly critical example of such a final filter function. Because the pore sizes of the final filter obviously govern its performance, their constancy over the entire duration of the filtration process requires being validated by before-and-after integrity testing.

Surface retention. Early on there was confusion concerning the reliability of membrane filters and the regularity of their pore structures. It was assumed that particles could not permeate pores because they were too large to enter the pores. Surface retention, therefore, had to be their mode or position of restraint. It is now known that membrane pores are not so regular. The particle-arresting pore restriction can be within the body of the membrane, thin as it is. This is particularly true for the anisotropic filters.

Nevertheless, the term *surface retention* is used in conjunction with membrane or final filtrations. It still often implies, incorrectly, an arrest of particles by membranes based exclusively upon sieve-type retentions, as distinct from the adsorptive captures within the interior of depth-type filters. The phrase *surface retention* also implies therefore, possibly incorrectly, a consequence of absolute retention to the use of membrane filters in pharmaceutical operations.

Absolute retentions. To the uninitiated, *absoluteness* means that the mere use of microporous membranes assures the removal of all microorganisms, or at least those larger than the filter's pore-size rating. At a somewhat more sophisticated level of comprehension, *absoluteness* implies a degree of filter efficiency, independent of the operational conditions of the filtration. The latter situation holds, however, only when the smallest particle of the particle-size distribution is larger than the largest pore of the pore-size distribution. In such cases, all the particles are sieve-retained by the filter, and such operational conditions as the number of particles, the differential pressure, and the characteristics of the suspending fluids have no effect on the completeness of the particle retention (the filter efficiency). Where, however, particles are small enough to enter and permeate the filter pores, the completeness of their removal does indeed depend upon the operating conditions of the filtration.

The term *absoluteness*, therefore, does not refer to an inherent property of filters. Rather it reflects the particle-size/pore-size distributions relationship present in any given filtration context.

Of course, given the finite size of any filter's largest pores, it is possible to stipulate a particle size that will be too large to permeate a membrane, even a depth-type filter of broader pore-size distribution. It is, therefore, possible to define a given filter as being *absolute* at a given dimensional rating. Such ratings may even have utilitarian purposes. They should not be permitted to cloud the issues of particle-size and pore-size distributions, which are seldom if ever known; and the contributions of particle and pore shapes, which are almost never known. Above all, the word *absolute* in conjunction with filters, membrane or otherwise, should not be permitted to suggest that validation of the filtrative exercise is not essential, at least in pharmaceutical usage.

There is no industry standard for rating membrane filters. There are, however, certain retention standards that, whether based on spherical latex particle or on organism retentions, bring some degree of order to the practice. This is lacking in the case of the depth-type filters. So much depends upon the types of particles used, the liquid vehicle employed, the particular operational parameters, and especially the testing protocol (as whether single or multipass), that the ratings are usually called *nominal*. Actually, the term *nominal* is extremely uncertain in its implications. It can come to mean whatever the filter manufacturer may want it to mean (Johnston, 1990).

For this reason, when one manufacturer's depth-type filter, say of a 1- to 20-μm rating, is being substituted for by the product of another, it may well be found that the pore-size ratings and functionalities do not correspond. Trial and error are necessary to effect such substitutions.

Particle Shedding by Filters

Since microporous membranes are not constructed of bits and pieces of polymer but are produced by the reverse-phase process in continuous film form, they have not been suspected of giving rise to fibers. Studies reveal, however, that such filters may indeed give rise to particles.

The very filters employed to retain the particles are, in themselves, to some extent the source of particulate matter. A distinction is here made between the downstream particle that escapes the filter action uncaptured, and the particle released from the filter structure itself. The shed particle could have been set free from the filter by the flow of the permeating liquid stream, as debris by a cleansing action. Conceivably, particles could also result from the deterioration of given filters as could be occasioned by the unsuitability of the filter medium for the application: a classical case of filter/fluid incompatibility.

With the exception of a notable paper by Krygier (1986), the published conclusions of most studies, whether correct or not, seem partisan. "The best filter" turned out to be the one being commercialized by the sponsoring laboratory (Hall, 1984a and 1984b; Grant et al., 1986). Importantly, one of these studies lacked background controls, and neither was based on statistical data involving replicates.

Particle shedding by filters, like filter efficiency, is not invariant. It too reflects the influences of the test parameters: the rates of fluid flow, the temperature ambiance, differential pressure levels. The particle counts themselves may reflect the noise level of the measurement as influenced by the rate of liquid flow through the instrument. Transient but hard-to-detect pump vibrations, electrical interferences (despite the use of "isolators"), and the very real influence of cartridge-to-cartridge variability, all also influence the particle counts. This latter point grows in importance when one imposes intrabatch filter variability upon interbatch variances.

Given the strong influences of the experimental test design upon the resulting particle counts, it can be questioned whether arbitrarily selected measurement conditions have other than arbitrary significances when directly comparing one filter type to another by way of comparative particle counting in test stands.

The proven utility of particle counters speaks for itself. The instruments are highly reliable when correctly employed, and the results they yield are correspondingly dependable (Krygier et al., 1985). As with all measurement devices, however, their findings reflect the influences of the test parameters. The interpretation of the results, especially in complex situations, may have validity only within the defined limits of the experimental design. Filter evaluations, whether on the basis of the counting of shed particles or otherwise, offer such complexities.

It is generally recognized, for example, that the measure of filter efficiency in terms of particle retention may be influenced importantly by the size and shape of the particle; its population density; the applied differential pressure; and very likely the nature of the fluid in terms of its pH, viscosity, temperature, and chemical makeup.

Particle shedding by a filter is only one measure of its performance. Particle retention, the reason for using the filter in the first place, is perhaps of greater importance. It is indeed conceivable that the filter that sheds more may better retain particles, to yield, on balance, a smaller downstream particle population.

A study was reported wherein four cartridges were investigated by particle counting and SEM examinations for their particle-shedding propensitites. The results were evaluated statistically using a Student's t-test. Confidence levels of greater than 99% were considered as being necessary to establish implicitly a statistical differentiation (Meltzer, 1987f).

The study established that variability among cartridges, at least of the filter brands examined in quadruplicate samples, was too large to permit differentiation to be made on the basis of particle shedding. Moreover, the sample size necessary for a statistical differentiation is probably too large for practical testing, especially if lot-to-lot variations are to be considered.

- All the filter specimens of each of the four filter types examined shed particles, and continued to shed particles throughout the duration of the test.
- Pulsing of the cartridge filters accelerated the rate and/or extent of shedding, and hence presumably can accelerate filter cleansing.
- On the basis of four samples for each filter type, no statistically valid differentiation based on shedding could be made among the filter types tested.
- To attempt to compare filter types on the basis of single samples is inappropriate.

However stated, to date no statistically valid differentiation among cartridge filter types has been established in any study on the basis of particle counting.

The purpose of filtration is to remove particles. On the basis of this action, differentiation among commercially available cartridges seems possible. As things presently stand, the utilitarian focus should not be on shedding, but on particle retention: a reduction in the number of particles downstream of the filter.

In a study relating to the preparation of high-purity water intended for high-performance liquid chromatography work, it was found that the particle counts of samples of deionized and distilled feedstock water were actually increased (fourfold) by filtration through microporous membrane filters. Particle counting and size analysis were performed by measurement of the angular scattering of laser light, as occasioned by its encountering interfering particles present in the water through which it was directed. Significantly, the relative volumes of particles, as obtained by addition of all particles within a given size range and the summing of the total of all the size ranges, was essentially the same regardless of the pore-size rating of the membrane used, whether 0.22 (0.2) µm-rated or 0.45-µm-rated. Interestingly, the results were essentially the same for each of four brands of membranes tested. The data are shown in Table 5-3. The implications of this study are clear. The subject particles are seen as arising from the shedding of the membrane filters, not from particulate matter unrestrained from passage through the filters (Decedue and Unruh, 1984).

Nowadays, particle shedding is quoted in filter validation guides. Filters should, in any case, be flushed before being committed to use.

The threat posed by particles in injectables has already been remarked upon. Often the particles shed by filters are spherical in shape. Smolders (1979) saw the phenomenon as being caused by the precipitation of polymer from very dilute solution, and presented scanning electron micrographs of such spheres generated in cellulose triacetate membrane formation. The prohibition against fibers in pharmaceuticals defines *fibers* as particles having an aspect ratio of at least 3 to 1, length as related to width. It would be ironic indeed if spheres were judged, on account of the 1-to-1 aspect ratios of their sphericity, not to be fibers.

To avoid such fiber release it is necessary to rinse such filters with an aqueous medium prior to product filtration. Alternatively, product can be filtered through the membrane to wash adhered dust particles from the membrane's downstream surfaces. The filtrate resulting from the product rinse can then be recirculated through the filter to free it of the entrained dust particles; or the first portions of filtrate (where feasible), can be discarded, or can be segregated to be refiltered with other product batches. The point being made is that microporous membrane filters may not, on account of their nonfibrous construction, be considered as necessarily exempt from the possibilities of being fiber-releasing.

Prerinsing the downstream side of small filters used in conjunction with syringe injections should also be made to avoid introduction of particles into the body, as in intrathecal injections into the subarachnoid space around the spinal cord between the fourth and fifth vertebrae, between the top of the spinal column and the base of the brain.

Possible Impurities

Microporous membranes potentially contain extractables, some more than others. These are most often residuals from the casting operation or are surface-active agents or other compounds added to the membrane to ensure its wettability by water. Promotional statements that such wetting aids are permanently anchored, fixed, or chemically grafted to the membrane may not always be accurate.

Acrylates and methacrylates, polar compounds capable of being grafted due to their vinyl unsaturation, are often joined chemically to membrane surfaces to render them hydrophilic. One filter manufacturer uses hydroxypropyl acrylate and tetraethylene glycol diacrylate for this purpose. However, homopolymers also form, to be available as extractables.

During steam sterilization certain nylons may undergo thermal depolymerization by a "zipping action" to generate small quantities of soluble polyamides.

Technologies for fabrication of these filters may introduce into their finished polymeric constructions solvent residues, pore-formers, quench-bath components, stabilizers, and/or processing aids. These may yield organic extractables during the service life of the filters, albeit perhaps at acceptably low diffusion-governed concentrations.

Most of the filter types used, including microporous, RO, and UF membranes, are manufactured by the reverse-phase process (Meltzer, 1987b). This consists of dissolving the constituent polymer in solvent(s) or cosolvents; frequently of modifying the resulting degree of solvency by the measured addition of an appropriate nonsolvent; followed by the subsequent exposure of the cast composition to a quenching or gelling solution consisting essentially of nonsolvent(s). To be sure, the membrane resulting after a succession of processing steps is usually subjected to the cleansing action of water extraction baths. Nevertheless, opportunity exists for avid retention of the organic solvents and nonsolvents within the membrane polymer. Their removal is usually dependent upon concentration-gradient driven diffusions. In such operations, time for diffusion is an important factor, and the rate of diffusion decreases with time as the concentration decreases. Complete organic removal is approached asymptotically. The quantity extracted and measured becomes defined by the duration of the extraction time as diluted by the extraction volume.

In applicational contexts where longer time intervals are involved larger quantities of extractables may manifest themselves, albeit at the dilute concentrations dictated by the quantities of water flowed through the filter per unit of time. Dilute or not, such extractables serve inevitably as sources of TOC.

Different polymers require different solvent and nonsolvent systems to become converted into membranes. Most of the processes are proprietary, but the relevant patent literature often discloses useful details.

According to patent sources, nylon (polyamide) membranes may involve the use of such solvents as formic acid or methyl formate and, in addition to water, may require the use of methanol nonsolvent.

Cellulose acetates (and their blends) may depend upon acetone, with or without dioxane, as solvent; or upon formamide. Polysulfone may require the solvating action of dimethylformamide. Polyvinylidene fluoride (PVDF) polymers, according to the patent literature, may be brought into solution by acetone or by dimethyl acetimide. Acetone and water or water alone serves in the forming or quenching bath.

It may bear repeating that the processing of the membrane filters subsequent to their formation does not in itself guarantee freedom from extractables; neither does the use of low-boiling materials such as of acetone or methanol. Dilute solutions, even of volatile materials, in high-molecular polymers exhibit low vapor pressures, rendering more difficult the removal of such substances.

In the manufacture of microporous PTFE, a lubricating agent that is a petroleum solvent (e.g., kerosene or naphtha) is added to the finely divided resin at the preforming stage. The resin and lubricant are formed into a billet, which is extruded through a die and calendered into a tape. The tape is then stretched in a controlled manner into a thin membrane, the rate of stretch being important; and is sintered (i.e., taken above its melting point, T_m, which is approximately 340 °C). The lubricant is removed by evaporation either before or after stretching. The presence of the lubricant may show itself in differential scanning calorimetry as an obvious peak at approximately 224 °C. The finished microporous PTFE membrane is of course intended to be free of the lubricant.

The availability of extractables from the track-etch membranes is less apparent, the membrane source being finished polycarbonate or polyester film. Films that are track-etched may contain process aids. Also, the etching process itself may be productive of TOC extractables.

Wetting Adjuncts

The desire for water-wettable filters necessitates the filter manufacturer's use of wetting adjuncts, with few if any exceptions. It is true that one nylon 66 filter manufacturer claims his product to be inherently hydrophilic. The relevant patent ascribes the "inherent" hydrophilicity to be caused by a favorable molecular arrangement of amide groups. This is said to have been made possible by the manufacturing manipulations covered by the patent. Be that as it may, no structural measurements are offered in support of the hypothesis. One could speculate that polyamide polymer may become wettable because it undergoes surface hydrolysis by the formic acid used in its preparation to yield hydrophilic amine and carboxylic acid moieties. Other explanations may be offered as well.

There is on the market a nylon 6 membrane that is formulated with polyethylene glycol (PEG) to enhance its handling properties. Interestingly, PEG serves, at least in other contexts, as a wetting agent for membranes. One inventor advocated PEG as a wetting adjunct in the production of PVDF membranes. The use was of high-molecular-weight PEGs; these are relatively insoluble in water, and are applied from alcoholic solutions. Water extractability, however, is not a quantum phenomenon. It manifests itself as differences in extents, not in kind. The patent literature also reveals that membranes may rely for their wettability upon the use of monofatty esters (e.g., palmitic) of polyethylene glycol. These also may be applied from their alcoholic solutions. Once applied, they are said to be water-insoluble, hence inextractable by water.

One particular PVDF membrane manufacturer claims to have converted its product to a hydrophilic nature by a grafting process involving the amino acid glycine. The term *grafting* is usually taken to mean a fixed joining to a surface, as through the creation of a chemical bond. The implication of the term is a permanent, nonextractable union of hydrophilic graft overlaying hydrophobic structure. The actual details of the subject manufacturer's process are proprietary. Another patent describes membranes composed of blends of PVDF and vinyl acetate. The latter component when hydrolyzed would yield polyvinyl alcohol, hydrophilic on account of its hydroxyl groups, presumably in sufficient quantity to render the entire polymer blend water-wettable. In any case, grafted membranes are not necessarily exempt from liberating extractables upon aqueous contacts (Meltzer, 1989b).

Among the water-extractable wetting adjuncts utilized by membrane manufacturers, the following are common: various ethylene oxide and/or propylene oxide adducts, such as Triton X-100 and similar nonionic surfactants; and ethylene oxide adducts to celluloses, such as the Klucels forthcoming from the Hercules Company, the Pluronic products of Wyandotte Chemical, and similar polyethoxylated substances. The widespread use of polyethylene glycols or of their polypropylene glycol counterparts has already been alluded to. Polyvinylpyrrolidone (PVP) is also widely used as a wetting adjunct. Glycerin and ethylene glycol also serve to reduce surface tension. Finally, the polar residues of the membrane casting and forming solutions present in the filters incline them to be hydrophilic.

TOC of extractables may find their genesis from any or all of the sources just referred to. Being organic entities, they are susceptible, with differing propensities, to oxidative alterations and degradations. All would be subject to attack by ozone.

Filter manufacturers copiously preflush cartridges with water having a resistivity of 18 megohm-cm to meet the needs of the semiconductor rinsewater market. All should be called upon to do as well for pharmaceutical applications regarding extractables. The standard for prerinsing, whether by user or manufacturer, should be by way of TOC measurements. Nor should performance of the USP toxicity tests serve to obviate the extractables test. These may or may not be adequate. The wetting agents used are often secret, and their means of grafting or anchoring are usually proprietary. The USP toxicity tests may or may not be enough. Even if the sensitivity of the Ames test were to be employed, the potential threat of unknown extractables should be eliminated by a preflush protocol.

Filter users are normally called upon to perform some kind of aqueous

Table 5-3
Relative Volume of Particles in Filtered Water

Size Class	*Unfiltered Feedstock*	*Filtered 0.22 μm*	*Filtered 0.45 μm*
0.39	—	—	294.26
0.45	—	305.62	—
0.53	47.49	—	—
0.76	11.64	—	164.77
0.91	—	112.20	—
1.21	60.52	—	—
1.51	—	80.88	94.42
2.11	—	26.24	37.49
2.87	8.84	51.06	26.04
Total relative volume	134.49	576.00	616.98

Decedue and Unruh (1984); Courtesy, *Biotechnics*

prerinse to ready the filter for its integrity testing. Such prerinses for the removal of organic extractables, while not required by regulations, will serve to dispose the filter towards a more advantageous performance without unduly burdening the filter user. The absence of an officially published Good Manufacturing Practice should not serve as a bar to consensus action based on common sense.

Extractables

Certain filter manufacturers have investigated the potential for extractables with great thoroughness, examining not just the membrane but also the other components of the filter construction. This suits the present requirements of the FDA investigators who are interested in the extractables forthcoming even from the O-rings. Long-term, the extractables will have to be specifically identified. Currently, the effort is being made by a series of different techniques but is often still at the mg/L measurement stage. However, useful information is also gleaned from reverse-phase high-performance liquid chromatography and by Fourier transform infrared spectroscopy. Heavy reliance is placed upon static soak techniques wherein the filter or components are imprisoned within a volume of extracting liquid at an elevated temperature or periods of time sufficient to complete the diffusive migration of the extractant from the polymeric material into the liquid medium. The static soak technique seems presently to satisfy FDA investigators. However, such extractions are concentration-gradient limited. Procedures involving Soxhlet extractions wherein fresh extracting fluid (solvent) encounters the polymer being extracted could possible offer a more thorough treatment. Present techniques seem adequate, however.

It would be ideal if in each case the the extractables study were conducted using as the liquid the specific drug preparation of interest. That proves to be impossible, however. Despite the fact that most drug formulations, some 80%, are primarily aqueous, the low concentrations of extractables relative to the high concentration of drug components frustrate analytical evaluations. In the event, "worst case" extraction studies were performed based upon a series of extraction solutions or solvents. In a study entitled a model stream approach, Stone et al (1994) utilized water, pH 2.0 HCl, pH 12.5 NaOH, 20% NaCl, 0.1 Tween (surfactant), and 100% denatured alcohol to elute extractables from a filter device. The extractables were analyzed gravimetrically as non-volatile residues, as TOC, by Fourier transform infrared spectroscopy, and by reverse-phase high-performance chromatography. What is of importance is that no significant extractables were seen in any of the extraction studies.

At the present time, extractable studies are not joined to toxicological testing. The latter still, rely largely upon the USP Class VI tests. The USP General Mouse Safety test, various cytotoxicity tests, and the Ames mutagenic test are also available for this purpose.

One filter manufacturer has investigated the subject of extractables for his product by determining the non-volatile residues (NVR) obtained using a wide spectrum of pure solvents. (See Table 5-4.) The NVRs secured using separately both water and 95% alcohol were analyzed using Fourier Transform Infrared Spectroscopy. Low molecular weight oligomers of nylon and polyethylene terephthalate polymers were identified. The NVR extractables passed the USP Class VI tests for biological safety. The quantities of extractables were "extremely low"; too low to permit their quantitation in the presence of the ingredients present in actual pharmaceutical preparations. Therefore, extractable studies using the modeling solvents approach provides a useful means of investigation. The data in Table 5-4 provides suitable guidance (Pall).

Reif et al (1996) performed a comparative study of competitive filters and prefilters on the market. Commendably, the rival filter manufacturers were not identified, signaling a responsible technical investigation rather than a market oriented exercise. The study identified the sources of filter-device extractables, e. g. membranes, drainage layers, O-rings, cap, core and supports. It discussed the various methods available for extract analysis and critiqued their advantages and limitations. An apparatus suitable for extraction studies was devised (Figure 5-13). It was employed in conjunction with water and ethanol.

Using gas chromatography, mass spectroscopy, and particularly reverse phase chromatography, the extractables from each of the four competitive filter types examined were found to be so minimal in quantity as to be influenced by extractables migrating from the wrappings used to package the filters themselves. (Reif et al. 1997).

Grow-Through

Unlike nonviable particles, organisms collected on a membrane can continue to grow and flourish as a function of time, perhaps to be found eventually on the other side of the filter. This can occur when the liquid flow is ongoing, as in dynamic water system applications, or during static periods when there is no flow but the filter is still wet in place. Though not all filters are susceptible, there is no disputing the phenomenon of the possible penetration of the filter as a function of time. This is usually referred to as *grow-through*. Some decry the use of the term *grow-through* and prefer *pass-through* or *penetration*. Filter structural differences and utilitarian implications are intended in these distinctions.

The condition is one in which filters, even those that can sustain 1 x 10^7 *Pseudomonas diminuta* ATCC-19146 and greater, may exhibit organism penetration in time. To rationalize the appearance of organisms downstream from a membrane presumably impervious to their filtrative passage, it is conjectured that the organism penetrates as it multiplies, and that this differs from ordinary organism pass-through or carry-through by the flowing stream. Most organisms divide by binary fission, a process wherein the entire contents of the parent cell are equally partitioned between two daughter cells. Grow-through assumes that in this process the new cells are able to negotiate the pore passageways that are too small to permit passage of the larger parent cells. This explanation supposes that even the largest cells of the membrane's pore size distribution are too small to permit passage of the "normal-sized" microbes, but that the organisms penetrate in their smaller sizes. (Christian and Meltzer 1986).

An opposing view is also held. It is known that microporous membranes possess pore-size distributions, some more extensive than others. It is argued that penetration by organisms occurs only for microporous membranes of wider pore-size distributions. In this view, eventual pass-through of a membrane takes place because the organisms so grow in number that the few larger pores come to be encountered and penetrated. The event is seen to reveal the existence of undesirable larger pores in the filter (wide pore-size distribution). No mysteries of binary fission need be invoked. Membranes of sufficiently narrow pore-size distribution should be exempt from this failing. Narrower pore-size distribution for equal-rated membranes would offer fewer larger pores. This would militate against grow-thorough. Therefore, it is advocated, such filters should be used in long-term applications. As shown by Pall and Kirnbauer (1978), certain nylon 66 membranes have unusually narrow pore-size distributions.

There are cases, however, where membranes of narrow pore-size distribution have been reported to exhibit penetration or grow-through (Howard and Duberstein, 1980).

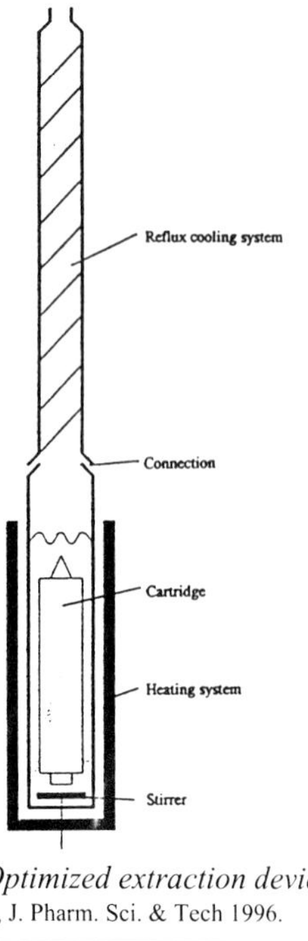

Figure 5-13. Optimized extraction device.
Courtesy, Reif et al, J. Pharm. Sci. & Tech 1996.

The result of grow-through of organisms to the downstream side of the filter is a recontamination of the solution itself, after purification by filtration. Grow-through is not capable of easy experimental standardization. Obviously, the sizes of the organisms and of the filter pores (normally represented as a filter pore-size rating) are important. As discussed, the pore-size distribution should be of influence, although this parameter remains totally unexplored. The inhibitory or stimulatory nature of the suspending liquid, its temperature, and the dynamics of the fluid flow, in addition to the number and types of organisms, all exert an influence on the rate of grow-through. Regarding the sustenance of organisms by the suspending liquid, it is of interest that Gram-negativess can flourish even in distilled water seemingly free of nutrients (Rubow, 1981).

Blow-Through. Wallhäusser (1983b) calls attention to what he names the *blow-through* or *blowgun* effect, a consequence of the grow-through process. During the filtration the bacteria cells collect on the upstream side of the filter. If the filtration process is interrupted, the bacteria proliferate, with some growing from the filter surface into the pores. Some make their way deep into the filter medium. When the filtration system is started up again, bacteria that are in a suitable position will be catapulted by the differential pressure out into the "sterile"

Table 5-4
Non-Volatile Residues Extracted from Autoclaved General Purpose Nylon 66 (ABINRP) Cartridge[a]

Solvent	*NVR(mg)*
acetone	270[c]
acetonitrile	240[c]
ammonium hydroxide	58
benzyl alcohol	290
n-butanol	52
n-butyl acetate	84
dimethyl formamide	263
ethanol, 3A	51
ethanol, absolute	44
ethanol, 50%	69
ethanolamine	264
ethyl acetate	220
ether (diethyl)	35
n-heptane	22
hydrochloric acid 10%	410
isopropyl alcohol	35
methanol	41[b]
methyl isobutyl ketone	180
propylene glycol	155
pyridine	310
water	22
xylene	230

a) 4-Hour reciprocating soak in 1.5 liters of the indicated solvent at room temperature.
b) Slight haze on dilution with water.
c) Haze or precipitate on dilution with water.

downstream side.

In one instance, as the Wallhäusser data show, instead of the customary passage of one to two bacteria per liter through a given filter, 29 per liter occurred after an overnight shutdown and system start-up the next day. Forty minutes later, after a 48-liter throughput, all bacteria were rinsed out and a normal bacterial passage was established. The blow-through effect was noticeably stronger after a system was put in service again after a weekend shutoff. The bacteria count of the first 2-liter sample was greater than 1,000 for the 2 liters. After passing a 58.5-liter rinse, the bacteria passage rate was still greater than 1,000 for 2 liters. That number remained unchanged until after an additional 52.5-liter throughput. After another stagnant period of 24 hours, the system was put in service again. The passage rate was greater than 1,000 for the 2 liters until after a 300-liter rinse.

Even with double-layer filters, long standstill periods contribute to a blow-through effect with bacteria-laden (*P. diminuta*) filters. More than 100 liters of water are necessary to rinse such filters free of bacteria, to become sterile effluent.

With ultrafilters, the tangential flow in normal operations retains bacteria along with the concentrate. With these filters, long stagnant periods followed by start-up also cause blow-through.

Blow-through is more dangerous than grow-through when a system is restarted, since the bacteria within a filter will be ejected into the downstream side. This blowgun effect is influenced by the filter thickness, the size of the filter pores, the differential pressure, and the presence of surface-active substances in the fluid to be filtered. Depending on the filter type and the standing time, an initial rinse may be successful in freeing the filter of bacteria. However, it is difficult to predict the quantity of water and rinse time necessary to accomplish this.

According to Wallhäusser (1983b), the interval for an intermittent system may be markedly reduced with filters grown through and blocked after just a few days. Therefore, intermittent filtration processes also necessitate sanitation after every shutdown to avoid blow-through contamination.

Influence of Pore Size and Organism Size

Leahy and Gabler (1984) tested both 0.22 (0.2) µm-rated and 0.3-µm-rated membranes with *P. diminuta* and with *E. coli* organisms for grow-through propensities. The test equipment consisted of a 47-mm-diameter test filter holder situated between two chambers. The downstream chamber exited by means of valve through a 47-mm analytical filter. The organism-suspending liquid at a challenge level of 10^8 organisms/cm^2 of filter area was passed through the test membrane. Periodically thereafter, soybean casein digest broth was put through the filter. The organism content of the effluent was analyzed for evidence of microbes, an indication that grow-through had occurred. Experimentation was carried out until either the filter clogged or grow-through took place. It was found that grow-through of the 0.22-μm-rated filters by *P. diminuta* took place after about 120 hours; and by *E. coli* after about 360 hours. (*E. coli* are somewhat larger than *P. diminuta*.) In the case of the 0.3-μm-rated membrane under the test conditions used, the grow-through rate for *P. diminuta* was some 24 hours, whereas that for *E. coli* was about 180 hours. As expected, grow-through required less time for the larger-pore-size-rated filter.

Howard and Duberstein (1980) examined the long-term effects (18 days) of the retention by various commercially available filters of organisms smaller than *P. diminuta* naturally occurring in Long Island well waters. They found that while there was variation among the different 0.2-μm-rated brands of filters tested, none was as impervious to grow-through as were the 0.1-μm-rated membranes that were examined. It may be that these findings serve as the basis for the advocacy that 0.1-μm-rated filters should be substituted for their 0.2-μm-rated counterparts where long-term usages involving periodic filter sanitation are involved.

Effect of Membrane Anisotropy

The flow-enhancing qualities of anisotropic filter structures have been discussed, as was the advantage of being thus able to offer tighter filters of greater retentivity than the conventional 0.2-mm-rated membranes without the sacrifice of usual rates of flow.

Simonetti and Schroeder (1985) investigated polysulfone membranes of such anisotropic constructions in both 90-mm-diameter disk and cartridge forms for their grow-through propensities as compared to those of conventional 0.2-μm-rated membrane filters. The *P. diminuta* challenge levels employed were in the neighborhood of 5×10^9 to 1×10^{10} organisms. In the case of the 90-mm-diameter disk filters, after verification of the integrity of the filter, 1 liter of the appropriate *P. diminuta* suspension was directed at the test filter at 50 psig. At periodic intervals, sterile lactose broth was passed through the filter and evaluated for the presence of organisms. In the case of the cartridges, the flowrates were initially set at 8 liters per minute, and were later reduced to 4 liters per minute. A slipstream of the filtrate was periodically assayed for its organism content. The duration of the test was set at a maximum of 10 days or 240 hours.

It was found that, with the exception of certain nylon and PVDF 0.2-μm-rated membranes, the conventional 0.2-μm-rated filters (of polysulfone, polypropylene, or cellulose) as well as the anisotropic polysulfone, resisted *P. diminuta* grow-through for the full 240-hour period. In the case of the 90-mm-diameter disks, some PVDF samples showed grow-through after 48 hours, some after 76, and some after 120 hours. Some nylon disk samples exhibited grow-through after 72 hours. The grow-through resistances of the cartridges manifested differences after a duration of between 48 and 72 hours. In occasional specimens, Simonetti and Schroeder (1984) found that the nylon and the PVDF cartridges did show evidence of grow-through after 72 hours and 48 hours, respectively.

These investigators privately reported that in the case of the anisotropic membranes, organism growth within the pores follows the path of least resistance, growing preferentially upstream toward the larger diameters of the pore passageways. Such a tendency, if generalized in the case of anisotropic membranes, could deflect organism growth from the grow-through tendency that seems inevitable in filters of more conventional isomorphic design.

Effect of Filter Hydrophobicity. Using variations of their techniques, Leahy and Gabler (1984) were able to demonstrate that in the case of air-vent filters, hydrophobicity is a factor that militates against the occurrence of grow-through. In these tests, aerosolized *P. diminuta* suspensions were used to challenge the test filter. It was found that in the case of the cartridges constructed of hydrophobic PVDF, grow-through became manifest only after some 21 days. Hydrophilic cartridges of similar ratings evidenced grow-through in 120 hours. Filter hydrophobicity discourages the permeation and intrusion of a filter by the water that is essential to organism proliferation, and thus serves to inhibit the grow-through phenomenon in air-vent filters.

In most pharmaceutical contexts, the filtrative removal of organisms from solutions seldom requires longer than a 12-hour period. Pyrogenicity is the concern of longer durations. Opinion seems generally inclined to the belief that 0.2-mm-rated membranes in continuous usage exhibit grow-through after 3 days.

Because some membrane filters come to contain flaws, (a possible occurrence in any manufacturing process) it is sometimes assumed that all filters are inevitably subject to grow-through. This is not true (Howard and Duberstein, 1980). However, there is disagreement, often commercially driven, regarding the pore-size ratings that are exempt, on account of their small pore dimensions, from grow-through. The need to integrity-test filters to ascertain their freedom from flaws is self-evident.

Even when a filter does not permit grow-through, its long-term use will permit the passage into its effluent waters of endotoxin arising from its retained Gram-negative organisms. Ultrafilters of 10,000-dalton ratings are usually employed to retain bacterial endotoxin, although as a practical matter, ultrafilters of 100,000 daltons may suffice where compendial water systems are involved (Sweadner et al., 1977).

Because of the possibilities of grow-through, continuous operations involving filters require a proper maintenance protocol, namely, periodic sanitizations. Otherwise organisms may appear downstream of the filter. Even when sanitizations keep the organisms under control, microporous filters will pass their metabolic lipopolysaccharides, and endotoxins. These are pyrogenic when introduced into the body by injection, and constitute objectionable, organic contaminants.

Pore-Size Ratings

In filtration practices, the emphasis is so heavily on particulate retention—for example, as in bacterial filtrative sterilizations—that it is sometimes popularly believed that filters are classified according to the actual physical dimensions of their pores, especially as these are idealized to be circular and retentive of spherical particles. This characterization can indeed be made of the track-etched membranes where scanning electron microscopy serves to measure dimensionally the shapes, almost always circular, and sizes of the pore openings. However, the pores of the more commonly used reverse-phase or solution-type membranes cannot so easily be defined in terms of shapes or sizes. Instead, they are convoluted apertures of complex and uncertain architecture (Williams and Meltzer, 1983).

Membrane pore-size ratings have not been ascribed from direct measurements or mensurations, but have been inferred from the rates of flow of air or water through them. Much ingenuity has been exercised in developing methods of measuring the size of filter pores by the flow of the fluids. Flow measurements both of air and water have been widely used (Jacobs, 1972; Erbe, 1933; Alkan and Groves, 1978; Yasuda and Tsai, 1974); and more recently vapor pressure analysis by Katz (1982), and new mathematical insights, (Johnston, 1983; Badenhop, 1983), have been brought to bear.

In the pore-size calculations based on fluid flow, certain simplifying assumptions must be made regarding pore shape or geometry. However necessitated by mathematical need, these assumptions result in numbers that are approximate rather than accurate. Worse, they may be imprecise to unknown degrees. The derived numbers are useful in comparative contexts, where relative magnitudes are being considered. They can be misleading, however, when used for their retention implications relative to particles whose dimensions have been ascertained by direct measurements.

Mercury porosimetry has also been used. In this technique, mercury is forced into the filter at successive increments of pressure. Measurement is made of the volume of mercury intruded into the filter at each pressure. The higher the pressure, the smaller the pore penetrated by the mercury. Obviously, the smaller the opening, the greater its resistance to the inward flow of the mercury; hence, the need for the progressively higher pressures.

This technique is useful for the measurement of total porosity (total void volume) and does offer insights into the pore-size distribution of the filter. An excellent discussion of this technique is available (Brock, 1983). Whatever its virtues, however, the method has serious shortcomings (Rootare, 1970). Indeed,

Badenhop (1983) concluded that the method is unsuited to the pore-size measurement of microporous membranes.

Given the utilitarian application of microporous membranes to the filtrative removal of particles, it may seem surprising that more plentiful efforts have not been made to describe filter pore-size in terms of the minimum size of particles removed from fluid streams. The subject is, however, a complex one. The particles' sizes and shapes are important, as are their chemical makeup and that of the conveying fluid. The operational conditions of the filtration (i.e., the differential pressure, and even the protocol of the test itself) may influence the rating accorded the pore-size of the filter. Above all, the complexities of the particle-retention mechanisms come into play. More than the straightforward simplicity of sieve-retention is operative. Adsorptive effects, electrical charge-involved phenomena, and noncharge hydrophobic influences complicate conclusions that would otherwise derive from the retention of given-size particles by given-size pores (Bowman et al., 1967).

Sizing by Particle Retention

Except for the use of bacterial challenges, if one may judge from the absence of accounts from the technical literature, membranes are not sized by their abilities to hold back particles of specific dimensions (Johnston, 1975). The most recent work has involved membrane sizing by the retention of polystyrene latex spheres. An exposition of the technique as well as of its practices and usage is described by Simonetti et al., (1986). In addition, specific particle-size segments of AC Fine Test Dust have been used to size certain polypropylene prefilters. From time to time, silica (in any of its colloidal forms), carbon, and various other finely divided solids have been experimented with (Stewart, 1987). However, the uncertainties of the particle size distributions as well as the use (necessarily) of highly arbitrary testing protocols diminish the usefulness of the conclusions reached.

What is notable from a comparison of the retention of specific bacterial challenges and of cross-linked polystyrene latex spheres is that all the so-called 0.2-μm-rated membranes of commerce (if one may generalize from the types examined) retain challenges of 1×10^7 *P. diminuta* per square centimeter of filter surface. As shown in Table 5-1, that is not true of 0.198-μm latex-sphere challenges. (Tolliver and Schroeder, 1983).

Krygier (1986) made a translation of the two retention phenomena in the case of one type of filter, showing that membrane rated 0.2 μm on the basis of *P. diminuta* retention is 0.46-μm-rated on the basis of minimum latex particle size retention. The 0.1-μm-rated counterpart (on the grounds of *Mycoplasma* retention), is 0.25-μm-rated on the basis of latex sphere retentions. Pall et al. (1980) had shown the same relationship.

Few among the microporous membrane manufacturers have expressed pore-size rating on the basis of the sieve retention of polystyrene latex spheres. It may be that the other manufacturers stress the retention ratings conventionally so as to be of interest to the filtrative sterilizations of the pharmaceutical field. Perhaps the greater sensitivity of bacterial measurements is seen as being of overriding significance. There may be other reasons. It is regrettable, however, that the numerical imprecisions of the microbial retention test, regardless of its pharmaceutical usefulness, are not ameliorated by a more universal application of the latex sphere retention technique.

Implications of Pore-Size Ratings

How the different filter manufacturers variously arrive at their pore-size ratings, filter users almost invariably consider them to be particle (organism) retention limits based on the sieve-capture mechanisms. With only rare exceptions, however,the pore-size rating does not designate a retention value. Some, from time to time, are puzzled by the observation that organisms, presumably of a given size, are not retained by filters presumably of an adequate pore-size rating. Also, there are those who expect 0.2-μm-rated membranes, usually utilized to effect filtrative sterilizations based on *P. diminuta*, to interdict the passage of all microbes. Thus, Howard and Duberstein, (1980) remarked upon the presence in Long Island well waters of organisms that escaped being arrested by 0.2-μm-rated membranes. They advocated, therefore, that 0.1-μm-rated filter, be used; but they were designated to be 0.28 μm on the basis of latex particle retention (Pall et al., 1980).

L-form bacteria. Thomas et al., (1991) reported that *Pseudomonas aeruginosa* organisms were found downstream of a 0.45-μm-rated microporous membrane; the implication being that they should have been retained. The downstream microbes had morphological characteristics similar to those of L-form cells known to exhibit wall-defective variants. (The appellation L-form derives from the Lister Institute of Preventive Medicine in London.) As a consequence, these organisms are irregularly shaped into a contorted rodlike configuration (Collentro 1993). It was postulated that these bacteria were in a stressed form in response to a nutrient-limiting diet, or to sublethal doses of ultraviolet light. Gould (1993), as also Kogure et al., (1975), state that organisms in such hostile circumstances undergo diminutions in size and changes in form as means of promoting their survival. As expressed by Gould (1993):

> When bacteria are introduced with the source water, they are in an environment that is relatively rich nutritionally compared to the environment that they may end up in further along in the water purification system. Bacteria invoke a number of survival mechanisms in the transition from feast to famine. They minimize cell size in order to maximize surface-to-

volume ratio. By becoming small round cells or very thin long cells, they minimize the amount of cellular material they need to synthesize, while maximizing their contact with scarce nutrients.

It is hypothesized that L-form organisms negotiate microporous membranes expected to retain them because their defective wall structures reduce their rigidity to the point where they can traverse the tortuous pores of the filter.

There may be some confusion regarding the passage of organisms through 0.45-µm-rated filters. It is true that on the basis of size restraints, certain microbes are too large to penetrate 0.45-µm rated membranes. A case in point are the *Serratia marcescens* organisms. Usually, however, when the complete retention of organisms is sought, 0.2-µm-rated membranes, the sterilizing filters, are employed. The 0.45-µm-rated filters are, however, used to capture organisms in the Recovery Method for eventual viewing under the microscope, as detailed on page 81. Some practitioners use 0.2-µm-rated membranes for this purpose, but the literature states that the 0.45-µm-rated filters yield higher Recovery numbers (Sladek et al., 1975 and Carter 1996). The Recovery Method is useful in revealing and comparing trends in organism populations. Except where complete retentions have been demonstrated in the case of specific membranes, it would be an unwarranted assumption to expect 0.45-µm-rated membranes to retain completely those organisms whose arrest is usually accomplished by way of 0.2-µm-filters.

Leahy and Sullivan (1978) did demonstrate that a particular mixed esters of cellulose membrane of the 0.45-µm-rating retained *P. diminuta* organisms grown on minimal saline lactose broth to the extent of 1×10^4 or $1 \times 10^5/cm^2$. It would be foolhardy in the extreme, however, to project this performance of other 0.45-µm-rated filters without experimental verification. Carter (1996) confirm this experience for certain hydrophilic PVDF filters on the market

Once-filtered organisms. Reti et al., (1979) report a study wherein organisms, *Pseudomonas diminuta* ATCC-19146, that negotiated one filter were not necessarily retained by an identical, repetitive filter downstream. While this can be explained on the basis of the organisms within the filtrate pool from the first membrane being hydrodynamically carried to the larger pores of the second, it does contradict the article of faith that the log reduction values of succeeding filters are necessarily additive.

These investigators found that retentions strongly bear an inverse relationship to the transmembrane pressure. This conclusion is hardly surprising where adsorptive particle retentions are involved. Reti et al. (1979) also report, however, that this inverse dependency of differential pressure and retention grows more marked the closer the size of the organism matches that of the pore. It is rationalized that when the particle is small, the differential pressure serves to increase the velocity of the suspending liquid. When the size of the organism approaches that of the pore, the transmembrane pressure is exerted largely on that particle itself. Conceivably, shearing forces may so distort the organism that it becomes forced through the filter. Permanent shear-caused distortions may account for such particles not being retained subsequently by repetitive filters.

Sterilizing Filter

The present unsatisfactory situation wherein the meanings of nonstandardized pore-size designations are uncertain, and where these may differ in their definition from one manufacturer to another, has been resolved in the important application dealing with filtrative sterilizations.

The FDA (1987) has defined a sterilizing filter as: "A filter, when challenged with the microorganism *Pseudomonas diminuta*, at a minimum concentration of 10^7 organisms per cm^2 of filter surface, will produce a sterile effluent." Any commercially produced membrane that meets this qualification may be labeled "sterilizing filter."

By this functional definition of a sterilizing filter, the FDA has eliminated the confusion connected with pore-size ratings. To be sure, the validation of such sterilizing filters in actual field applications is to be done for "worst-case conditions." These "worst-case conditions," not being specified, can invite troublesome interpretations. But that is a detail. The FDA's functional definition of a sterilizing filter addresses succinctly the needs of the filtrative sterilization application.

Retention Values

It should be noted that the FDA's definition of "sterilizing filter" refers to an organism challenge per square centimeter of filter surface. It is an area challenge, not a total challenge. Thus, a filter cartridge may be challenged with a total of 5×10^{10} *P. diminuta*. If the cartridge comprises 5 ft^2 (5,000 cm^2) of effective filtration area (EFA), then the area challenge will be equivalent to $5 \times 10^{10}/5{,}000 = 1 \times 10^7/cm^2$. This cartridge will qualify as a sterilizing filter provided it yields sterile effluent. However, if the filter cartridge is composed of 7 ft^2 (EFA), then $5 \times 10^{10}/7{,}000 = 7.1 \times 10^6/cm^3$. This cartridge will not qualify as a sterilizing filter according to the FDA guidelines. However, Johnston and Meltzer (1979) discussed the inadvisability of interpreting retention data legalistically. The danger is that borderline performance may come to be regarded as being acceptable. What is important is the cm^2 area challenge, not the total challenge.

Bacterial retention by a filter is expressed as its LRV (log reduction value). If the filter instrument or device, such as flat disk or cartridge, retains, say, a total challenge of 1×10^{10} *P. diminuta*, then its LRV is defined as log $1 \times 10^{10}/1$, or 10. A filter with an LRV of 10 means thereby that it withstands a total challenge of 1×10^{10} to yield sterile effluent. A filter with an LRV of 10 is not necessarily a sterilizing filter. To calculate whether a filter device with LRV of 10 is a sterilizing filter, it is necessary to divide the total challenge by the EFA of the subject filter.

The origins of the numbers $1 \times 10^7/cm^2$ are obscure. It is popularly, if erroneously, believed that this number represents the quantity of pores present in the surface of the 0.2-μm rated sterilizing-grade membrane. Over time, this number achieved respectability, although the mathematical assumptions underlying its derivation rendered the actual value questionable. Indeed, independent calculations involving other simplifying assumptions have placed the number of pores at approximately 200 times as many (Meltzer, 1987g). Actually, the number of pores of any size is unknown. However, an important ramification of the $1 \times 10^7/cm^2$ figure was the support it gave to the assumption that challenging a sterilizing filter with a like number of *P. diminuta* would ensure that each pore would be confronted by an organism. In this way, each pore would be tested for its adequacy of retention regardless of size. This could serve to alleviate concerns associated with the uncharted area of pore-size distributions. Challenge levels larger than $1 \times 10^7/cm^2$ would be unnecessary because the additional organisms would presumably be retained by the filter cake formed from the $1 \times 10^7/cm^2$ challenge rather than by the filter itself. Higher challenges would, therefore, be meaningless. However, the pore number calculations were shown to be erroneous on statistical grounds (Juran, 1974). Thus, an effort to lay down a uniform coating of, say, 2 organisms/μm^2 of surface would result in 15% of the pores remaining vacant while another 15% would contain three or more microbes.

The absurdity of defining the challenge level on the basis of the calculated number of pores/cm^2 is shown by consideration of the repetitive pore layering. A membrane filter can be considered to consist of a layered construction of individual filter planes, each with its own pore-size distribution (Piekaar and Clarenburg, 1967). The overlapping of these planes yields a series of pore paths whose individual pore-size distribution, above a certain critical filter thickness, begins to approach the overall pore-size distribution of the filter (Pall and Kirnbauer 1978). Even if the thickness of a single such hypothetical plane is the dimension of its largest pore, and if the largest pore of a 0.2-μm-rated membrane is approximately 0.4-μm (double the mean flow-pore value) and is too large to retain P. diminuta, then a 150-μm thick membrane will contain a series of some 300 to 400 such planes. However rough this arithmetic, it suggests a high redundance of successive pores to the permeating liquid. This manifold pore layering would serve to ensure the sterilizing retention by the filter despite its larger pores. It seems irrelevant, therefore, to be concerned with challenging surface areas having dimensions as small as 1.0 μm^2.

Be that as it may, the $1 \times 10^7/cm^2$ challenge was stated by the Health Industry Manufacturers Association as defining sterilizing filters (HIMA, 1982). Whatever its limitations, it was elevated to a status beyond protest when FDA stipulated it as the microbiological test of a sterilizing filter "under worst-case conditions" (Food and Drug Administration, 1988).

Actually, in its guidelines on aseptic processing, FDA states that sterilizing filters should withstand challenges of at least $1 \times 10^7/cm^2$. Some regard this as suggesting that larger challenges would provide additional safety margins. Although it represents a minimum level, the stipulation of $1 \times 10^7/cm^2$ is a sufficient level. Implications that it is inadequate because it is a minimum value are in fact untrue. Indeed, if a drug preparation were to contain an organism population even approaching $10 \times 10^7/cm^2$ of *P. diminuta*, one would be advised to decrease this number by prefilter action to optimize the retention by the final filter. The filtered solution, sterile though it would be, would undoubtedly be too high in endotoxin content to qualify as an injectable.

Nevertheless, there are those who advocate the use of higher challenge levels. Whatever such justification, intimations that filters are confronted at lower challenge densities because they cannot withstand the higher levels, or the companion claim that the more strongly challenged filter inherently retains better, is unwarranted. Such implications are the product of marketing efforts, not of responsible filter characterization.

It is difficult to avoid the conclusion that challenges greater than $1 \times 10\text{-}^7/cm^2$ are unnecessary. In fact, the $1 \times 10^7/cm^2$ value enjoys credibility only because it has been specified by the FDA. For most pharmaceutical preparations undergoing final filtration, it is absurdly high. In any case, the challenge level is more than enough and will suffice until FDA revises the limits to levels that more realistically match actual bioburdens (Mouwen and Meltzer 1993). Usually found bioburdens are on the level of $1 \times 10^3/cm^2$.

Smaller-than-0.2-µm ratings

The utility of the FDA definition of *sterilizing filter* is that in the pharmaceutical practice of filtrative sterilizations, the uncertainty of 0.2-µm-ratings is replaced by the sure meaning of *sterilizing filter*.

Efforts have been made to give utilitarian definition to other filters by means of organism retentions. Presumably, 0.1-µm-rated membranes will completely retain *Mycoplasma*, and 0.45-µm-rated membranes will completely retain *Serratia marcescens*. Such retention definitions may indeed have useful value, as in the case of *Mycoplasma*-retaining membranes, for fetal calf serum filtrations. Nevertheless, however useful the applicational definition, it does not constitute a measurement of actual pore size, although it bears, of course, some relation. An extreme example is shown by some membrane manufacturers who confer a 0.04-µm-rating upon certain of their ultrafilters because they retain bacteriophage. The bacteriophage may well be 0.04 µm in size. Whether the filters retain them because the pores are of a corresponding size begs the simplicities of sieve retentions. It is certain that the exclusivity of the sieve mechanism of capture by such filters has never been validated.

The pore-size rating of membrane filters is a complicated matter, far exceeding the matching of the pore-sizes of the filter to retained particles of appropriate size. In the circumstances, recourse is had to utilitarian or performance definitions, wherein a filter is "pore-sized" in accordance with its retention of specific particles of utilitarian or applicational interest.

The problem of how to assign pore-size ratings to membrane filters on the basis of their retention of particles of a given minimum size would seem forthcoming from the use of spherical latex particles. What the implications of such numerical ratings would be in various filter applications is a separate matter. This approach has, however, not been endorsed by filter manufacturers. It merits greater consideration than it has thus far received.

Pore-Size Distribution

Pore structure is complex and little understood (Meltzer, 1988; American Filtration Society, 1991). The pore sizes, however defined, are relatively narrow in the distribution of their degree of spread. Certain of these membranes have narrower pore-size distributions than others. This may or may not be advantageous to the user, depending upon the circumstances. (See Figure 5-14a and 5-14b,

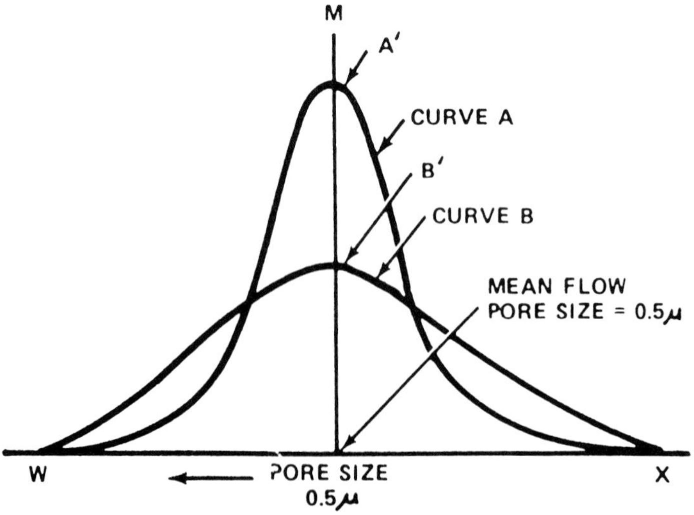

Figure 5-14a. Hypothetical pore-size distributions A. Two different-shaped curves representing identical bubble points, equal flow porosities, and the same mean flow pores. Filter B would retain 0.5-μm particles less completely than would filter A.

Marshall and Meltzer (1976); Courtesy, Parenteral Drug Association
Meltzer (1987b); Courtesy, *Ultrapure Water* journal

Meltzer, 1987h). Where the pore-size rating does not reflect the largest retentive pore size present in the filter, a narrow pore-size distribution is desired. This means that fewer pores larger than the pore-size rating will be available for particle passage, the filter presumably having been selected on the basis of the matching of its pore-size rating with the size of the particles to be retained. In any case, a Gaussian distribution of pore-sizes is not necessarily best. A long spectrum of smaller pores would promote the retention of particles smaller than the pore-size rating.

This is of obvious importance in applications where no particle is too small to be ignored. As complete a removal as possible of particles is also advisable in pharmaceutical production. Present USP standards for large-volume parenterals specify that these may not contain more than 5 particles per milliliter of sizes greater than 25 µm, and not more than 50 larger than 10 µm per milliliter. These standards may perhaps reflect the practicality of reliably detecting smaller particles by present technologies, for it is well known that even smaller particles can be harmful to the human system in terms of myocardial damage; injury to such organs as liver, lungs, and, kidney; and capillary blockage in general. Moreover, smaller particles in colloid form may lose their mutual electrical repulsions as a function of time. Their agglomeration into larger particles would then take place. Thus even very small particles constitute an area of potential concern, as the small particles may grow larger with time.

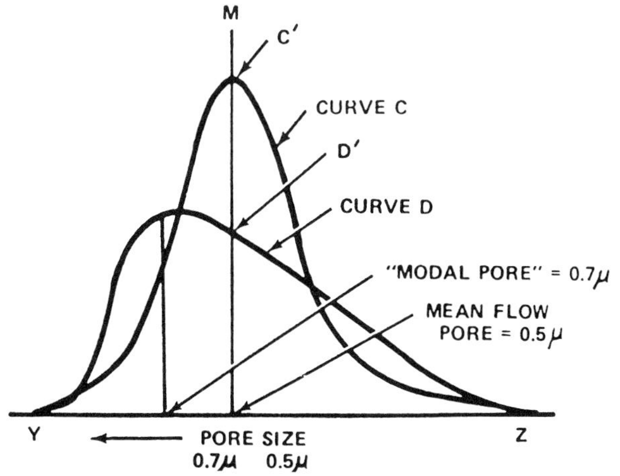

Figure 5-14b. Hypothetical pore-size distributions B. The modal pore in clogging. Two different-shaped curves representing identical bubble points, equal flow porosities, and the same mean flow pores. The filtration of 0.7-µm particles will clog filter C more slowly than filter D. Both filters will exhibit identical flowrates with clean fluids.
Marshall and Meltzer (1976); Courtesy, Parenteral Drug Association

Maximization of Filtrative Particle Removals

It is generally comprehended that particles are retained by filters in sieve fashion wherein they are restrained simply because they are too large to fit through pore passageway constrictions; additionally, they may become adsorptively sequestered onto filter surfaces, whether by charge-involved forces or by hydrophobic effects. The adsorptive captures serve to remove particles small enough to permeate the filter pores. The charge-involved phenomena that may be operative may include the ionic charges common to the charge-modified filters of commerce, or may derive from factors such as hydrogen bonding or Van der Waals forces, etc. Hydrophobic adsorptive effects, essentially charge-unrelated, are a result of free surface energy minimization. Whatever the adsorptive sequestration mechanisms, they result in the filtrative removal of particles too small to be sieved from conveying fluids.

Where particles are arrested by a filter because they are too large to pass through its pores, their retention is complete. The filter's absoluteness is independent of the number of particles; is not influenced by the chemistry or physics of the fluid medium; and is not a function of the transfilter pressure, except as this may so distort shapes of particles and/or of pores as to alter the geometry that compels sieve retention. (These latter occurrences are seldom alleged.)

The direct pressure effects upon particles whose dimensions approach those of the pores undoubtedly have different retention consequences than those upon much smaller particles being carried by the fluid in the pores (Reti et al., 1979). However, so little is known about particle and pore shape and size distributions as to render speculation on this point unprofitable. What is known with certainty is that higher applied differential pressures, albeit conducive to higher initial rates of flow, serve to compress the particle layer positioned at the filter surface. This may decrease fluid permeation through this polarized layer and, especially where the particulate matter is deformable, may earlier compromise the useful service life of the filter (Figure 5-15).

Attempts at maximization of filtrative removal thus require the minimization of the transfilter pressure. The quantitative imperatives in any particular case can be established only by experiment.

Temperature

For operations wherein temperature management of fluid being filtered is practical, elevated temperatures are generally believed to be promotive of particle retention. Higher temperature increases the vigor of the Brownian motion, which through collisions of the fluid molecules with particles enhances the chances of particle/pore-wall encounters. Higher viscosities are an impediment to the amplitude of the Brownian motion. Temperature elevations proportionately decrease liquid viscosities, allowing for longer Brownian motion pathways. This makes for enhanced small-particle capture (Johnston, 1990).

A filter operating in circumstances wherein sieve retention is the only operative mechanism of particle removal is invariant in its filter efficiency. In such situations, the reliability of the filter is independent of such filtration conditions as applied differential pressure, particle challenge level, and temperature; and of such fluid properties as pH, ionic strengths, viscosities, and surface tension.

Any or all of these factors may govern the filter action, however, where adsorptive particle removals are concerned. In such cases, filter efficiency is not invariant. It is subject to the filtration conditions. These must, therefore, be so selected and managed as to maximize the filtrative particle removal efficiency. In any actual filtration, the particle retention mechanisms are largely unelucidated. Hence, prudent filter operation necessitates that a given operational practice be conducted with a view towards the positive enhancement of small-particle removals by adsorptive effects. (Brose and Hendricksen, 1994).

Applied Differential Pressure

Figure 5-16 depicts the alternative possibilities open to a particle small enough to enter and permeate a filter pore system. It may traverse the filter passageways and emerge unscathed with the convective fluid; or it may experience a pore-wall encounter to become adsorptively sequestered from the fluid stream. The longer

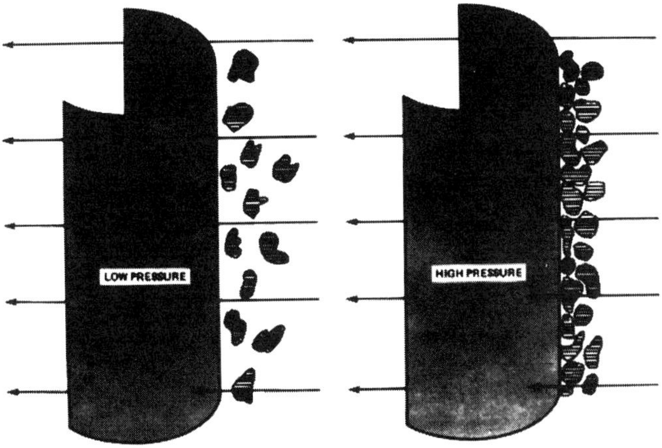

Figure 5-15. Effect of differential pressure on throughput volume.
Meltzer (1987a); Courtesy, Marcel Dekker, Inc.

the particle is resident within the pore system, the greater its probability of pore-wall encounter. The particle's duration within the pore is governed primarily by the velocity of the suspending fluid. This, in turn, is a direct function of the applied differential pressure. The lower the transfilter pressure, therefore, the higher the filter efficiency and the more likely the particle removal (Tanny et al., 1979; Leahy and Sullivan, 1978) (Tables 5-5 and 5-6). The requisite diminution in the applied differential pressure may require the use of more extensive filter surface to maintain desired rates of flow. An added benefit of lower ΔP is the formation of less compacted filter cake, permitting greater total throughput. As in most engineering optimizations, the key to the practicality of the approach involves economic considerations.

What is a safe maximum differential pressure to utilize? The answer is obscured by the site-specific definitions of the particle sizes and pore-channel diameters and lengths that are involved. The former are very seldom known, the latter almost never. In pharmaceutical practices where particle removal is usually modeled by the *P. diminuta* organism as raised on a minimum diet (0.3 × 0.7 - 1.0 μm in size), applied differential pressures not to exceed 30 psig (2 bar) are usually relied on; although many pharmaceutical filtrations are performed at 20 psig or even lower. This differential pressure level is mirrored in the HIMA protocol for defining sterilizing filters (HIMA, 1982). In semiconductor rinsewater applications, differential pressure levels are selected on the basis of the rates of flow that eventuate. Systems are often oversized so that 2 to 3 psig often suffice. In some cases the pressures may attain 30 psig (2 bar). Hango (1990) expects flows of 2 to 4 gpm (7.6 to 15 Lpm) from a 10-inch (25-cm) microporous cartridge. This can generally be realized using less than 2 to 5 psig of differential pressure. Similar flows from a 0.04-μm-rated filter could require 12 to 15 psig. The use of finer pore-size-rated filters in conjunction with lower pressure differentials would necessitate the installation of added filters to avoid the sacrifice of flowrate. This highlights the economic development in system design, an ever-present consideration.

Higher differential pressure results in increased rates of flow. This, in turn, minimizes the residence time of the particle in the pore passageway, leading to a reduction in adsorptive particle arrests. Overall, increased temperature promotes adsorptive sequestrations.

Neither increased fluid velocities nor higher viscosities are seen to promote particle desorption. The particle once in contact with the pore wall is not "dragged" from its fixed site by a viscous fluid. Nor do higher stream velocities serve to remove it. This is so because within pores having the diameters common to microporous membranes, the fluid flow is laminar and it is slowest adjoining the pore walls. Once adsorbed to the pore walls, therefore, the particles remain independent of stream velocity or viscosity effects.

Particle Challenge Densities

A study of Figure 5-16 reveals why filter efficiencies are dependent on the particle challenge levels where adsorptive sequestrations are involved. It is a matter of probabilities. A given particle entering the pore may become adsorptively captured; as also may a second, third, etc. Inevitably, however, the more particles involved, the greater the possibility of particles escaping arrest (Elford, 1933). Thus, to maximize particle capture, the number of them confronting the filter should be minimized. (Wallhäusser, 1975, 1976).

Prefiltration, as is shown in Figure 5-17, is usually used to prolong the service life of a final filter. It does so by having the prefilter sacrificially assume some of the particulate burden. The final filter, spared this portion of the particulate load, has its service life prolonged. Even when the length of the filter system's useful service is not the concern, however, the employment of prefilters (or of repetitive filters) results in a lower particle challenge density confronting the final filter. This serves to increase the filter efficiency of the final filter.

Repetitive Filters

Obviously, where particles are small enough to penetrate the filters they may do so, except as they may be restrained by adsorptive captures. Were there to be repetitive final filters, or even prefilters, particles penetrating the first layer would have also to permeate a second barrier before emerging uncaptured by the filter system. In essence, a thicker filter is created, one offering added particle/pore-wall encounter likelihoods. Therefore, the use of repetitive final filters maximizes the removal of smaller particles. It also has a salubrious effect in situations where the particles are large enough to be sieve-retained except that the filters may possibly be flawed (Figure 5-18).

Where the repetitive filters are physically separated, the permeating fluid can form a pool. Under low applied differential pressures, a particle penetrating a large pore or flaw in the first filter may within the liquid pool become directed to flaws in the second filter. The conveying liquid, taking the path of least resistance, preferentially seeks out the larger pores available to it (flow through these orifices being a function of the pore radius to the fourth power). Where the transfilter pressures are high, the fluid is impelled to flow in straighter lines, normal to the repetitive filter's surface. Orientations, within the liquid pool between the filters to larger pores are foreshortened or eliminated by the higher rates of flow (Reti et al., 1979). Elimination of the interfilter fluid pool and of its heightened particle-passage effects can be had by the contiguous positioning of the repetitive filters so that no space separates their surfaces, rather than disposing them in serial filter fashion (Wrasidlo and Mysels, 1984). With such repetitive filter arrangements, low applied differential pressures may advantageously be used.

In summary, four practices should be invoked in order to maximize particle captures by filters, particularly small-particle removal. The first of these, the use of elevated water temperatures, may find economic justification difficult, given the energy costs associated with the heating of large volumes of water. The practice of using heated water for its greater effect in rinsing operations is, however, presently finding its advocates within the semiconductor industry.

Prefilters should be utilized to reduce the particle challenge density. Repetitive, contiguously arranged final filters should be employed to provide additional possibilities for adsorptive sequestration and to shield against possible filter flaws. Above all, low applied differential pressures should provide the motivation to the fluid flow.

With attention given to such operational details, the use of filters should lead to the maximization of particle removals, especially of smaller particles, from fluid streams.

Nanofilter Usage

Filters are counted upon to remove particulate matter, including bacteria, and to reduce the organic content (TOC) of the water. Nanofilters, RO filters of a more open construction, are used at 97% or so recovery levels. These are appropriate when bivalent ions are to be removed. They, as also RO filters, generally remove organic molecules of sizes larger than 200 in molecular weight, and effect organism reductions to below 3 per 100 mL. In Japan, Neodenko uses filters of

Table 5-5
Pressure-Dependent Retention Performance

Operating Pressure psig)	*Total Filtration Time for 2,000 mL (min:sec)*	*Organisms Passing After 500 mL*	*1,000 mL*	*1,500 mL*	*2,000 mL (org/100 mL)*	*Average Number of Organisms in Filtrate/mL*
5	189:30	0	0	0	0	~0
5	75:00	4	12	7,200	7,200	—
5	304:00	0	0	0	0	—
15	108:27	0	13	19	39	—
15	69:30	3	2	0	7,200	10-20
15	43:58	6	15	12	11	—
30	18:35	93	91	61	66	—
30	16:12	38	34	39	52	50-100
30	50:02	7,200	7,200	7,200	7,200	—

Cellulose triacetate 0.45-μm-rated membrane challenged with *P. diminuta* suspension of 10^5 org/mL 2,000 mL over 9.6 cm^2 available surface (47-mm disc). Total organism challenge level 2×10^2 org/cm^2

Tanney et al. (1979); Courtesy Parenteral Drug Association

polyvinyl alcohol laid down upon a polysulfone backing at a differential pressure of about 150 psig. Toray employs a polyamide upon a polysulfone at differential pressure levels of about 300 psig.

In some quarters there is a reluctance to use pleated cartridges at points of use. It is feared that the flexing of the pleats may abrade the filter medium, with the creation of particles. Since POU filters for gases are seldom changed, pleated filter use is avoided by some in such applications.

Integrity Testing of Filters

When a filter is removed from its package prior to installation and use, the only way to determine whether its specifications are met, short of actually employing it, is to inspect its performance in an integrity test. For this reason, integrity tests are important.

The practice of integrity testing derives from requirements in pharmaceutical filtrations wherein a surety of retention of a particular organism, *P. diminuta*, is sought. This is assumed to be indicative of the retention of the other organisms normally encountered in pharmaceutical processing. In the pharmaceutical industry, there are certain regulations that stipulate the performance of integrity testing.

The bubble-point method of integrity testing is the only one with a theoretical basis that is linked directly to the largest pore-size of the filter. The linkage, although existing, is inexact, however; and its importance is usually exaggerated.

Bubble-point values become increasingly uncertain as the effective filtration

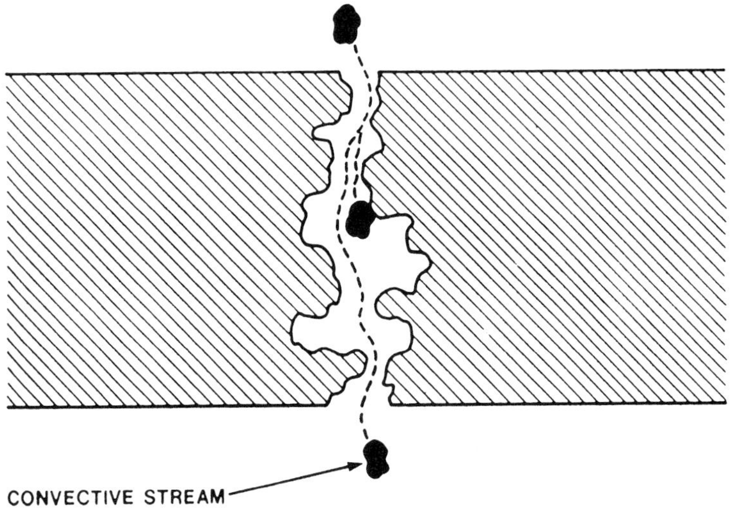

Figure 5-16. Alternative paths for particles entering pores.
Meltzer (1987a); Courtesy, Marcel Dekker, Inc.

area of the filter increases. This is because air diffuses across the filter during the performance of the bubble-point test. Obfuscation of the true bubble point may result. The larger the effective filtration area (EFA), the greater the diffusion and the more likely its interfering effect in creating the "continuous stream of bubbles" that defines the bubble point. Use has been made of the diffusive airflow itself to devise an integrity test. The diffusive airflow test is an integrity test method based upon empirically established correlations of diffusive airflow values to organism retentions. As usually performed, it is a single-point measurement wherein the rate of diffusive airflow is measured at a given applied differential pressure. Single-point measurements can be highly unreliable.

Nevertheless, the established practice is to perform single-point measurements. This should be changed to full-curve plotting by an automated test device (Meltzer, 1992). At the very least, a diffusion point and the bubble point should be measured.

To perform either the bubble-point test or the diffusive airflow test (unless one employs automated testing devices), it is necessary to invade the equipment area downstream of the filter. In pharmaceutical practices, this poses a risk to the sterility of the filtered product. Reliance is often set instead on the pressure-hold test. In this procedure, an unaccustomed loss of pressure upstream of the filter in its sealed housing is taken as evidence of excessive air diffusion across the filter and/or of an improperly sealed system. Either case indicates a failure, the causes of which can then further be explored.

The virtue of the pressure-hold test is its noninvasion of the system downstream of the filter. It avoids, therefore, an important shortcoming of the bubble-point and diffusive airflow methods. Employing given housing and filter combinations, it would be possible to develop a history wherein unusually rapid

Table 5-6
Effect of Pressure on the Passage of *P. diminuta* through Membranes of Various Pore Sizes

		β Ratio		
Filter Type	*Pore Size (μm)*	*0.5 psid*	*5 psid*	*50 psid*
GS	0.22	$>10^{10}$	$>10^{10}$	$>10^{10}$
HA	0.45	10^{8}	10^{7}	10^{6}
DA	0.65	10^{4}	10^{4}	10^{3}
AA	0.80	10^{2}	10^{1}	10^{0}

Leaby and Sullivan (1978); Courtesy, *Pharmaceutical Technology* losses in pressure within the filter vessel could reliably be taken to signal sealing leaks and/or filters with excessive diffusion rates. In pharmaceutical contexts, there is the additional problem of correlating pressure losses with exact levels of organism retentions. Where knowledge of the volume of the filter housing and of its occupying filters is known, the free volume can be deduced. Based upon this and the perfect gas law, the diffusive airflow rate can be calculated for the filters involved. Knowing this, excessive pressure losses can be judged as signaling integrity test failures. These would differ, however, for different housing/filter combinations. While such calculations are possible, there have been few published pressure-hold histories, and these are not generally transferable to other systems.

It may be helpful to review the various integrity tests and to explore their areas of application as well as their imitations.

The Integrity Tests

The integrity tests have been devised by the various filter companies to permit the non-destructive assaying of filter integrity. They are not products of the FDA, nor is their use a subject of FDA imprimaturs or disallowances. The appropriateness of any integrity test rests solely upon its demonstrated, documented correlation to organism retention levels, and is only as good as the extent and reliability of the experimentally established correlation.

In the case of the bubble-point integrity test, soon to be discussed, the organism retention level, expressed as log reduction value, is correlated with specific bubble point values, Figure 5-19 (Johnston and Meltzer, 1971). Integral filters, usually in cartridge form, are shown to pass the subject integrity test, while nonintegral filters that fail to withstand 1×10^7 organism challenges per square centimeter of filter surface do not pass the integrity test. This empirically established correlation is accepted. Filter manufacturers generally do not correlate an entire range of integrity test values, both above and below the failure point, with specific levels of organism retention. For one thing, filter manufacturers try to avoid producing failed filters. Therefore, a well-defined series of such failures is not easily available for testing.

Each integrity test derives its authority from the empirically established correlation just mentioned. While useful in presenting the same conclusion regarding filter integrity, the various integrity tests are independent of one another. They have not been shown to correlate with one another. This holds even for the diffusive airflow (forward flow) test that is performed at a pressure level approximately 80% of the bubble point. It is not required to correlate to the bubble-point values of filters. Each test rests its own worth upon its own correlation to a sufficiency of organism retentions.

Because the correlation sanctioning its use is empirically established, the causal relationships involved are muted. Thus, the bubble-point test does presumably derive from the largest pores present in the filter. Cause and effect are self-evident. However, the diffusive airflow (forward flow) test does not measure the largest pores. It reflects only the filter's total porosity. Yet, on the basis of empirical correlation, it too is an accepted integrity test. The water intrusion test (also called the water pressure integrity test) also relates to the largest pores. Being newly devised, it undergoes greater challenges. Its acceptance, however, is validated by the correlation of its test values to suitable organism retention values.

The Bubble-Point Capillary Rise Phenomenon

If a glass capillary has one of its ends placed into a pool of water, the water will rise into the tube. The height of its rise will reflect the inner diameter of the capillary: the narrower the dimension, the greater the rise. More importantly, the narrower the capillary diameter, the greater the air pressure required to force the liquid out of the tube. The water rises in the tube because attractive hydrogen bonding forces acting between it and the glass lift it along the glass surfaces until the mass of the risen liquid equals the force of gravity. (Thus water will not rise in a wax tube nor mercury in a glass tube because no attractive forces are operative.) The physics involved in this event, as elucidated by Laplace, are expressed by the equation:

$$P = (4\gamma \mathrm{Cos}\theta) / D \qquad \text{Eq. 5-1}$$

Where P is the pressure necessary to expel the water; d is the diameter of the tube; γ is the water's surface tensions expressive of the cohesive force operative among

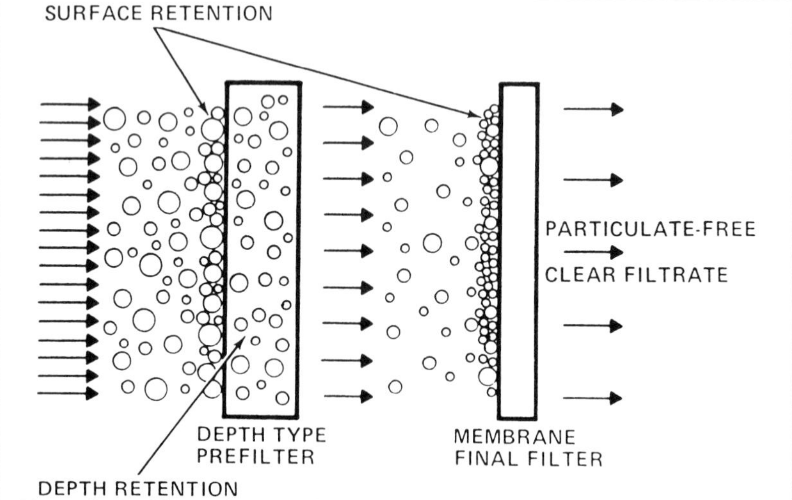

Figure 5-17. The mechanism of prefiltration.
Meltzer (1987g); Courtesy, Marcel Dekker, Inc.

water molecules; and Cos θ, where θ is the angle of wetting, describes the adhesive forces operative between the water and the glass molecules.

What is important to note is that P and D are inversely proportional. That is, the smaller the capillary diameter, the greater the pressure needed to expel the water.

The Bubble-Point Test

If a water-wettable membrane disk is dropped horizontally onto a pool of water, the liquid will be imbibed into its pores, replacing the air. The disk can then be positioned between supporting screens in a suitable holder, and can be overlaid by a pool of water. Air pressure can then be applied to the bottom of the lower screen. Nothing visible occurs initially as the air pressure is raised. At some level, however, a continuous stream of bubbles will be seen issuing from the face of the membrane. The membrane's bubble point has been reached, and is described in terms of the air-pressure value needed to achieve it. In principle, this is the basis of the bubble-point integrity test.

The above occurrence can be interpreted in terms of the capillary-rise phenomenon. The water is attracted into the membrane pore walls, thus displacing the air. As the applied air pressure reaches a high enough level, it expels the liquid from the set of largest pores present in the filter, and passing through, the air is seen as a continuous stream of bubbles. The attractive wall-effect is least per volume of water for the widest capillaries. Therefore the bubble-point test is a measure of the set of the largest pores present in the filter. (It is taken as unlikely that there would be only one largest pore among the millions of pores present.) As popularly expressed, the bubble point measures, in psig (pounds per square inches of pressure gauge) the largest pore(s) charac-

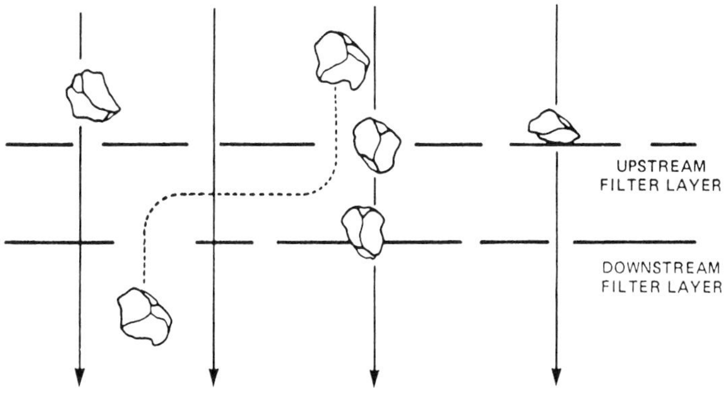

Figure 5-18. Effect of repetitive filter layers on particle retention and integrity testing.
Meltzer (1987b); Courtesy, Marcel Dekker, Inc.

terizing the filter.

Miscalculation of Pore Dimensions

Indeed, given Laplace's equation, it ought to be possible to calculate the exact diameter of these largest pores. Such calculations would assume, however, that the pores have the circularity of round capillaries. Actually, the pores of the reverse-phase membranes have unelucidated shapes. Their complexities are shown in Figure 5-20. There is reason to believe that the pores are polygonal in shape. In any case, they are not circular, and calculating their areas on the basis of (πr^2) and their perimeters on the basis of ($2\pi r$) (the proper expressions for circular capillaries) leads to misleading numerical results. Indeed, this one of the reasons that the much-used 0.2 (0.22) μm rating is erroneous (Williams and Meltzer, 1983).

Effect of Vehicle

The surface tension of the wetting liquid is one of the terms in the Laplace equation, and it affects the bubble-point value of the filter. The use of drug product or vehicle as the wetting fluid, therefore, probably gives different values than those yielded by water, and accordingly differs from the manufacturer's values based on water.

Some filter users perform both initial and final bubble-point tests in water, washing out the product with. water before the final reading. Others believe that the final product cannot be sufficiently removed, and prefer the initial bubble point using the drug vehicle. In this case, a comparison of the initial bubble points

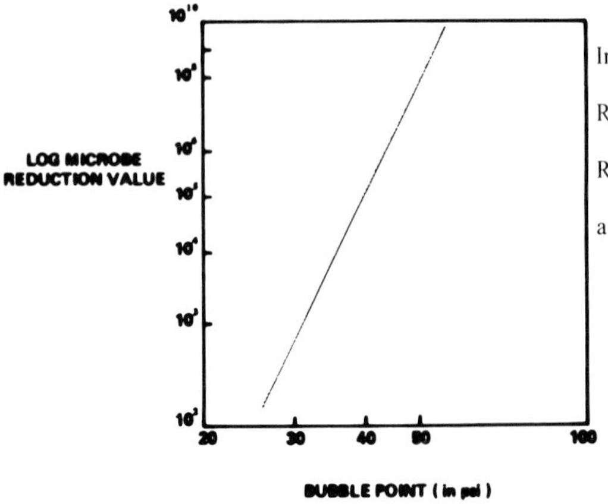

In In R = In a + 2 In P

$R^2 = e^{aP}$

$R = 10^{aP}$

a = experimental constant reflecting how the bubble-point is measured, volumetric flow rate, differential pressure, filter area, duration of the filtration, the types and numbers of the microorganisms being filtered, etc...

Figure 5-19. General curve relating microbe retention to bubble point.
Johnston and Meltzer (1971); Courtesy, *Pharmaceutical Technology*

is made using first water then product. This permits the numerical difference between the two liquids to be calculated. It is then used to translate the final bubble point, that taken with products, directly into that which would presumably have been yielded by water.

The acceptable minimum bubble point can be determined with the help of using product as the wetting liquid (Parker 1986, Desaulniers and Fey, 1990).

$$P_p = P_o \div P_w \times P_m \qquad \text{Eq. 5-2}$$

where P_p is the mirdmum acceptable bubble point with product,
P_o is the average of the bubble points observed using product,
P_w is the average of the bubble points observed using water, and
P_m is the manufacturer's stated minimum bubble point.

Enough samples are run with both water and product in ol- der to give an acceptable average value.

All the above assumes that the vehicle is so compatible with the filter that it does not alter its bubble point, through a plasticizing action, for instance.

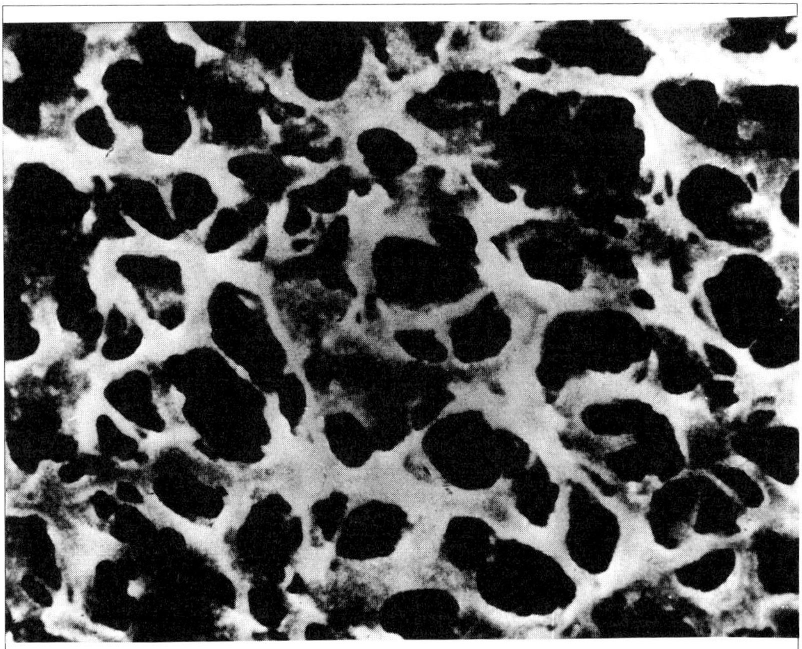

Figure 5-20. The unelucidated shapes of reverse-phase membrane pores.
Meltzer (1987b); Courtesy, Gelman Sciences, Inc.

Correlation with Organism Retentions

Whatever the earlier practices, bubble-point values now derive their authority not from any fancied translation to particular pore sizes, but because they have been shown to correlate empirically with organism retention levels. Figure 5-19 shows a generalized relationship of such a plot. It bears repeating that bubble-point readings do not signal filter integrity because they equate with a particular size pore, whether 0.2, 0.22 μm, or whatever; but because these readings in psig units have been established experimentally as correlating with specific organism retentivities. This correlation reflects the transmembrane pressure level of the organism challenge test. It requires being validated for higher levels.

Proper Performance of the Bubble-Point Test

The various filter manufacturers use somewhat different manipulative protocols in performing the bubble-point test. Since the membrane user is seeking to imitate an experimental procedure, it is required that the precise protocol being used be that of the manufacturer of the filter being tested when manual tests are being made. If subsequently another manufacturer's filter is being used, that very manufacturer's bubble-point procedure should be substituted. There is, as yet, no standardized manual bubble-point procedure. A faithful duplication of the manufacturer's experimental protocol is called for. Bubble-point testing by way of automated test machines does not require an imitative protocol.

In pharmaceutical practices, an acceptable and even preferred alternative is for the user to employ a single bubble-point protocol for all filters, coupling that procedure with one's own determination for the filter type's organism retention levels. This practice simplifies the training of integrity test personnel. Moreover, it offers the advantage of independence from reliance upon filter manufacturer retention data.

In the semiconductor industry, a single protocol may be adopted and become sanctioned for use for all filters. Numerical dislocations become keyed in as a use history develops. In the electronics industry, numbers need not precisely translate to exact organism retentions. The integrity test serves rather as an identification of the filter type and rating; however, the pore-size rating is not necessarily an expression of the filter's particle retention capability.

Diffusive Airflow Testing

In the bubble pointing of the filters, gradually increasing air pressure is applied to one side of a wetted filter. The other side of the filter, exposed to the outside atmosphere, is at a lower level of pressure, namely atmospheric. In accordance with the physical law governing the solubility of gases in liquids, more air is dissolved at the higher pressures present in the upstream portions of the thin water layer wetting the filter than in the downstream portions. This is so because Henry's law says that the amount of a gas dissolved in a liquid is a direct expression of that gas pressure over the liquid. As a result, as the dissolved air (forced into solution by the higher pressure) diffuses to the downstream lower pressure regions of the water layer, it comes out of solution. The amount of air thus diffusing across the wet membrane can be detected as bubbles before the bubble point is reached. It can be collected as a function of the time and can be measured.

When the bubble-point test is being run, the air pressure on the upstream side of the filter is raised slowly, so as not to overshoot the actual bubble point. Meanwhile, air is diffusing across the wet layers of the filter. If the filter is large enough in area, the amount of diffused air can form a detectable stream of bubbles. This may be confused with the steady stream of bubbles that emerges at the true bubble point, the frank or viscous airflow that takes place through the largest pores vacated of their liquid content. Therefore, for larger-area filters such as cartridges, the reliability of a bubble-point determination may become compromised by the diffusive airflow.

The rates of diffusive airflows differ so much from the more rapid passages of air at the bubble point, however, that the automated integrity test devices can reliably detect the differences. Regardless, filter manufacturers have found it possible to correlate the amount of air diffused across a wetted filter, at a pressure below that of the bubble point, with the organism retention propensities of that filter. This empirical correlation forms the basis for the diffusive airflow test to

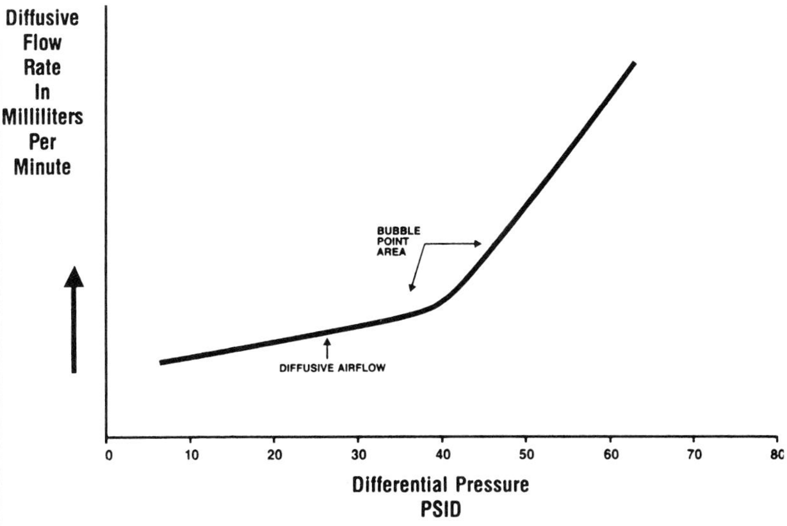

Figure 5-21. Diffusive flowrate in milliliters per minute.
Meltzer (1989c); Courtesy, *Ultrapure Water* journal

be used as an integrity test. In its performance, a pressure is maintained on the upstream side of the wetted filter at one pressure point (40 psig for example, at about 80% of the bubble-point value); and the volume of air diffused across the filter over, for example, a 5- to 15-minute interval is collected and measured. If the total volume does not exceed a given maximum (experimentally established by the filter manufacturer as correlating with a minimum of organism retention), the filter is judged integral.

As explained, the capillary rise phenomenon described by the Laplace equation forms the basis of the bubble-point test. However imperfectly translated, the bubble-point value is related to the size of the filter's largest pores; which, in turn, relates to organism retention. However, the diffusive airflow is governed by Fick's Law of diffusion, which, while influenced by the total porosity, has no direct relationship to the size of individual pores. It is therefore more complex to explain the correlation of diffusive airflow with organism retention. It can be accepted and used for what it is, an experimentally established relationship. Its utility is derived solely from this empirical connection. The correlation is limited by the accuracy and reliability of the experimental work performed by the individual filter manufacturer in demonstrating its existence. It is generally not known just how and with what detail the various filter manufacturers have established such correlations for each of their filter types. Not each filter manufacturer has necessarily done a thorough job.

The Diffusive Airflow Curve

The curve describing the passage of air through a wetted filter is shown in Figure

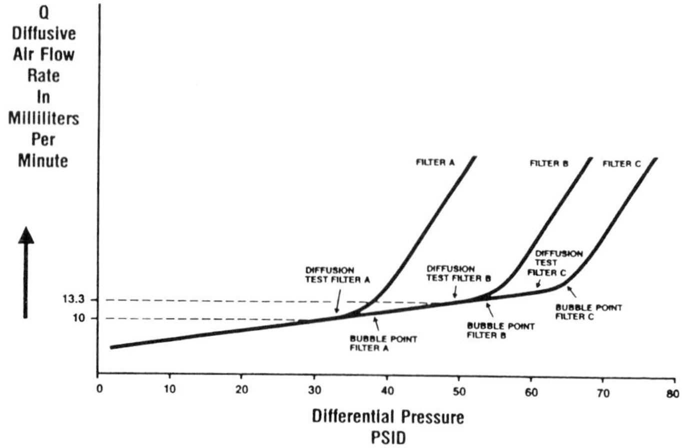

Figure 5-22. Diffusive airflow rate in milliliters per minute; bubble points and diffusive airflows at 80% of the bubble points.
Meltzer (1989c); Courtesy, *Ultrapure Water* journal

5-21. It consists of a straight line of gradual slope, followed usually a curved region within which lies the bubble point, and that is succeeded by an abruptly rising straight line denoting bulk airflow through the pores blown free of water. The left portion of the curve, the straight line of more gradual slope, represents the diffusive airflow.

Filters having larger pores exhibit lower bubble-point values. Thus the larger the pores that are present, the earlier the diffusive airflow line will be broken by the onset of the bubble point. This is shown in Figure 5-22 where filter A, containing larger pores than filter B, exhibits its bubble point at a lower differential pressure similarly for their relationships to filter C.

Until the bubble point of filter A is reached, the diffusive airflow curve is the same for all three filters. To distinguish between filters by means of diffusive airflow testing, it is necessary to perform the measurement at a differential pressure level between their bubble points: lower than one bubble point, higher than the other. No differentiation can be made among filters whose bubble-point readings are higher than the diffusive flow test pressure. In Figure 5-22 are depicted filters A and B. Filter A has a bubble point of 37 psig, and when tested at 30 psig, yields a diffusive airflow of 10 mL/min. By comparison, filter B shows a bubble point of 50 psig, and when measured at 40 psig, shows a diffusive airflow of 13.3 mL/min. If measured at 30 psig or below, filter B would exhibit the same diffusive flow as filter A. Differentiation between these filters must therefore be made at pressures above 30 psig. This is one reason that diffusive airflow measurements are made at as high a differential pressure level as

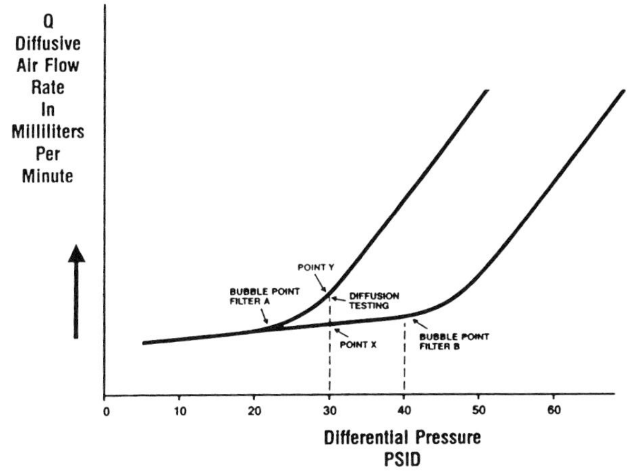

Figure 5-23. Diffusive airflow rate in milliliters per minute; diffusive airflow passing and failing.
Meltzer (1989c); Courtesy, *Ultrapure Water* journal

possible, consistent with avoiding the "knee," or curved area, of the airflow-versus-applied-pressure curve where measurement is difficult. The earlier practice of performing diffusive airflow measurements (or forward flow determinations) at lower differential pressures is to be avoided.

Consider Figure 5-23 as showing the air permeation curve of filter B as a wet sterilizing filter, traditionally 0.2-µm rated. The bubble point is shown as occurring at 40 psig. If a single-point diffusive airflow test is performed at 30 psig, the rate of air diffusion, as measured by collection of the air over a given time interval, would be found to fall on the diffusive airflow line (Figure 5-23, filter B, point X). If, however, it were found to be in excess of that rate, it would be taken to mean that instead of the supposed 0.2-µm-rated filter, a more open membrane was being tested (Figure 5-23, filter A, point Y).

Single-Point versus Multipoint Determinations

The bubble-point method of filter integrity testing assumes that filter pores may be regarded as capillaries, whatever their actual shapes, in that the air pressures necessary to evacuate them of imbibed water are inversely proportional to their diameters, however imperfectly defined by their pore-size rating. This accords with the rise of water in capillaries as elucidated by Laplace. It follows then that when a filter is bubble-point tested, the first set of pores emptied is composed of its largest pores. Regardless of how many pores may characterize a filter, its inherent bubble point reflects only the presence of its largest pores. The bubble point is independent of a filter's total porosity (Meltzer, 1989a; Schroeder and DeLuca, 1980).

By contrast, the diffusive airflow test reflects, in the volume of air that diffuses

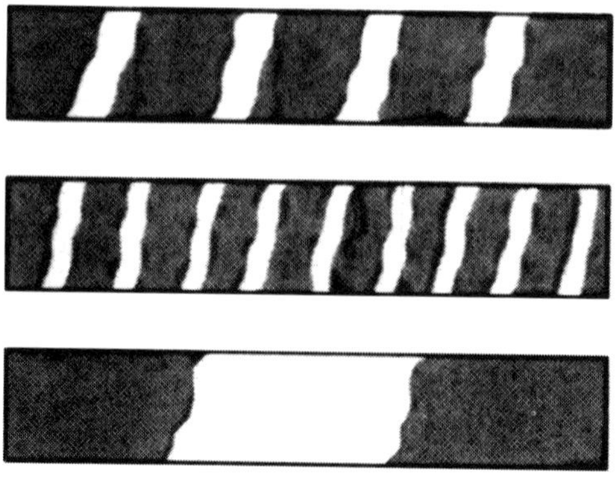

Figure 5-24. Rate of diffusion is a function of total porosity, not pore size.
Meltzer (1989c); Courtesy, *Ultrapure Water* journal

through a filter per unit time at a given pressure, the total porosity of the filter. It does not reveal the presence of the largest or of any other particular size pores (Meltzer, 1989c).

To be sure, in accordance with Fick's Law of diffusion, when a diffusive airflow integrity test is performed, the quantity of diffused air collected will be a function of the diffusivity of the air in the liquid medium, the solubility coefficient of the gas, the thickness of the filter, the transfilter pressure, and the extent of the filter area; all this in addition to the total filter porosity.

As Figure 5-24 illustrates, many small pores, fewer larger pores, or even a single very large pore can equally comprise an identical total porosity value. This would in each case represent ρ in the integrated form of Fick's equation describing the diffusion phenomenon (Reti, 1977):

$$N = DH\,(P_1 - P_2)\rho/L \qquad \text{Eq. 5-2}$$

where N is the permeation rate, D is the diffusivity of the gas in the liquid, H is the solubility coefficient of the gas, (P_1-P_2) is the transfilter pressure, L is the thickness of the liquid in the membrane, and ρ is the total void volume of the filter, its total porosity.

It bears being repeated that the authority of the integrity test values derives from empirically established correlations of these values with organism retention levels. The reliability of an integrity test for a given filter type directly reflects the quality of the experimental work performed by the individual filter manufacturer in establishing the underlying correlation.

The filter manufacturer specifies the lowest bubble-point value (the largest pore size) acceptable for that particular type of filter. Lower values imply the presence of larger pores that could be lacking in the sufficiency of their retentions. The upper acceptable limits of the manufacturer's diffusive airflow are also based upon experimentally demonstrated correlations of their levels with dependable organism retentions.

Filter manufacturers characterize a given filter type by a single acceptable maximum diffusive airflow level. A lower-than-the-maximum diffusive airflow value is acceptable. To avoid the experimental difficulty of comparing data points in an area of change (i.e., on a curve), single-point diffusive airflow tests are carried out on the straight-line portion of the curve. This is done at pressures as close to the bubble point as is feasible, usually at about 80% of the bubble point. This tie of the customary single-point testing pressure level with the bubble-point pressure references the diffusive airflow test to pore size. Therefore, higher than the maximum allowable diffusive air flows signifies the presence of too large pores.

Where single-point diffusive airflow determinations are made at a given pressure, as recommended by the filter manufacturer, the maximum allowable diffusive rate level may be used as a go/no-go integrity test criterion, and indeed often is. This is proper for the initial testing of filters of the types whose pores have been demonstrated to be adequately retentive by the established correlation between the diffusive airflow rates, a manifestation of the total porosity, and organism retentions. This sanction does not extend, however, to postfiltration diffusive airflow testing. The occurrence of pore-size changes during the filtration, a possible (if remote) development of flaws, must be entertained.

In the single-point determination, a too-high value is prudently rejected as signaling the possible presence of flaws. However, a value lower than the stipulated maximum is accepted. This latter reading is ascribed to a lower total porosity. But could it not also reflect a total porosity low enough to mask in its diffusive airflow rate the existence of pores large enough to compromise the filter's integrity? The filtrative accretion of retained material, viable or not, must inevitably come to block or diminish the size of the pores. This results in decreased total porosity, directly expressed in lower diffusive airflow values. A sufficient drop in such final airflow values may mask the presence of a flaw developed in the filter subsequent to its initial testing. For this reason a filter's entire airflow permeation curve, particularly including its bubble point, must be characterized. It is this measurement and this measurement alone that is capable of unambiguously revealing the existence of insufficiently retentive pores. The inquiry into such presences is the very purpose of filter integrity testing.

The plotting of a filter's complete air permeation history (as a function of increasing transfilter pressure), leading up to and even beyond its bubble-point, is most conveniently performed using an automated integrity test device, of which there are several in the market. Such electromechanical testing is more reliable than the relatively arduous manual exercise, its readings being less subjective.

The bubble-point integrity test and the diffusive airflow test are not in conflict. Each has its proper area of application. The more certain implications to retention based upon definition of the largest pores present in a filter may be had where bubble point testing is possible. Where diffusive airflows interfere with bubble point determinations, the diffusive airflow measurements themselves, correlated to organism retentions, serve as integrity tests.

Diffusive airflow measurements have their advantage in addition to serving as indicators of filter integrity. They can more precisely reveal filter incompatibilities. They can be used to gauge the completeness of a filter's wettablity, and they are more revealing of a filter's clean water flow properties.

In almost all its applications, however, diffusive airflow integrity testing requires defining the diffusive airflow curve by way of multipoint measurements using the liquid product in question. This is especially true in filter validation contexts where product-specific testing is necessitated.

Once the full diffusional airflow curve has been elucidated, single- point diffusional flow testing is warranted, as in production integrity testing settings.

Single point diffusive flow testing can be used as a standard integrity test method for use in the pharmaceutical production environment. (Weibel et al, 1986).

Anisotropic Filter Effect

Pore anisotropy, present to some small extent in most conventional isotropic membranes, results in an exaggeration of the diffusive airflow rate. Obviously, then, this exaggeration becomes magnified in the case of true anisotropic membranes. These show very pronounced diffusive airflow rates whose magnitude, although proper and appropriately correlated with organism retentions, would be indicative of failure in the case of the conventional isotropic membranes. The investigator must take care not to automatically translate a high rate of diffusion into a condemnation of the filter. The only point to be addressed is whether the diffusional airflow value accords with the filter manufacturer's correlation of organism retention.

The exaggerated diffusional airflow rates of the anisomorphic (anisotropic) filters serve also to interfere with their bubble points. The anisomorphic diffusional flows manifest themselves as a stream of bubbles, which may be confused with those generated at the bubble point. The diffusive airflow begins earlier (at lower differential) and is more vigorous because of the thinner water layer contained within the funnel-shaped anisotropic pore. The results are apparent low bubble points, "continuous streams of bubbles," that incline the uninitiated to conclude that a failed filter is at hand. Anisotropic membranes are characterized by lower bubble points than those exhibited by isomorphic filters, but they accord with the requisite organism retentions notwithstanding. Anisotropic membranes are often incorrectly condemned as having bubble-point failures. Once again the filter manufacturer's information regarding the particular filter being used must serve as the inspector's reference point. The significance of the bubble point for any filter lies not in the magnitude of its number, but in its empirical correlation to $1 \times 10^{7}/cm^{2}$ *P. diminuta* retention as established by the filter manufacturer and as attested to by available documentation.

Multicartridge Testing

With larger area filters (generally anything bigger than a 10-inch cartridge) the diffusive airflow rate is sufficient to obfuscate the bubble-point measurement. However, some filter users ingeniously perform the bubble point even on multicartridge assemblies by rapidly raising the air pressure to just below the bubble point and then proceeding slowly. Less diffusive airflow takes place in the shorter time and the bubble point is therefore not masked. The practice seems to be successful but is not widespread.

Since the bubble point signals the presence of the set of largest pores present, it serves as an integrity test even when multiple cartridges are involved. Presumably the set of largest pores, even if present in only one cartridge, still manifests correlation with the organism retention of the entire assemblage of filters.

Nevertheless, because diffusive airflow in multicartridge arrangements can interfere with bubble-point measurements, most users of such devices undertake their integrity testing by way of diffusive airflow measurements. At least two problems inhere. Unlike the bubble-point measurement where the airflow presumably marks a single area or cartridge out of an entire array, the diffusive airflow averages the air volume coming out of the entire collection of filters. The excessively high airflow emanating from one filter may therefore be masked where low flows come from another (or others). In other words, a given out-of-specification filter may not necessarily be revealed by diffusive airflow testing where multicartridge arrangements are used.

In the semiconductor industry, large-scale final filters, as distinct from point-of-use filters, often comprise multicartridge arrangements that are 21 cartridges round and 30 inches high. This is equivalent to 63 ten-inch cartridges. The diffusive airflow issuing from such an assembly can be 63 × 24 mL/min, or 1,512 mL/min of air. The collection of so much air in a diffusive airflow test is not conveniently performed. The tendency, therefore, is to resort to integrity testing by the pressure-hold test, wherein the collection and measurement of large volumes of air are not required.

Diffusive Airflow versus Time

Ordinarily, a filter subjected to integrity testing is examined in only two instances, once just before use and once just after use. It has been reported that in large-volume parenteral production, filters may be integrity-tested periodically during production runs of longer duration. Filters used in air filtrations (whether as vent filters or for the purification of fermentation air) are integrity-tested, presumably after every batch operation; are sterilized; and are again integrity-tested prior to yet another reuse. This practice is relatively widespread because air streams are usually so clean as to impose only small particulate loads upon the filters. Indeed, some filter manufacturers claim that their filters are capable of withstanding some 100 hours, or so, exposure to steam, for just such applications. Be that as it may, most users will prefer a new filter after ten uses or so. There is, after all, some accumulation of particulates whose subtle influences may somehow not be alleviated by steam nor be revealed by customary analyses.

More recently, diffusive air testing has received diligent application in the semiconductor industry. Some users have compiled a history of daily and/or weekly testing of the same filter: an experience rare until now. Interestingly, more than one has reported a diminution, sometimes to an apparent leveling off, from an initial high (albeit acceptable) diffusive airflow value.

It is rationalized that the filters, all inherently hydrophobic and brought to a state of wettability by the use of wetting adjuncts, reflected in their first reading an incompleteness of wetting. Thus, while all pores contained water enough to block bulk airflow (as at a bubble point), the liquid layers in some may have been thin enough to yield high diffusive airflows. With time, it is hypothesized, the wetting improved; the narrower pores became more filled with water as a function of time; and this occasioned gradually decreasing diffusive airflows as the water thicknesses increased and became fuller.

As regards the integrity implications of this situation, the filters could be judged integral as long as the initial single-point reading was not excessive in value. (How revealing it would have been for the entire air diffusion curve to have been elucidated!)

What is of additional interest is that a periodic daily plotting of diffusive airflows may serve to indicate to filter manufacturers the thoroughness with which their wetting-agent treatments serve to modify the inherent hydrophobicities of their filters.

Pressure-Hold Test

In the performance of the diffusion airflow integrity test, a wetted filter sealed into its housing is subjected to a continuously maintained level of air pressure on its upstream side, and the volume of air that diffuses during a stated time interval is collected and measured. If the housing is improperly sealed, air will leak out. Small leaks may even go undetected, although providing opportunities for contaminative entry into the system. If the pressure level is sufficiently maintained, which is not too difficult in the case of small leaks, the volume of air collected downstream will not be affected.

The pressure-hold test is a variant of the diffusive airflow test. All is arranged as in the diffusion test except that when the stipulated applied pressure is reached, the pressure source is valved off. The decay of pressure within the holder is then observed as a function of time, utilizing a sensitive gauge affixed to the upstream side of the holder. The decrease in pressure can come from two sources, the first being diffusive loss across the wetted filter. Since the upside pressure in the holder is not maintained, it decreases progressively all the while diffusion takes place. The rate of diffusion is, therefore, progressively decreasing. As a result, the volume of air collected is less than in the diffusive airflow test. The second source of pressure decay is that caused by faulty filter/housing assembly. Indeed, one virtue of the pressure-hold test is that it tests the integrity of the plumbing. That is why it is often used as the initial integrity test. As laudable as the intention is, however, the pressure-hold measurement is not an integrity test in that it does not correlate the organism retention capabilities of the filter with any precise measure of air-pressure diminution.

The pressure-hold test measures the loss of air from within the holder that houses the filter(s). The perfect gas law governs the air loss measurement.

$$PV = nRT \qquad \text{Eq. 5-3}$$

where n is the moles of gas, R is the universal gas constant, T is temperature, V is gas volume, and P is the gas pressure.

Two points are made. First, the decrease in gas pressure measured by an upstream gauge is influenced strongly by the volume of the filter holder. It would depend upon the particular holder/filter combination. Second, to be an integrity test reflective of a filter's organism retention capabilities, the test measurement, as of pressure decay, must be demonstrably correlated to that property. If the pressure-hold test has been correlated with organism retentions, then it has been done so largely and only privately by users who have developed their own historical basis after ruling out the existence of housing leaks caused by improper sealing. More recently, some filter manufactures have offered to furnish filter users with curves describing the loss of airflow under pressure-hold conditions. The user, of course, must furnish the filter supplier the exact details of the filter and housing being used. (Even the placement of the valve and any tubing volume involved must be considered, because this can affect the total volume within which the pressure decay takes place.) Changing either the filter or the housing necessitates a redetermination of the diffusive airflow loss under the pressure-hold conditions, for this may change the total volume surrounding the filter in its housing.

Hango et al. (1989) published on the use of the pressure-hold method as an integrity test under conditions of having the exact volume of the holder/filter and the relevant diffusive airflow defined by the filter supplier (Figure 5-25). Under

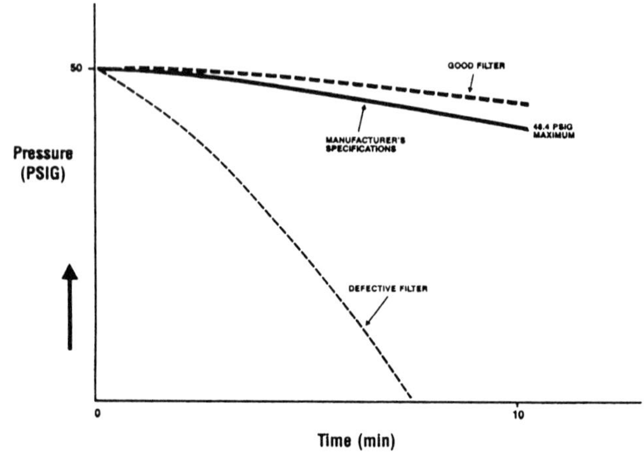

Figure 5-25. Filter integrity testing; pressure hold.
Hango et al. (1989); Courtesy, *Ultrapure Water* journal

these circumstances, the pressure (volume) decay measured under pressure-hold conditions (in the absence of plumbing leaks) can be correlated to ordinary diffusive airflow data that are in turn correlated with specific organism retention values.

Usually data on the pressure decay ensuing from the pressure-hold tests cannot be correlated with organism retentions. In this sense it is not a nondestructive assay of the filter for its organism retention capabilities. In the semiconductor industry, however, where the integrity tests are used to signal conformation to the filter's specifications (rather than to reflect precise organism retention levels as required by FDA regulations in pharmaceutical processing), the pressure-hold test can serve very well, provided that the measurement of the pressure decay is sensitive enough, and that a use history is developed for the given holder/filter employed.

Characterization of the Pressure-Hold Test

One advantage of the pressure-hold test is that it is capable of revealing imperfections in the assembly and sealing of the housing and filters as well as of disclosing flaws in the filters. This is useful particularly in initial integrity testing for the early disclosure of filter seating failures or of housing sealing leaks, enabling prevention of a profitless undertaking of the filtration in the first place.

A second advantage is that the pressure (volume) decay reading central to the pressure-hold test can be made on the upstream side of the filter, on the housing itself, without compelling invasion of the downstream side of the system. Aseptic invasions and connections are common; they are successfully made every day. They do, however, portend risk to the system and are best avoided where possible.

The use of automated test devices also permits avoidance of downstream invasions during the performance of the more conventional integrity tests.

In measuring the pressure or air volume losses from the filter housing, it is not necessary to measure the large air volumes (or their water displacements) that are so burdensome to the use of the diffusive airflow test on multicartridge housings. Most of the automated integrity test devices use mass pressure transducers to measure the flow of air into the housings to replace the air lost, or else they measure the in-line gas flow. These measurements can be made with great accuracy. Pressure transducers have a sensitivity of ± one millibar. That is why the automated instruments have requisite detection sensitivity. Such a sensitivity is required because the pressure-hold test, even more than the diffusive airflow method, is strongly influenced by temperature. In the former case, temperature is a factor in the perfect gas law. In the latter, the gas solubility and its diffusivity (as well as the volume it occupies) are influenced by temperature.

Determinations of the pressure (volume) decays by means of the gauges normally employed in the manually performed pressure-hold tests are woefully inadequate. According to Schroeder, pressure gauges commonly require pressure losses of at least 40 mbar/min in order to record the event. Such a loss in a 10-inch cartridge would be forthcoming from a flaw 50 μm in size (or an aggregate of flaws to that size) at a pressure level of 40 psig. Conventional pressure gauges lack the requisite sensitivity for application to the pressure-hold test. Nevertheless, at least one filter manufacturer believes it is adequate to use gauges of 1 1/2 inch diameters. If there are no sealing leaks, the pressure in the housing will decline about 1 psig over a 10-minute period. After 20 minutes, hopefully, such a drop can be noticed even on 1 1/2 inch gauges. In the event of system leaks, the pressure drops more precipitously. Such small pressure-drop readings may be of value in determining whether filter seating or housing O-ring leaks exist. Such readings are too insensitive to reveal much about the filter.

Larger-diameter gauges would be more useful, but these and their periodic calibration are expensive. Even more expensive are the automated integrity testing devices, often referred to as electromechanical testing machines. Yet it is these very instruments that should be used in performing the pressure-hold (and other) integrity tests.

IBM, a semiconductor manufacturer, conducted pressure-hold testing using an automated testing device at 50 psig (Hango et al., 1989). The pressure decay was measured over a 10-minute interval, although sometimes it was foreshortened to 1 minute and extrapolated to 10.

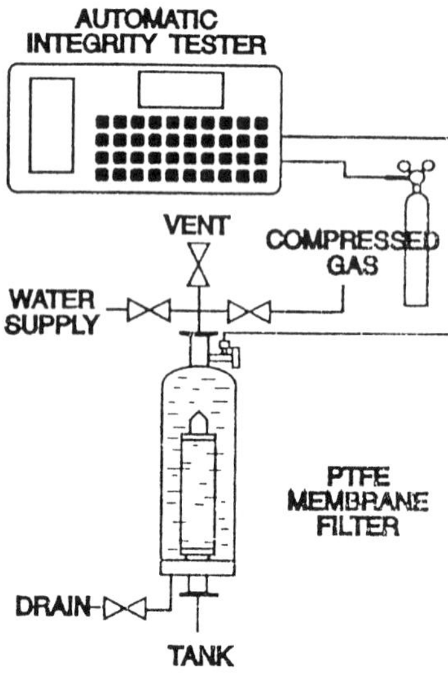

Figure 5-26. Water intrusion test setup.
Tarry et al. *Ultrapure Water* (1993).

Water Intrusion Integrity Test

For integrity testing the hydrophobic vent filter it can be wet out with alcohol, and an alcohol bubble point performed. Isopropyl alcohol in 60% aqueous solution or 25% aqueous tertiary butanol are both satisfactory. The alcohol is then removed by drying prior to the filter being autoclaved. Polysulfone filters may stress-crack under alcohol drying. For such polymers, removal of the alcohol by water flushing is indicated. The sterilized vent filter is then installed aseptically.

It is also possible to define

the largest pores of a hydrophobic membrane by the pressure needed to force water into such pores. Obviously, as is known from mercury porosimetry work, for instance, higher pressures are required to intrude a nonwetting liquid into pores of narrower diameter. Therefore, a measurement of water intrusion into a hydrophobic membrane will reflect the entrance, or incipient entrance, of water into the largest pores of the filter. The upstream side of the hydrophobic filter cartridge housing is flooded with water. Nitrogen gas pressure is then applied by way of an automatic integrity tester to a level of 2.5 bar (36 psig). A period of pressure stabilization takes place over some minutes during which the cartridge pleats adjust their positions under imposed pressures. After the pressure drop thus occasioned stabilizes, any further pressure drop in the upstream pressurized gas volume, as measured by the automatic tester, signifies a beginning of water intrusion into the largest (hydrophobic) pores, water being incompressible. The automated integrity tester is sensitive enough to detect the pressure drop (Figure 5-26). A correlation has been demonstrated between the observed pressure drop and the organism retention characteristic of the hydrophobic membrane (Tarry et al., 1993; Dosmar et al., 1993, and Tingley et al., 1995) (Figures 5-27 and 5-28). It is this empirically established correlation that serves as the validating authority for the water intrusion test. By way of this procedure, hydrophobic vent filters can be integrity tested in-situ without the use of alcoholic solutions and

Table 5-7
Retention LRV as a function of water intrusion pressure (10-in. Aervent filter cartridges).

Water intrusion point pressure (psi)	*Retention LRV*
21.5	9.42
22.5	9.45
23.5	10.0
25.0	10.5
25.5	9.01
27.0	9.81
27.0	10.8
32.5	10.9
32.5	>11.3
36.0	>11.3
26.0	>11.4
37.0	>11.3

Challenged with *p. diminuta* per HIMA methodology. >= sterile effuent
From Tingley et al. 1995; Courtesy *Pharmaceutical Technology*.

without risk to downstream-filter asepsis.

Tingley et al. (1995) confirmed the suitability of the water-flow methodology to the in-line testing of hydrophobic filters. These investigators confirmed correlation between their water intrusion point pressures and log reduction values for organism retentions, as shown in Table 5-7. The test, as also the other integrity tests, is sensitive to temperature and to the water purity in terms of surface tension. It is, however, less sensitive to temperature variations than the bubble point and forward-flow (diffusive air flow) measurements because of the large thermal mass represented by the water in the housing. Tingley et al. (1995) demonstated that the water intrusion or water-flow test was as robust as the alcohol-based bubble point measurement test.

The basis for this integrity test is as already discussed above. Correlations have been established between the organism retentions exhibited by a filter and the rates of pressure drop from a given pressure level as caused by water intruding into a hydrophobic filter (Figure 5-29). The larger the rates of pressure drop, the greater the extent of water intrusion into the pores, as measured by pressure drop over a given time interval. The lower the pressure drop, the narrower the pore, the more retentive the filter. The principle underlying this integrity test is the same as that which is the basis for mercury intruding a nonwettable (to mercury) glass capillary, except that pressures too low to cause polymeric pore distortions are involved. Nonintegral filters will actually have water intruded into them. Integral filters will not. The automatic test machine

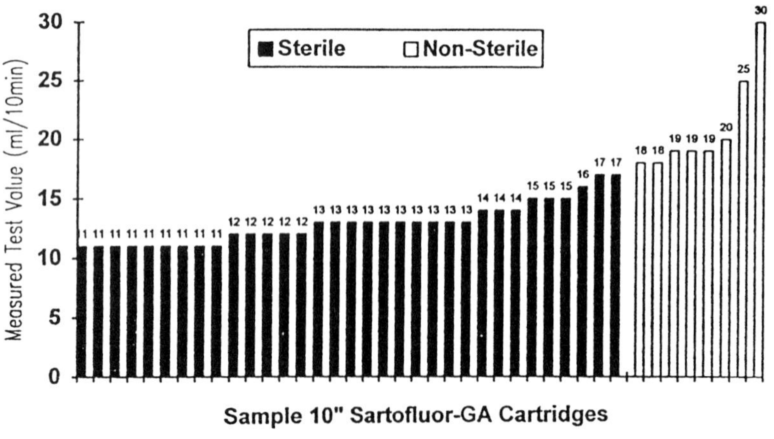

Figure 5-27. Bacterial challenge correlation in the Water Intrusion Test.
Tarry et al. (1993); Courtesy, *ULTRAPURE WATER* journal.

is sensitive enough to detect the small pressure-decrease rate attendant upon incipient water entry into integral filters.

Since the water pressure intrusion test involves wetting phenomena, it will reflect, in common with the other integrity tests, the influences of surface tension (therefore, water purity), temperature, and pore wettability. The importance of these factors in the operations of the bubble-point, diffusive airflow (forward flow), and pressure-hold integrity tests has been detailed by Scheer et al. (1993).

The pore-wettability bears being noted. The wettability of a polymeric surface by water depends upon its critical surface tension. Water has a surface tension of 72 dynes/cm at ambient temperatures. To be wetted by water requires a polymer to have a high CST, one that approaches the surface tension of water. Polytetrafluoroethylene (PTFE) has an extremely low CST. It will have extreme reluctance to be wet by water; aqueous alcoholic solutions have lower CSTs than water and, therefore, more readily wet PTFE filters. Vent filters made of PVDF and of other hydrophobic polymers have higher CST values than PTFE. They will more readily be wetted by water. Therefore, filters composed of less hydrophobic substances can be expected to exhibit water pressure integrity test values different than those given by PTFE filters. Even more, polymers having CSTs of between 19 and 21 can be expected to vary greatly in their wettability. Some authorities believe the CST values of 45 dynes/cm are required for wetting. In any case, because of the lower CST value of PTFE polymer(s), filters of this composition may show more steadfastness of water intrusion test (WIT) values

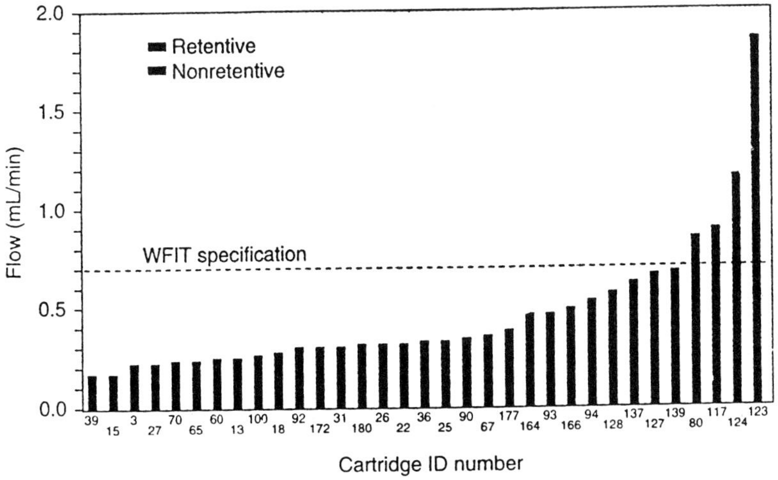

Figure 5-28. (a) Water flow values correlation to bacterial retention (Aervent cartridges ar 38 psi test pressure); (b) test value-LRV correlation achieved with a flow specification of 0.7 mL/min water (Aervent cartridges at 38 psi test pressure).
Tingley et al. (1995), Courtesy, *Pharmaceutical Technology.*

than vent filters of not so low CST.

Air Filter Hydrophobicity

As stated, the condensation of water within the pores of vent and air filters would block the flow of air. To minimize this interference and its untoward consequences, hydrophobic membranes are used for this purpose. Water is more easily expelled from such filters. However, a film of moisture, not necessarily enough to block the pores, may still be present. Air filters undergo repeated use because they are ordinarily little consumed in a single processing operation. Before reuse they are steamed to resterilize them. They are then integrity tested for their continuing suitability to retain organisms. Steam sterilization can leave a film of water upon local portions of the hydrophobic filter surface rendering them hydrophilic.

This can lead to organism penetration of the air filter as a function of time. It would be wise to ensure the proper drying of the steamed air filter. This achievement can be tested by use of the very water intrusion test used to establish the integrity of hydrophobic filters.

The water intrusion test depends upon and measures the hydrophobicity of the filter. Only the experimentally demonstrated correlation of its values with the entrance of water into the hydrophobic pore structure establishes it as an integrity test. But the basic measurement of filter hydrophobicity is itself an inherent requirement in its pertinence to air filter reuse. Consider an integral air filter than contains hydrophilic accretions or deposits upon its surface. Their presence may

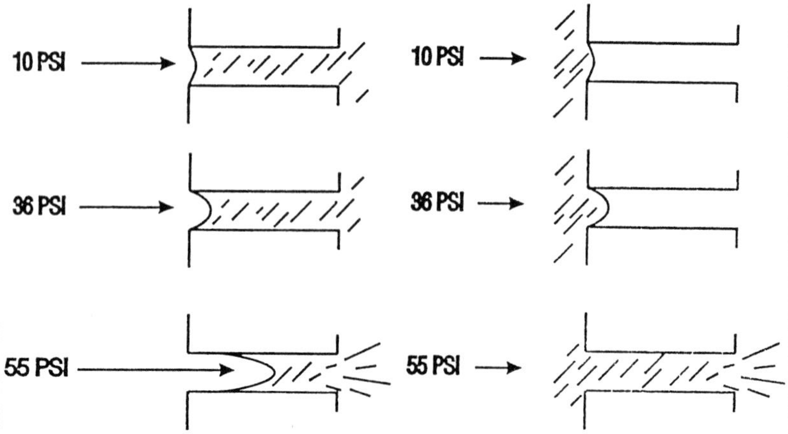

Figure 5-29. Water bubble-point test (left), and water pressure integrity test (right), 0.2 μm pore.
Tarry et. al. (1993); Courtesy, *Ultrapure Water*.

encourage microbial growth and, ultimately, organism penetration. Solely ensuring air filter integrity, however essential, is not enough in air filter usage. The filter's full hydrophobicity must also be assessed to ensure freedom from compromising hydrophilic impurities.

As previously stated, in the usual air filtration or vent filter applications, the filter is so little exhausted by the depositions it collects that its reuse is compelled for economic reasons. Hence the need periodically to repeat its integrity verification before and after each individual use—ideally without removing it from its installation and usually after steam sterilizations. The filter may remain integral, but if it collects, as it well may, deposits of hydrophilic matter, then as localized and limited as these may be, they can serve as loci for organism growth and penetration, defeating the very purpose intended by the use of a hydrophobic filter. If the intention of the integrity test in air filtration applications is solely to assess filter integrity, then the water intrusion test may, on occasion, mislead and be responsible for the discard of integral filters. If, however, the purpose of examining the filter is to gauge its suitability as a longer-term air filter, as in fermenter operations for example, then the water intrusion test is sovereign for the purpose because it simultaneously measures the integrity and the hydrophobicity of the subject filter. Both of these operations are required in a filter dedicated to longer-term air filtration applications.

When the water intrusion test indicates an integral filter, it may be used (or reused) with confidence, even in long-term air applications. Failure to pass the water intrusion test signals a need for further filter assessment. A bubble-point test subsequently performed and passed successfully may indicate that the filter

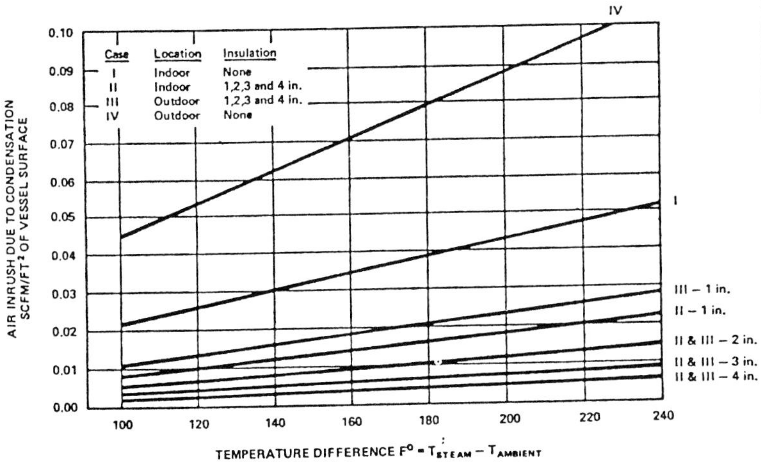

Figure 5-30. Air inrush characteristics caused by steam condensation.
Cole (1977); Courtesy, *Pharmaceutical Technology*

is not sufficiently free of deposits to permit its safe reuse, albeit integral. Then, if considered desirable, a suitable filter-refurbishing effort may be undertaken. (Meltzer et al. 1994)

As regards the water-flow, water intrusion test technique (Tingley et al 1995) conclude: "The ultimate goal of developing a practical water-flow integrity test was to obviate the use of alcohol in filter testing and to incorporate the alcohol-free test into product batch-release protocols."

"Quality control requirements for water-flow integrity testing will be met by functional validation as well as by historical trending. As part of the in-plant validation process, a water-flow test can be conducted routinely, before an off-line alcohol test. This will provide process-specific correlation between the two test methods. Until the water-flow test is qualified, the alcohol integrity test values can still be used for release protocols."

"When filters are not tested poststerilization, the water-flow technique can be initiated for evaluation before formal inclusion in the process. An added benefit of this trial is the identification of non-integral filters that might otherwise affect batch quality."

Present Status of Integrity Testing

The integrity tests are by far most reliable and least ambiguous when performed using an automated test device. These instruments have the additional considerable advantage of not requiring the invasion of the system downstream of the filter.

- The integrity testing of a given filter should be carried out in conformity with its manufacturer's protocol.
- The bubble-point test is the only integrity test with theoretical underpinnings to the largest pore size. It loses reliability as the effective filtration area increases.
- The diffusive airflow test derives authority only from its experimentally demonstrated (empirical) correlation to organism retention levels. It should be performed full scale.
- As commonly performed without benefit of automated instruments, both the bubble-point and the diffusive airflow measurements necessitate invasion of the system downstream of the filter, risking asepsis.
- The pressure-hold test does not violate downstream system integrity. It can be a useful indicator of system leaks, whether of seals or filters or both. Its readings require being correlated with retention levels. Its performance needs the sensitivity of automated testing devices.
- The water intrusion test is suitable for the determination of hydrophobic membrane integrity.

- Integrity testing can be used to investigate filter compatibility.
- Initial integrity tests should be performed. As a matter of practicality, the pressure-hold test can serve the need of initial integrity testing when performed by automated devices.
- In common with all test methods, the various integrity-test procedures have their limitations. Where their positive implications are not overstated they provide useful and dependable indications of a filter's suitability. That is their purpose. They should be used nonritualistically, however, with an understanding of their limits. So performed, they provide dependable conclusions.

Integrity Tests for RO and UF Filters

Basically, there are no established integrity tests for RO and UF membranes, certainly not of the type that directly correlate to organism retentions.

Red Dye Test for RO Membranes

A solution of rhodamine dye of no particular concentration is prepared in aqueous solution and is circulated throughout the RO filter being tested. The filter is then taken apart and examined. The rhodamine of molecular weight 700 to 800 permeates even pinholes to become evident as red marks. This test is not a performance test. It is used as a membrane construction guide. Thus a spiral-wound RO arrangement when postmortemed may show a red streak where folds have damaged the membrane. Crossover patterns due to damage caused by the polypropylene spacer layers become evident, and pinholes show up. Radiating "spider webs" can be seen at faulty glue lines.

Comparison of Chloride and Sulfate Rejections

Reverse osmosis membrane rejects sodium chloride and sodium sulfate to different extents. This can be used as an in-service integrity test for these filters. A solution of low osmotic pressure containing equal parts of sodium chloride and sodium sulfate to the total concentration of about 500 ppm is passed through the RO unit. At 60 psig, about 89% of the sodium chloride and 99% of the sodium sulfate are rejected. At 400 psig and with a total salt concentration of 200 ppm, about 95% to 97% sodium chloride and 99.9% of sodium sulfate are rejected. Where leaks are present, the percentage rejections will be less, and their differences will be minimized in accordance with the size of the membrane flaw.

The above test conditions apply to cellulose acetate type ROs. Thin-film composite RO membranes will require a variation on the above test values.

Many variations of this type of rejection test exist. In essence, rejection measurements are made periodically. As the values are seen to decline, the RO membrane is replaced. The end point signaling replacement is subjectively arrived at. There is no established standard.

Ultrafilter Cutoff Verifications

The integrity testing of ultrafilters is even more difficult. The different commercial UF filters have their own particular cutoffs. It is the maintenance of the given cutoff ability that is ascertained in the "integrity testing." Thus, UF filters with cutoffs of 10,000, meaning that larger sizes of molecules are held back by these filters, can be tested for their abilities to retain cytochrome of molecular weight 12,500. To measure the cytochrome, a colorimeter is used. Alternatively, Cibacrom Blue, a blue dye, can be measured visually to see whether it passed through the membrane intended to retain it. This testing, repeated periodically, serves as an integrity test. When the larger indicator molecules pass through the membrane, it is judged to have degraded to the point where its replacement is indicated. In this vein, UF filters characterized by higher cutoffs are variously tested with appropriately sized molecules. Most of these are proteins, and their detection may require the use of a spectrophotometer.

At least two complications are involved. First, size is important, but shape is even more so. Unfortunately, few good models for both shapes and sizes are known.

In addition, it must be ascertained that the dye or protein being used as a size model is not prevented from going through the filter by becoming adsorbed to the polymer constituting the membrane. For instance, cytochrome will adsorb to cellulose acetate and would therefore not be likely to permeate UF membranes made of that polymer, regardless of the cutoff limit.

Bioengineering users are not happy with the testing of ultrafilters using proteins such as albumin. They fear the adsorption of the test protein by the filter, followed by its at least partial elusion to contaminate the very protein they are preparing.

One UF filter manufacturer is developing an "integrity test" based on the detectable passage of air through the filter when it is subjected to a pressure of 20 psig. The air is discerned in the form of bubbles; the pressure is then reduced to 5 psig and the bubbles stop. Regrettably, this test is lacking in delicacy. It differentiates only between UF membranes of molecular weight cutoffs of 10,000 and 100,000. It is useful, however, in detecting flawed filters wherein the UF membrane has become separated from its supporting scrim.

Nonstructured Depth Filters

The removal of particles from the fluids containing them can often be accomplished by contacting the suspension with finely divided solids onto whose surfaces the particles adsorb or within whose layers they can become sieve removed (Fiore et al., 1980). Thus, deep-bed filters of substances such as sand (Ogedengbe, 1984), garnet, anthracite, coal, or charcoal, perform the particle-removal actions desired of them in water purification contexts. Particle capture in such instances occurs throughout the deep-bed filter, hence the term depth filter (as distinct from surface or screen filter) to describe the loci of particle removal. Such nonstructured depth filters are devised also by stirring finely divided solids such as diatomaceous earth, perlite, fumed silica, and/or various other filter aids into the suspension, followed by the filtrative removal of both the purifying particle and the particles it has entrapped by adsorption.

Thus in pharmaceutical manufacturing, diatomaceous earth finds application in serum purification, antibiotics manufacture, and in-vitro diagnostics preparation. Granulated activated carbon is used for color removal in large-volume parenteral manufacture and in antibiotic manufacture. Fumed silica is used in the preparation of certain therapeutic blood fractions. Since these finely divided solids are often used in the form of layers supported on a septum, or in the form of deep beds, they are defined as nonstructured filters or prefilters, the latter term stressing their customary usage. The term *prefilter*, in turn, implies a filtrative action involving adsorptive removals (as well as sieve retentions), especially of the particles of impurities small enough to enter the filter pores (the interstices among the solid granules) along with the permeating liquid.

Filter Aids

Yet there is a group of granulated solids among these materials that, because of their sizes, shapes, and mode of disposition, form layers whose filtrative action differs from the conventional unstructured depth filters such as sand or carbon. These nonstructured filter materials are given the appellation of *filter aids* in the industrial filtration field where they are most widely used. Actually, however, they are not filter aids in the sense that flocculating agents may be said to assist in the filtrative removal of fine particles. Rather, they constitute the primary filter material. Although the filter aid particles are capable of adsorptive capture, their cakes, when properly composed, are believed to be tight enough to restrain particles chiefly by sieve retention. The nonstructural depth filters or filter aids can provide a high particle-loading capacity even while permitting high rates of flow. Filter aids are useful industrially in the filtrative breaking of oil emulsions by the removal of stabilizing solids; and in the removal of solids from aqueous streams even when the solid contents are too low for flocculation, (namely, below 5 ppm) reducing them to as low as 0.1 ppm. Filter aids in conjunction with a rotary vacuum drum have been used to remove particles too fine to be separated by most fixed media. An example is 6% or higher of solids from antibiotic fermentation broth filtrations where the median particle range is only some 1 to 2 μm.

General Properties of Filter Cakes

There are a number of properties of the filter cakes or layers built of the various nonstructured depth filters that determine their suitabilities for particular filter applications. Thus the pore sizes of their interstices govern their sieve retentivity and influence their rate of flow. Flowrate, however, is also dependent on the number of pores. Pore size is more important, as shown by the following Kozeny-Poiseuille equation.

The volume average pore diameter, D, as distinct from the flow or number average pore diameter, is inversely related to the surface-to-volume ratio of the particles constituting the nonstructural filter, S.

$$D^2 = 16E^2 \div S^2(1 - E)^2 \qquad \text{Eq. 5-4}$$

Where E represents the void volume porosity (Carman, 1937).

The volume average pore diameter thus derived is smaller than that obtained from flow average calculations because the flow average number reflects the fourth-power flow relationship to the pore radius as in the Hagen Poiseuille equation. In any case, S, the ratio of surface to volume, becomes increasingly larger as the particle size declines; the smaller the filter aid particles, the smaller the volume average pore diameter.

Therefore, as is the general rule in filtration, one aims for a minimum but adequate retention in order to avoid the undue penalizing of the rate of filtration by retention of smaller than required particles. Within the context of the nonstructured depth filters, however, protection of the septum against fouling must also be ensured. Consequently the cake must be tight enough to keep the impurities from penetrating to the septum or support layer. Cain (1973) showed that the highest filter aid efficiency will be yielded by a filter aid whose median pore size most closely matches the median particle size of the suspended solids whose removal is desired.

The cake permeability to liquids is, therefore, dependent on the number of pores but especially on their size. The density of packing, and the cake incompressibility in turn, define the pore sizes; for it is the dimensional stability of the cake structure that governs the permanence of the pore sizes, the retentivity, and the flowrates achieved under the applied differential pressures over the duration of the filtration.

The permeability of the filter aid cakes also defines the accessibility of the suspension being filtered to the filter cloth, pad, or septum on which the cake is constructed by deposition of the discrete filter aid particles. This is important when cleaning operations are involved. It is desired that the impurities not penetrate the filter cake to foul the septum. It is found that some 3% of larger particles, above 150 mesh in size, should be in the particle mix. This serves to bridge over the septum openings and helps, therefore, to form a stable precoat. Low cake densities make for good permeabilities. The densities should be on the order of 160 to 320 kg/m^3(10 to 20 lb/ft^3), depending on the filter aid. Small and more regularly shaped particles have higher normal packing densities and lower permeabilities. This makes for the retention of finer particles by sieving, but may unduly penalize the rates of flow. Generally speaking, the more narrow the particle-size distribution, the more efficient the filter-aid cake, for the more regular its degree of packing and the smaller its interstices. The median particle sizes of filter aids will range from 6 to 30 μm or more.

Following formation of the precoat, the liquid can be mixed with a body feed of filter aid and be presented for filtration. With batch-type operations it is satisfactory to add the filter aid to the liquid in a tank and to agitate the mixture as it is fed to the filter. Unfortunately, the body feed, usually of the order of 0.1%, serves to abrade the pump surfaces, and it itself undergoes physical degradation while being pumped.

Most usually, therefore, a slurry containing as high as 18% of filter aid is prepared and, by means of an injection pump designed to avoid abrasion (usually of a plunger type or diaphragm [tube] type), is added to the system just before the filter, thus sparing the filter feed pump needless abrasion.

When the change is made from precoating to filtering the liquid with the body feed, a continuous flow with the minimum pressure variation should be maintained in order to support the precoat in position against the septum.

The finer grades of filter aid will yield greater retention efficiencies along with lower flowrates, because of the closer packing and the smaller pores that result from the use of smaller particles. This is in accord with Kozeny's teaching.

Those who are interested in the details concerning precoats of the various filter aids, the management of their formation and removal, and their areas of application are directed to Chapter 1 of *Filtration in the Pharmaceutical Industry* (Meltzer, 1987a). The immediate interest centers upon water purification applications, especially where precoats of powdered ion-exchange resins are constructed upon septa for the purposes of condensate polishing waste removal in the power generation field.

Septa

String-wound media, usually polymeric, and metallic mesh compositions, whether sintered or not, are currently used as septa in powdered resin precoat systems. Weissman (1988) called attention to the Darcy equation governing the flow fluid through filters:

$$Q/A = K\Delta P \div ut \qquad \text{Eq. 5-5}$$

where Q is flowrate in gpm, A is effective area in ft^2, ΔP is differential pressure in psid), u = viscosity in centipoise, t is thickness in inches, and K is the permeability factor

Weissman (1988) described the requirements of the septum media upon which the precoat is deposited. Because the precoat undergoes periodic removal upon its exhaustion and replacement, effort is made to preserve the underlying septum in a clean condition. Therefore, it is not intended to act as a filter, but only as a support for the precoat. The precoat is the filter medium. It is meant to retain the objectionable particles. If these penetrate the precoat, they should not be retained by the septum lest the porosity characteristics of the latter be altered to a point where the next precoat to be formed may be inadequate. If particles become lodged in the septum, they should be amenable to removal by backwashing. Weissman (1988) says the following regarding the ideal properties of septa:

> For optimal surface filtration the medium should be as thin as possible yet strong enough to withstand repeated back-wash without distorting the pore size distribution; it should provide a high void volume to ensure long life between back-wash (maximum resin utilization) and the medium should retain precoat solids only on the surface to facilitate back-wash. The filtration medium should function as a barrier to precoat solids. Powdered resin particles should not pass into the pore structure; rather they must collect as a porous cake on the septa.
>
> By design, the pore-size distribution of the septa should closely match that of the porous cake, in order that the precoat does all the filtering. Solids that pass through the precoat should, by design, pass the filtration septa to limit fouling of the septa by corrosion products and to ensure consistent service life, cycle after cycle.
>
> If the septa are too coarse, resin fines will pass into the effluent. If the septa are too fine, corrosion products will be retained and some fraction will remain embedded in the filter medium even after backwash. The available open area is then gradually reduced (after each cycle) and the pressure differential across the filter medium is progressively increased. In time, the pressure drop across the medium becomes significant and the total allowable pressure differential across the precoat plus medium is reached in a shorter period of time, reducing service life, forcing wastage of resin, and increasing waste handling costs.
>
> For each precoat formulation, there will be some optimum medium construction that permits consistent service life. That medium should have a pore structure that is as uniform as possible to provide a sharp particle size cutoff, as this too reduces the probability that the medium will become fouled by corrosion products.
>
> As the pore-size distribution of the medium is more uniform, a more uniform precoat is produced along the length of the septa, and localized "thinning" is avoided.
>
> As the medium is made thicker, there is a higher probability that the fine corrosion products that pass through the precoat will impinge onto the walls of the pore structure and be retained by the septa. To minimize the

capture of fine particles and to make it easier to "clean" elements that become fouled by particulate matter, the optimal medium should be as thin as possible.

There is some reason to believe that metallic septa offer advantage. They can be constructed to have a more narrow pore-size distribution (i.e., a more regular mesh pattern than the interstices of their string-wound counterparts). This, in turn, may influence the more even deposition of the precoat, making for its more uniform pore characteristics.

Metallic septa are comprised of two types: woven wire elements, and those prepared by the sintering of metal particles. Often used in original equipment offerings, the wire septa are of open construction (ANRT, 1966) and may easily be damaged either mechanically or by pressure surges. As a result, their initial pore-size regularity may become distorted. Wire septa have a narrow pore-size distribution that, however advantageous, has its shortcomings in that it is less retentive of smaller particles. For these reasons, such septa may pass powdered resin into the effluent, to the corrosive detriment of reactors or generators. Typically, the mean pore size is used to rate filter retention. Most filters are characterized by some pore-size distribution.

It is generally believed that a narrow pore-size distribution is beneficial since it avoids the situation where pore sizes larger than the desired removal rating are present. On the other hand, a broader pore-size distribution, at least at pore sizes smaller than the removal rating, improves retention of the smaller particle sizes.

Importance of Wire Diameter

A greater degree of porosity results from the use of fibers (thinner metal constructions). For example, given two woven wire compositions, the one comprised of thinner-diameter wire has less space per unit area occupied by metal. The result is more open space per unit area (higher porosity). Regulation of the available open space into pores of proper size adequate to prevent powdered resin penetration is a function of the thinness of the wire making up the media. Unfortunately, the practicality of wire screens becomes limited by the degree of wire thinness necessary to secure the high porosities requisite for low-pressure-drop septa.

On a more fundamental basis, the Kozeny equation relates a filter's average pore diameter, its porosity, and the diameter of the constituent particles or fibers (Carman, 1937), to larger pores. Matting layers of fibers superimposes small pores over large and visa versa, thus reducing the average pore-size distribution. The greater the extent of matting, the more uniform the pore-size distribution becomes.

Fiber metal media, by variation of their aspect ratios and their degree of matting, can be made to exhibit porosities from 50% to 80%. By proper management of the fiber metal aspect ratios and degree of matting, a desired balance of dirt-holding capacity, particle removal efficiency, and pressure drop can be achieved. This versatility makes fiber metal media eminently suited for condensate polishing. Fiber metal media can be tailored to operate at optimum efficiency with a wide spectrum of resin powder types. In sum, fiber metal septa offer exceptionally high total porosities and advantageous low pressure differentials (Goeminne et al., 1974).

Sintered metal particles have extremely short aspect ratios (i.e., the ratio of length to width, typically 2:1 to 4:1). As a consequence, there is a limit to how thin the media can be made. Thus, they have low porosities (30% to 40%), resulting in lower dirt-holding capacities and higher pressure drops. In efforts to improve this situation, different manufacturing techniques such as the use of polymeric adjuncts are sometimes used in order to make possible more uniform pore-size distribution.

Technology makes possible fiber metal septa. These are composed of stainless steel fibers drawn exceedingly fine and formed into nonwoven mats. Woven wire media may be thin as 0.001 inch (25.4 μm); metal fiber media may be as thin as 2 μm, with aspect ratios of 1,000:1. As a result, these media have a high porosity, high dirt-holding capacity, and a broader pore-size distribution; and they filter fine.

The random deposition of fibers in the nonwoven mats yields a filter of broad pore-size distribution. As previously stated, finer filtration is the result. However, there may be concern regarding the retention capabilities of the larger pores. These larger pores are moderated into smaller entities by the process of matting the fiber metal media. According to Piekaar and Clarenburg (1967), a filter can usefully be considered as consisting of repetitive planes of filter media, each with its own pore-size distribution. The superimposition of one plane on another serves to juxtapose smaller pores with larger ones.

Ideally, the pore-size distribution would consist of few or no pores larger than the removal rating of the filter (i.e., a pore-size distribution skewed in the direction of smaller pore sizes). The extent of this departure from a narrow pore-size distribution should not be at the expense of desired flowrates, the rate of flow being the fourth power of the pore diameter.

Septa based on sintered metal particles, although generally more robust, have limitations. The disposition of metallic particles of less than uniform size does not necessarily form a sintered septum of uniform pore sizes. Where this is the case, powdered resin particles may not be be restrained by the larger pores. In addition, the total porosities, their degrees of openness, can be rather restricted since they are formed largely of irregularly shaped particles. Total porosity (void volume) is the ratio of open space to the volume taken up by the filter medium. This open space, suitably divided into pores, constitutes a filter. Liquid permeation and particle retention both occur at the pore sites. Clearly, the larger the number of pores, the greater the particle-loading capacity of the filter and the longer its useful service life (the time interval until its eventual clogging). In addition, total porosity is inversely proportional to pressure drop (i.e., the higher the porosity of the septum, the lower the initial pressure drop and the longer the useful service life as defined by the selected terminal pressure drop). See equation 5-6.

$$d^2 = (d_f)^2 E^2 \div (1\text{-}E)^2 \qquad \text{Eq. 5-6}$$

where d is the average pore diameter (assuming a circle), E is the porosity of the medium, and d_f is the diameter of the fiber.

From the direct relationship of d to d_f, it follows that the thinner the fiber, the smaller the interstice or pore diameter.

In the case of sintered particles rather than wires or fibers, the effect is more gross, and the Kozeny equation becomes:

$$d^2 = 16E^2 \div (1\text{-}E)^2 \div (S/V)^2 \qquad \text{Eq. 5-7}$$

where S/V is the surface to volume ratio. (See page 275 for slightly different expressions.)

Finely drawn metal fibers are matted into random filter compositions (septa). Random packing is ordinarily characterized by a broader pore-size distribution. Matting is a process that successively imposes a progressive modification of the pore-size distribution to where it is relatively narrow while exhibiting a high total porosity.

The fine diameters of metal fibers yield a septum of high void volume (porosity). Matted septa exhibit relatively narrow pore-size distributions, low initial pressure drops, and high particle retentions. Low pressure drops and loading of the powdered resin precoat at lower feed velocities are made possible with fiber metal septa. This reduces the possibility of progressive septum blockage by resin particles becoming so impacted into the metal structure as to resist backwashing. Overall, fiber metal septa should exhibit more consistent powdered resin coatings and longer on-stream service lives.

The septa themselves may be so sufficiently fine in their pore structures as to serve advantageously in power generation filtrations without precoats. In such usages they are referred to as "naked" filters. An example of such an application would be the removal of the fine crystalline particles of magnetite, the ferrous oxide of iron, accompanied by the fine particles and gels of its red (ferric) oxide and/or hydrated oxides (these solids being the products of carbon steel corrosion). Such a filtration might be sought at a differential pressure of about 20 psig. Desired could be a flowrate of 3,000 to 6,000 gpm. For the sake of practical economy, the filter(s) should have a service life of at least a 2-year period of intermittent functioning. This ought be made possible by the backwashability of the filter.■

CHAPTER 6

SPECIFIC IMPURITIES

SUSPENDED MATTER, SILICA, OXYGEN, ORGANIC SUBSTANCES

Specific substances in water are considered contaminants in particular applications. Methods for purifying a source water from these ingredients will be considered. However, for these methods to be carried out effectively and practically, certain other feedwater components must first be eliminated or controlled. This is done in a pretreatment stage, shortly to be discussed. Microbiological contamination (considered in Chapter 2), and also suspended matter, silica, organic substances, oxygen, and soluble iron and manganese are among the specific impurities that require being dealt with. The nature and removal requirements of certain of these merit a more particular examination.

Suspended Matter and Its Management

Nature of suspended solids. Water in contact with the earth, with the rock and soil over which and through which it flows, may pick up solid particles that can become suspended in it. By definition, it is these suspended particles that constitute TSS, the total suspended solids component, of a water.

The suspended matter can originate from many sources, and may represent a wide variety of substances. Various organic materials, such as lignins and tannins; silica from any of its many sources, particularly at lower pHs; alkaline earth ions encountering higher pH environments; clay, often containing metallic entities, whether in conjunction with organic matter or not; suspensions of organisms, viable or not; inorganic salts and minerals precipitated in discrete forms, as a result of the exceeding of their solubility products; insoluble carbonates converted from soluble bicarbonates by the loss of carbon dioxide; soluble ferrous and manganous salts rendered insoluble by the oxidative conversion to their higher valence states, all may contribute to the TSS of a water.

Different kinds of suspensions. When the volume or body of the suspending water becomes quiescent, as when the velocity of a stream subsides, a portion of the suspended solids may separate out. The suspended solid particles that separate out do so because they are large and heavy. These settleable solids may be collected and weighed, or they may be assayed volumetrically by means of settling cones, devices designed for the very purpose. (A quantity of water with its suspended matter is placed into a volumetrically graduated cone. After a suitable period of time allowed for settling, the volume occupied by the settleable solids at the bottom of the cone is recorded.)

Some of the solid particles will, however, remain suspended even over significant periods of time. The solids that are not settleable, those that remain suspended in the supernatant liquid, are called its turbidity. Such particles are fine in size. They may also be collodial; that is, they may bear electrical charges on their surfaces. (The significance of this phenomenon will shortly be considered.)

Turbidity

Turbidity in water is measured by the effect of the fine particles upon a light beam directed through the water sample. The intensity of the light source is standardized for analytical purposes. The interference of its transmission through a standard dimension of water by the light-scattering and -blocking action of the suspended particles is measured in different ways using different instruments. It is quantified in various terms such as Jackson turbidity units (JTU) or nephelometric turbidity units (NTU). The JTU is measured with a transmitted light beam; the NTU, by light scattering. Unfortunately, there is no correlation among the various units of turbidity measurement that holds for all waters, but some useful relationships do exist. Thus, turbidity standards prepared from suspensions of 325-mesh diatomaceous earth give an NTU reading of 100 and a JTU reading of 40.

Silt Density Index

The silt density index (SDI) is a measurement of the total suspended solids (see page 530). The assessment is made by measuring the effect that the TSS within a water specimen has upon the clogging rate of a 0.45-μm-rated membrane filter. Unfortunately, the standards whereby microporous membranes are rated differ from one manufacturer to another. Moreover, there is some variability for a given type of membrane even as prepared by a given manufacturer. However, while flawed by this lack of ideality, the SDI test is still a very useful procedure. The test is of American Society for Testing and Materials origin, ASTM D-4189-82. It is applied in so many modified forms, however, that its original protocol is almost irrelevant.

The ASTM D-4189-82 method utilizes filtration of the water specimen through a 47-mm-diameter 0.45-μm-rated microporous membrane under a constant pressure of 30 psig (207 kilopascals [kPa]). The rate of plugging of the filter is measured, and the SDI is calculated from the rate of plugging.

The time required to flow 500 mL of the water being assayed, t_i, is noted. After another interval, T (usually 15 minutes) of water flow, another 500 mL is filtered and the time required, t_f, is noted. The SDI value is calculated from the formula:

$$SDI = 100(1 - t_i/t_f) \div T \qquad \text{Eq. 6-1}$$

Depending upon the filter-clogging propensities of the water, the sizes of the filter and/or of the water sample; and the interval, T, between the samples may be altered. The sensitivity of the method is increased by using a larger interval between samples, and by larger-sized samples. Heavily laden waters, those with high TSS values, will require smaller samples. Obviously, the filter type will influence the test results (Simonetti and Schroeder, 1985).

In effect, the reduction in the flowrate of the second 500-mL portion of water through the 0.45-rated microporous membrane after the flow interval of 15 minutes is taken as a measure, however crude, of that water's fouling potential. Presumably , 0.45-μm particles and larger are seen as the problem. Smaller particles are guarded against agglomeration by the addition of dispersing agents.

Because of the mathematical relationships in the SDI equation, for a water sample having an SDI_{15} of 5, the flowrate of the second 500-mL sample will take 4 times longer to flow through the membrane than a specimen having an SDI_{15} of 1. Thus, an SDI_{15} reading of 3 bespeaks a water that flows more than twice as fast as one showing an SDI_{15} of 6. A water with an SDI_{15} of 2.5 is far better than one with an SDI_{15} of 3.

Reverse osmosis unit manufacturers will guarantee a minimal life to their instruments, usually from 3 to 5 years, provided the feedwaters do not exceed specified SDI limits. These are commonly set at 5 for spiral wound devices, and less than 3 for hollow-fiber units.

In addition, since the quality of feedwater is affected by seasonal changes, SDI tests should be performed routinely to monitor the adequacy of the prefiltration system.

Another protocol for performance of the SDI is described by Crits (1989). Utilizing 47-mm 0.45-μm-rated microporous membrane at 30 psig, the time is recorded when 100 mL is collected at the beginning, and again after 5, 10, or 15 minutes. There is not any accepted relationship between the SDI values developed at 5 and, say, 15 minutes. The 5-minute interval is the shortest used; 20 is the longest. The membrane itself flows 450 milliliters per minute (mL/min) for clean water. Usually the second interval is set for 15 minutes or to give 75% to 80% plugging. Initially, the test is run for 5 minutes to obtain indications regarding the water quality. When the two measured flows are equal, the SDI, their ratio minus one, is zero. Waters with SDIs of 3 are acceptable for use with hollow fibers. Ultrafilters or RO remove the TSS responsible for the SDI values, but become clogged in consequence. Waters with high SDIs usually require treatment with alum and/or polyelectrolytes followed by filtration (deep-bed) to reduce their clogging propensities. Interestingly, waters with high SDIs do not necessarily cause fouling. Perhaps the zeta potential of the particles is the important factor.

A counterpart to the ASTM silt density index test is called the silting index (Bratby, 1980). It is determined by the formula:

$$SI = \frac{\frac{\text{time to filter}}{\text{2nd 5-mL sample}} - \frac{\text{time to filter}}{\text{1st 5-mL sample}}}{\text{time to filter 1st 1-mL sample}} \qquad \text{Eq. 6-2}$$

Procedural variations make it difficult to employ such tests in interlaboratory work. However, when performed in a consistent manner by the laboratory utilizing it, such a filter-plugging type assay is highly suited to comparative testing.

The SDI is a useful indicator of a water's TSS content. It can be used to determine the effectiveness of various processing procedures upon clarification of the water. Although not an absolute measure of TSS (given the influence of different particle sizes, shapes, and characters), it can be applied to waters exhibiting turbidities of as low as 1.0 NTU; and it is, therefore, usually suited to the analysis of well waters, filtered waters, and clarified effluent waters.

Kaakinen et al. (1994) discussed the need for the SDI test and set for its operational protocols. These investigators also described two different automated SDI instruments that they consider improvements over manually performed SDI tests.

For a test to be indicative of the actual practice, its operation protocol must be closely as possible imitate the specific use conditions. This is not so for the SDI determinations. They utilize flows normal to the filter face, dead-end filtrations, not the tangential flow common to RO operation. Also, they employ microporous filters, usually 0.45-µm-rated, rather than RO membrane types. In an effort to devise an SDI type test more identical to and therefore more significant to the RO operation it is intended to prognosticate, Durham (1991) devised what he called the crossflow fouling index. This test procedure establishes a fouling index value utilizing crossflow separation. The colloidal fouling is quantified by measuring the decrease in permeate flow over time.

Katz and Clay (1986) pointed out that there are cases where high SDIs do not foul, and where low SDIs do. For any SDI value there may be a large variation in the size, size distribution, chemical nature, and electrical charge on the particles involved; therefore, colloidal material would not be retained by 0.45-µm-rated membrane filters, but may be retained by charge attractions to other particles that are captured. Thus the nature of the particles that are restrained by the filter may importantly influence the SDI. The fouling potential of the particles will reflect their zeta potential, and this is responsive to the pH and ionic strengths of the feedwaters.

Not all investigators consider the implications of the SDI test helpful, citing that the effects of a given filter upon a particular water can be judged only in an actual use context.

Nevertheless, despite limitations and exceptions, SDI measurements are important tools in assessing membrane demineralizer performance, and in evaluating pretreatment efficacies for such purposes. Some attribute relevant SDI values to the presence of small particles. Goozner and Gotlinsky (1990) relied upon the SDI determination to assess the effectiveness of prefiltrative activity on RO units.

Vaughan et al. (1989) observed that the quality of the water being fed an RO is critical to the performance and service life of the unit, and that SDI assays serve to characterize the water suitability. Pretreatment of the water to reduce its SDI to acceptable values may entail softening, descaling, and filtrative purification. With Dallas city water, Vaughan et al. found that a certain 10-μm-rated spun-bonded polypropylene prefilter served to reduce the original SDI values of 6 to 20 to an acceptable level of less than 5. They also utilized SDI measurements in the selection of prefilters for RO operations. (See Chapter 9, Page 531).

The practical aspects of performing the SDI test were discussed by Elstad (1992) in terms of the necessary apparatus and procedural protocol. That the SDI test results may be dependent even upon the actual test equipment used, whether plastic or stainless steel, was demonstrated by Walton (1987).

Colloids, usually containing silica, iron, and some organics, can be kept under control once the SDI is reduced to 5 or less by the use of coagulation and flocculation, if necessary. Silt density index values greater than 5 may require the feeding of coagulant polymers. Such polymer treatments are generally unwelcome in pharmaceutical settings, but polymer feeds can reduce SDI readings from 15 or 20 to 1 or 2 in high-silt waters. Such polymer feeds are made in advance of the multimedia filters. The polymeric coagulant may leak through the deep beds. Its removal by ion-exchange beds is reliable, though its removal from such beds may be difficult.

Multimedia beds can reduce a water's SDI to 3 and provide turbidity of less than 0.2 NTU (Gagnon and Rodriguez 1994). It would be useful to be able to estimate in advance just how "filterable" a water is; how long a service life it would permit a filter. It would then be possible to determine whether it would pay to treat the water to lower its TSS in order to prolong the filter life. The required filter area could, perhaps, also be estimated from learning a water's filterability, as also the frequency of filter changeout.

Colloid destabilization may eventuate from the colloid concentration that results from the reverse osmosis operation itself. Colloid coagulation at the RO membrane surface may result in the fouling of the membrane. The silt density index is one of the measurements appropriate to the determination of colloid concentrations. Its measurement carries implications important to RO membrane fouling.

The silt density index is a very important factor as relates to the design of RO systems. Plotting the flux rate in gallons per day of an RO, versus the SDI of the water to be processed, can often be used to size the system.

Stokes' Law.

Let us examine why solid particles may remain suspended in water, and what may cause them to settle out. The suspension and the settling out of solid particles in a liquid, such as water, is described by Stokes' Law.

$$V_{stokes}=(d_1-d_2)a^2g/18\eta \qquad \text{Eq. 6-3}$$

Where V is setting velocity, a is diameter radius of particles, d_1 is density of particle, d_2 is density of medium, h is viscosity of medium, and g is the gravitational constant

There are two main components to the settling out of suspended particles. The first is the difference in the densities of the solid particles and that of the liquid. The greater the difference in the densities, the solid usually being the more dense, the faster the speed of the settling out; the quicker the separation of the two phases, liquid and solid. The second consideration in the settling out of particles from a liquid depends upon the size of the particle. Settling occurs because gravitational forces act upon the suspended particles. The gravitational influence varies with the square of the particle diameter. Therefore, smaller particles remain in suspension longer than do larger particles. It is often possible, however, to cause smaller particles to agglomerate into larger units, hence speeding their removal from the suspension. The diminution of the water's TSS is the result.

Brownian Motion

A certain degree of agglomeration may inevitably occur over time. Discrete suspended particles may collide with one another. The flowing of the water may itself cause such occurrences, so that small particles may adhere together to form units of larger sizes that are now more influenced by the force of gravity. Even in quiescent waters the suspended particles are in movement, constantly buffeted by ions and water molecules that themselve are in the perpetual, erratic motion common to all molecules above absolute zero. (Indeed, the significance of absolute zero is that only at that temperature and below do all molecular and atomic movements cease. Increasingly at higher temperatures the amplitude of these movements becomes greater.) As a result of sustaining collisions with the ever-moving water molecules and ions, the suspended particles may themselves be caused to undergo movement. This is the phenomenon known as Brownian motion, more apparent with smaller particles consituting colloids. The result is that smaller particles may become joined into larger entities that sooner settle out of suspension. These reductions of TSS can occur over time.

The collisions of smaller particles may result in agglomerations because the mutually attractive Van der Waals forces can operate over the smaller separation distances among the collided particles.

The Collodial State

Colloids consist of particles of from 0.005 to 0.2 mm in size, too small to be visible under an optical microscope. In its simplest form, the colloidal state is a suspension of discrete particles that resist settling out for several reasons. Each particle bears a surface charge. These charges can arise from the adsorption of ions into the solid surface, from ionization of molecules on the surface, or from dissolution of ions from the solid into the liquid. Since like charges repel, and since all the particles bear the same charge, the discrete particles repel one another and do not agglomerate to form a sediment.

Because of their small size, collodial particles are also subject to Brownian motion. They are bombarded by the movement of the ions in the solution, ions that are in motion because of their thermal energy. These collisions give erratic motion to the colloid particles, and help to prevent their settling out.

Even though colloidal particles present in water themselves undergo collisions, these do not result in agglomeration because the particles, swathed in their double layers, are too distant from one another, even in collision, to permit the Van der Waals attracting forces to be effective. The influence of these secondary valence forces obeys the inverse square law. These forces decrease inversely as the square of the distance over which they operate. They diminish very rapidly with distance. When the charge layering is reduced by charge neutralization the distance between the core particles is reduced. Collisions become productive of agglomeration, building to particle sizes that may be responsive to Stokes' Law.

Even if the charges were neutralized (that is, if the colloid were destabilized), the particles (as described by Stokes' Law) could each be too small (in size and hence in mass) to respond to the law of gravity. For such uncharged particles to settle out, they would first have to be coalesced into larger entities. This could happen spontaneously upon charge neutralization in response to the particles' Van der Waals attractive forces.

Electrical Double Layer

Collodial phenomena are complex. The colloidal particle bears a charge. In aqueous media it is generally positive. This charge layer attracts a layer of largely negative charges that, in time, attracts yet another layer of largely positive charges, and so on. Thus each core particle is surrounded by a series of charged layers. After the first layer, successive charge layers are progressively less firmly held. The first two layers are the important ones and constitute what is known as the colloid's electrical double layer. The second layer is less firmly held. Also, it is less regular in the homogeneity of its charge character. It is therefore possible to separate the core particle and its surrounding first charge layer from the second of the two layers constituting the double layer.

Zeta Potential

The core particle and its tightly adhering first charge layer can be separated from the more diffusely held second charge layer by its movement toward an electrode in responses to an imposed electric current. The separation of the two charge layers reflects the potential at their plane of shear. It is called the *zeta potential* and is measurable by a zeta meter. Its magnititude relates inversely to the ease of coagulation of the colloid particles, an exercise that involves double-layer separation and charge neutralization. The zeta charge is opposite to that of the particle itself.

According to Cohen's rule, a particle suspended in water takes on a zeta charge that reflects both its and the water's dielectric constants. Water has a dielectric charge of 72. If the particle has a higher dielectric value, its zeta potential in water is positive. (Asbestos is a case in point.) If the dielectric charge of the particle itself is lower, its zeta potential is negative. Most particles suspended in water bear negative zeta charges. These become fixed to and can be agglomerated among other means, by positively charged sites and ions.

The measurements of zeta potential, even by the zeta meters devised for that purpose, are time-consuming to a degree that reduces their practicality in assaying the quantity of alum needed for the clarification of a water.

Streaming-Current Potential

In the measurement of zeta potential, the core particle surrounded by its first sheath of charges is caused to separate from its second charge-envelope by being moved electrically through the suspending water towards an electrode. The same separation of the electric double layers can be obtained by anchoring the particles, as by adsorption to surfaces, and causing the liquid to flow past them. This technique is called streaming current potential. It is easier to perform than zeta potential measurements, and also measures the voltage necessary to separate the double layering and hence the ease of colloid destabilization.

Streaming-current potential is useful because it provides measurement of the net surface charge of the collodial particles. This correlates with how much coagulant needs to be added to the collodial suspension to cause it to agglomerate. The coagulant, such as alum, supplies multivalent cations to neutralize the negative charges of the first electrical layer. This charge neutralization destablizes the colloidal suspension, permitting the particles to agglomerate and to become large enough to be responsive to gravitational settling.

Streaming-current detectors have been found suitable for controlling coagulation chemical additions in on-demand systems to prevent under-or-over dosing. These devices have also been found useful in allowing better control of reverse osmosis fouling as caused by collodial depositions.

Carling and Roy (1989) described a streaming-current detector (SCD) suitable for controlling coagulation pretreatments as regards coagulation chemical addition to on-demand systems to prevent either under- or overdosing. The SCD is an on-line electrokinetic charge analyzer with measuring, recording, and control functions. It controls chemical addition in response to a measurement of the net surface electrical charges derived from the particles present in the water sample. It is these charges that require neutralization for particle agglomeration to occur. The chemical added in response to the charge measurement serves to neutralize these charges, thus causing the desired agglomeration.

Veal (1990) described a suitable instrument and reported on the use of streaming-current potential measurements to assess the coagulation requirements of waters containing colloids. In potable water treatment plants, such devices are relied upon to gauge the amount of alum needed. The findings are, however, usually confirmed by coagulation jar tests.

Curcie (1989) utilized a streaming-current detector in a study on the fouling of polyamide hollow-fiber RO devices. He found that the SCD measurements generally correlated with zeta potential measurements and the SDI. Curcie applied streaming-current potential measurements to a successful control of coagulant addition. His studies directed him to the use of finer sand in the monomedia sand filter. Continuous in-line measurement by the SCD device of the water entering the sand bed permitted better control of the RO fouling caused by wide swings in SDI quality.

Removal of Colloidal Impurities

Colloidal organics will frequently be associated with such metallic entities as iron, aluminum, manganese, and titanium; and with silicon. Organometallic colloidal matter often manifests itself as a coloration on membrane filters when these are part of the water purification system.

Unless removed from the water stream undergoing processing, colloids may come to foul RO membranes, stills, and deionizing resin beds. (See page 531).

Kunin (1984) spoke of the "universal colloid," a widely encountered composition of silica, organic material, and metallics. One may speculate about its origins: possibly metallic ions or atoms from claylike sources, chelated by the hydroxyl and carboxylic acid groups induced into otherwise covalent organic structures by some degree of oxidation, the overall structure too weakly ionic to be removed by ion exchange. Such colloids could permeate ion-exchange beds to deposit upon boiler tubes. Their carbonization to metallic residues would cause corrosion (Foster, 1991). Such corrosion could be attributed incorrectly to an insufficiency on the part of the ion-exchange resins to remove metal ions, when in reality the un-ionized metallic atoms find transport by means of organic-group chelation. Foster speculated additionally that the destruction of the organic material, as by encounter with ultraviolet light or ozone, could remove its chelating abilities, resulting in the sudden release of metallic ions where previously none could be detected. For such reasons, colloidal matter should be removed from feedwaters, as by coagulation or by membrane processes such as ultrafiltration or reverse osmosis.

Colloid particle stability. The greater the electrical charge between both layers (i.e., the greater the zeta potential), the higher the stability of the colloid, because of the greater repulsion between the particles. These repulsive forces can be neutralized by adding ions bearing charges opposite to those of the particle itself.

The stronger the neutralizing charges, the greater their effect. It has been reported that trivalent ions such as aluminum and ferric are about 30 times as influential as divalent ions, which in turn exert approximately 16 to 40 times the effect of ions bearing single charges (Luttinger, 1981). Substituting monocharged cations for multivalent cations, as occurs in water softening, will have the opposite effect; and will therefore serve to stabilize the colloid.

Colloidal particles may not spontaneously separate from a watery suspension, regardless of the time interval allowed. These must be treated apropriately to effect their separation and removal.

The separating out of suspended colloidal particles may involve the neutralization of mutually repulsive electrical charges, followed by agglomeration and flocculation of the suspended particles, as by alum pretreatment. Alternatively, the colloids usually encountered in water sources can be filtered out by ultrafilters of 100,000 daltons or less. It would be economically wasteful, however, to utilize ultrafilters in a pretreatment mode. They are appropriately used for colloid removal in polishing operations.

The treatment of waters containing colloids has as its objective the destablization of the colloid so that the suspended particles can agglomerate and settle out. This is managed by the addition of ions of opposite charge to neutralize the colloid's mutually repelling charges. The neutralization of this charge permits agglomeration or coagulation of the particles. The larger the charge (zeta potential) the more coagulant needs to be added to destabilize the colloid.

Coagulation. Some preliminary discussion of the coagulation and flocculation phenomena has already been made, as also of the role of alum in these actions. Additions of alum, or of ferric chloride and lime combinations, often serve economically to remove colloids from waters (Bratby, 1980). Copperas, hydrated ferrous sulfate, has also long been used for this purpose. The bivalent ferrous ions (transformed into trivalent ferric by air oxidation) and the trivalent ferric or aluminum ions serve to neutralize the negative colloidal charges. The zeta potential of the suspended material having been brought to zero, the particles will tend to settle out (but slowly, in accordance with their small size and mass). Alum in this role is a coagulant. If very much charged material is present, excessively high alum doses may be required. In such cases, polyelectrolytes in polymer form may prove efficacious, if expensive. They are charge neutralizing, as is the polyvalent aluminum ion. Polymer reduces the amount of alum required.

The polymeric polyelectrolytes act similarly to the alum. They may be either polycationic or polyanionic. The are constituted of long-chain polymers bearing a multiplicity of like-charge ionic sites. Most particles have negative zeta potentials in water.* Therefore, the polymers coagulants used, usually from 10,000 to 1,000,000 g/moles in molecular weight, are cationic in nature. They are usually either polyquaternary amines or polyamines. In the latter case, the charge density will vary with pH. Being polyfunctional, they serve to contact and bridge many particles. This causes the particles to settle out by being joined into aggregates large enough to respond to gravity, in accordance with Stoke's law. They are usually effective in small dosages, from 0.5 mg/L to double that concentration at the most.

Flocculation. Alum plays another useful role in suspended-solids control. It readily dissolves in warm water. After a short while, a precipitate forms. Depending upon the pH, the precipitate changes in character, but in essence forms any of a series of hydrated aluminum oxides. What is important is that these tend to be flocs, rather than more densely crystalline. Alum will form flocs best at pH 5 to 7. As the floc, filamentous and diffuse, settles in the water, it gathers within its diffuse structure the many small charge-neutralized particles (formerly colloids). In its aggregate form, the floc speeds the settling out of the particles and, incidentally, of itself. In this action the alum serves as a flocculant (Dwyer, 1966).

A flocculant bridges the surfaces of separate charge-neutralized particles or their agglomerations (also called flocs), building up to a large-size aggregate or floc. Flocculation is promoted by slow mixing; high mixing shears may disrupt flocs. The proper rate of mixing and the amount of alum required for a given water is determined by jar tests in the laboratory, wherein the flash-mixing of the plant treatment is imitated for 30 to 60 seconds, followed by slow mixing for 20 minutes, followed by a 1-hour settling period. What is sought is a maximum diminution in the water's turbidity.

Polymeric flocculants are of high molecular weight, from 1 to 20 million. The higher the molecular weight, the greater the particle-bridging capacity. Almost all are copolymers of acrylamide or modified polyacrylamide. Where polyelectrolyte is used to induce flocculation, excess should be avoided in order to not

* When a colloid is described as being negative it is meant that it has a negative zeta potential or a negative streaming-current potential. This means that the first charge-layer, that immediately surrounding the core particle, is negatively charged. The opposite is true for a positively charged colloid.

unnecessarily burden the subsequently used ion-exchange resins, or require the task of polyelectrolyte removal.

Removal of TSS particulates. It is absurdly wasteful to treat water with a coagulant or flocculant just prior to its being filtered. Coagulation and sedimentation are time-involving processes. Their action requires a suitable storage venue, commonly a settling tank. Up to 10 hours may be allowed for sedimentation. The process can utilize clarifiers (see below) when flows of up to 1,000 gpm are required. Concrete basins can be used where larger flows are involved. Smaller flows can be accommodated by the use of deep-bed filtration.

Where alum or polyelectrolyte cannot possibly be accorded the required destabilizing and settling time, removal of the colloids or of only partly destabilized colloids may be attempted by deep-bed filtration. The colloids may not be retained, being too small. The flocculated destabilized portion will be retained. Some operators advise the use of diatomite and pressure leaf filters in such situations. Others eschew the use of diatomaceous earth in pretreatments, believing it introduces greater problems than the colloids themselves pose. The alternative is the recurrent expense of using string-wound cellulosic, glass, or polypropylene fiber cartridges. Charge-modified microporous membranes can arrest and retain colloids that would otherwise penetrate ion-exchange beds to threaten the fouling of RO membranes and stills.

Good colloid reduction is required. The matter involves judicious handling, however, as in many cases the practice of flocculation can cause more problems than do the untreated waters.

Waters exiting coagulation and flocculation treatment contain a quantity of aluminum ions. Although it is now becoming of concern to the EPA for potential health reasons, aluminum is not yet analyzed for in potable water treatments. Rendering aluminum-containing waters acidic (as when they are being prepared for reverse osmosis treatment by cellulose acetate RO membranes) causes filter-blocking deposits, described as "peanut butter" fouling. Such deposits are particularly persistent with regard to polyamide membrane surfaces. (See Potable Water Treatment, Chaper 1.)

The chlorination of such waters also renders them acidic and liable to such fouling:

$$Cl_2 + H_2O \longrightarrow HOCl + H^+ + Cl^- \qquad \text{Eq. 6-4}$$

Clarifiers. Clarifiers are usually circular structures, in essence large chambers; the diameters of which may range from 8 to 325 feet (Purchas, 1981). Into a center well is pumped the water to be treated along with an addition of, for instance, alum and polymer. (Alternatively, the water may be treated externally, and the mixture then pumped to the clarifier.) Recirculation assures intimacy of mix. As the sediment settles, an overflow of clear water exits through ports at the top of the clarifier. Scraper arms and blades move the settled solids toward the clarifier bottom, from which they are removed through a sludge outlet. Such clarifiers can be operated in batch or continuous fashion.

In primary sewage treatment, the overflowrate is about 0.3 gpm/ft^2; the detention time is 2 hours. Water clarification generally provides an overflowrate of 0.3 to 0.45 gpm/ft^2 (18 to 27 gph/ft^2), utilizing a detention time of 3 hours. Lime and lime-soda softening treatments yielding an overflowrate of 1.2 gpm/ft^2 require a detention time of 2 hours.

Some suggest that when a water's TSS is above about 100 ppm, a clarifier should be used because with so heavy a load the time required for deep-bed backwashing would be excessive. A typical example of a clarifier use at a semiconductor plant follows: An upflow clarifier is used in conjunction with an alum floc blanket. (Alum forms an aluminum hydroxide floc at pH 6 to 10). The clarifier consists of 12 inches of anthracite over 12 to 16 inches of sand overlying gravel. The bed is self-grading after backwashing. The first 6 inches of anthracite performs all the retention, and successive layers serve as supports for the anthracite and sand, respectively.

The need for backwashing is signaled by the increase in resistance to flow through the deep-bed clarifier. This is done by means of two sight glasses (gauges would do as well). The first glass connects with the water layer above the anthracite; the second, with the bottom of the clarifier. In a case when no water flows, both gauges read the same. When water is permeating the bed, the resistance to the permeation causes a lowering of the water level in the sight glass at the clarifier bottom. This is an expression of the pressure drop across the deep-bed filter.

The backwash flow must be vigorous enough to disrupt the structure of the particle-retaining layer and set loose the retained particles. Therein lies the advantage of using anthracite, which is lighter than sand. It therefore requires about 50% less backwash flow to expand to its disrupted state. This is important to the economics of pumping, the water used, and the volume dumped to the sewer.

The inner contents of the 20-foot-diameter clarifier, dark with the alum floc and its associated particles, are circulated counterclockwise. The up-welling water is clear, and flows out of the clarifier through "launderer" channels that are part of the instrument's periphery. The exiting water from the clearwell flows to the next stage of the pretreatment operation.

Whether following its residence in a clarifier or in place of one, the water treated appropriately to its colloidal contents is freed of its suspended matter by exposure to deep-bed filtration. This is described in Chapter 7, "Pretreatment of Waters."

Silica

Integrated circuit manufacture requires water with a silica content of less than 5 ppb of silica (ASTM Electronic Grade Water, Type E-1). So low a silica content is not required of waters used for compendial purposes in pharmaceutical applications. Nevertheless, the preparation of pharmaceutical waters by means of reverse osmosis and particularly by distillation may require the attainment of very low levels of silica lest RO membranes become unduly fouled and still surfaces become functionally compromised.

Stills stipulate a level of less than 1 ppm of silica concentration in the feedwaters (less than 0.01 ppm for boiler feedwaters). Waters often contain in excess of 5 to 10 ppm of silica. The silica must be removed or it may deposit as a vitreous coating on the still surfaces, for it is present in steam in volatile form. It should be pointed out, however, that in certain stills, once a thin surface vitreous glaze has formed, further silica depositions do not adhere, but flake off. Interference from silica is thus limited. In one case, the vapor-phase compressive distillation of a water containing 18 to 20 ppm of silica content (no strongly basic anion-exchange silica removal was involved) produced a thin glaze where the only untoward effect was to diminish somewhat the heat transference of the cooling coils. Instead of producing 3,000 gallons per hour (gph), the still yielded 2,800 to 2,900 gph. The trade-off against the savings in strongly basic anion-exchange resin was considered acceptable. There is, however, a condition to be guarded against. In situations where the efficiency of the still blowdowns may become impaired, the build-up of silica deposits in the still, adhering or not, may cause silica entrainment in the steam.

Silica can also foul RO membrane surfaces. Its removal is best accomplished by the use of strongly basic anion-exchange resins, from which, incidentally, the silica is difficult to remove in the regeneration process. Fouling of RO membranes is especially bad when the water also contains aluminum ions, presumably remaining from an alum flocculation treatment. A similar problem results if magnesium ions are incompletely removed.

Almost all natural waters contain silica in combinations of ionic, colloidal, and suspended forms. Well waters in many parts of the country are rich in silica. In the U.S. there are two areas of high silica; in the Pacific Northwest the water is very clean except for about 30 ppm silica: in the Southwest silica contents of 100 to 120 ppm have been reported, although silica solubility is about 60 to 70 ppm. At these levels the silica problem is handled by the use of dispersants in conjunction with operating RO units at only 50% to 60% recovery, a major expense of water consumption.

A major source of silica is diatoms, single-celled plants that exist in natural waters and flourish in warmth and sunlight. Their cell walls are composed almost exclusively of silica. Diatoms bloom in the spring; in the late spring in the Los Angeles area. Usually, they are removed from the feedwaters by sand bed filtration. Silt is also a source of both soluble and colloidal silica. Silica in the water is a big problem in Mexico.

The chemistry of silica is complex, and its removal from water is therefore complicated. Silica may exist in ionized forms that are responsive to strong anionic exchange. It may be present in colloidal forms, often accompanied by organic matter and even by heavy metals. As such it is removable by membranes having a tightness equivalent to a molecular-weight cutoff of 100,000 daltons or less. However, Bates et al. (1988) said that colloidal silica is difficult to remove by RO (or by ion exchange). Silica may also exist in a granular or suspended form.

The colloidal or polymeric form of silica is too slightly ionized to be removed by ion exchange or to be detected by the classical molybdate (blue) color test. Hence it is referred to as non-molybdate-reactive silica. An example of the complexity of silica's chemistry is the fact that it exists in an equilibrium condition among its three forms. Higher pH waters tend to dissolve the silica. Being essentially nonionic, the polymeric or colloidal form is difficult to measure and to be alerted against. However, colloidal silica of very low molecular weight is adsorbed on ion-exchange resin (Nakamura et al., 1988). In essence, the control of silica in high-purity water depends upon how well the colloidal form can be determined by analysis leading to its removal (Lerman and Scheerer, 1988).

Silica leakage from DI beds. Curiously, ionic silica contains silica that is not, on account of its size, adsorbed by conventional anionic-exchange resins. Hence this form of silica is called giant silica, being about 10 μm in size, about 10 to 1,000 times larger than the standard silica colloids, which are approximately 10 to 2,000 angstroms (0.2 nm) in size.

Because all ionic silica is not removable by anionic exchange, it cannot be said that the analytical differences between ionic silica and the total silica is colloidal silica. Colloidal silica is not totally adsorbable by anion exchange. However, large-pore anion exchangers can remove colloidal silica. Colloidal silica is difficult to remove either by ion exchange or by RO (Bates et al., 1988). Ionic silica is measured by the standard molybdenum blue standard method, which has a detection limit of 3 ppb.

Nakamura et al. (1988) traced giant silica to suspended or colloidal silica not removed by coagulation/sedimentation, or by filtration preceding ion exchange. It need not necessarily be removed in mixed-bed operations if the macroreticulated resin pores are too small to admit entry of these giant particles. This may cause silica leakage from mixed resin beds. An anion-exchange resin having pore sizes of 8 to 20,000 angstroms was not complete in its silica trapping; one with a pore-size range of 25,000 to 230,000 angstroms (23 μm) yielded no silica leakages. All too often there is a silica breakthrough or leakage from mixed-bed operations.

Fortunately, giant silica is destabilized in the acid or alkaline pH ranges, leading to its removal by strongly basic anion exchange. Nakamura et al. (1988) stated that silica is only weakly ionized at the pH of most waters. Therefore, its removal by ion exchange may be imperfect where giant silica is involved: in essence, where the effect of its ionic charge is minimized by the bulk of the charge-bearing particle. However, its level exiting mixed beds is lower than that of effluent waters from twin beds. There is a window in the solubility of silica, between 68 and 85 °F (20 to 29.5°C), that enables the use of reverse osmosis to minimize the silica effect.

It was concluded by Nakamura et al. (1988) that complete silica removal, even of the giant silica, the large-size form of slightly ionized silica, can be achieved by a water purification system comprised of coagulation/filtration, twin-bed ion exchanges, and mixed-bed polisher. The two-bed system works because the water issuing from the cationic unit is pH 2 or 3. This serves to depolymerize the giant silica, enabling its removal in the anionic exchange bed following. Abrams (1991) disagrees, citing Ilar's *Chemistry of Silicates* in reference. A RO unit can be substituted for the twin beds. It removes the colloidal silica, giant or otherwise, and ionized or otherwise, on the basis of size, much better than does a two-bed DI system. On the other hand, from a soluble silica standpoint, the two-bed arrangement is likely to be far better than a cellulose-type RO, and somewhat better than a thin-film-composite RO. To spare the RO against fouling, the coagulation/filtration step is included. In this step, the raw water pH is adjusted to the acid side to enable giant silica removal by the alum floc.

Pittner et al. (1986) stated that a polyamide double-pass RO unit may reduce a pH-neutral or acidic water's silica content more completely than either ion exchange or cellulose acetate RO, to below 20 ppb. This is so because at these pHs, silica is too little ionized to invite effective rejection by either ion exchange or RO. Double-pass RO using PA membranes to achieve silica reduction should therefore be of interest. It would be of value to compare double-pass RO with RO and ion exchange in combination, in terms of silica removal and comparative costs. Some believe that total silica concentrations would be lowered more by the RO/DI combination.

Colloidal silica is at equilibrium with dissolved silica. The pH of the water strongly influences the equilibrium. Neutral pHs favor the formation of colloidal silica (Sinha, 1990). There are no on-line instruments that measure either total or colloidal silica. Only reactive silica can be measured by on-line instrumentation. Strongly basic anion exchange in the hydroxyl form is counted upon to remove colloidal silica. To accommodate the large sizes of colloidal silica particles (tens of micrometers [μm]), macroporous resins of from 5 to 10 μm are used. The use of ion exchange for this purpose requires measuring silica uptake efficiency by comparing influent and effluent levels, flowrate influences, silica leakage levels, and frequency of regeneration.

Some electronic high-purity water users rely ultimately upon charge-modified filters for silica colloid removal. Ultrafiltration serves usefully in this application as well (Sharpe, 1985). In power utilities, UF may be used after mixed-bed DI as prefilter to RO. Usually, however, the RO is placed upstream of the ion-exchange beds. (See page 500).

The maximum allowable silica level has been set at 0.005 mg per liter as SiO_2 in electronics. Automatic silica analyzers detect only ionizable silica, not the un-ionized colloidal form. According to Nakamura et al. (1988), silica in any of its several forms can be determined by the following steps: (1) Ionic silica is assessed by the colorimetry of acid molybdate, (2) ionic and colloidal silica are determined colorimetrically after digestion with sodium bicarbonate, and (3) Total silica is assayed colorimetrically after sodium bicarbonate digestion. Thus, ionic silica can be measured directly; colloidal silica, by subtracting the ionic value from the total silica; and the suspended silica represents the difference between the total silica and step 2, the sum of ionic and colloidal silica. Lerman and Scheerer (1988) commented upon analytical protocols and sensitivities.

Organic Matter

The common practice of referring to organic substances as TOC is really incorrect because TOC refers to organic matter as defined by an analytical technique, the TOC measurement. Be that as it may, in this writing the common practice is continued. The term TOC as used here should be taken to mean organic materials.

The presence of organic substances in waters intended for high-purity applications is objectionable. They cause corrosion problems in boiler operations. For the Water for Injection used by the pharmaceutical industry, the organic content must be below the detectable limit of the *USP* Oxidizable Substances Test performed with acidic potassium permanganate solution. A new standard of 500 ppb as measured by a TOC analyzer will be in place.

The TOC compositions present in the waters being treated are generally not known. Indeed, they may arise from the very operations inherent in water purification practices. The TOC may originate as extractables from PVC pipe, as plasticizer, stabilizers, or even unconverted monomer. In contrast, piping of PVDF is satisfactory in its very low level of extractables. Inevitably, TOC will leach from ion-exchange resins in the form of styrene, divinybenzene and any of the normal impurities of these monomers. Accordingly, only low-leachable resins should be employed. Filters, too, may serve as sources of TOC leachables. The TOC maay here be constituted of casting solvent and polar pore-former residues. Some filters contain wetting adjuncts as well. Therefore, new RO membranes, and other filters as well, should be rinsed to drain before being put online. Microbial sources of TOC should be eliminated, or at least minimized, by the proper maintenance of air filters on degasifier air-intakes, an operational practice too often observed in the breach. Additionally, the use of good nitrogen blanketing on water storage tanks should be made. Also advised is the use of the activated carbon filters on decarbonator air intakes to avoid the introduction of TOC along with the air (Pate, (1991).

Organic materials of the most varied types may be present in source waters, emanating from a spectrum of origins encompassing farm runoffs and industrial pollutants. While small in quantity, the presence of these organics may pose large problems. Upon chlorination they may give rise to such substances as carcinogenic trihalomethanes. They may adsorb onto the surfaces of deionizing resins, thereby reducing ion-exchange capacities. Their deposition upon RO membrane surfaces will result in diminution of effective filtration area. Their existence in waters presented for distillation may cause foaming and the carryover of impurities. Also, organics in conjunction with silica and heavy metals seem to constitute the "universal colloid" (to use Kunin's terminology) so troublesome to primary water treatment procedures.

The EPA has identified some 1,500 molecular species of organic low-molecular-weight nonionic compounds in Mississippi River water at New Orleans. These are all candidates for inclusion in the potable waters derived from the river water, as well as being components of industrial source waters originating in the municipally treated waters.

Largely, the organic entities present in raw or even potable waters are of vegetative origins. At one end of the scale, the existence of organics may be below the levels of chemical detection, its presence only inferred (as from the influences of the water in tissue culture work). At the other extreme, the decaying remnants of vegetation may plainly be visible in the water source.

Organic materials originating from vegetative sources are usually described generically. Humic acids comprise a loosely bound association of compounds of above 2,000 molecular weight. Their polar functional groups, including carboxylic acids, the products of oxidative degradations, are insufficient in their ratio to the molecular mass to permit water or alkali solubility. The fulvic acids, similar in structure to humic acids but possessing smaller molecular weights and hence greater polar-functional-group-to-mass ratios, are defined by their water and/or alkali solubility. The fulvic acids, which like the humic acids contain phenolic as well as carboxylic acid structures, are about 500 to 2,000 in molecular weight. (Lee et al., 1981).

Soluble organics that may be present are proteins, sugars, and fulvic acids, among other simple or polymeric molecules. Insoluble organics that may be encountered are organisms, oils, tannic acids, and humic matter.

Organics in treated waters derive from microorganisms and their metabolites; from oleophilic substances forthcoming from pumps and from the air streams of forced draft-degasifiers; from organics extracted from resins, filters, and pipes; from decomposition products of humic origins; and from the degradation components of the water treatment devices themselves, such as derive from the action of chlorine or other oxidants on resins, RO membranes, or other polymeric articles.

A more detailed account of organic matter present in waters was given by O'Brien (1987) as a result of his examination of the relevant literature. Measured analytically as total organic carbon, virtually all the organic material in surface water derives from humic matter. This, O'Brien characterized as a nondescript mixture of compounds formed by microbial and enzymatic actions upon vegetative and animal matter present in soils. Existing in a wide range of molecular weights, these organic molecules are constituted of polymerized amino acids, peptides, proteins, sugars, tannic acid, and gallic acid components. The smaller-molecular-weight polymers are the more soluble. The larger, less soluble substances may achieve molecular weights of hundreds of thousandths.

The humic material in its complexity may vary from location to location and from season to season, and may be constituted of such elements as nitrogen, sulfur, and phosphorus in addition to carbon, hydrogen, and oxygen. It will contain a preponderance of phenolic and carboxylic acid groups, and will therefore be responsive in anion exchange. It may also contain sizable amounts of anions. The basicity of such groups, coupled to the acidic phenol and carboxylic acid structuring, impart an amphoteric nature to the humic material. The spatial arrangements of amine groups, carboxylic acid moieties, and hydroxylic entities endow the humic material with chelating properties; therefore, it is often associated with heavy metals. Given the presence of multivalent cations, such as the ferric ions common to many clays, the humic material forms colloids, often of a complex nature, and contains silica as well.

Organic substances present in waters are commonly referred to as total oxidizable carbon (TOC). (DOC) *Dissolved oxidizable carbon*, is differentiated from TOC in that it contains no suspended (insoluble) TOC. Given the narrow lumens of the needles used in sampling waters for analyses of organics by TOC analysers, the distinction between DOC and TOC may often not be too significant.

Organic Removal

Given the wide variety of organic materials that constitute TOC, no single means of removing them all suffices. Consquently, different removal methods are applied in different contexts. Adsorption onto activated carbon is one method. Although lacking the specific "activated sites" of activated carbon, the extensive surface areas of ion-exchange resins provide regions for non-charge-related hydrophobic adsorptions. Anionic-containing TOC (in the form of carboxylic acids groups) can also be removed by anion-exchange reactions. Indeed, the relative surety of these removals over the less certain adsorptive binding mechanisms inclines to the oxidative alteration of the TOC so that it comes to be characterized by carboxylic acid groups that permit their anion-exchange removal. As a result of their oxidiative degradations, large-molecular-weight TOCs of whatever character become transformed into polar low-molecular-weight entities. The desired TOC modifications can be caused by interaction with ozone, or with hydrogn perioxide and/or ozone as catalyzed by 185-nm ultraviolet light (see page 160). The anion-exchange removal is usually accomplished using acrylic anion-exchange degasifiers. That should also be the preferred route for removing the trihalomethanes, these being only slowly adsorbed by carbon, and being relatively inert to oxidation.

It may be profitable to elaborate on the above methods of TOC removal. Organics, with some notable low-molecular-weight exceptions, can generally also be retained by RO membranes. Certain organic compounds are low enough in their molecular weights to be *volatile organic carbon* (VOC). (See page 32). Such compounds may be removed simply by a proper application of heat. These volatile organics are also called *purgable organic carbons* (POC) and may be removed from their aqueous solutions by air sparging.

When the organic entity possesses even a weak charge (e.g., carboxylic acid groups) as a result of having undergone oxidation, the process invokes the actual ion-exchange function of the resins. The organics may also be removed by an undifferentiated general adsorption onto the extensive bead surfaces. The removal of organics by the use of ion exchange is more dependable than that by adsorptive techniques, whose efficacy may be compromised by factors such as excessive rates of flow.

When the trace removal of organics is made in the latter stages of pure water systems, as distinct from pretreatment operations, even the use of mixed ion-exchange resins may generally be economically feasible.

Ion-exchange resin beds with their large surface areas and ionic charges invite the depositions of organic molecules. The extent of attraction and adherence differs with different organics.

There are two extremes in the removal of organics by ion-exchange resins. Where the organic is completely nonpolar, it will not be removed, except as oleophilic materials may coat surfaces by hydrophobic absorptions. The influent and effluent water will essentially both reveal the same TOC content. In the other extreme, the organic may be so polar and so binding to the resin as to absorb irreversibly. It is this type of organic molecule that is responsible for resistivity drops. In attaching to the anion-exchange sites, the organics prevent the resin's intended ion removal by ion exchange.

To really assess the effect of organics, broad classifications like TOC are not enough. Ideally, their precise identification should be available. In any case, the adsorption of organics onto the resin bead surfaces serves to remove them from the water. However, the effect upon the resin bead is one of fouling. With a clean resin there is no dip in resistivity as a function rate of flow. Such a dip occurs, however, when organic fouling is occurring because the functional groups on the resin become preempted or masked by the organics. Ordinarily, a resin bed can be restored by a 10-bed-volume rinse. Because organics are harder to remove, an organically fouled bed may require a 20-bed rinse volume. The organics, having been oxidatively altered, contain carboxylic acid groups (and also often phenolic groups). These, being anionic, exchange with the anion-exchange resin. Elution of the organic is better achieved with sodium chloride solution than with caustic because the affinity of strongly basic resins is greater for chloride ions than for hydroxyl ions. By the same token, the chloride ion will more easily compete with organic acid groups for the anion-exchange site and will therefore better serve to displace the organic foulants.

To forestall organic fouling of the resin beds, scavenger resins are used sacrificially upstream of the beds dedicated to ion exchange. Weak aliphatic resins, acrylic acid types, are used for this purpose. Acrylic macroreticular resins serve best as reversible traps for organics because the acrylic polymer chain desorbs better.

Organic traps consisting often of activated charcoal and of cross-linked polystyrene resin beads, reticulated but not bearing ionic functions, are found to be economically acceptable. An organic colloid containing silica and heavy metals may also be removed by ion exchange. Its charges are presumed to arise from the ion-bearing clay particles and the oxidatively altered organic composing it, to which is appended (possibly in ion-exchange fashion) the heavy metal atoms.

Colloidal matters, whether partly organic or not, usually have their removal effected by the use of ultrafilters having dalton ratings of 100,000 or less, or by the action of charge-modified microporous membranes.

O'Brien (1987) found that, while no single removal techniques served totally to remove the wide variety of organics constituting humic matter, reverse osmosis and mixed-bed ion exchange retained 90% of the TOC. (This high percentage of removal may, however, not always be attained. The effectiveness of ion-exchange resin varies with its age and regeneration history. Also, the nature of the raw water has its influences.) Coagulation with alum and RO caused a 50% TOC reduction. The latter treatment was especially efficacious on molecular-weight entities above 500, and most effective on even higher molecular weights (e.g., greater than 100,000). O'Brien suggested that where the TOC is relatively low, the removal process dependent upon RO membranes be used after the DI beds, to remove also the soluble organics extracted from the ion-exchange resins.

Collentro (1987) championed the use of ultrafiltration for the removal of organics. He pointed out that the accumulation of retained matter upon such filters comes to constitute a dynamically formed filter in its own right. This serves progressively to remove smaller organic molecules from the liquid stream. In this view, the ultrafilter functions primarily as septum upon which a true organic-removal membrane dynamically forms. Indeed, Collentro made the interesting suggestion that organic removal be minimized upstream of ultrafilters in order to speed the in situ deposition of this filter layer. The phenomenon Collentro alluded to is common in the ultrafiltration of protein solutions and is well substantiated in such practices (Gabler, 1987).

Dvorin and Zahn (1987) found that the use of a hollow-fiber ultrafilter operating on a water having TOC values of 100 to 250 ppb yielded effluent of 30 ppb of TOC on average. However, ultrafilters having dalton ratings of 10,000 were required; ratings of 50,000 or 80,000 were not fine enough. Concomitantly, chloride and sulfate values as measured on autoclaved samples, originally at 60 to 400 ppb, decreased to an average of about 15 ppb each. The conductivity decrease was attributed to the removal of organically bound minerals. Collentro (1987) pointed out that colloidal materials appear to contribute low levels of conductivity to waters. Their removal is effected by ultrafiltration. The use of ultrafilters both in the removal of colloids (ion-associated) and of organic material (also ion-associated) serves to reduce conductivities, even though the intersegmental distances of ultrafilters are too large to restrain the passage of ions themselves.

Some stills incorporate digestion chambers wherein organic matter can be destroyed by oxidative treatments such as by potassium permanganate or by hydrogen peroxide, before the water containing the organic is distilled.

The present most usual method of organic removal, largely based upon economics and convenience, relies upon adsorption by carbon beds. This practice, however, incurs the contributions by the carbon beds, or at least by less-than-optimally operated carbon beds, to elevated microorganism and pyrogen levels.

Reduction of TOC by the use of carbon has yielded mixed results. It is effective in some waters but not overly helpful in others. Frequent testing is required to determine when and whether carbon replacement is necessary, and the carbon beds shed particles and bacteria. Therefore, such TOC removal is largely limited to the pretreatment step.

The removal of TOC in the water polishing stages wherein low TOC levels are further reduced to state-of-the-art limits relies upon processes such as RO, and UV/ozone combinations.

Organic molecules may be removed, or be rendered more amenable to removal, by oxidative degradations. Ozone ultimately converts organic entities to carbon dioxide and water (Francis, 1987). Such complete ozone destructions of the organic molecules are not easily or economically attained. It is usually more feasible to oxidize the organic to its carboxylic acid form, whereupon it may be removed by ion exchange. Curiously, the ion-exchange resins themselves may serve as sources of extractable organic compounds. Perhaps for this reason the destruction of organics by ozone is often performed in the return loop of the water main, where ion exchangers are positioned. There is no unanimity on this point, however. Ozone may be used in the pretreatment section primarily to remove organic matter. More often it is used in a polishing treatment either before or after ion exchange. If used before, it is employed intermittently for short times and is removed by the use of ultraviolet light before it may enter and damage the ion-exchange resins.

An elaboration of how ozone and/or UV, sometimes synergized by the presence of hydrogen peroxide, are used to remove organic matter by means of oxidative degradations has been described in Chapter 3, page 160.

Cohen (1995) made comparisons of TOC removal from municipally treated waters using three different methods of purification: mixed-bed DI resins, granular activated carbon (GAC) plus the mixed-bed, and reverse osmosis in addition to the mixed-bed. Resin deionization by itself gave water with a TOC reading of 1,200 ppb. The addition of activated carbon resulted in TOC levels of 600 ppb. However, the carbon bed required backflushing and steam regeneration to remain effective over long periods of time. The combination of mixed-bed deionization and reverse osmosis reduced the TOC level to 200 ppb, as shown in Figure 6-1. As is illustrated in Figure 6-2, the salubrious influence of 185 nm ultraviolet light upon TOC reduction, from less than 100 ppb to greater than 10 ppb, is effected by subsequent removal of the oxidized TOC by the anion-exchange moiety of mixed-bed resins.

Trihalomethanes. The very chlorination or other biocidal treatment of water intended to render it microbiologically potable or otherwise microbiologically controlled or acceptable can create reaction by-products from organic substances present (e.g., those of humic acid origins). The new organic molecules may be objectionable in their own right from health points of view. In any case, at least for semiconductor operations, being TOC, they require being removed from the water.

Chlorine, being a powerful oxidant, initiates free-radical attacks upon organic molecules such as humic acids. Such reactions are abetted by the visible light spectrum. The resulting oxidative degradation produces chlorinated structures of progressively smaller molecular weights as the longer carbon-to-carbon chains of more complex molecules undergo successive free-radical chain scissions, and as hydrogen substitutes upon the carbons are replaced by chlorine. One consequence of this degradative chain reaction is the formation of chloroform ($CHCl_3$), frequently found in such treated waters.

Bromine, like chlorine a halogen, is also often found present in waters; usually through admixture with seawater, as in the San Francisco Bay area. Bromine is set free from its compounds by the action of elemental chlorine, which replaces it by substitution. The liberated bromine attacks organic matter in much the same way chlorine does, albeit not as vigorously. The result of oxidative degradations caused by bromine is bromoform ($CHBr_3$). Where both chlorine and bromine are present, the halogenated single-carbon entities of interest that are present are chloroform, bromoform ($CHBr_3$), bromodichloromethane ($CHBrCl_2$), and dibromochloromethane ($CHBr_2Cl$). This group of compounds, known as the trihalomethanes, are of concern in drinking water contexts because of their reputed carcinogenic properties. If waters containing THMs are subjected to UV light, a drop in resistivity will occur. The THMs contribute to the clumping of mixed-bed ion-exchange resins and resist removal by resin regeneration. Analyses for THMs are not commonly performed on chlorinated waters intended for subsequent primary processing.

The EPA safety standard for trihalomethanes in drinking water is presently set at a maximum of 100 ppb; this standard is pending reduction to 25 and may be decreased further to 5 ppb, as occasioned by the carcinogenicity of these compounds to laboratory animals. Some semiconductor manufacturers seek TOC levels of less than 2 ppb. The formation of THMs from TOC is stated to be (grossly) 20 ppb per 1 ppm of TOC (Singer, 1989; Chawla et al., 1983).

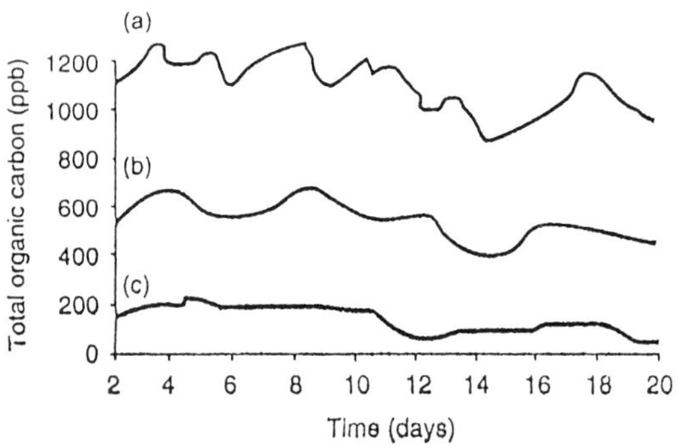

Figure 6-1. Measurements of TOC after various water pretreatment schemes using (a) ion-exchange resins only, (b) ion-exchange resins and GAC; and (c) reverse osmosis and ion exchange.
Cohen (1995); Courtesy, Pharmaceutical Technology.

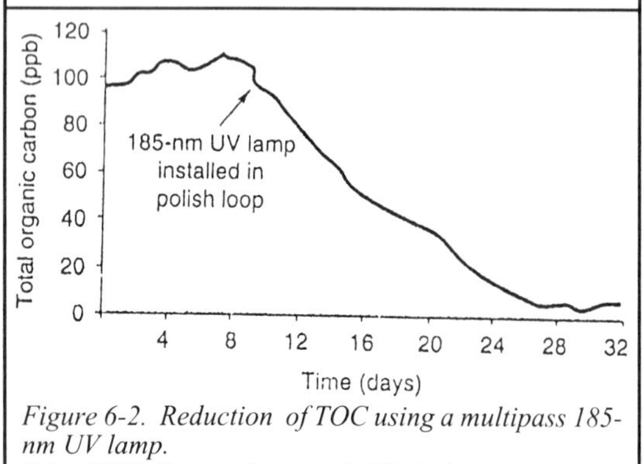

Figure 6-2. Reduction of TOC using a multipass 185-nm UV lamp.
Cohen (1995); Courtesy, Pharmaceutical Technology.

Krasner et al. (1989) examined waters from some 35 water treatment facilities. On a weight basis, trihalomethanes were the largest class of disinfection by-product (DBP) found to be present. Halogenated organic acids were the next most prominent group of compounds found. That the chlorination of organic compounds is an oxidative free-radical degradation, as of humic acid substances, is shown by the fact that formaldehyde and acetaldehyde are also produced (Table 6-1). These compounds also result from the ozonation of organic-containing waters. Chloramination of municipally treated waters is being practiced to avoid trihalomethane formation. Chlorine dioxide has also been advocated for the same reason. But these disinfectants produce other by-products. Krasner et al. (1989) found that chloramination produces cyanogen chloride. The removal of the chloramine from waters by activated carbon adsorption or by breakpoint chlorination is discussed. (See pages 52 and 316).

The diversity of DBRs found in drinking waters is shown in Figure 6-3. Table 6-2 shows median values for DBPs for a year in one study. Where bromine is present in the water, or becomes present when displaced by the added chlorine, the brominated disinfection by-products can have the variety shown in Table 6-3. Of the THMs, some 90% is chloroform, with the remainder containing bromine substituents (Singer, 1989).

THM removal. The THMs, being of low molecular weight, do not reliably undergo removal by RO filtration. They are too small in size to be retained by the RO membranes to any dependable degree. Their removal by adsorption to surfaces, such as those of activated carbons, membranes, or resin beads, is too dependent upon the vagaries of flowrates, concentration-to-surface considerations, and the general influences governing absorptions to be reliably effective. However, Chawla et al. (1983) did report 70% removals of THMs by carbon columns. (The actual amount obtained in any case will of course reflect the flowrates; the ratio of THM to adsorptive sites; the relative concentration of other molecular species competing for adsorption; and such influences as pH tand emperature) The conversion of the THMs by 185-nm UV irradiation to ionic

Table 6-1
Formaldehyde and Acetaldehyde Concentrations Produced by Batch-Scale Ozonation and Chloramination of State Project Water

		Ozonated Water Ozone Dose — mg/L					
By-product	*Raw*	*1.1*	*2.1*	*3.2*	*4.2*	*Ozonated* and Chloraminated*	*Chloraminated***
Formaldehyde-μg/L	ND	2.2	3.2	3.9	7.5	7.0	ND
		(0)+	(0.1)	(0.1)	(0.5)	(0.7)	
Acetaldehyde-μg/L	ND	ND	ND	ND	4.5	4.5	ND
					(0.4)	(0.1)	

* Ozone dose, 4.2 mg/L; ** Chloramine dose, 1.5 mg/L.
+ Average deviation of duplicate determinations; ND-Not detected
Krasner et al. (1989); Courtesy, American Water Works Association.

species whose removal can be effected by anion exchange has been discussed (see page 186). However, chloroform, the nonbrominated THM, cannot be modified by 185-UV treatment to yield an ionic entity capable of ion-exchange removal.

The carbon/chlorine bond is more stable than the chlorine/bromine bond. The THMs containing bromine are decomposed by the action of UV radiation. The resulting bromide ions lower the resistivity of the water.

Being of low molecular weight, the trihalomethanes are among those organic compounds classified as volatile organic compounds. Their boiling points are close enough to that of water to render them difficult to separate from water by distillation, particularly at trace levels. (See Chapter 10.) However, the use of deaerators in conjunction with the stills can be of help. Table 6-4 from Tom (1989) sets forth the molecular weights and boiling points of trihalomethanes normally encountered in water purification.

According to Tom (1989), vapor-compression stills consistently gave better THM removal when they were designed with the tube bundles (wherein the water is boiled) in a horizontal rather than a vertical position. Using THM feedwater

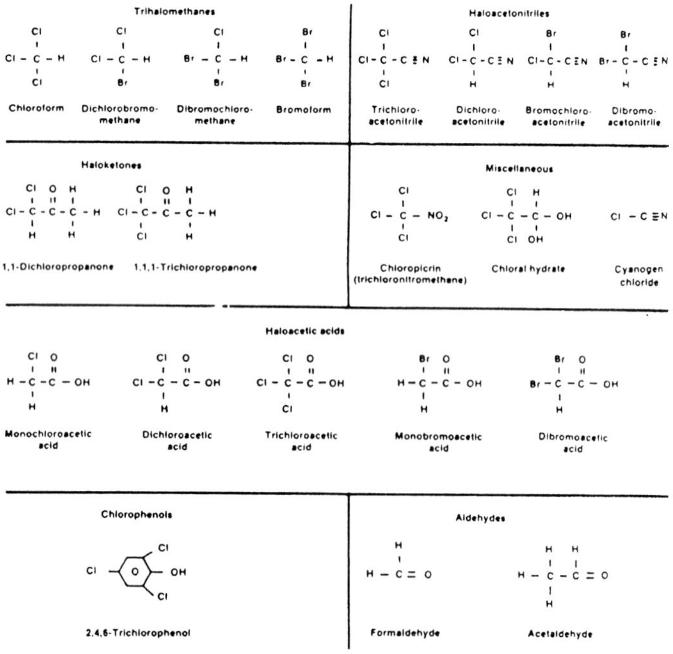

Figure 6-3. Structural formulas for disinfection by-products.
Krasner et al. (1989); Courtesy, American Water Works Association

Table 6-2
Quarterly Median Values of DBPs in Drinking Water

	Concentration — µg/L*			
Quarter	*1st Quarter*	*2nd Quarter*	*3rdQuarter*	*4th*
Disinfection By-product	*(Spring 1988)*	*(Summer 1988)*	*(Fall 1988)*	*(Winter 1989)*
Trihalomethanes				
Chloroform	15	15	13	9.6
Bromodichloromethane	6.9	10	5.5	4.1
Dibromochloromethane	2.6	4.5	3.8	2.7
Bromoform	0.33	0.57	0.88	0.51
Total trihalomethanes	34	44	40	30
Haloacetonitriles				
Trichloroacetonitrile	<0.012	<0.012	<0.029	<0.029
Dichloroacetonitrile	1.2	1.1	1.1	1.2
Bromochloroacetonitrile	0.50	0.58	0.70	0.59
Dibromoacetonitrile	0.54	0.48	0.51	0.46
Total haloacetonitriles	2.8	2.5	3.5	4.0
Haloketones				
1,1-Dichloropropane	0.52	0.46	0.52	0.55
1,1,1-Trichloropropanone	0.80	0.35	0.60	0.66
Total haloketones	1.4	0.94	1.0	1.8
Haloacids				
Monochloroacetic acid	<1.0	1.2	<1.0	1.2
Dichloroacetic acid	7.3	6.8	6.4	5.0
Trichloroacetic acid	5.8	5.8	6.0	4.0
Monobromoacetic acid	<0.5	<0.5	<0.5	<0.5
Dibromoacetic acid	0.9	1.5	1.4	1.0
Total haloacids	18	20	21	13
Aldehydes				
Formaldehyde	NA	5.1	3.5	2.0
Acetaldehyde	NA	2.7	2.6	1.8
Total aldehydes	NA	6.9	5.5	4.2
Miscellaneous				
Chloropicrin	0.16	0.12	0.10	0.10
Chloral hydrate	1.8	3.0	2.2	1.7
Cyanogen chloride	0.45	0.60	0.65	0.80
2,4,6-Trichlorophenol	<0.3	<0.4	<0.4	<0.4
Halogenated DBPsum§	64	82	72	58
Total organic halide	150	180	170	175
Plant influent characteristics				
Total organic carbon—mg/L	NA	2.9	2.9	3.2
Ultraviolet absorbance—cm^1	NA	0.11	0.11	0.13
Chloride —mg/L	NA	28	32	23
Bromide — mg/L	NA	0.07	0.10	0.07

* Except where otherwise indicated (plant influence characteristics)
Total class median values are not the sums of the medians of the individual compounds but rather the medians of the sums of the compounds within that class.
NA — not analyzed
§ The halogenated DBPsum median values are not the sum of the class medians for all utilities but rather the medians of the halogenated DBPsum values for all utilities. This value is only the sum of XDBPs measured in this study.

Krasner et al. (1989); Courtesy, American Water Works Association

levels of from 9.7 to 102 ppb, the distillate concentrations were found to be below 0.5 ppb, the sensitivity limit of gas chromatography used to analyze for these substances (Tom, 1989). The advantage in THM removal afforded by this type of still was ascribed to the enhanced possibilities permitted by the design details for the deaerative removal of volatiles such as the THMs.

Chu (1989) confirmed that the 185-nm UV irradiation of water containing THMs resulted in a resistivity drop. Since other molecules were likewise affected, the contribution of THMs required being confirmed by gas chromatographic analysis. Also confirmed were the suppositions that vacuum degasification would more effectively remove the lower-molecular-weight THMs. Thus 70% of the chloroform, 50% of bromodichloromethane, 30% of dibromochloromethane, and 19% of bromoform were removed, volatility usually being a direct function of molecular weight.

As regards the removal of THMs by ion-exchange resins, Chu (1989a, 1989b) found the larger-surfaced macroreticulated bead form to be almost twice as effective as the gel-type bead. Cation-exchange resins removed less than 10% of the chloroform, 15% of the bromodichloromethane, 35% of the dibromochlo-

Table 6-3
DBP Concentrations at Utility with Seasonal Change in Bromide Levels (utility 12)*

Component	*Summer 1988*	*Fall 1988*	*Winter 1989*
Plant influent—*mg/L*			
Total organic carbon	2.6	2.2	2.8
Chloride	111	215	202
Bromide	0.41	0.78	0.79
Clearwell effluent—*µg/L*			
Chloroform	4.7	1.4	0.86
Bromodichloromethane	13	7.5	6.5
Dibromochloromethane	28	25	24
Bromoform	26	72	53
Total trihalomethanes	72	106	84
Trichloroacetonitrile	<0.012	<-0.029	<0.029
Dichloroacetonitrile	0.74	0.24	0.19
Bromochloroacetonitrile	1.6	0.96	1.4
Dibromoacetonitrile	4.6	7.0	11
Total haloacetonitriles	6.9	8.2	13
Monochloroacetic acid	<1.0	<1.0	<1.0
Dichloroacetic acid	2.9	1.7	0.9
Trichloroacetic acid	1.6	1.2	0.8
Monobromoacetic acid	1.0	1.6	1.3
Dibromoacetic acid	14	17	13
Total haloacetic acids	20	22	16

* Data for spring 1988 were not included because bromide was not measured that quarter.
Krasner et al. (1989); Courtesy, American Water Works Association

romethane, and 50% of the bromoform. The same trend favoring the removal of the more brominated THMs was shown by anion-exchange resins in the chloride form, albeit to a greater overall extent. The above figures were obtained from measurements after 5 bed volumes (20 minutes after sample loading). Measurements taken after 64 bed volumes (4 hours after sample loading) showed a decrease in THM removal efficiency to less than 15%. Clearly, the resins' capacities for THM were speedily exhausted. These data indicate that only small THM volumes were removed overall, since the resins have a service life of days as makeup resins and a useful life of weeks as polishing resins. Anion-exchange resins in their hydroxide forms showed an almost 100% removal efficiency for the brominated THMs even after 700 bed volumes (44 hours after sample loading). The chloroform removal was less than 50%. However, Chu (1989) demonstrated that the THM removal was not caused by adsorption by the resin, but resulted from chemical reaction with hydroxide ions.

Stevens et al. (1989) found that the mixture of disinfection by-products produced during chlorination was most significantly affected by the pH of the treated waters. These investigators elucidated a direct relationship between trihalomethane control, occasioned by low pH; and the control of most of the other DBPs, at higher pHs, as revealed in Table 6-5. Whatever the significance of these various compounds to potable water ingestion, they demonstrate the complexity of organic removal from chlorinated waters, and by extension, to ozonated waters.

Studies by Singer and Chang (1989) showed that surface waters subjected to chlorination at near-neutral pHs contain a ratio of total organic halides to trihalomethanes of 3.4 to 1. On a chlorine-equivalent basis, the total THMs constituted about 26% of the total organic halide disinfection by-products.

Wiegler and Anderson (1990) considered possible alternatives for the removal of THM. Among the qualifications and concerns to be met were the safety of the RO/DI system and the economics involved. The use of ozone followed by

Table 6-4
Physical Properties of Some THM Members

	Molecular Weight	*Boiling Point*
Trichloromethane (Chloroform)	119.4	143°F (61.7°C)
Bromodichloromethane ($CHCl_2Br$)	116.8	194°F (90°C)
Dibromochloromethane ($CHBr_2Cl$)	208.3	246°F (119°C)
Tribromomethane (Bromoform)	252.8	301°F (149.5°C)

Tom (1989); Courtesy, *Ultrapure Water* journal

its removal upstream of the RO/DI was rejected because the ozone equipment manufacturer would guarantee no THM levels lower than 10 to 15 ppb. The capital costs would have been $400,000, although the operating costs would have been low. Use of ozone in a storage tank venue was unattractive because the mixed-bed resins in the recirculation loop would have been affected. Moreover, studies showed ozone to be inefficient in degrading the carbon/chorine bond. Actual data concerning the removal capability of ozone on THM does not exist.

The removal of THMs by adsorption onto carbon seemed to promise success, being used by many. However, no reliable, relevant data concerning THM removal efficiency existed. Vacuum degasification was considered. It seemed

Table 6-5
Conditions of Formation of DPBs

<table>
<tr><th></th><th colspan="3">Conditions of Formation</th></tr>
<tr><th>By-product</th><th>Chlorination at pH 5</th><th>Chlorination at pH 7</th><th>Chlorination at pH 9.4</th></tr>
<tr><td>TTHM</td><td>Lower formation</td><td></td><td>Higher formation</td></tr>
<tr><td>TCAA</td><td colspan="2">Similar formation</td><td>Lower formation</td></tr>
<tr><td>DCAA</td><td colspan="3">Similar formation - perhaps slightly higher at pH7</td></tr>
<tr><td>MCAA</td><td colspan="3">At concentrations <5 μg/L, trends not discernible</td></tr>
<tr><td>DBAA</td><td colspan="3">At concentrations <1 μg/L, trends not discernible</td></tr>
<tr><td>CH</td><td colspan="2">Similar formation</td><td>Forms within 4 hours; decays over time to <5 μg/L</td></tr>
<tr><td>CP</td><td colspan="3">At concentrations <1 μg/L, trends not discernible</td></tr>
<tr><td>DCAN</td><td>Higher formation</td><td>Forms within 4 hours; then decays over time to <5 μg/L</td><td>At concentrations <2 μg/L, trends not discernible</td></tr>
<tr><td>BCAN</td><td colspan="3">At concentrations <2 μg/L, trends not discernible</td></tr>
<tr><td>DBAN</td><td colspan="3">At concentrations <0.5 μg/L, trends not discernible</td></tr>
<tr><td>TCAN</td><td colspan="3">Not detected</td></tr>
<tr><td>111-TCP</td><td>Higher formation</td><td>At concentrations <2 μg/L, trends not discernible</td><td>Not detected</td></tr>
</table>

TTHM - total triahlomethane
TCAA - trichloroacetic acid
DCAA - dichloroacetic acid
MCAA - monochloroacetic acid
CH - chloral hydrate
CP - chloropicrin
DCAN - dichloroacetonitrile
BCAN - bromochloroacetonitrile
TCAN - trichloracetonitrile
TCP - 2,4,6-trichlorophenol

Stevens et al., (1989); Courtesy, American Water Works Association

Table 6-6
Summaries of TOC and THM Readings (in ppb) from Initial Tests of UV Lights

		Sample Point			
Sample Date	*Parameter*	*Pre-UV*	*Post-UV*	*Post-Degas*	*Post-Mixed Bed*
9/5/89	TOC	330	140	100	60
	$CHCl_3$	19	18	4.6	7.2
	$CHCl_2Br$	34	30	13	2.8
	$CHClBr_2$	27	13	8	.6
	$CHBr_3$	7.8	1.6	1.1	ND
9/6/89	TOC	300	130	75	60
	$CHCl_3$	17	16	4.5	7
	$CHCl_2Br$	32	28	13	3.9
	$CHClBr_2$	27	14	8.9	1.2
	$CHBr_3$	8.3	1.7	1.3	ND
9/7/89	TOC	260	140	70	45
	$CHCl_3$	17	17	4.4	6.3
	$CHCl_2Br$	31	28	12	5.7
	$CHCLBr_2$	25	14	8.1	2.7
	$CHBr_3$	8.2	1.8	1.1	ND
9/8/89	TOC	240	130	100	35
	$CHCl_3$	15	14	4.1	7
	$CHCl_2Br$	32	27	13	2.7
	$CHClBr_2$	30	14	9.5	.7
	$CHBr_3$	10	2.3	1.9	ND
9/11/89	TOC	170	140	120	80
	$CHCl_3$	17	16	4.6	7.1
	$CHCl_2Br$	34	25	14	.2
	$CHClBr_2$	27	13	9.6	ND
	$CHBr_3$	7.2	1.7	1.1	ND
9/12/89	TOC	150	140	140	63
	$CHCl_3$	4	14	3.4	6.2
	$CHCl_2Br$	33	28	13	5.5
	$CHClBr_2$	30	14	9.0	2.4
	$CHBr_3$	9.7	1.9	1.2	ND

ND - Not detected (<0.5 ppb)

Wiegler and Anderson (1990); Courtesy, *Microcontamination*

promising for the lighter THMs, those with fewer bromine atoms, but less encouraging for their heavier analogues. The capital costs would have been about $120,000, with low operating and maintenance costs. Militating against this method was the lack of actual THM removal efficiency data.

The use of added ion-exchange capacity to manage the THM removal was entertained. It would have entailed $200,000 as a mid-range capital cost, but would have involved very high operating costs. While THM removal by ion exchange is efficient, the saturation level is too low; regeneration or replacements would have been needed at too-frequent intervals. On-site regeneration, every 2 to 3 weeks, would have been too cumbersome for the actual circumstance.

The best possibility for THM removal was judged to be the use of 185-nm UV lamps. The capital costs involved were expected to approximate $160,000, with very low operating costs. It was estimated that 85% of the THM would be destroyed. However, chloroform is immune to UV-initiated decomposition and could therefore accumulate to some level. A desired goal of 15 ppb maximum can be obtained provided the THM concentration does not exceed 100 ppb. To optimize the effect of the 185-nm UV lamps, they should be preceded by an RO unit to remove as much UV-adsorbing substances as possible. A subsequent ion-exchange mixed-bed polishing would remove the ion-bearing entities created by the UV irradiation. Table 6-6 illustrates the findings of Wiegler and Anderson (1990) concerning the TOC and THM levels incidental to their 185-nm UV work on THM reductions. Table 6-7 sets forth the resistivity readings at various

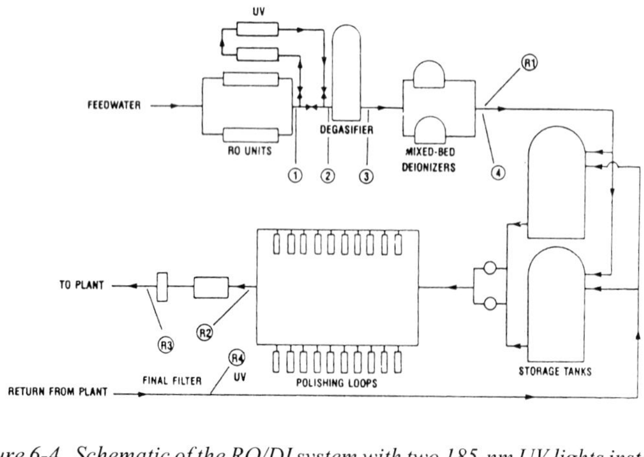

Figure 6-4. Schematic of the RO/DI system with two 185-nm UV lights installed for testing purposes. Sample points for THM measurements are numbered 1 to 4; sampling points for resistivity readings are shown as R1 to R4.
Wiegler and Anderson (1990); Courtesy, *Microcontamination*

positions within their water purification system relative to the 185-nm UV irradiation. Figure 6-3 depicts the water purification arrangement involving the UV installation.

Avoidance of THMs. Given the difficulty of controlling the microbial population of waters, the availability for industrial usage of chlorinated municipal waters may be judged to be advantageous. Yet it is specifically this chlorination that produces the THMs as the end products of the oxidative degradation (by chlorine) of the organic molecules present. It would be far better, at least from this point of view, to avoid microbial control by chlorine. Ozone would be a better choice. True, the organic impurities would still become oxidatively degraded and the end products too could be harmful and contaminating. However, they would not be characterized by the recalcitrance of the stable carbon/chlorine bond and could be removed at the carboxylic acid stage of their oxidative degradation by the use of the ion-exchange resins. Where possible, the chlorination of waters, whether for potable or municipal purposes, should be avoided.

Table 6-7
Summaries of Resistivity Readings from Initial Tests of UV Lights

		Sample Point			
Date	*Time*	*Post-Mixed Bed*	*Post-Polish*	*Post-Final Filter*	*DI Water Return*
9/5/89	10:30	17.6[a]	18.8	18.7	19.1
	3:00	18.5	19.0	19.5	19.2
9/6/89	8:00	18.5	18.6	18.5	18.8
	1:30	18.6	18.8	19.1	19.0
	5:45	18.6	18.6	18.6	18.9
9/7/89	8:00	18.5	18.7	18.5	18.8
	12:00	18.7	18.8	19.0	19.0
	5:30	18.6	18.7	18.8	18.9
9/8/89	8:00	18.5	18.6	18.5	18.7
	5:00	18.4[b]	18.7	19.2	19.2
9/11/89	8:00	12.0[c]	18.7	18.8	19.0
	12:00	18.2	18.8	18.9	19.1
	5:00	18.2	18.8	19.0	19.0
9/12/89	8:00	18.6	18.8	19.1	19.0
	4:00	18.5	18.9	19.2	19.1
9/13/89	9:00	18.6	18.9	19.0	19.0
	12:00	18.6	18.9	19.3	19.1

[a] Bed B. [b] Switch to Bed A. [c] Bed B on.
Wiegler and Anderson (1990); Courtesy, *Microcontamination*

Chloramine removal. The formation of chloramines by the interaction of the chlorine introduced during the preparation of potable water and the ammonia subsequently added to prevent the formation of trihalomethanes has been discussed (Morris and Wei 1969; Wei and Morris, 1974). (See pages 52.) The existence of chloramines in water used in hemodialysis practice is a cause of hemolytic anemia, as is also the presence of copper, nitrates and nitrites.

The chloramines are not removed by reverse osmosis treatments. The chloramines can be removed by adsorption to activated carbon (Komorita and Snoeyink, 1985). Interestingly, mono- and dichloramines react with activated

Table 6-8
Some Physical Properties of the Volatile Pollutants

Systematic and Trivial Name References	*Formula*	*m.w.*	*D o/rl*	*m.p. °C*	*b.p. °C*	
Trichloromethane (chloroform)	$CHCl_3$	119.38	1.446	-63	61.0	a
1,1,1-Trichlorethane	CH_3CCl_3	133.41	1.338	-50	75.0	a
Tetrachloromethane	CCl_4	153.82	1.594	-23	77.0	a
1,1,2-Trichloroethylene	$ClCH{=}CCl_2$	131.39	1.464	-87	86.9	a
Bromodichloromethane	$CBrCl_2$	163.83	1.980	55	87.0	a
Bromotrichloromethane	$CBrCl_3$	198.28	2.012	-6	105.0	a
Chlorodibromomethane	$ChBr_2Cl$	208.29	2.451	-22	119.5	a
1,2-Dibromoethane	$BrCH_2CH_2Br$	187.64	2.160	8	131.5	a
Tetrachloroethylene	$Cl_2C{=}CCl_2$	165.83	1.623	-22	121.0	a
Tribromomethane (bromoform)	$CHBr_3$	252.75	2.894	8.3	150.5	a
Benzene		78.12	0.879	5.5	80.1	a
1,3-Dimethylbenzene		106.17	0.864	-47.9	139.1	a
1,4-Dimethylbenzene (p-xylene)		106.17	0.861	13.3	138.4	a
1,2-Dimethylbenzene (o-xylene)		106.17	0.850	-25.2	144.4	b
Methylbenzene (toluene)		92.15	0.867	-95	110.6	c

a. Griesinger and Banks (1986) b. Weast (1976) c. Roller (1965)
Kroneld (1991); Courtesy, *J. Parenteral Science and Technology*

carbon in a two-stage conversion to yield ammonia and nitrogen gas (Scaramelli and DiGiano, 1977).

Breakpoint chlorination can be used to destroy the chloramines. When the ammonia nitrogen reacts with the chlorine to produce the chloramines, part of it is oxidized to nitrogen gas and nitrate ions. The utilization of this reaction is promoted by further (breakpoint) chlorination to convert the chloramines into nitrogen gas and nitrate ions (Saunier and Selleck, 1979).

Saunier and Sellack (1979) investigated the above reaction in pilot plant studies involving flowrates of 0.12 L/sec (2 gpm). The water was pumped from a fiberglass-lined steel tank by way of a positive-displacement pump into a chlorine-contact chamber wherein the chlorine was added by venturi action. Contact times of various durations, up to 5 minutes, could be arranged. Ammonia nitrogen was added in the form of ammonium chloride. The conversion of the ammonia nitrogen into chloramines and the subsequent oxidation of these into nitrogen gas and nitrate ions is by way of a complex chain of chemical reactions involving postulated intermediates.

Breakpoint chlorination increases with the chlorine-to-ammonia ratio. The speed of the oxidizing reaction of the chloramines is greatest at pH 7.5. Mono-

Table 6-9
Different Methods Used in Eliminating Some Volatile Hydrocarbons from water.

	After Treatment		
Substance mg/L n = 20	*Tap Water*	*Distillation, Traditional*	*Water Softening*
$CHCl_3$	67.7 ±0.6	69.1 ±0.9	44.9 ±0.6
$CHBrCl_2$	10.8 ±0.5	11.1 ±0.6	9.7 ±0.5
$CHBr_2Cl$	2.4 ±0.4	2.5 ±0.3	1.6 ±0.3

	After Treatment			
Substance mg/L n = 20	*Active Charcoal Filtering*	*Reverse Osmosis*	*Paper Filtering*	*Used Dialysis Fluid*
$CHCl_3$	47.1 ±0.7	38.1 ±1.2	37.9 ±0.8	37.3 ±1.3
$CHBrCl_2$	9.8 ±0.5	7.8 ±0.5	7.9 ±0.4	7.5 ±0.5
$CHBr_2Cl$	1.7 ±0.4	1.4 ±0.3	1.4 ±0.3	1.4 ±0.3

Crane et al. (1991); Courtesy, *J. Parenteral Science and Technology*

and dichloramine may disappear in a matter of minutes at high ammonia concentrations; other organic nitrogen compounds, more slowly. Nitrogen trichloride is also a reaction product, but is itself subject to conversion, presumably through labile intermediates, into chlorine and nitrogen. By means of breakpoint chlorination, then, the chloramines may be removed from waters containing them. Indeed, this practice is used in the pharmaceutical industry.

Volatile organics. (See page 32). Volatile contaminants such as the lower hydrocarbons, their chlorinated derivatives such as the trihalomethanes, and various benzene compounds can each and all be present in high-purity waters. As shown in Table 6-8, the EPA presents a list of volatile organics. These compound are described as being "organics which readily volatilize, or travel from the water into the air." Hence, they are also called *purgeable organic compounds* (POC).

Kroneld (1991) illustrated in Table 6-9 different methods used to eliminate volatile organics from aqueous solutions. He found most efficacious the use of an airstream flowing countercurrent to the feedwater being cleansed. He found that this method efficiently removed the fugacious organics, as shown in Table 6-10. The coupling of this "eliminator of volatile pollutants," EVP, is advocated as a pretreatment to water being directed to distillation. The temperature of the water being treated was at 130 °C under 5-bar pressure (72.5 psig), and the water-to-air ratio was 1.5.

Carcinogenic, mutagenic, and teratogenic properties have been imputed to volatile organics in pharmaceutical contexts; as has their interference in cell culture work.

Measurement of Organics

BOD. In its historical context, the measurement of organic substances contained in waters probably stems from the biological oxygen demand (BOD) determinations of wastewaters (*Standard Methods 1989,* part 5000). The BOD test is an empirical determination of the oxygen consumed (demanded) by a water sample undergoing incubation under specified conditions of time and temperature. The oxygen consumed is largely that utilized by the bacteria present in the water sample. Since oxygen has only a limited solubility in water, a sufficiently small aliquot sample of the water must be taken so as to permit a complete bacterial digestion to take place. An empirical determination is made of the proper sample size, the proportion of its organic content to the microbial digestion capabilities. The presence of chemical reducing agents such as sulfides and ferrous iron will also cause an oxygen consumption. The BOD measurement provides an estimate of the environmental effects of water effluents. It is more usually confined to wastewater examinations. The specifics of the BOD procedure are given in *Standard Methods 1989* (part 5000).

COD. As water may contain organic substances such as may not readily be detected by the oxygen uptake attendant upon bacterial digestions, the assay of such organics may be made by the use of chemical oxidants. Measurement of the consumption of the oxidant (chemical oxidation demand, COD) leads to an estimation of the organic matter that is present in the water.

In general there are two methods of determining COD. The first uses hot chromic acid solution to oxidize organic matter. It analyzes for both biodegradable and nonbiodegradable organic matter. When the analytical technique uses permanganate, the test measures the susceptibility of organic matter to oxidation by permanganate alone. It is not so strong an oxidizing agent as chromic acid, but is still a very useful control test.

Various oxidizers have various differing oxidative strengths, and different organic molecules have their individual propensities for undergoing oxidations. Some favor a COD measurement based upon potassium permanganate oxidations. Ordinarily a COD procedure based upon the more aggressive oxidizer action of acidic potassium dichromate is favored (*Standard Methods 1989,* part 5220, pp 5-10). The COD measurement is used as a gauge of the oxygen equivalent of the organic content of a water sample. It is possible to relate the COD to the BOD by empirical correlation. The COD test is useful for monitoring and control of organic matter, usually in wastewaters.

Potassium permanganate test. The details of the Oxidizable Substance Test used to detect oxidizable organic materials present in Purified Water are given in the *USP 23* (p. 1636). As previously stated on page 27, the test may become obfuscated by suspended matter or colors other than pink. The end-point detection can be improved by the use of UV-visible spectra to detect the presence

Table 6-10
The Average Reduction (%) of Some Volatile Hydrocarbons and Benzene Derivatives During Elimination Tests with the EVP Equipment

Model Compounds Tested n = 12	*Distillate with one EVP Equipment*	*Distillate with Two EVP Equipment*
Volatile hydrocarbons		
$CHCl_3$	98.4	99.1
$CHBrCl_2$	99.8	99.7
$CHBr_2Cl$	98.9	98.8
$CHCl_3$	77.4	86.5
Benzene derivatives		
Touene	41.7	85.8
Total	96.0	97.1

Kroneld (1991); Courtesy, *J. Parenteral Science and Technology*

of permanganate, or by the filtrative removal of haze-forming particles of manganese dioxide and other colloids (Kenley et al., 1990).

As previously discussed in Chapter 1, page 29, the organic compounds originally selected by the Water Quality Committee of the Pharmaceutical Manufacturers Association to serve as standards for the TOC method of analysis, as recommended by the Japanese Pharmacopeia, were potassium hydrogen phthalate (potassium biphthalate), for its high degree of purity, its water solubility, and its ease of oxidation; and sodium dodecylbenzene sulfonate, a surfactant frequently used in the cleaning of water systems, and more difficult to oxidize. However, both these reference compounds include ionic moieties whose presence in the water would interfere with the accurate measurement of carbon dioxide by conductivity. In order not to exclude from the instrument selection process any TOC analyzer that operated by conductivity measurements, the standard materials were changed. Sucrose replaced the potassium hydrogen phthalate. Pare benzoquinone is the suitability reference substituted for the sodium dodecylbenzene sulfonate. These reference compounds are well described and characterized in the pharmaceutical compendia, and are, therefore, suited to serve as standard reagents.

In practice the TOC instrument will be calibrated by reference to a 0.5 mg/L (500 ppb) solution of sucrose NF prepared by a 4 hour drying at 105 °C and weighed to yield a concentration of 1.19 mg/L; equating to 0.5 ppm or 500 ppb of TOC. The 1,4-benzoquinone will be computed to 500 ppb TOC for testing.

Proof of the instrument's system suitability will be its detection of the reference quantity of 1,4-benzoquinone within the range of a high of 15% and a low of 20%. The latitude of this range is set to accomodate the different oxidation chemistries of the various TOC analyzers.

Detection of the presence of those oxidizable organics responsive to permanganate is limited by the sensitivity of the test to only parts per million (ppm). (Table 6-11). In contrast TOC analyzers are routinely used to detect 20 ppb of organics in semiconductor rinsewaters. Certain of these instruments are speci-

Table 6-11
Levels of Carbon in Various Combined Forms at Which Water Will Still Pass the Oxidizable Substances Test

Compound	*Maximum Level (mgC/L)*
Acetonitrile	>5000
Methanol	2500
Potassium hydrogen phthalate	500[a]
Glucose	5
Sucrose	2.5
Sodium dodecylbenzenesulfonate	1

Crane et al. (1991); Courtesy, *J. Parenteral Science and Technology*

fied to measure as little as 5 ppb when properly maintained.

TOC analyzers. Several devices are available on the market for the analytical determination of dissolved organic compounds. Euphemistically entitled *total carbon analyzers*, they should more accurately be called *total oxidizable-carbon analyzers*. Most of the available devices use different oxidation chemistries, not equally efficient in the oxidation of given organic molecules. Indeed, some organic compounds (e.g., cyanuric acid) are very different to oxidize; and difficulty is encountered even with the simple alcohols such as methanol and isopropanol.

The various TOC analyzers can be divided into high- and low-temperature oxidizers. Some depend upon high-temperature combustion of the sample.

One actually utilizes combustion at 680 °C; another manages combustion at 950 °C by way of cobalt oxide catalyst. These high-temperature instruments are usually bulky, but should be more aggressive in their oxidation of recalcitrant organic compounds. Two other TOC analyzers depend upon the oxidizing power of potassium persulfate as augmented by ultraviolet light. Yet another claims improved results using persulfate oxidation in the presence of the visible or near-visible wave lengths of 200 to 300 nm. Presumably, hydroxyl free radicals are more plentifully generated at these wave lengths. Persulfate alone at 100 °C is utilized in another design; while yet another depends upon persulfate under titanium dioxide catalysis to effect the oxidation of organic substances (Table 6-12).

The several TOC devices also differ in how they detect the carbon dioxide, CO_2, that is the product of the organic oxidation, and in how they measure its

Table 6-12
Oxidation and Detection Methods of Principal Models of Total Organic Carbon Analyzer, for High-Sensitivity Applications

Oxidation Method	*Detection Method*
Laboratory (batch) analyzers	
UV + persulfate[a]	NDIR[b]
Hot persulfate	NDIR
UV	Conductivity
Process (on-line) analyzers	
UV + persulfate	NDIR
UV	Conductivity

[a] Method used by the Dohrmann DC-80, employed in this study.
[b] Carbon-dioxide-specific nondispersive infrared detector.
Crane et al. (1991); Courtesy, *J. Parenteral Science and Technology*

extent. Many quantify it by nondispersive infrared analysis, NDIR. In the case of the carbon dioxide, concentration is derived from conductivity readings, CO_2 being the acid anhydride of carbonic acid, which, however feebly, dissociates into hydronium and bicarbonate ions, HCO_3^-. However, the presence of nitrogen, phosphorus, chlorides, or sulfates in the water also gives rise to ionic species. These mask the true carbon dioxide values. Therefore, this TOC analyzer is rather restricted to TOC analyses of waters where interfering elements are absent. The other TOC device also collects the carbon dioxide as it dissolves in water. However, the carbon dioxide passes into the water through a hydrophobic microporous membrane under the impetus of its concentration gradient. Water and its contained ionic impurities cannot permeate the hydrophobic membrane. Therefore, no interferences with conductivity result. This TOC instrument may, therefore, be employed even in the analysis of wastewaters. To date, only the last two described TOC analyzers can be used as on-line instruments (Table 6-12). (Crane et al., 1991; Godec et al., 1992).

One actually uses oxygen at 800 to 900 °C. Two others utilize the oxidizing power of potassium persulfate as augmented by ultraviolet light. Another claims achievement of better oxidations by the avoidance of UV light, using persulfate and heat instead. These analytical devices also differ in how they detect the products of the oxidation, and in how they measure its extent. Some trap the carbon dioxide that is evolved and measure it by NDIR. Others utilize colorimetric end points in titrations. Conductivity measurements are also used (Crane et al., 1991). (See Table 6-12.)

It is recommended by the WQC/PMA that the TOC analyzers be capable of

Table 6-13
Comparison of TOC and Oxidizable Substances Tests for Various Concentrations of Potassium Hydrogen Phthalate (KHP)

		Average TOC Found		*Average Abs. Units*		
Sample	*KHP Spike mgC/L*	*mgC/L*	*SD*	*528 nm*	*SD*	*Solution Color*
1	0	0.123	0.006	0.0875	0.0025	pink
2	0	0.110	0.010	0.084	0.001	pink
3	0	0.110	0.011	0.084	0.003	pink
4	0	0.117	0.006	0.085	0.003	pink
5	0	0.113	0.006	0.084	0.001	pink
6	12.5	10	0	0.078	0.001	pink
7	100	97	3	0.069	0.001	pink
8	250	243	6	0.055	0	pink
9	500	490	10	0.013	0.006	faint pink
10	1000	960	21	0.013	0.006	faint orange
11	2000	2030	60	<0.0025	—	colorless

Crane et al. (1991); Courtesy, *J. Parenteral Science and Technology*

measuring TOC to levels at least as low as 50 ppb (0.05 ppm). Since the acceptible TOC level is set at 500 ppb, the higher sensitivity of the instruments offers a prudent margin of safety to the procedure. As a matter of interest, some pharmaceutical water systems produce WFI with TOC contents as low as 10 ppb (Cohen, 1995). As commendable as this may be, it is questionable whether standards aimed for in semiconductor contexts have reality as goals in pharmaceutical applications (Collentro, 1994). They may be excessive and wasteful to attain.

As shown in Table 6-13, the TOC analyses are much more sensitive than the *USP* Oxidizable Substances Test.

Anderson (1986) reported a study of several commercially available TOC analyzers. This investigator made it plain that only those organics are measured that are oxidized and detected by the specific instrumental technique used. Analysis by TOC does not identify specific compounds. Results were reported in terms of micrograms of carbon per liter. Anderson illustrated (Table 6-14) that a water sample containing 84 x 10^{16} molecules of hexane or 250 x 10^{16} (three times as much) acetic acid would yield the same TOC value, namely, 100 ppb. Yet, while 84×10^{16} molecules of hexane or of benzene sulfonic acid would both yield TOC values of 100 ppb, the mass concentration of the benzenesulfonic acid would be twice as great.

Not surprisingly, the analytical results given by different types of devices do not necessarily agree. It may reflect upon the objectivity of users that the most popular of these instruments yields lower TOC readings that its next most popular competitor; and this in contexts where low TOC levels are being sought!

Sakamoto and Miyasaka (1987) stated that TOC analyzers based on wet chemistry involving persulfate oxidation combined with UV irradiation, as specified by *Standards Methods,* 16th Edition, are capable of detecting lower TOC levels than are those dependent upon combustion, as adopted by Japanese

Table 6-14
Comparison of Number of Molecules/Liter and Mass/Liter for Certain Materials at 100 ppb as TOC

Compound	*Equivalent Molecules/liter*	*Equivalent Mass Concentration (μg/L)*
Hexane (C_6H_{14})	84×10^{16}	119
Acetic acid ($C_2O_2H_4$)	250×10^{16}	250
Benzenesulfonic acid ($C_6H_6SO_3$)	84×10^{16}	220

Anderson (1986); Courtesy, Semiconductor Pure Water Conference

Table 6-15
TOC Determination of Various Organic Compounds

Organic Compound	*Chemical Formula*	*TOC by Combustion Infrared Oxidation (mg C/L)* 1	2	3	4	5	Av	*TOC by Persulfate UV Oxidation (mg C/L)* 1	2	3	4	5	Av	*Average Rate of Oxidation* (%)
Methanol	CH_3OH	1.8	1.7	-	-	-	1.8	1.70	1.71	-	-	-	1.71	95.0
		3.7	3.7	-	-	-	3.7	3.45	3.38	-	-	-	3.42	92.4
Ethanol	C_2H_5OH	1.7	1.7	-	-	-	1.7	1.59	1.65	-	-	-	1.62	95.3
		3.5	3.4	-	-	-	3.5	3.27	3.29	-	-	-	3.28	93.7
2-Propanol	$(CH_3)_2CHOH$	2.1	1.7	1.9	1.9	1.8	1.9	1.77	1.82	1.87	1.85	1.81	1.82	95.8
		3.7	3.8	3.8	3.9	3.6	3.8	3.65	3.65	3.70	3.72	3.67	3.68	96.8
Citric acid	$C_6H_5O_7Na_3$	2.0	1.9	2.0	-	-	2.0	2.06	2.00	2.01	-	-	2.02	101
		3.9	4.0	4.1	-	-	4.0	3.98	3.95	4.00	-	-	3.98	99.5
Benzoic acid	$C_7H_6O_2$	2.3	2.3	2.2	2.1	2.1	2.2	2.04	2.02	2.02	2.09	1.99	2.03	92.3
		3.9	4.0	4.1	-	-	4.0	4.02	3.98	3.95	-	-	3.98	99.5
Potassium hydrogen phthalate	$C_8H_5O_4K$	2.0	2.0	1.9	-	-	2.0	1.99	2.02	2.00	-	-	2.00	100
		4.0	4.0	-	-	-	4.0	3.98	3.99	-	-	-	3.99	99.8
Acetone	C_3H_6O	1.9	1.8	1.9	-	-	1.9	2.00	1.95	1.93	-	-	1.96	103
		3.9	3.8	-	-	-	3.9	3.87	3.78	-	-	-	3.83	98.2
L-Sodium glutamate	C_5H_8ONNa	2.0	2.0	-	-	-	2.0	1.99	1.99	-	-	-	1.99	99.5
		3.9	4.0	-	-	-	4.0	3.96	3.99	-	-	-	3.98	99.5
4-QAmino-benzene sulfonate	$C_6H_7O_3NS$	2.0	2.0	2.2	1.9	2.0	2.0	1.92	2.00	1.97	2.03	2.00	1.98	99.0
		4.1	4.1	4.2	4.2	4.1	4.1	3.94	3.91	4.02	3.99	4.01	3.98	97.1
D-Glucose	$C_6H_{12}O_2$	1.8	1.7	-	-	-	1.8	1.82	1.70	-	-	-	1.76	97.8
		3.8	3.8	-	-	-	3.8	3.79	3.80	-	-	-	3.80	100
8-Quinolinol	C_9H_7ON	2.0	2.0	-	-	-	2.0	2.02	1.97	-	-	-	2.00	100
		4.0	4.1	-	-	-	4.1	4.02	4.02	-	-	-	4.02	98.0
4-Amino-antipyrine	$C_{11}H_{13}ON_3$	1.9	1.9	1.8	-	-	1.9	2.07	2.00	1.93	-	-	2.00	105
		3.9	4.0	4.2	-	-	4.0	3.96	3.97	3.96	-	-	3.96	99.0
2,4,6-Tri (2-pyridil) 1,3,5-triazine	$C_{18}H_{12}O_6$	1.9	1.8	2.0	1.9	2.0	1.9	1.69	1.61	1.59	1.58	1.59	1.61	84.7
		4.0	4.0	3.9	3.6	3.7	3.8	3.48	3.50	3.30	3.28	3.15	3.34	87.9
1,10-Phen-anthroline	$C_{12}H_{10}ON_2$	2.0	2.0	1.9	-	-	2.0	1.94	1.90	1.92	-	-	1.92	96.0
		3.9	4.1	4.0	-	-	4.0	3.75	3.89	3.84	-	-	3.83	95.8
Methylene blue	$C_{16}H_{18}N_3$-cis	1.8	1.8	1.7	-	-	1.8	1.72	1.80	1.77	-	-	1.76	97.8
		3.6	3.4	3.5	-	-	3.5	3.51	3.50	3.54	-	-	3.52	101
Methyl orange	$C_{14}H_{14}O_3N_3SNa$	2.3	2.4	2.3	-	-	2.3	2.25	2.18	2.20	-	-	2.21	96.0
		4.4	4.3	4.4	-	-	4.4	3.92	4.07	4.00	-	-	4.00	90.9
Orange II	$C_{16}H_{11}O_4N_2SNa$	1.5	1.5	1.5	-	-	1.5	1.48	1.51	1.41	-	-	1.47	98.0
		3.0	2.9	2.9	-	-	2.9	2.93	2.81	2.77	-	-	2.84	97.9

Sakamoto and Miyasaka (1987); Courtesy, *Ultrapure Water* journal

Table 6-15 (cont.) TOC Determination of Various Organic Compounds

Organic Compound	*Chemical Formula*	*TOC by Combustion Infrared Oxidation (mg C/L)* 1	2	3	4	5	Av	*TOC by Persulfate UV Oxidation (mg C/L)* 1	2	3	4	5	Av	*Average Rate of Oxidation* (%)
Decyl sodium sulfate	$C_{10}H_{21}O_4SNa$	2.1	2.1	-	-	-	2.1	2.03	2.04	-	-	-	2.03	96.7
		4.0	3.9	-	-	-	4.0	3.89	3.84	-	-	-	3.87	96.8
				(2.2)						(1.83)				(83.2)
Dodeyl sodium sulfate	$C_{12}H_{25}O_4SNa$	2.0	2.0	-	-	-	2.0	2.01	2.06	-	-	-	2.04	102
		4.0	3.9	-	-	-	4.0	3.97	3.92	-	-	-	3.95	98.8
				(2.0)						(1.34)				(67.0)
Tetradecyl sodium sulfate	$C_{14}H_{29}O_4SNa$	2.0	2.1	-	-	-	2.1	2.04	2.00	-	-	-	2.02	96.2
		3.8	4.0	-	-	-	3.9	3.90	3.85	-	-	-	3.88	99.5
				(2.1)						(0.84)				(40.0)
Ethane sodium sulfonate	$C_2H_5O_3SNa$	1.9	1.9	-	-	-	1.9	2.00	1.96	-	-	-	1.98	104
		3.6	3.6	-	-	-	3.6	3.79	3.80	-	-	-	3.80	106
				(3.7)						(3.60)				(97.3)
1-Butane sodium sulfonate	$C_4H_9O_3SNa$	2.0	2.0	-	-	-	2.0	2.04	2.05	-	-	-	2.05	103
		3.7	3.7	-	-	-	3.7	3.97	3.95	-	-	-	3.96	107
				(3.7)						(3.59)				(97.0)
1-Hexane sodium sulfonate	$C_6H_{13}O_3SNa$	1.7	1.8	-	-	-	1.8	1.98	1.94	-	-	-	1.96	109
		3.4	3.2	-	-	-	3.3	3.74	3.68	-	-	-	3.71	112
				(3.4)						(3.25)				(95.6)
1-Octane sodium sulfonate	$C_8H_{17}O_3SNa$	2.0	1.8	-	-	-	1.9	2.01	2.02	-	-	-	2.02	106
		3.6	3.9	-	-	-	3.8	3.86	3.84	-	-	-	3.85	101
				(3.9)						(3.62)				(92.8)
1-Decane sodium sulfonate	$C_{10}H_2O_3SNa$	1.9	1.8	-	-	-	1.9	2.03	2.04	-	-	-	2.04	107
		3.7	3.5	-	-	-	3.6	3.90	3.89	-	-	-	3.90	108
				(3.8)						(3.54)				(93.2)
Dodecyl benzene sodium sulfonate	$C_{18}H_{29}O_3SNa$	1.9	1.9	-	-	-	1.9	1.92	2.15	-	-	-	2.04	107
		3.7	3.7	-	-	-	3.7	3.75	3.71	-	-	-	3.73	101
				(-)						(not measurable)				(-)
Peptone	-	2.5	2.2	2.3	-	-	2.2	1.99	2.04	2.03	-	-	2.02	91.8
		4.3	4.3	4.2	-	-	4.3	3.99	4.07	4.03	-	-	4.03	93.7
Humic Acid	-	2.7	2.6	-	-	-	2.7	0.75	-	-	-	-	0.75	27.8
		4.9	4.9	-	-	-	4.9	1.45	-	-	-	-	1.45	29.6
		4.6	4.3	4.5	-	-	4.5	2.41	2.33	2.20	-	-	2.31	51.3
Fulvic acid	-	3.5	3.0	3.2	3.3	3.2	3.2	1.86	1.68	1.69	1.72	1.60	1.71	53.4
		5.8	5.3	5.5	5.3	5.1	5.4	3.30	2.98	2.99	3.02	3.13	3.08	57.0

Sakamoto and Miyasaka (1987); Courtesy, *Ultrapure Water* journal

Industrial Standards. Additionally, wet chemistry analyzers permit continuous on-line measurements to be made. Such instruments are limited, however, by the completeness with which the particular wet chemical oxidation can affect the specific organic compounds being dealt with.

The Japanese investigators compared one instrument based upon combustion of organic compounds at 950 °C over cobalt oxide catalyst, with another that utilized persulfate UV irradiation to convert the organics into carbon dioxide. In both methods the carbon dioxide was quantified by NDIR. Numerous organic compounds were subjected to these comparative TOC analyses. Some examples of the findings of Sakamoto and Miyasaka (1987) are shown in Table 6-15. It can be seen that the different organic compounds were oxidized with various degrees of efficiencies, as measured by rates of oxidation. Thus acetone was oxidized 100%; alcohols, on the order of 95%; and 2,4,6-tri(2-pyridyl)-1,3,5 triazine, about 85%.

Moreover, the results obtained from the two different TOC analyzers differed, particularly where humic and fulvic acids were involved. The wet-chemistry persulfate/UV method gave lower results than did the combustion method. Sakamoto and Miyasaka (1987) concluded that the TOC instrument based upon persulfate/UV irradiation is relatively unsuitable for determining the TOC in natural waters.

The TOC analyzers are especially valuable in indicating trends and in discerning comparative levels of organic contamination. Baffi et al. (1991) found TOC analysis a suitable tool for validating the cleansing procedures designed to remove residual biotechnology products at various stages of a manufacturing process. Traditionally, enzyme-linked immunosorbent assays (ELISA) and Lowery protein assays have been used for this purpose, and TOC analyses are found to be highly complementary. The detection limit approximates 0.1 ppm. Its quantitation limit is 0.5 ppm. Baffi et al. stated the TOC accuracy to be 50% to 70% or greater in the 0.5- to 1.0-ppm range, while its variability was only about 5%.

As discussed in Chapter 2, page 75, studies may have established a direct correlation between organism counts and TOC levels (Dawson et al., 1988). Such a correlation might conceivably be expected to exist for waters that are highly purified except for their organism contents.

Oxygen Removal in Pharmaceuticals.

In the pharmaceutical production and utilization of high-purity water, the presence of oxygen is generally of minor concern. It is understood that it may favor proliferation of aerobic organisms, and may promote the oxidative degradation of organics, such as polypropylene and ion-exchange resins, particularly when catalyzed by near-ultraviolet light and/or heat. Such concerns are not of great practical moment, however. They are easily accommodated within normal high-purity water production practices, and seldom call for specific efforts at oxygen removal.

The adverse effects of oxygen on the stability of drug formulations are comprehended. Where necessary, these formulations have been stabilized by the use of antioxidants and the displacement of air by an inert atmosphere such as nitrogen (De Rudder et al., 1989). Charge-modified microporous membranes,

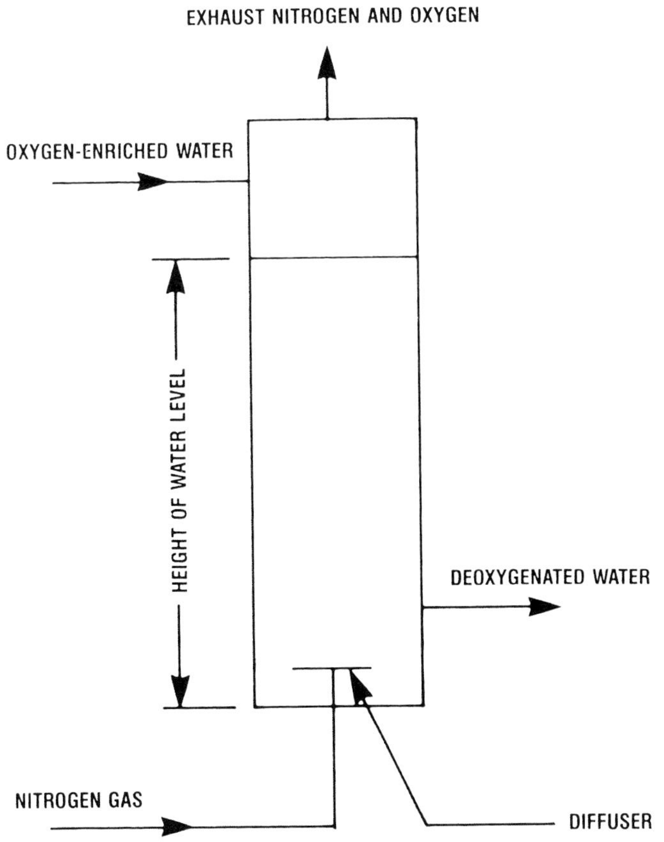

Figure 6-5. Schematic of a nitrogen gas purging system for DI-water deoxygenation.
Sinha (1991); Courtesy, *Microcontamination*

polyamides bearing quaternary amine groups, had their charge functionality destroyed by oxygen at 30 °C. The exposure time was not stipulated. Oxygen could be removed from the system by use of a two-stage vacuum degasifier.

The corrosive effects of oxygen on the surfaces of stills at the high temperatures of distillation can be avoided by the removal of this gas from the water. Deaeration is one means. Both vacuum deaerators and those involving the use of steam are available. The devices employing steam to break the liquid water into spray, followed by a sweep through the thin aqueous spray or film, are the more effective. By such means the oxygen content of the water can be brought to its bounds of analytical detectability, some 0.005 mL per liter (Strauss, 1973; Cotton, 1980). Chemical scavenging of oxygen, such as by sodium sulfite and sodium bisulfite, can be used in conjunction with deaeration. Usually, however, oxygen removal is not too important in water purification for pharmaceutical purposes. It is of greater significance in the power generation field.

Zoccolante (1987) stated that the use of vacuum degasification can reduce oxygen to 0.1 ppm, while simultaneously removing carbon dioxide. He cited as an alternative the use of a palladium-doped ion-exchange resin through which the oxygen-bearing water is flowed. Hydrogen gas is added. The palladium oxide catalyst combines the hydrogen and oxygen into water, removing both. The oxygen is removed to less than 0.1 ppm by this method. It has the added advantages of requiring only minimal energy and very little floor space. Oxygen removal is of great concern in the semiconductor field. The method used in this connection may be of interest to pharmaceutical processors.

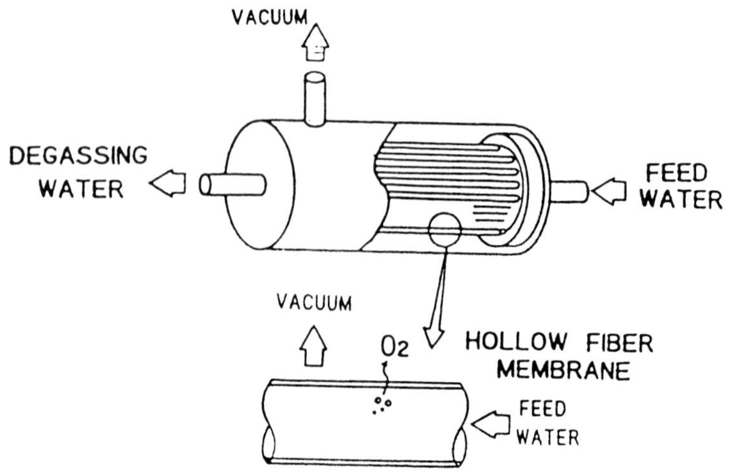

Figure 6-6. Module of membrane degasser.
Imaoka et al. (1991); Courtesy, Semiconductor Pure Water Conference

Sato et al. (1991) advanced two methods for minimizing the concentration of oxygen dissolved in water; a nitrogen gas bubbling method, and a membrane degassing method. In the former, nitrogen gas, in the form of fine bubbles, is sparged into the water. In keeping with Henry's law, the dissolved oxygen adjusts its concentration downwards to accord with its lower partial pressure in the nitrogen atmosphere now overlying the water. The principle of using gas to remove a different gas dissolved in a liquid is time-honored in its successful application.

Nitrogen may be forthcoming from cryogenic sources. Alternatively, a source of pure nitrogen gas under pressure may be used. One of two techniques is generally involved. A constant flow of nitrogen is supplied to the storage tank and then out by the way of a vent filter. This method may not be sufficient if a large rate of water withdrawal should suddenly exceed the rate of nitrogen flow. A balanced-pressure method seems generally more satisfactory. It involves the maintenance of a small positive pressure of nitrogen in the headspace above the stored water. A nitrogen pressure of from 2 to 10 inches of water is usually employed. During tank discharge, the inflow of nitrogen gas is controlled to equal the egress of water from the storage tank (Sinha, 1991).

In the membrane degassing method, a membrane that is hydrophobic and is hence not permeable to liquid water transmission separates the water containing the dissolved oxygen from a vacuum source. A suitable membrane may be composed of PTFE, or of silicone gum rubbers that are known to be amenable to oxygen permeation. The imposition of the vacuum tends to aspirate dissolved

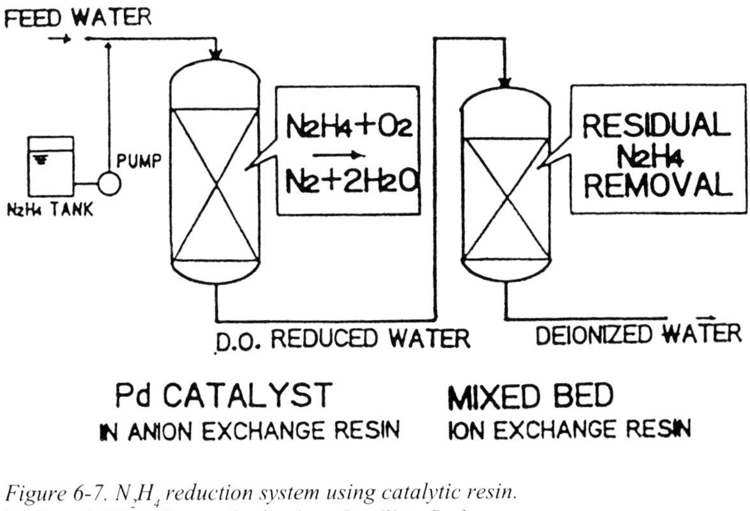

Figure 6-7. N_2H_4 reduction system using catalytic resin.
Imaoka et al. (1991); Courtesy, Semiconductor Pure Water Conference.

oxygen from the water. Obviously, the rate of oxygen removal mirrors the gas permeation constant of the film barrier, reflects directly its area, and expresses the concentration of the gas in the water, the process being concentration-gradient driven.

Sinha (1991) advocated the deoxygenation of water by the sweep of a nitrogen gas stream, as shown in Figure 6-4. According to Sinha, in most DI water systems a nitrogen blanket is used to overlie the contents of the water storage vessels. The concern is with the effects of carbon dioxide upon the pH of the water, and the contamination by impurities such as organisms, and hydrocarbons. commonly present in the air.

Sato et al. (1991) advised that the use of membrane degassing to reduce the dissolved oxygen concentration to 500 ppb, followed by nitrogen gas sparging, gives superior results. Dissolved oxygen can be reduced to 5 ppb using the protocol and the equipment described by Sato and his collaborators (1991).

Two different methods were used by Imaoka et al. (1991). In each, the oxygen concentration, usually at 9 ppm, was reduced by vacuum degasification, the high-purity water being purified as it passed in an evacuated chamber through hollow fibers amenable to oxygen permeation. At 50 torr, the dissolved oxygen content of the water was reduced to between 300 and 400 ppb. Each of two different methods characterized the second stages of the two different oxygen-removal methods. In one, palladium deposited upon the surface of anion-exchange resin beads catalyzed the combination of the remaining oxygen with hydrazine. In the other, hydrogen was used in place of the hydrazine. The use of the catalyzed oxidation/reduction with either hydrogen or hydrazine to remove oxygen has long been employed in the power industry. These two-stage oxygen-removal methods reduced the dissolved oxygen levels to 5 ppb (Figures 6-5 and 6-6).

Imaoka et al. (1991) also referenced the nitrogen-sparging technique as reducing the dissolved oxygen concentration to 10 ppb or less, depending upon the number of spraying towers used (i.e., upon the thoroughness of the nitrogen sparging). The oxygen-removal devices were coupled with more conventional purification units to produce high-purity waters with total residue levels, including TOC and silica, of 1 ppb or less. This level of purity approaches the limits of detection for all analyzers.

Oxygen Removal by palladium-catalyzed hydrogen. Techniques for the removal of oxygen from water may usefully be forthcoming from the power generating industry. Oxygen is removed by a palladium-catalyzed combination with hydrogen. For this process, hydrogen from storage cylinders is fed into oxygen-containing waters that encounter palladium-doped, anion-exchange resins. The two dissolved gases combine stoichiometrically to produce water. The resin vessel is a typical rubber-lined, carbon steel ion-exchange tank. In one case it held some 50 ft^3 of resin and had a 100% freeboard for backwash expansions (Sloane and Hernon, 1990). The dissolution of hydrogen is the rate-limiting step. Usually used is a static in-line mixer wherein the hydrogen gas is dispersed by way of a 0.2-µm-rated porous sparger. Undissolved hydrogen enters the resin vessel, to be bled into a forced-air purge tank. This prevents hydrogen buildup and its associated dangers.

The amount of hydrogen injected is based on an algorithm that considers four factors: the oxygen level influent and effluent, the resin bed, the resin-bed effluent hydrogen level, and the water flowrate. The hydrogen feed is varied in direct proportion to the water flow and its oxygen content. It was found that at water flowrates of under 120 gpm, less than 50% of the hydrogen was dissolved. At double that rate, 90% to 95% was dissolved; and at 360-gpm flows, 100% entered solutions (Sloane and Hernon, 1990). The attaining of complete deoxygenation to 1 ppb levels required flows of 240 and 360 gpm. A satisfactory high flowrate through the mixer also achieved with consistency the desired deoxygenation limits of less than 1 ppb.

The safety of the hydrogen chemistry operation is ensured by appropriate use of interlocking switches, automatic relief valves, pressure switches, and external hydrogen pressure relief valves within the general fail/safe design (Sloane and Hernon, 1990).

Ammonia

Ammonia (NH_3) is a natural product of the decay of organic nitrogen compounds. As part of the nitrogen cycle, it is influenced by biological activity and is a transient consitutent in water supplies. Proteinacious material, whether of plant or animal origin, return to the environment as waste products or through decay partly in the form of ammonia. Such biological processes occur also in sewage treatment plants. Therefore, ammonia is a common consituent of sewage plant effluents; to concentrations usually of 10 to 20 mg/L (Nalco, 1988).

Surface waters also acquire ammonia through the decomposition of agricultural runoff containing fertilizers and animal wastes, as from farms and feedlots. The ammonia from such origins may find its way into underground aquifers.

Ammonia is often added to chlorinated waters in water treatment plants in order to convert the free chlorine into the chloramines (page 52) that are less productive of objectionable trihalomethanes through the oxidation of organic molecules, TOC. The removal of chloramines from water supplies by breakpoint chlorination and adsorption to activated carbon may generate ammonia (Komorita and Snoeyink, 1985):

$$NH_2Cl + H_2O + C \dashrightarrow NH_3 + H^+ + Cl^- + C_{oxidized} \qquad \text{Eq. 6-5}$$

Ammonia, normally a gas at room temperatures, is extremely soluble in water because of its high propensity for hydrogen bonding. The form in which it exists in aqueous media depends upon the pH of the solution. By itself, ammonia is the base anhydride of ammonium hydroxide:

$$NH_3 + H_2O \text{ ----> } NH_4^+ + OH^- \qquad \text{Eq. 6-6}$$

Additionally, it is highly likely that free ammonia is present in waters to which it was added in order to transform chlorine into chloramine. Such additions are almost unavoidably excessive.

This dissociative equilibrium accounts for the high pH of ammonia solutions. In the presence of neutralizing pHs, ammonia exists as the ammonium ion (NH_4^+). In the form of its ammonium ion it can be removed from the water by cation-exchange resins. Ammonium compounds may also result from the thermal decomposition of the quaternary ammonium radical of strong anion-exchange resin. Despite its volatility, ammonia, because of its high solubility, can only incompletely be removed from water by degasification. For the same reason its distillative separation from water is not completely possible. It should, therefore, be absent from feedwaters intended for stills lest high- conductivity product waters result.

Disi (1995) stated that 1 ppm of ammonia causes a reduction of 8 microsiemens (μS) in the resisitivity of water. Therefore, its presence in amounts permitted by the USP chemical tests, namely, 0.1 mg/L, may nevertheless be too high to pass the new conductivity tests.■

CHAPTER 7

PRETREATMENT OF WATERS

CHLORINATION, MULTIMEDIA FILTRATION, SOFTENING, DEGASIFICATION, AND CARBON BEDS

The preparation of water of the qualities required for application in the power-generating industry, for semiconductor rinsewaters, or for pharmaceutical purposes is generally divided into three stages: pretreatment, a principal purification, and polishing or point-of-use treatment.

The principal purification is generally one of or a combination of the following: ion exchange, reverse osmosis, and distillation. To render the principal purification process practical (*practical* being defined usually in economic terms), pretreatment of the source water is almost always required. It is this pretreatment that makes realistic the service life and performance of the principal purification steps. Otherwise the achievements of ion exchangers may be lessened by prematurely abbreviated service lives; RO units may operate substandardly, at excessive costs; and stills may corrode or become dysfunctional. The purpose of the polishing or point-of-use purification stage is to preserve the quality of the water as prepared in the principal purification step over the time interval prior to its actual use; and, if possible, to bring it to the peak of its quality by a final refining treatment at its point or time of use.

Each of the three purification stages is necessary to ensure the final quality of the high-purity water (although "high purity" is a term little used in the pharmaceutical industry). An inadequate pretreatment inevitably results in an uneconomical process, however, and may actually frustrate the ultimate achievement of the desired quality of the production water.

Certain objectives sought in the pretreatment phase, such as the removal of colloidal and organic materials, are also the goals of the subsequent polishing activities wherein regulatory or state-of-the-art purity levels are intended for already highly purified waters. The refinements of the polishing activities can differ markedly from the pretreatment steps even though similar types of activities may be involved. Thus fine filtrations, such as may be obtained from membrane devices, may be used in water polishing. They could be inappropriately costly, however, in pretreatment contexts where more extensive particulate burdens are more economically accommodated by deep-bed filtrations. Similarly, ozone may be used in pretreatment efforts to reduce or eliminate organic matter. It may also be employed, but differently, for the same purpose in a polishing mode.

Pretreatments generally deal with higher levels and quantities of impurities; polishing activities are more concerned with accomplishing subtle but significant refinements. The distinction deserves recognition. Chapman et al. (1983, Part IIa) define pretreatment as encompassing all measures taken to improve the quality of the water entering the plant (as from a municipal treatment facility), through its final deionization. Posttreatment or polishing includes all measures designed to improve the quality of the water after its final deionization and before its use.

As the *U.S. Pharmacopoeia* (1995) stipulates, and as the Food and Drug Administration therefore requires, pharmaceutical waters for compendial purposes must derive from sources suitable in their quality for drinking water. Where a water agency has converted raw waters into potable waters by conventional procedures, or where natural waters reflect drinking water quality, the pharmaceutical manufacturer may utilize them to prepare compendial waters. To do this there will be invoked such primary treatments as ion exchange, RO, and/or distillation, possibly in concert with electrodeionization, electrodialysis, and/or ultrafiltration adjuncts. Before these primary purification methods can be applied, however, the water may first require further pretreatment, for the exercises performed to achieve compliance with EPA regulations will not be rigorous enough to prepare a water for, say, distillation.

In any case, pharmaceutical processors who do not rely upon potable water sources will first have to perform a purification operation to produce potable-quality water.

The origin of the raw water is generally from either surface sources (lakes, ponds, rivers, and reservoirs) or ground sources (wells and aquifers). Surface waters originate essentially as rainwater that gathers as runoff. Consequently they are usually soft but with high total suspended solids. Groundwaters tend to be distinctly different, as they are much more likely to be hard (albeit with lower TDS levels). Analytical characterizations of these differing sources are required in order to know which of the radically different pretreatment strategies are needed.

Each of the pretreatment operations will be examined in detail, in terms of aims, procedures, and limitations. It may not be amiss, however, to consider a broad overview of what may constitute the pretreatment regimen in a given situation.

The water pretreatment train generally, but not invariably, consists of:

Raw water —> chlorination —> iron and manganese removal —> coagulation and settling —> deep-bed filtration —> water softening —> activated carbon treatment.

In the pretreatment regimen to prepare a water for primary purification processes, the organism population is reduced to acceptable levels and microbiological management is assured by the early addition of a biostat/biocide, usually chlorine.

The water is chlorinated as soon as possible, often at the wellhead, to control the microbiological growth. Where municipal water supplies are used, these have usually already been chlorinated. Nevertheless, it is not uncommon to add more chlorine to bring the water up to the plant's stipulated chlorine level. Total reliance regarding chlorination is not placed upon the municipality's performance.

Finished, injectable pharmaceutical products are limited by federal regulations from exceeding specific numbers of given-size particles. Large-volume parenterals (those administered in single doses larger than 100 mL, usually in IV infusions) may contain no more than 5 per mL of particles larger than 25 μm, and not more than 50 per mL larger than 10 μm. In addition, they may contain "no visible particles." Small-volume parenterals administered in conjunction with a large-volume parenteral (LVP), in doses up to 100 mL, may contain only up to one fifth of these numbers per dose, regardless of volume. An ample medical literature has attested to the health threat posed by particles even smaller than those stipulated (Plumer, 1970; Turco, 1981; DeLuca, 1983).

The incoming water often needs to be freed of its suspended solids. Table 7-1 illustrates the findings of Goozner and Gotlinsky (1990) regarding the silt density index values of certain source waters.

Deep beds of sand or of multimedia are used to remove particulate matter

Table 7-1
SDI Values for Raw Water in Various Locations

City	*Water Source*	*SDI*
Albuquerque, NM	Deep wells	3-5
Lubbock, TX	Lake Meredith	6-20
Dallas, TX	Mixed well/ reservoir/river	6-20
Juarez, Mexico	Wells	4
Long Island, NY	Deep well	1-2
Milton Keynes, England		>20
Central Indiana	Mixed well/reservoir/creek	5
San Diego, CA	Reservoir	13
Suburban Los Angeles	Colorado Delta/California Reservoir	>20
Suburban Boston, MA	City	3
Santa Clara, CA	City	3
Portland, OR	City	14
Seattle, WA	City	18

Goozner and Gotlinsky (1990); Courtesy Ultrapure Water Journal.

(suspended solids) from the incoming feedwaters. This is intended for coarse particles of from between 30 and 7 µm in size. Particle types, sizes, amounts, and the temperature and flowrate of the water affect the filter efficiency.

Water softening is intended to remove mostly the scale-forming alkaline earth, divalent ions; although other interfering metallic ions such as iron, manganese, and aluminum may be removed as well. The reliance is upon cation-exchange resins in the sodium form. An exchange is made; the objectionable bivalent ions are removed from the water, to be replaced by sodium ions. The TDS contents of the water remain unchanged.

Carbon beds may follow. They are very effective in chlorine removal, less so in organic removal. They may require frequent replacement. Their chief problem is that they usually endow their effluent waters with high organism and endotoxin contents. For this reason chlorine is often removed instead by the chemical injection of reducing agents such as sodium bisulfite; and organics are removed by the action of macroreticulated anion-exchange resins in their chloride form.

Finally, cartridge filters in the form of nominally rated depth-type filters, microporous membrane filters, or even ultrafilters are used to protect ion-exchange beds, RO units, and stills from incompletely removed or newly introduced microorganisms; and from particles sloughed off from deep beds and even from ion-exchange columns.

Schematic of water pretreatment facilities (Figures 7-1 to 7-3) to produce water intended for pharmaceutical purposes were given in a report by the Deionized Water Committee of the Pharmaceutical Manufacturers Association. (Chapman et al., 1983, Part II). Its treatment steps parallel those that would be used in the pretreatment of water designed for the semiconductor or power industry as well:

The raw water is passed through an activated carbon filter to remove chlorine and organic adsorbents; and then through a water softener to remove calcium, magnesium, and other cations that cause water hardness. The softened water is then deionized by passage through ion-exchange resin beds, of two-bed and/or mixed-bed configuration.

It is possible to disagree with the specifics of this pretreatment outline. For instance, it may be better to soften the water before removing the chlorine. However, it is in the very nature of water treatment that alternate modes of practice may be considered and implemented. There is room for technical disagreements and different viewpoints.

Chlorine Treatment

Most often, chlorine is added to a water supply until a residual concentration of 0.5 to 2 ppm is achieved. Muraca et al. (1990), whose focus was the biocidal removal of *Legionella pneumophila*, referred to chlorine residuals of 2 to 6 ppm.

L. pneumophila, relatively resistant to chlorine, required chlorine concentrations greater than 3 ppm to be inactivated and suppressed. Chlorine concentrations in potable water supplies are generally below 1.0 ppm. Chlorine being a strong oxidizer, some of the initially added chlorine becomes consumed in destroying oxidation-susceptible molecules. On occasion, therefore, an initial chlorine quantity of 50 ppm is added as a shock pretreatment. The large quantity added provides for a chlorine residue after the loss of chlorine through chemical reaction, as with ferrous or manganous ions, or by the oxidation of labile organic molecules. Stable residuals of chlorine may be difficult to establish initially. The levels may fluctuate because of variations in incoming water quality, flowrates, consumption by oxidizable impurities, or interaction with indigenous biofilms (Muraca et al., 1990). Therefore, the chlorine concentration is sometimes added, beyond an existing residue. The practice is referred to as hyperchlorination.

Chlorine is generally added to the waters directly as a gas from storage cylinders, where it is contained under pressure. Naturally, suitable precautions and controls figure in the handling of this toxic element. Gaseous chlorine addition is used principally in larger installations. Smaller chlorinators rely upon "active" chlorine as derived from liquid sodium hypochlorite solutions (household bleach), metered by a chemical pump into the water, or batch-fed periodically (Cruver, 1990). The use of the liquid hypochlorite solutions avoids the capital costs and hazards associated with chlorine gas storage and handling. It is enabled by the more modest flowrates and water usages of the smaller systems.

Carmody and Martyak (1989), in dealing with an IBM high-purity water system, utilized sodium hypochlorite as their source of chlorine. Even-smaller water systems may rely upon the periodic addition of calcium hypochlorite pellets.

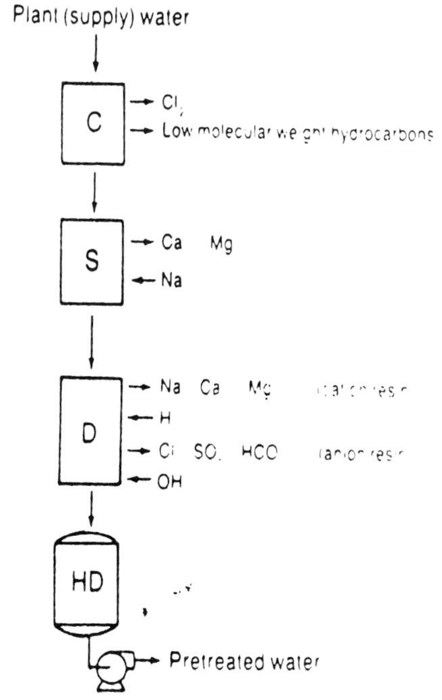

Figure 7-1. A basic pretreatment system (C = carbon filters, S = softener, D = deionizer, and HD = holding (distribution).
Chapman et al. (1983 Part II);
Courtesy, *Pharmaceutical Technology*

The reason chlorine gas and hypochlorite solutions are identical in their actions is because chlorine dissolves in water to give hypochlorite ions.

$$Cl_2 + H_2O \longrightarrow HOCl + H^+ + Cl^-$$

$$HOCl \longrightarrow H^+ + OCl^- \qquad \text{Eq. 7-1}$$

The amount of hypochlorous acid (HOCl) and hypochlorite ions (OCl^-) present depends upon the pH, as Cruver (1990) showed in Table 7-2. The higher the pH, the greater the degree of HOCl dissociation into OCl^-. Cruver (1990) stated that HOCl is 100 times more powerful an oxidant and disinfectant than is the hypochlorite ion. The concentration of hypochlorous acid is higher at low pHs, its dissociation being suppressed by high hydrogen ion concentrations.

The pK_a at 25 °C for hypochlorous acid, the point where it exists half in undissociated form and half as H^+ and OCl^- ions, is at 7.4, as stated on page 108. The significance of the pK_a finds practical expression in application (Beckwith and Moser, 1933; Conley and Puzig, 1987; Sergent, 1986).

Chlorine combines readily with the nitrogen in cellular proteins. Gross cell changes caused by this chloramination of cell protein renders chlorine toxic to all living systems.

Iodine, like chlorine, is a halogen and as such exerts a biocidal/biostatic influence. It is, however, not so powerful an oxidizer. It has not been implicated in trihalomethane formation, and does not require carbon adsorption or chemical reductive reactions for its neutralization, although it can be neutralized by sodium bisulfite or removed by ion-exchange (see page 387). It can be removed from waters by volatilization, as during distillation processes. In one case, microbial counts in an RO permeate tank were 100 to 300 cfu/mL. An injection of iodine in liquid form was made in the return loop to the permeate tank to provide a concentration of 0.3 to 0.56 mg/L. Microbial counts were reduced to fewer than 0.2 cfu/mL. The iodine was removed from the RO permeate without further effort when the water was ultimately distilled. The distilled water contained no detectable organisms (Nyakanen and Cutler, 1990).

The presence of the chlorine residual is usually retained as long as possible within the water stream as it undergoes processing, in order to provide a bacteriostatic umbrella against ever-present threats of microbial recontamination.

Water that has been chlorinated to control the microbiological growth is next generally treated to get rid of its suspended solids. Coagulation and flocculation, already discussed in Chapter 6, may be indicated. Whether so or not, the feedwater is usually subjected to deep-bed filtration.

Deep-Bed Filtration

Sand bed filters are used to remove total suspended solids in the preparation of potable water. When this water flows into a plant for processing, it may yet contain suspended solids as revealed by its silt density index. The same may be the case for non-municipally treated feedwaters. Deep-bed filtration, or media filtration, as it sometimes is called, is employed to remove or at least significantly reduce the TSS.

What is required of the deep-bed filter is that it must prevent passage of the suspended matter; be capable of accommodating a reasonable volume of suspended material; and hold the retained solids so loosely as to be amenable to easy cleansing by backwashing.

The deep-bed filters are contained within a steel pressure vessel coated to withstand the corrosive effects of water and to resist the abrasions of the sand (or

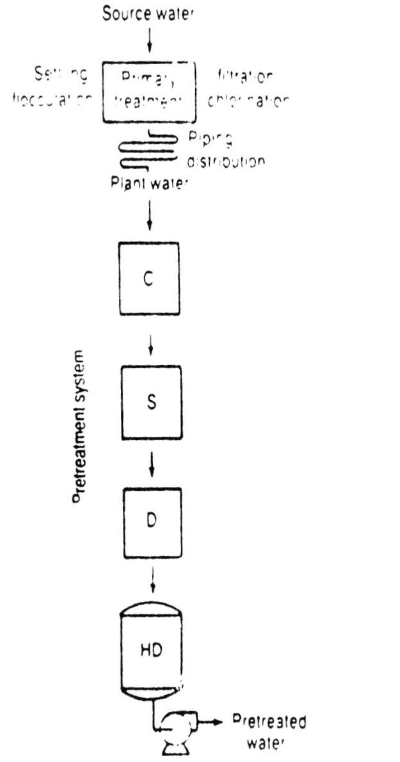

Figure 7-2. Typical primary treatment plus pretreatment.
Chapman et al. (1983, Part II);
Courtesy, *Pharmaceutical Technology*

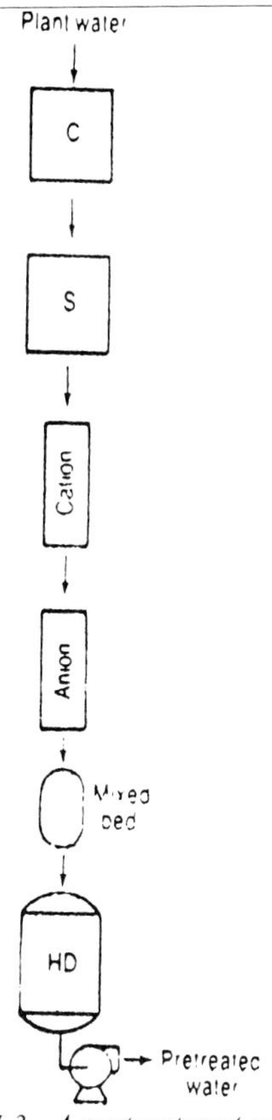

Figure 7-3. A pretreatment system with a combined two-bed/mixed-bed scheme.
Chapman et al. (1983 part II);
Courtesy, *Pharmaceutical Technology*

other) particles that constitute the bed. The coating is usually of PVC or of epoxy. The sand overlies a bed of gravel, usually consisting of several layers of different sizes, above a water distributor/collector.

Deep-bed filters may themselves serve as havens where organisms can proliferate. For this reason also the water is chlorinated before it enters the deep beds. This practice serves to keep the beds sanitized. A superchlorination treatment is often invoked (e.g., 5 ppm for 30 to 40 minutes, or 10 ppm for 15 to 20 minutes. Recirculation through the sand beds, as through other deep beds, is sometimes used to discourage planktonic organism growth. This should not be done with waters that have been dechlorinated.

Chlorine added automatically to water on demand may alter the pH to lower levels, thereupon resolubilizing the aluminum hydroxide floc. This may prove to be a cause of RO membrane fouling, and should be guarded against by careful control and adjustment of the pH.

Three common types of media are generally used in the construction of deep beds, and are controlled in their variation by two screen analysis tests. The effective size (ES) is the mesh size of a screen that accumulates 90% of the sample. The size of screen mesh that retains 40% is also measured. The uniformity coefficient (UC) is the size of that mesh divided by the ES (Allen, 1975).

The ES and UC relationships for anthracite (density 1.5), silica sand (density 2.5), and calcium carbonate (density 2.7 to 2.95), are as follows:

1. Fine sand of an effective size of about 0.4 to 0.64 mm and a uniformity coefficient of 0.64/0.4 or 1.6 (meaning that 10% of the sand is finer than 0.4 mm and 60% is finer than 0.6 mm).
2. Fine anthracite (No. 1) of ES 0.65 to 0.8 mm and UC of 1.85.
3. Calcium carbonate of ES 0.5 (0.4 to 0.7 mm) and UC of 2.

Calcium carbonate beds are sometimes used in home water purification, but not in centralized treatment plants. The intention in home systems is not that of deep-bed filtration but to neutralize waters of low pH in order to minimize the corrosive effects upon plumbing and heating systems. That purpose is usually served in centralized water treatment plants by lime or slaked lime. Obviously, this usage adds calcium ions to the water. The practice is therefore avoided where this would be of concern.

Garnet or illminite, density 3.5 to 4.5 (average 3.8), is also used, particularly in multibed constructions. The sand used has a density of 2.5; and the bituminous coal, 1.5 to 1.8.

Interestingly, diatomaceous earth cannot be used. It is rapidly blinded by alum floc.

Anthracite is generally used where silica could be leached and would be found objectionable. Deep-bed filters of anthracite offer the additional advantages of extended filter runs, therefore requiring less backwashing; and the possibilities of higher filtration rates. The reasons are that the anthracite particles are more sharply angular, producing larger voids than does the sand, with higher dirt-holding capacities for certain types of suspended particles.

Anthracite beds are used to remove 40-μm particles such as are visibly present in runoffs.

Silica sand is the commonly used medium for constructing deep-bed filters (Ogedengbe, 1984). Such beds have nominal porosities of about 10 to 40 μm. New beds tend to have the lower porosities. While relatively cheap and effective, such beds can leach silica in situations characterized by high heats and alkalinities.

Sand, because of its relatively high specific gravity, can be backwashed at higher rates of flow than can crushed anthracite with only one half of the sand's bulk density. Comparable flowrates would carry off too much of the anthracite.

Such beds, some 30 inches in depth, trap the particulate matter within only a relatively thin layer, to a depth of about 6 inches. The remainder of the depth of the bed moderates the rate of water permeation through it. The flow volumes attained at the moderated rate of flow derive from the extent of bed surface.

The size of the grains determines the packing density. That and the depth of the bed define the velocity of the water being filtered. Coarse-grained filters, making for larger intergranular spaces (the filter pores), must be used in deeper beds than are those of finer grains in order to yield the same rate of flow. In turn, the coarser grains require a greater backwash velocity to lift the particles for proper cleansing. An American Water Works Association (1969) publication on wastewater plant design treats fully on the subject of deep-bed design.

In the construction of deep beds, two considerations apply: the permeation of the water downward, and the passage of water upward during backwash. What is desired, ideally, is to prevent any floc from passing through the bed, but for the

Table 7-2
Effect of pH on Dissociation of Hypochlorous Acid at 30 °C (86 °F)

pH	*%HOCl*	*%OCl⁻*
5.0	99.7	0.3
6.0	96.9	3.1
7.0	75.9	24.1
7.2	66.5	33.5
7.4	55.6	44.4
7.6	44.2	55.8
8.0	23.7	76.3
9.0	3.0	97.0

Cruver (1990); Courtesy, Membrane Planning and Technology Conference floc to be held as loosely as possible to permit easy release upon backwashing. The floc is trapped almost completely at or near the bed's surface. The extent of the floc penetration should be checked by tests of the water passed through pilot filters of various depths. The depth of the bed serves chiefly to moderate the downward velocity of the water. The bed's performance is, therefore, described in terms of its face area (i.e., in square feet) rather than in terms of its cubic foot contents. (This holds also for the active carbon beds shortly to be discussed.) Gravel beds are often used as support and to keep the granular media out of the underdrains.

Slow sand beds, formerly widely used, flow at rates of under 2 to 3 gpm/ft^2. Presumably, they retain particles by a sieving action, being tightly packed. They require being backwashed after 24 to 48 hours. Slow sand beds could cover 2 to 3 acres. At flows of 0.2 gpm/ft^2, miles of such filter fields are needed to accommodate the "Schmutzdecke," the slimy layer of organisms that accumulates on top of the sand bed.

Rapid sand filters, less prodigal of land use, yield permeation rates of 4 to 16 gpm/ft^2. They require backwashes after 4 to 6 hours. They are reputed to better retain the alum floc, presumably through particle adsorption as well as sieving, down to 1 ppm of turbidity. Flows are usually at 4 to 6 gpm/ft^2.

The more rapid filtration is the result of utilizing coarser sand granules in conjunction with pump pressures rather than gravity. A less clear water results because they are not so effective as the slow beds. They may require the upgrading conferred by polymeric coagulants (Purchas, 1981).

Sand beds pre-RO would require flows of about 1 gpm/ft^2. Actual flows will very much depend upon the silt density index of the water. Very small suspended particles could require coagulation by polymer addition prior to entering the multimedia bed. Reductions of SDI can thus be effected, from 15 to 20 down to an SDI of 2 to 3. Only 30-second retention times may be needed, but polymer enhancement is most likely at temperatures of 70 to 75 °F (21 to 25 °C). Unfortunately, some polymer may emerge in the effluent waters to create problems downstream. These can involve irreversible combinations with the ion-exchange resins, or very persistent deposits upon RO membranes. The use of cartridge filters may have to be made to remove finer particles when these characterize the SDI. Hango (1990) described an operation involving the use of polymer in conjunction with multimedia beds.

Most RO units require media (deep-bed) filtration down to about 5 μm. Typically, for larger RO units, multimedia filters are used, followed by cartridge filtration to restrain the passage of the multimedia particles from depositing upon the RO. For small ROs, 10 gpm or so, the use of cartridge filters alone may not create an unreasonable expense. Turbidimeters used on-line can be used to measure the effectiveness of the filtrative treatment.

As is shown in Figure 7-4 of single-medium filters, the medium grades itself by hydraulically floating the smallest particles to the top where they form the densest layer. Within its successive depth, the bed becomes increasingly more open; the "pores" are funnel-shaped in principle, with the largest dimension downstream. The bed retains particles only within its top few inches. A particle permeating this top layer may well escape capture altogether. An ideal filter would be of the opposite construction. It would have its largest opening upstream. The spacings among its granules would become progressively smaller throughout the depth of the bed.

Such a bed results from the use of multimedia wherein the lightest is ground the least fine; the densest material, the most fine. Thus, water permeating the anthracite encounters sand, a finer but heavier material below the anthracite. The finer sand packs closer, filtratively retaining particles that were too fine to be removed by the anthracite layer. The water then encounters the even more finely crushed garnet rock. Finer particles yet are removed from the water (Figure 7-5). Such beds can usefully be thought of as being a sand bed given an extended service life by the prefiltrative action of the anthracite layer. The percolating waters emerge to be polished by the finely ground garnet layer.

Actually, multimedia beds can also be constructed solely of sands: of as many as five layers of different sizes of sand, each layer having different retention properties. Sands of different densities are used. Normally, multimedia beds have retentions of 10 μm. Their flowrates are usually about 5 to 10 gpm/ft^2. when serving the critical function of RO pretreatment. The flowrates can be higher, about 8 to 15 gpm/ft^2, in the less critical posture of prefilter for ion-exchange functions.

The use of multimedia beds serves the particle-retaining purpose of slow sand beds without their concomitant restrictions to flow. These beds permit higher flowrates without sacrificing retention. Their acceptable flowrates are about 15 to 20 gpm/ft^2 when ahead of applications such as cooling towers and heat exchangers, where gross particulates are the concern. Vendor catalogues tend to be somewhat optimistic on multimedia flowrates. As prefilters to ion-exchange systems, such filters can run at up to 10 gpm/ft^2. Rates double that are sometimes stated, but at a drop in efficiency. The actual rate to use depends of course upon the specific water supply and its total suspended solids burden. Prefiltrations to reverse osmosis are more critical. On a low-colloid well supply, 10 gpm/ft^2 could be good. On a surface supply with a high TSS, 5 to 8 gpm/ft^2 would be more suitable.

A three-layer bed can be structured of large, least-dense granules of anthracite; medium-size, more-dense sand; and finest-size, most-dense garnet. The chief components of garnet, a rock, are oxides of yttrium, iron, and aluminum (Sinha, 1990). When such a multimedia bed settles down, the most closely packed layer is at the bottom, the least tightly packed is on top. More of the multimedia bed thus serves to retain particles, essentially in three layers. For this reason, multimedia beds have largely replaced sand filters. The use of finely ground garnet alone would cost too much, and its dense packing would occasion high pressure drops and too-frequent backwashing. The deep-bed pretreatment is very important. It influences all the purification treatments and units downstream, and it should not be skimped on.

When the retention of particles so accumulates as to build up a back pressure against water flow through the bed, say 15 psig of differential, the bed is backwashed to a "quicksand" consistency. In the process it becomes expanded, freeing the trapped particulate for removal by the backward liquid flow. The backwash water from such beds is considered sanitary waste, not chemical waste. Its disposal is, therefore, not too onerous. Backwashing is instituted periodically, signaled by the need to reduce the pressure drop (Purchas, 1981) or to rejuvenate the flow. A study of the backwashing of rapid granular media filters was reported by Addicks (1991).

The backwash rate is critical. Consider a pre-RO system where flowrates of 5 gpm/ft^2 are desired. This would require a 24-inch filter for 15 gpm, and the water supply pipe may be sized accordingly. However, backwashing to the quicksand consistency may require 15 gpm/ft^2. The water pipe must therefore be sized to supply at least 45 gpm. Fluidizing the bed is necessary to backwash out the trapped particulates. When the feed source is not equal to the backwash rate, multiple filters may be employed in parallel. This enables the reduction of the diameter of each filter so that the available water can supply the needed backwash rate.

When the backwashing is terminated, the bed settles down and reconstructs itself. The finest particles (garnet) are the heaviest and so settle at the bottom. The lightest (anthracite) gravitate to a position above the grains of intermediate density and size (sand).

Deep beds, particularly those of layered construction, the multimedia beds, are excellent filters capable of trapping substantial quantities of suspended matter. They usually remove particles in the 10- to 40-μm range; some say in the 7- to 12-μm range. They are rejuvenated by back flushing.

In an installation in Virginia, the multimedia beds operate from 2 to 6 gpm/ft^2 of bed surface. They operate for about 50 to 100 hours before the head-pressure loss necessitates backwashing. The backwash operation, which carries off the trapped particulates, takes about 15 minutes.

Adin and Hatukai (1991) offered a model for the optimization of deep-bed filters, to serve as a substitute for the commonly performed empirical pilot plant studies. These investigators indicated that process optimization based upon such performance indicators as run length and volume of water produced per run may contradict economic optimization, even where the finished water qualities are equal. Filtration rate is the main variable influencing the filter costs. Interestingly, Adin and Hatukai (1991) concluded that single-media filters can be as effective as dual- or mixed-media beds in retaining turbidity, and can produce least-cost water. Single media of basalt or tuff produced least-cost water, compared with single or dual media of sand and/or anthracite. The highest volume cost results from the use of sand, anthracite, and granulated carbon.

The construction and devising of depth media beds is still largely empirical in its nature. However, a matrix of scientifically based understanding underlies the artful attempts at new designs.

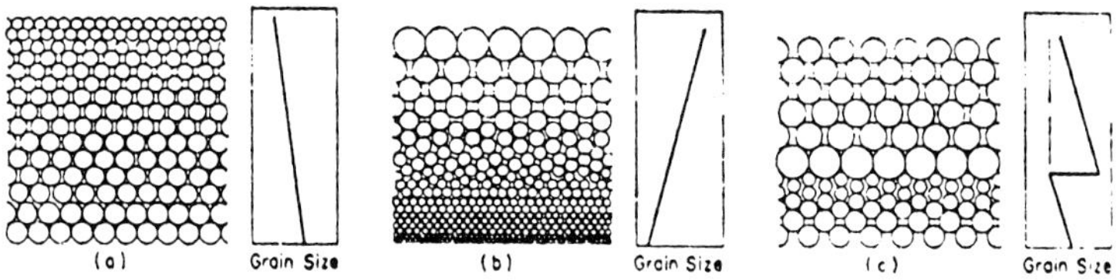

Figure 7-4. Cross sections of representative filter particle gradations. Diagram (a) represents a single-medium bed such as a rapid sand filter. The bottom half of a filter of this type does little or no work. Diagram (b) represents an ideal filter uniformly graded from coarse to fine from top to bottom. Diagram (c) represents a dual-media bed, with coarse coal above fine sand, which approaches the goal of the ideal filter.
Courtesy; American Water Works Association

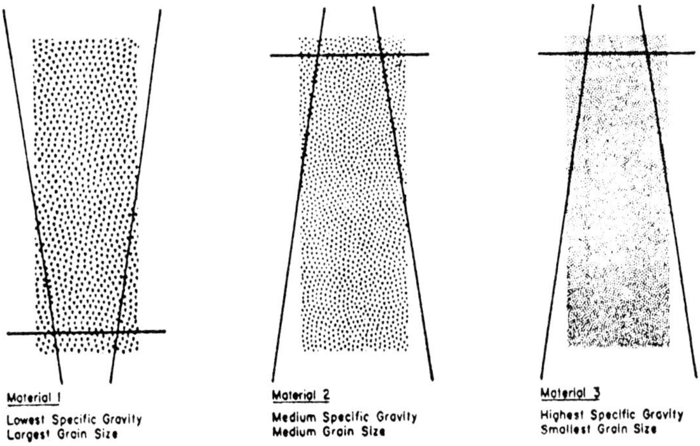

Figure 7-5. Cross sections through three different filter materials as expanded during filter backwashing. The diagrams show the relative vertical positions that might be assumed by three different commercial filter materials in water flowing upward at a rate of 15 gpm/ft², a usual backwashing rate.
Courtesy; American Water Works Association

Traps To Remove Colloids

Colloids that escape capture by alum treatment, or that are not so treated, may be removed by ion-exchange resin traps, albeit at a higher cost than by the use of alum. These traps consist of reticulated (i.e., porous) cross-linked polystyrene, bearing ion-exchange groups. They offer a larger internal area for colloid removal. The colloids, being bulky, are not very tightly held by these resins. The important question is which ion to put onto the resin upon regeneration to exchange with the colloid. In regeneration, caustic is very effective. However, when the hydroxyl ion is subsequently replaced by a colloid, the liberated ion serves regeneratively to replace a colloid held further down in the resin bed. In essence, one has a self-regenerating bed that is not too efficient at removing (i.e., retaining) colloids. If, however, the regeneration is done with a caustic brine solution (or with simultaneously introduced solutions of caustic and brine), then the hydroxyl ion of regenerated resin is replaced by a chloride ion that is not self-regenerating.

A standard water softening device can serve as a resin trap. It normally contains a cationic-exchange resin in its sodium form. It is used along with an anion-exchange resin regenerated with brine, which is introduced through an eductor. A pump is used to introduce caustic at the same time to give a combination type of regeneration. To prevent complicating precipitates from forming, the two solutions are introduced in diluted form.

Iron and Manganese

Iron is one of the more abundant elements in nature, manganese less so; although both appear together, being constituents of rocks and soils. They are sometimes found dissolved in natural waters, usually from deep wells. Both elements are found in both of their states of oxidation. The trivalent ferric state is usually low in amount because ferric salts are usually insoluble. It is possible, however, for the ferric iron to form soluble complexes with organics and with other salts, as through chelation. The tetravalent manganic combinations are very insoluble. The lower manganous state, although more stable than the bivalent ferrous state, is more complicated in its oxidation to insolubles. The removal of both of these elements usually consists of oxidation to insoluble forms, usually their hydroxides, followed by their filtrative removal. As such, they are subject to removal in the coagulation/flocculation step involving alum. Should they be present in surface waters, they would likely become oxidized to their higher valences by contact with air, and then converted to their insoluble hydrated oxides, a reaction that precipitates a rust-colored deposit from what had been a clear, colorless water.

Iron causes difficulties, usually uncontrolled depositions that block surfaces and restrict pipe passageways, when its concentrations reach 0.30 mg/L; in some industrial situations, 0.10 mg/L (American Water Works Assoc., 1969, p. 231). Manganese can be troublesome at concentrations as low as 0.05 mg/L; sometimes as low as 0.01 mg/L.

The alkaline earth elements (Ca^{+2}, Mg^{+2}, Ba^{+2}, Sr^{+2}) are usually considered responsible for permanent water hardness. Iron and manganese also belong in this grouping, however, for they too form mineral deposits. They are destructive of soaps because many of their salts, usually in some hydrated oxide form, are insoluble (Applebaum, 1968).

When iron and/or manganese are found in waters in their soluble form, their removal in the water purification scheme requires some promptness. Otherwise they become oxidized by contact with the oxygen in air to form their insoluble, higher-valence compounds. Since the insolubilizing oxidation takes time, the precipitated iron (ferric) and manganic deposits may form anywhere along the water purification train. To control this occurrence and to remove iron and manganese ions, managed oxidations followed by precipitate removal are staged at selected places and times, early in the pretreatment protocol.

Contact with air causes the oxidation of the ferrous iron, and at pHs above 8 of manganous ions, with the concomitant formation of the insoluble ferric and/or manganic oxide in their colloidal hydrated form, whereupon the colorless water turns red or brown. Aeration is the most direct approach to this problem, serving also to remove dissolved hydrogen sulfide gas (as it would also remove ammonia and carbon dioxide). The rate of the oxidative reaction using aeration is, however, not too rapid. The use of permanganate oxidation in conjunction with a filter bed of greensand (a zeolite containing manganese), in combination with a multimedia filter of anthracite and sand, serves effectively to speed the process. The oxidation by the manganic oxidizer within the greensand, itself transformed to an insoluble form, or so maintained within the zeolite structure, requires renewal by periodic applications of potassium permanganate. The bed, serving both as an oxidative catalyst and as a filter, is subjected to periodic regeneration. Ion-exchange resins can of course be used to remove the ferrous and manganous ions. Unless oxygen is excluded, however, ferric and manganic hydroxide will form as precipitates within the resin bed. The application of weakly acidic cation-exchange resin to the removal of iron from high-iron, high-alkalinity, high-hardness well water was described by Aronovitch and Ford (1995). Alkalinity and hardness were removed as well; iron from 20 mg/L to 5 µg/L; alkalinity, from greater than 400 mg/L to less than 125 mg/L. These investigators also advised concerning the advantages of regenerating the resin with hydrochloric acid rather than sulfuric acid. The latter acid cannot be used in high regenerating concentrations without risking the precipitation of insoluble calcium sulfate.

Chlorine is an even stronger oxidizer than oxygen. Its addition to waters containing iron and manganese can serve to insolubilize these two elements. At one pharmaceutical company in the Midwest (an area particularly rich in soluble iron and manganese), the chlorine added as biocide at the wellhead also precipitates these elements. Removal is promptly managed by multimedia bed filtration. The chlorine thus consumed is not available for microbial control, however, so that more must be added. If unmanaged, haphazard iron and manganese precipitates can build to thick layers within water pipes to restrict water flows and to provide shelter to ensconced organisms.

Comb and Fulford (1991) added chlorine (to an already chlorinated water) to a concentration of 0.8 ppm of free chlorine to oxidize the soluble iron present to an insoluble ferric precipitate. The chlorine was supplied by 12.5% sodium hypochlorite solution, and provided a residue of 0.4 to 0.6 ppm of chlorine for the sanitization of subsequent downstream cellulose acetate ROs. The precipitated iron was removed by filtrative action of a dual-media bed of anthracite atop greensand, the naturally occurring manganese zeolite itself utilized to oxidize soluble ferrous to insoluble ferric iron. The precipitated iron formed a "Schmutzdecke" layer upon the anthracite, easily removed by the backwashing rejuvenations of the dual-media bed. The greensand underlayer served to ensure the oxidation of ferrous or manganous ions that escaped conversion by the chlorine. In turn, the free chlorine present regenerated any greensand that became reduced during its desired conversion action of the soluble ferrous and manganous salts to their insoluble, filtratively removable analogs.

The use of lime, or of lime and soda ash, in the softening process (soon to be discussed) upon a previously aerated water will serve to remove the soluble iron as insoluble ferric hydroxide. Residual iron or manganese as ionic forms are removed by hydrogen-cation-exchange resins.

From an economics point of view, if low amounts of iron and/or manganese are to be removed, cation-exchange resins are to be preferred. For high amounts, greensand oxidations are better.

Zeolites

Silicates and aluminum silicates are molecular structures based on coordination lattices of large anions about small cations. Silicon is present as Si^{+4}; the anions are, in general, O^{2-}. These, being much larger than the positive ions, determine the general skeleton of the structure. These structures are called zeolites. Aluminum can be an isomorphous replacement of silca in these crystalline arrangements. Although the three-dimensional silicon-oxygen framework is electrically neutral, the replacement of Si^{4+} by Al^{3+} leads to an unbalanced anionic charge that leads to an association with cations. Such cations may become interchanged, but are so small relative to the zeolite structure that their exchange does not disrupt the physical, fixed arrangement of the silicon, aluminum, oxygen skeleton. These zeolites function, therefore, in the manner of the ion-exchangers. In greensand, the manganic ion is available to oxidize ferrous or manganous ions. It itself is reduced to manganous ions within the zeolite. No disruption of the zeolite structure results, and it is amenable to regeneration to the manganic valence state for repeated use.

Water Hardness

Calcium, magnesium, and bicarbonate are usually present in all waters. Essentially, water hardness is due to calcium and magnesium ions; however, barium, strontium, iron, and manganese ions also contribute to water hardness. The concentration of these latter ions in most raw waters is usually too low to merit them consideration. The term "permanent hardness" refers to the presence of calcium and magnesium ions, as in sulfates and chlorides: the noncarbonate hardness. Calcium and magnesium ions usually exist in waters in the ratio of 2:1.

Temporary hardness refers to the presence of carbon dioxide in the form of bicarbonate or carbonate, depending upon pH. It is ephemeral in its nature because it is destroyed by being heated. Thus calcium bicarbonate, soluble in water, is transformed by heat into insoluble calcium carbonate and evanescent carbon dioxide.

Water Softening

Water-softening pretreatment generally precedes dechlorination of feedwater in order to prolong the biocidal action of chlorine throughout the softening process as long as possible.

Softening is the sovereign way of removing calcium and the other elements that create scale. It is, therefore, usually used in-line with reverse osmosis systems to get rid of calcium and magnesium. It also removes aluminum, copper, and other troublesome trace metals. Aluminum, from the alum used as a coagulant in municipal potable water treatment plants, can have a ruinous effect upon RO membranes.

Water softening refers to treatments that remove the causes of water hardness with its concomitant threats of water management problems. *Water softening* is not the same as *demineralization* (a term more evocative of a broader spectrum of ion removal such as is effected by RO or by ion exchange). This ambiguity should be avoided (Chapman et al., 1984).

There are two general methods of water softening. The first involves the precipitation of calcium and magnesium as their carbonate and hydroxide forms, respectively, by the use of calcium hydroxide and sodium carbonate. This method, in its various manifestations, is called the lime-soda process, and it serves to reduce the water hardness by about one third. The second method is by the removal of the objectionable ions by ion exchange.

Lime-soda process. The addition of a mixture of lime (calcium hydroxide) and soda ash (sodium carbonate) reduces water hardness. The added lime converts the soluble bicarbonate salt to insoluble carbonate, which precipitates out.

$$Ca(HCO_3)_2 + Ca(OH)_3 \longrightarrow 2CaCO_3^- + 2H_2O \qquad \text{Eq. 7-2}$$

The hydroxyl ions supplied by the lime also serve to convert the magnesium to insoluble magnesium hydroxide, thus reducing that source of permanent hardness.

$$Mg^{2+} + 2OH^- \longrightarrow Mg(OH)_2 \qquad \text{Eq. 7-3}$$

The calcium ion portion of the permanent hardness is removed in the form of precipitated calcium carbonate by the carbonate ion supplied by the soda ash.

$$Ca^{2+} + CO_3^{2-} \longrightarrow CaCO_3^- \qquad \text{Eq. 7-4}$$

The lime-soda ash process has been detailed by Applebaum, (1968). Despite the economy of its operation, the lime-soda process of hardness removal by precipitation is declining in use. Overall it increases the total dissolved solids content of the water, and it requires much floor space. Its present use seems limited to softening activities made in conjunction with clarifiers.

Sodium cation exchange. The objectionable calcium and magnesium ions can be removed by ion-exchange reactions. The use of a sodium-cation exchanger will exchange the sodium ions of the resin for the calcium and magnesium ions in the water, thereby removing the water hardness. The TDS is unchanged. Regeneration of the sodium ion exchanger involves three steps: (1) A strong backwashing flow upward through the bed serves to remove foreign particulate matter, and loosens and regrades the bed. (2) A solution of salt is passed through the bed, causing the removal of the resin-bound calcium and magnesium, and recharging the bed by substituting ions in their place. (3) A downward rinse through the column with raw water washes out the excess brine along with the displaced calcium and magnesium, and readies the column for reuse. (See Figures 7-6 and 7-7).

Regrettably, the water-softening operation provides opportunity for the invasion of the water-processing system by organisms. Brine is used to regenerate the water softener. Not only is brine not a sanitizer, but the brine makeup tank may itself serve as a haven for organism proliferation. To minimize this latter possibility, the brine should be maintained in a clean area under closed conditions, at a saturated concentration, agitated (preferably by recirculation), and should periodically be prepared fresh. In an european practice, an electrolyzing current generates chlorine in the stand-by brine for sanitization. Just prior to use the chlorinated brine solution is washed from the sanitized resin. Calcium or sodium hypochlorite can be added to the brine for the same sanitizing effect (Weitnauer 1996). An argument can be made for the use of a softener

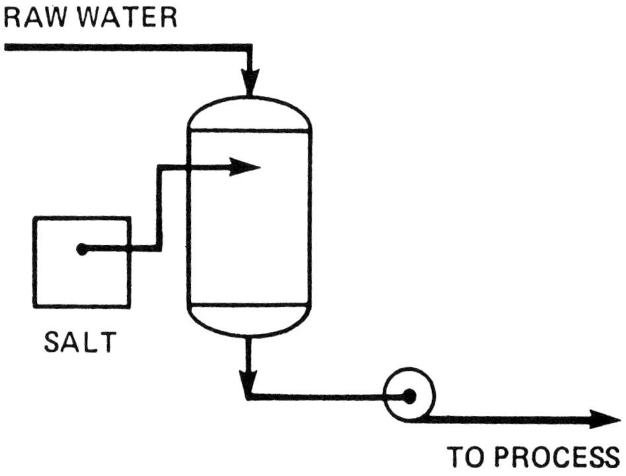

Figure 7-6. Water softening by cation exchange.
Meltzer (1987a); Courtesy, Dr. Robert Kunin

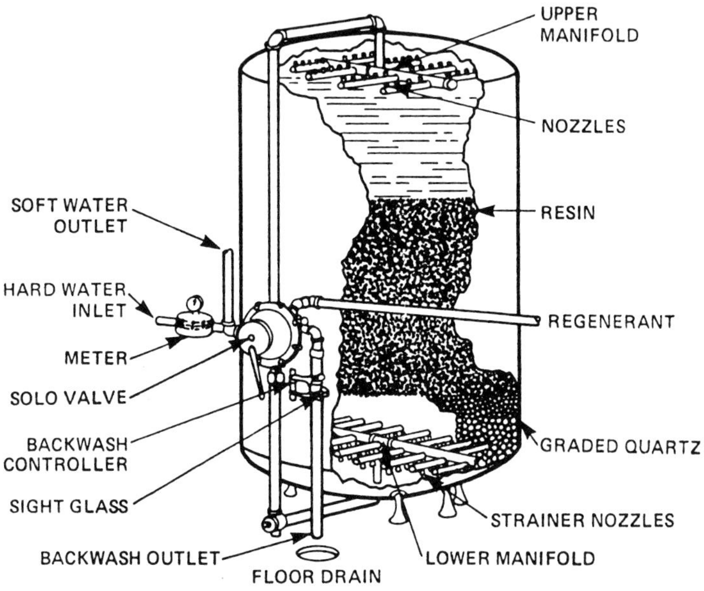

Figure 7-7. Typical commercial ion-exchange unit.
Meltzer (1987a); Courtesy, Dr. Robert Kunin

before the carbon bed, the latter intended to accomodate any remaining active chlorine not washed out of the softening resin. The cation-exchange resin used for water softening can be sanitized by way of hot (80 °C) water.

Where brine-regenerated softening is used, it is good practice to use two softeners that are out of phase by design, so that one is being regenerated while one is operative. To avoid organism growth, softeners not in use should be kept in recharged condition with 26% brine, ready to be flushed free of the brine and thus made water operative on signal. As a practical matter, commercially available water softeners can benefit from the addition of duty-cycle controls. The addition of calcium hypochlorite to the salt supply helps to keep the latter sanitized. Also, wherever possible, hot-water sanitization of the water softener should be performed at 65 to 90 °C. The cation-exchange resin survives heating at 90 °C.

Water contaminated with organisms derived from the water-softening operation will inoculate the ion exchangers that follow in sequence. For this reason, use is made of ultraviolet light units and of organism-retaining filters to minimize such possibilities.

The substitution of sodium ions for those of calcium and magnesium makes more difficult the subsequent deionization of the water by ion exchange, for sodium ions are the more difficult to remove. Therefore water softening is not used as a pretreatment before deionization, but is used before reverse osmosis.

But water softness may be used on aside operations, as in the removal of magnesium ions from water being used to prepare sodium hydroxide solutions. Upwards of 95% of water softening is used for the water conditioning involved in boiler and heat-exchanger usage. The use of the sodium form of ion exchange for this purpose obviates scale formation without the need for acidification. Additionally, as the water issuing from this type of softener is not acidic, it is therefore not very corrosive.

Hydrogen cation exchange. The use of conventional hydrogen-cation exchange resin substitutes hydrogen ions for the calcium and magnesium ions removed from the solution. The enrichment of the treated water with hydrogen ions (its acidification) converts the bicarbonate and carbonate ions to carbonic acid. This acid decomposes readily to release carbon dioxide.

$$\begin{aligned} H^+ + CO_3^{2-} &\longleftrightarrow HCO_3^- \\ H^+ + HCO_3^- &\longleftrightarrow H_2CO_3 \\ H_2CO_3 &\longleftrightarrow H_2O + CO_2 \end{aligned} \qquad \text{Eq. 7-5}$$

The liberated carbon dioxide is removed by use of degasifiers, soon to be discussed. The process is sometimes called *dealkalizing*. Objections to it center on the risk of bacterial contamination attendant upon removal by aeration, and its capital expense as occasioned by vacuum degasification. Besides, the use of certain RO devices permits the removal of carbon dioxide/bicarbonate more expeditiously. Whatever its limitations, the hydrogen-cation exchange method of softening (in effect, the use of the cation-exchange bed of the conventional twin DI bed arrangement), does lower the treated water's TDS, and is reported to have been used with great success for more than a decade (Marquardt et al., 1987). (See Figure 7-8).

Carbon Dioxide/Bicarbonate/Carbonate Alkalinity. As has been remarked upon (page 57), there is a pH-dependent equilibrium among carbon dioxide, and the bicarbonate and carbonate ions. Viewed another way, carbon dioxide in water can exist in any of three manifestations, depending upon its pH environment. The gas itself dissolved in water yields a solution of about pH 4, the end point revealed by methyl orange indicator or, more noticeably, by bromphenol blue at pH 3.7. Waters having lower pHs do so by dint of the presence of stronger acids than carbonic acid, whose acid anhydride is carbon dioxide. The Nalco Water Handbook (1988) states that distilled water, pH 7, completely saturated with carbon dioxide, approximately 1,600 mg/L, achieves a pH of about 4. (Other sources give values as high as pH 5.65).

From that pH upward to a value of about 8.3, at the color change detected using phenolphthalein, the carbon dioxide exists in equilibrium with the bicarbonate ion in response to the equations:

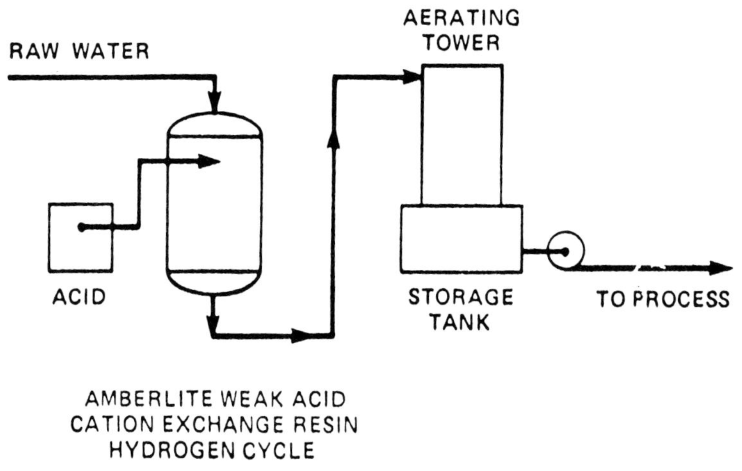

Figure 7-8. Elimination of water hardness and of carbon dioxide.
Courtesy, Dr. Robert Kunin

$$H_2O + CO_2 \text{<---->} H_2CO_3 \text{<---->} H^+ + HCO_3^-$$
$$OH^- + HCO_3^- \text{<---->} H_2O + CO_3^{2-}$$

Above pHs of approximately 8.3 to about 9.6 to 9.8, carbon dioxide exists as the carbonate ion. Above pH 9.6, hydroxyl ions appear increasingly (Nalco, 1988). The total alkalinity of a water is described as the sum of its titratable bases. It is a measure chiefly of the bicarbonate, carbonate, and hydroxyl ions present; contributions by phosphates, silicates, or borates being ignored. Because the pHs of natural waters seldom exceed 8.3, water alkalinity is seen to be the product of carbon dioxide and bicarbonate ions, a combination whose end point is below that of phenolphthalein (Nalco 1988, page 4.7). The strength of the bicarbonate concentration can be measured by titrating a water with acid to bring it to the "methyl orange" or M end point of approximately 4.4. The end point is called the methyl orange end point regardless of the actual indicator used (Standard Methods 1989, page 235). Below this pH, free carbon dioxide will increasingly appear in the aqueous solution. Whether in its free or combined form (bicarbonate), carbon dioxide requires being removed to deny its pH-influencing presence. Furthermore, the existence of carbon dioxide defines temporary hardness with its implications to potential scale formation.

Bicarbonate Removal

Bicarbonate ion may be removed by acid dosing to liberate carbon dioxide. Its removal will require the use of a degasifier or decarbonator, soon to be discussed. Bicarbonate ions can be rejected by RO membranes. However, their substantial formation from CO_2 necessitates pHs of about 8 or 8.5 , a level at which cellulose acetate membranes hydrolyze too rapidly for practical use. (Figure 7-9).

In RO pretreatments, acid addition can be used to convert bicarbonate/carbonate into CO_2. At pH 6, some 80% is converted into CO_2. Where it is desired to remove these entities as CO_2, as a rule of thumb, pH is adjusted to 6. This technique suffices for water systems above 100 gpm in size of flow. Smaller systems may find water-softening treatments more optimal. Removal of the CO_2 is necessary because it will otherwise permeate RO units. Equilibration of CO_2 with water will yield resistivities of about 250,000 ohms and pH of 5.65. Carbon dioxide can be removed from its aqueous solutions by the use of strongly basic anion-exchange resins (at significant cost, however, if the volume is substantial). Yet there are those who prefer this practice to the use of degasifiers. (See Figure 7-10).

Polyamide RO membranes are resistant to hydrolysis between the pHs of 4 and 11. At pH 8, these RO filters exhibit a high rejection of bicarbonate ions. Therefore it is possible to remove the CO_2 in the form of bicarbonate ion using polyamide RO membrane at pH 8 (Kraft, 1985). Depending upon the calcium ion concentration in the water, however, calcium carbonate scale formation on the membrane surface is a possibility at this pH. The probability can be ascertained by determining the Langelier saturation index of the water (See Chapter 9, page 528). The most economical method of controlling calcium carbonate scale formation is by acid dosing. Unfortunately, the polyamide RO membrane suffers a reduction in its bicarbonate ion rejections below pH 8. An alternative is to utilize additions such as sodium hexametaphosphate, 20 mg/L in the RO feedwater (Kraft, 1985). These additives promote the stability of supersaturated solutions of calcium carbonate, thereby preventing its deposition as scale upon the membrane surface. The use of such antiscalants in conjunction with a pH of 8 enables the use of polyamide RO membrane units to eliminate temporary water hardness.

High pH Hard Water

As stated, above pH 8 polyamide RO membrane can reject carbon dioxide in the form of bicarbonate. At higher pHs the CO_2 increasingly appears as carbonate ions. This too can be rejected by the polyamide RO but at the risk of precipitating calcium carbonate in excess of its solubility product. This problem can be avoided if hard waters at high pH are acidified, not to the point where carbon dioxide is released, but to pH 8 where it is in the form of bicarbonate ions. Minimizing CO_2 formation obviates as well the need for degassing devices.

Such acidifications can be achieved using the customary mineral acids, HCl, H_2SO_4, but the use of phosphoric acid, or even carbon

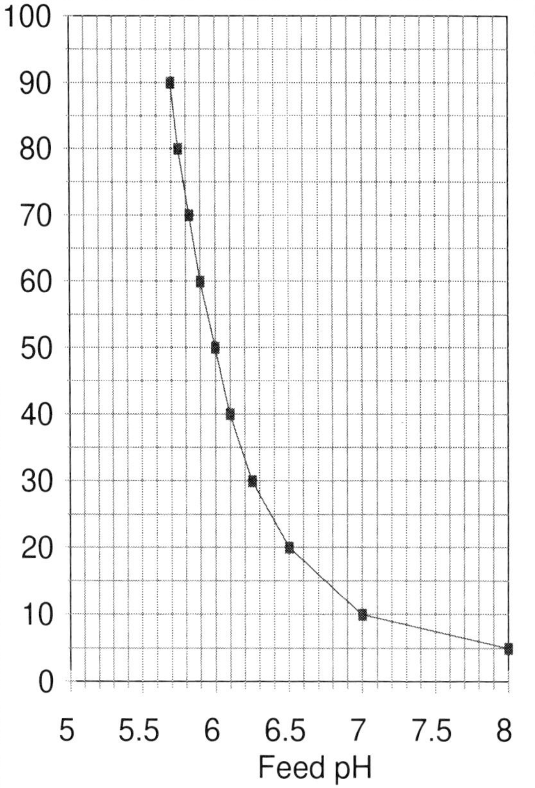

Figure 7-9. Effect of pH on bicarbonate passage.
Courtesy, Anderson Water Ltd.

dioxide (carbonic acid) also suffices, and makes less likely overdosing to the point of CO_2 generation. Letzner (1995) prefers the use of carbon dioxide, a technique used in the food industry. The hard waters thus treated are softened without the need for handling and disposing of large amounts of sodium chloride, as used in common softening operations. This addresses an environmental concern.

The waters thus treated may contain carbon dioxide whose presence could cause unacceptably low pHs. The carbon dioxide could be swept from the water by a nitrogen stream. The utility of this practice may depend upon the size of the installation.

Degasifiers

When utilities manufacture high-purity water for steam production, the carbon dioxide exiting the acidic waters that leave the cation-exchange beds is gotten rid of by blowing it out with an airstream. In the preparation of pharmaceutical waters where microbiological contamination is a major concern, such a purging airstream would require purification by HEPA filtration. Unfortunately, HEPA filters are not intrinsically sanitizing filters. That is the problem with forced-draft degasifiers (decarbonators). Applebaum (1968) described the construction of these and other degasifiers. In essence, they comprise towers packed with Raschig rings or other ceramic or nonceramic fill, which provide large surface areas over which the waters being freed of carbon dioxide trickle as they are being swept by a counter-current of air. In accord with Henry's law of gas solubilities, the carbon dioxide, being at low partial pressures, is released by the water to be carried away by the airstream (Figure 7-10).

Vacuum degasifiers substitute vacuum for the sweeping airstream to remove the carbon dioxide from the thin films of water permeating the packing of the deaeration towers. This removes the threat of microbial contamination but substitutes other disadvantages, among them the high capital and energy costs of pumps, the need for ASME-code vessels to withstand the vacuum, and requirements for the stainless steel construction and piping necessary to avoid contamination by substances such as iron.

As stated by Dietrich (1991), there are several types of vacuum degasifiers. The most common are tray-type deaerating heaters that use steam to strip dissolved oxygen from heated feedwater; and the vacuum degasifiers that operate near vacuum conditions to strip dissolved oxygen and carbon dioxide from water at ambient temperature. The tray-type deaerators are found mostly in power plants where steam is in sufficient quantity and readily available. Vacuum degasifiers are found in applications where steam is not available or where there is a need for degasified water and/or bacterial control at temperatures ranging from 35 °F to over 100 °F, such as electronics manufacturers or remote locations in power plants.

Dietrich (1992) discussed the ancillar equipment necessary for vacuum degasifier operations, such as the tower packing materials, the vacuum pumps, the product pressurization pump, instrumentation and controls. Vacuum degasifiers, while importantly directed towards carbon dioxide removal, are also suitable for the elimination of oxygen from waters. Degasifiers that rely upon the removal of gases by air stripping cannot remove oxygen because of the high oxygen content in the air. They are, therefore, more commonly referred to as decarbonators.

A degasifier is usually intended to remove carbon dioxide. Therefore, degasifiers are often used after cation-exchange beds because acidification of the water by cation-exchange reaction may release carbon dioxide. When RO is being utilized, the presence of a degasifier in a water purification system almost certainly bespeaks a prior decision to utilize an RO unit composed of cellulose acetate to eliminate bicarbonate in the form of carbon dioxide generated by acid addition. The hydrolytic stability of this polymer requires acid adjustment to pH 5.5 to 6, causing the release of carbon dioxide from carbonate or bicarbonate. It is the released carbon dioxide whose removal the degasifier is intended to accomplish.

The degasifier may be placed into the water purification train at any of several positions. It may be upstream of the RO unit, which in turn, precedes the ion-exchange facility (Figure 7-11). A less-expensive forced-air draft degasifier may be used here because any organism cross-contamination occasioned by impure air will find a barrier in the subsequent RO unit (at a concomitant cost in RO fouling, however). This arrangement gets rid of the carbon dioxide before it permeates the RO, thus avoiding its encounter with and consumption of anion-exchange resin. The maximum effect would be gained by using so low a pH as to convert

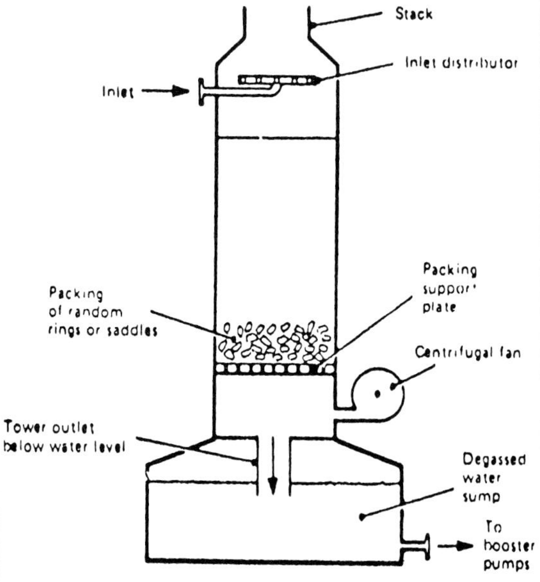

Figure 7-10. Degassing tower.

all bicarbonate present to carbon dioxide. Removal of the carbon dioxide may raise the pH of the water by some 1.5 units. To allow for this rise while maintaining a pH level of 5.5 to 6, the original pH of the water may require being brought in advance to possibly pH 4 to 5, or reacidification to pH 5.5 to 6 may be made. The latter alternative would, however, entail repumping.

Alternatively, the acidified water including the carbon dioxide may permeate the RO unit, to be degasified before entering the ion-exchange beds (Figure 7-12). In this position, a vacuum degasifier is indicated to minimize the risks of organism contamination common to forced-draft degasifiers. The water subjected to this arrangement may be set at a higher pH than in the previous example. However, any bicarbonate present may permeate the RO to be released as carbon dioxide. The thus-generated CO_2 will consume anion-exchange resin. This will require an unbalanced sizing of the cation- and anion-exchanger bed, resulting in a more complicated bed operation.

Waters exiting RO treatment can bear a higher anion than cation load because of the presence of carbon dioxide, silicate ions, or borate ions. When this is so, unbalanced ion-exchange resin bed requirements result, and necessitate being addressed. This is particularly worth noting for the arrangements utilizing RO followed by mixed-bed ion exchange.

The above complication can be minimized if the degasifier is placed downstream of the RO between the cation- and anion-exchanger beds (Figure 7-13). A vacuum degasifier is still required to avoid microbial contamination, but in this position it can remove almost all of the CO_2, even that generated by the acidity imparted to the water in the cation-exchange reactions. Some carbon dioxide, about 5 to 50 mg/L, will remain in the water exiting the cation-exchanger. This will consume some anion-exchange resin; but this arrangement does render the ion-exchange operations somewhat less complicated (Kraft, 1985). It is very infrequently that one encounters twin-bed deionizers downstream from an RO unit.

The problems associated with degassing equipment often compel the removal of CO_2 in the form of bicarbonate by polyamide RO membranes; most thin-film composite RO membranes are of this type.

The teaching is that it is more economical to use degasifiers to remove carbon dioxide than to utilize strongly basic anion exchange. At the Upjohn Company, however, a change was made from degasifiers to the ion exchange to eliminate the labor and time costs associated with the steam-sanitizing maintenance of the degasifier and the risks of microbiological contamination that persistently attended.

It should be pointed out, however, that despite the undoubted problems associated with degasification operations, as with all other water purification equipment, degasifiers are and have been used long and successfully (Hango, 1986).

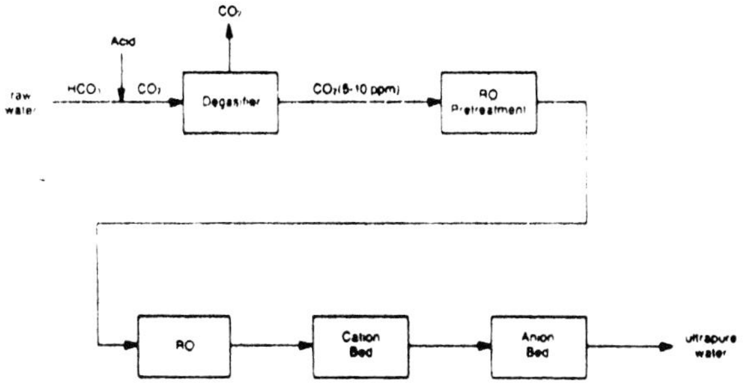

Figure 7-11. Simplified high-purity water system with a degasifier located before the RO system.
Kraft (1985); Courtesy, *Ultrapure Water* journal

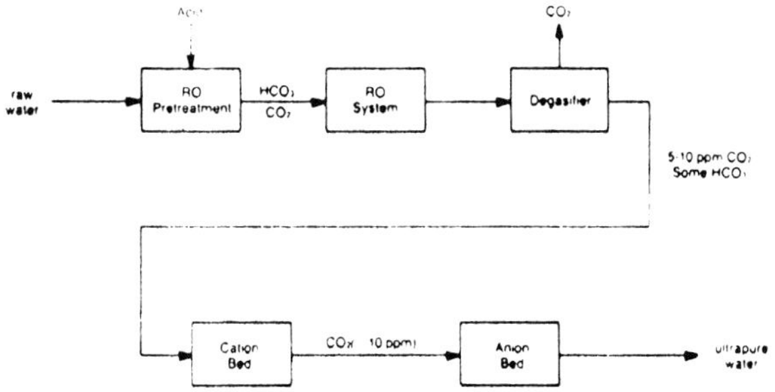

Figure 7-12. Simplified high-purity water system with a degasifier located between the RO and ion-exchange sections.
Kraft (1985); Courtesy, *Ultrapure Water* journal

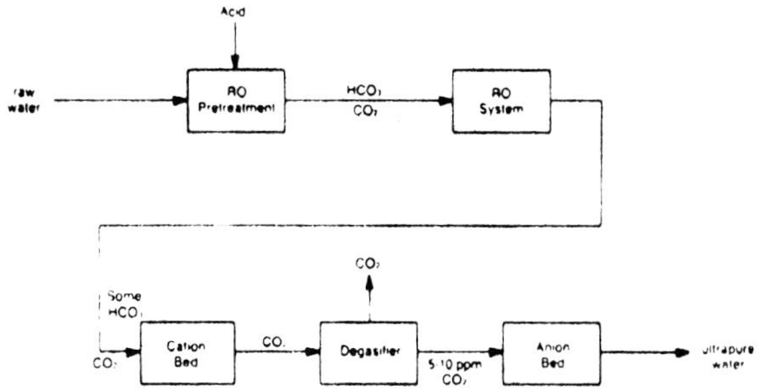

Figure 7-13. Simplified high-purity water system with a degasifier located between the cation and anion exchangers.
Kraft (1985); Courtesy, *Ultrapure Water* journal

Pasteurization of water, its being heated to 60 °C (140 °F), is practiced in order to reduce organism (principally Gram-negative) populations. Pasteurization tends also to free the water (degas it) from volatile gases such as carbon dioxide.

Also, as waters emerge from an RO system into the ambience of atmospheric pressure, their more volatile components become decreased in concentration, in accordance with Henry's law governing the solubility of gases. In this sense, storage tanks are degasifiers, particularly so for carbon dioxide when the water storage is under a nitrogen blanket.

Hardness Removal by Open RO Membranes

It is possible, by manipulative operations during membrane formation, to enlarge somewhat the intersegmental spacings beyond the distance truly representative of the bulk state. As a result, the prepared RO membrane is more open; thermodynamically metastable, but steadfast and permanent in the practical sense.

Such a thin-film composite RO membrane is available. It is functional in its rejection of divalent ions such as calcium, magnesium, barium, and strontium. It also reduces or eliminates the aluminum problem, aluminum ions being trivalent. However, it is too open to discriminate against sodium, potassium, and other monovalent ionic species. As a result, it can be used to effect water softening. Moreover, the openness provides membranes with respectable water flows at very low applied differential pressures. (See page 246).

Membranes of this type are variously referred to as nanofilters or as membrane softeners. They have not yet found strong industrial applications. They do effect hardness rejections in the 80% to 90% range and are even rated to reject about 10% of sodium. However, they constitute a high capital outlay. Moreover, rejecting calcium, they are also prone to calcium scale formation. An acid feed is therefore required to protect them. Additionally, being RO instruments, they do produce reject water. They avoid the use of salt, however, unlike the anion-exchange salt-form softeners. Large municipal softening systems are possible application for membrane softeners. Waste water from RO could be reused here, and the avoidance of adding sodium to the water, unlike anion-exchange softening, has desirable health implications for drinking water. Salt-free diets are desirable for hypertensive individuals.

Water Softening by Ion Exchange

As will be set forth in Chapter 8 "Ion Exchange," removal of the divalent alkaline earth elements responsible for water hardness can be accomplished by the use of weakly acidic cation-exchange resins to the extent that an adequate proportion of alkalinity is present.

Water Softening by Reverse Osmosis

If scale-forming conditions (shortly to be discussed) are absent, water can also be softened by reverse osmosis. Figures 7-14 and 7-15 show that there is a constant ratio between alkalinity and CO_2 as a function of pH. Thus, at pH 8.2 the ratio of methyl orange alkalinity to CO_2 is almost 100 to 1; there is no free CO_2.

As the pH drops to 5.3, the ratio becomes 0:1; there is 10 times as much CO_2 as bicarbonate. At pH 5, it is all CO_2. Therefore, after a cation exchange where the only cation left in solution is the proton, H^+, there is no bicarbonate present, only CO_2. After most RO operations, the effluent water is about pH 5 to 5.5, because most ions except the proton fail to pass through the RO membrane. There is some proton leakage. Therefore, the bicarbonate is almost all in the form of CO_2. Degassing or the use of strongly basic anion-exchange resin will be required. To utilize an RO device in conjunction with lowest-cost downstream operation, the pH requires being raised. This would enable the CO_2 to be rejected by the RO as bicarbonate ion. Where dual-pass product-staged RO units are used, one can either adjust the pH between the stages, or make an adequate initial pH adjustment using caustic before the first stage is joined.

One way or another, the presence of carbon dioxide must be eliminated if high-purity water with a resistivity of at least 2 or 3 megohm-cm is to be obtained.

Water softening provides an alternative to the use of acid in removing bicarbonate. With cellulose acetate RO units, acid must in any case be used to minimize hydrolysis of the polymer. Acidification is also employed when the capital costs of softening are being avoided. Just as cellulose acetate can be protected against scaling by the addition of acid, so too can polyamide RO units. However, polyamide RO can also be shielded against scaling by softening rather than by acidification.

Water Softening Applications

Where Purified Water is being prepared for nonsterile compendial formulations, water softening is usually not a required pretreatment step, since the ion-exchange demineralization that is usually employed accomplishes calcium and magnesium ion removal as well. When reverse osmosis is used to prepare Purified Water, or when Water for Injection is prepared using RO or distillation, water hardness and scale formation may be involved.

When the raw water enters mixed beds, however, there is concern about the presence of high concentrations of magnesium ions, a component of permanent hardness. Upon regeneration of the bed, the dilute sodium hydroxide used may precipitate magnesium hydroxide, $Mg(OH)_2$. This forms very gelatinous deposits, causing blockage of the resin bead surface.

Where WFI is being prepared, water softening is necessary. The avoidance of mineral scaling on RO membranes and upon still surfaces, as caused by water hardness, is clearly necessary.

The avoidance of mineral scale formation within boilers, heat exchangers, and pipes is sought in industrial water softening practices.

Water softening is a required pretreatment for RO. If the RO is below about 100 gpm, and/or the water is not extraordinarily hard, then water softening is indicated to prevent scaling. Otherwise, acid feeding should be used.

Water Softening Summary

The use of RO membranes for water softening, as indeed for any RO purpose, is capital-intensive. Additionally, the reject water stream equals about 25% of the feed volume. Its disposal entails a cost consideration, given sewage taxes and escalating water costs. Mitigating these costs is the pH neutrality of the softened waters. Carbon steel piping ought to suffice, except that the dissolving of iron into the water may be of some concern even at neutral pHs. Stainless steel piping would be more corrosion-resistant. In a softening RO application at low pressures, plastic piping may be the best choice economically.

It is best not to oversize water softening units. Oversizing, and thus underutilization, are their greatest problems. When not in use, they constitute dead-legs. It is advantageous to use two units in tandem. When used in series, they are both hydraulically active. Also, they can be arrayed in parallel via a bypass system. In such arrangements, it is best that the two devices be staggered in terms of their regeneration. Such regeneration is usually performed on a maintenance schedule. Hardness meters, although available, are seldom used.

Water softening may be performed before chlorine removal. This is done to keep the water in a biocidal condition as long as possible, even though the chlorine entering the DI resin beds does cause some resin degradation. Those who prefer to remove the chlorine prior to softening do so in order to avoid DI resin loss as well as loss of resin function through reaction with chlorine. Water softeners generally are followed by cartridge filters downstream. These serve automatically, therefore as prefilters for the RO unit that follows.

Activated Carbon Beds

It is common to treat raw water supplies with chlorine in order to control microorganism growth. Indeed, municipally prepared potable waters are thus treated before being distributed. Usually, the chlorine residual is retained as long as possible in order to discourage organism growth. Eventually it must be removed, for it can degrade ion-exchange resins, can be ruinous to RO membranes composed of polyamide polymer, and can corrode and stress-crack stainless steel stills. Beds of activated carbon are widely used to remove chlorine from the water. (Collentro, 1985a and 1985b).

Activated carbon reliably removes chlorine at flowrates of 2 to 3 gpm/ft^3 (not ft^2, because contact time rather than extent of filter surface is at issue). Ordinarily, an activated carbon bed suffices for a 1-year duration. In pharmaceutical usage, carbon beds are replaced when they evidence excessive particle shedding, or when the bacteria counts in the effluent from the bed cannot be controlled by appropriate means of sanitizing (hot water or steam). Carbon beds inevitably nurture bacteria in the bed regions below those wherein the chlorine is adsorbed and/or reacted.

Organic removal requires a far longer contact time. Flows of 1 gpm/ft^3 or less are needed. Some commercial accounts on the remediation of groundwaters

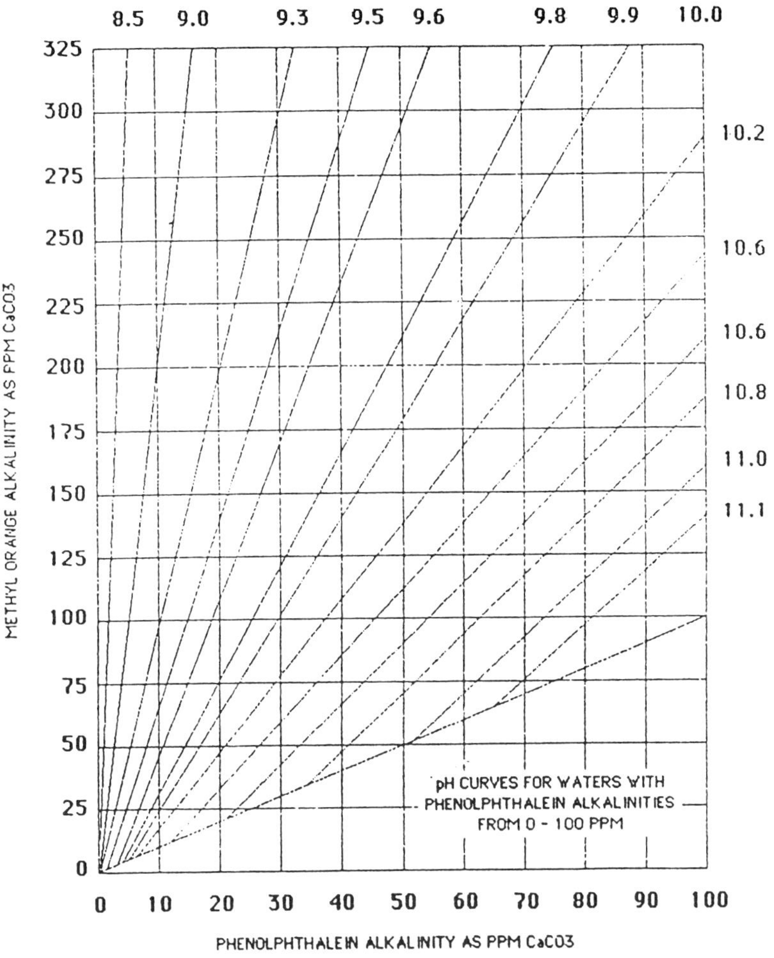

Figure 7-14. Effect of carbonate and bicarbonate alkalinity on pH.
Courtesy, Penfield Continental Water Systems

indicate that contact times of 60 to 120 minutes are required for organic removal. The adsorptive process for organics is slow. Measurements of carbon compounds—at least general TOC analyses on the influent and effluent waters—are necessary to direct the effort.

It is simply not known when a carbon bed, its organic adsorptive capacities exhausted, will become nonfunctional. Another objection to carbon-bed use is the leaching of inorganic ions from their ash components into the treated water.

The state-of-the-art detectable level of organic material by total oxidizable carbon methods is in the vicinity of 5 ppb. That value automatically becomes the standard for dense-circuitry rinsewater in the electronics industry, although many line geometries utilize waters with TOC levels of 20 ppb. Low as they are, TOC levels are trending downward.

The presence of organics above 2 to 3 ppm poses problems where ion-exchange usage is involved. The presence of organics in water may have deleterious effects on RO membranes, as well as depositing on them as coatings to interfere with their flux. If acidic organic materials gain entry into distillation units, volatile acids may become generated, to the corrosive detriment of the stills.

It should be noted that activated carbon not only removes chlorine by adsorption, but also reacts with it and becomes consumed thereby. According to Applebaum (1968), 1 pound of carbon reacts with 6 pounds of chlorine. Thus waters containing 1 ppm of chlorine will contain 8.3 pounds of chlorine per 1,000,000 gallons and will consume 1.4 pounds of carbon.

Michaud (1988), however, stated that each pound of activated carbon reacts with and is consumed by 2 to 3 pounds of chlorine. The dechlorination reaction is rapid, of a few seconds duration. In less than 60 seconds it is 99% complete. By contrast, organic adsorption by carbon requires a retention time of several minutes. A carbon bed designed for organic removal will therefore be overdesigned for chlorine uptake. The chief influences upon chlorine removal by activated carbon are temperature and pH. As for most chemical reactions, each 10-degree rise in temperature doubles the reaction rate between the carbon and chlorine. The carbon bed design should allow for the lowest temperatures expected to be encountered. At pHs below 7, free chlorine in aqueous solutions exists principally as hypochlorous acid (HOCl). Activated carbon very effectively accomplishes its removal. At pHs above 8.5, however, the chlorine is in the form of hypochlorite ion (OCl^-), whose removal rate is much slower, requiring some 3 minutes to effect 99% removal. As a consequence, chlorine breakthroughs may result when the pH rises on water supplies with fluctuating seasonal pH levels.

Since the adsorbency of carbon is a surface phenomenon, the surface area of the activated carbon is important. The smaller the activated carbon particles, the more the total surface area in the bed, and the faster the adsorption. In designing the carbon bed, however, the pressure drop across it must be considered. Once a certain maximum pressure has been reached, whether defined by pump limitations, tank strengths, or other parameters, the bed will require backflushing or replacement. The carbon bed may accumulate particulate matter through acting as a depth filter. This will progressively increase the pressure drop across it. Therefore, the smaller the activated carbon particles, the higher its clean,

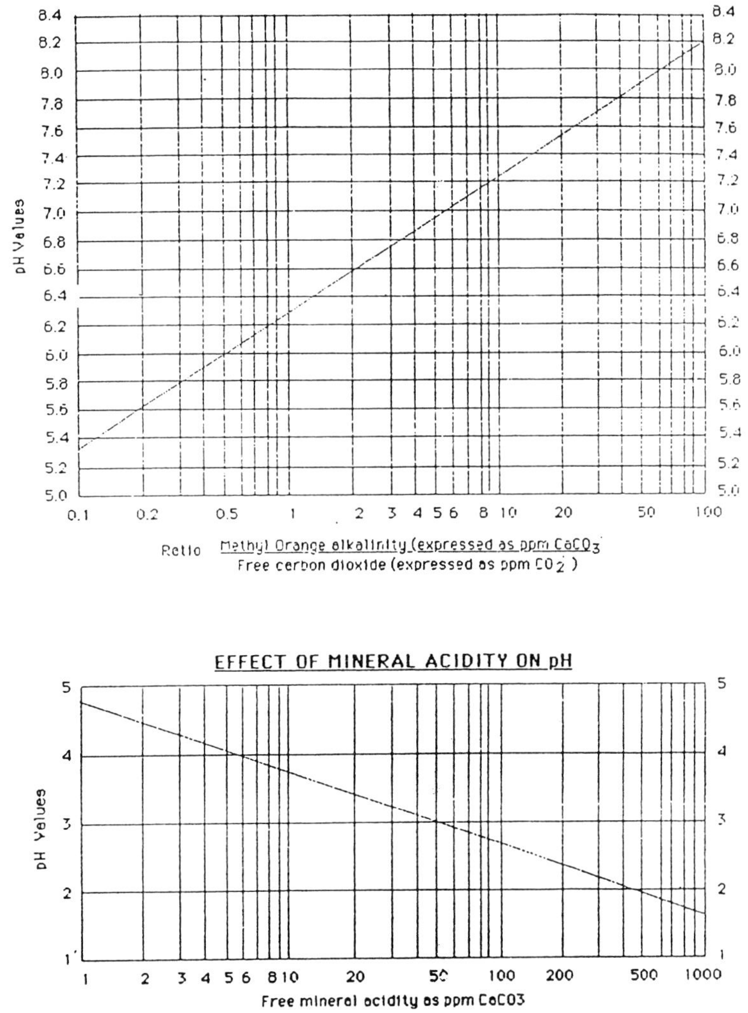

Figure 7-15. Effect of bicarbonate alkalinity and CO_2 on pH (top), and effect of mineral acidity on pH (bottom).
Courtesy, Penfield Continental Water Systems

initial pressure drop and the briefer its useful duration. Proper design balances both considerations.

The relationship of the height to the diameter of the carbon bed should be designed to yield the particular face velocity of water necessary to the treatment. If the water is relatively free of organics, as from deep wells, and needs only to be dechlorinated, then a face velocity as high as 4 gpm/ft^2 (15 Lpm per 929 cm^2) of cross-sectional bed area can be used (Collentro, 1985a and b). If chloramine (more frequently used by municipalities to avoid the generation of carcinogenic trihalomethanes by chlorine) requires being removed along with low organic levels, then a carbon bed depth of some 24 inches (60 cm) is needed. This would provide a face velocity of about 2 gpm/ft^2 of cross-sectional area. Waters containing greater quantities of organics along with trihalomethanes and chloramines require carbon bed depths of at least 4 feet. The corresponding liquid face velocity would be as low as 0.5 to 1 gpm/ft^2 (Collentro, 1985 a and b).

Applebaum (1968) stated that activated carbon beds are usually 2 to 5 feet deep and function at 1.0 to 1.5 gpm/ft^3 of carbon; large amounts of organic matter could require beds having depths of from 5 to 10 feet.

There is evidence that carbon adsorbs more efficiently at lower pHs. Therefore, carbon beds are sometimes preceded by a cation-exchange bed. The exchange of hydrogen ions for the cations originally in the water lowers the pH going into the carbon bed. Where this design is used, the cation-exchange column does not substitute for the cation-exchange bed, where it is used in subsequent twin-bed deionization. One shortcoming of this arrangement is the degradative action on the cation-exchange resin beads by the chlorine that is present.

There are those who advocate the placement of the carbon bed (the granular activated carbon, GAC) before the deep-bed silica or sand so that it can better serve to remove organics from the water (Nebel and Nebel, 1984). The arrangement is usually the reverse. The carbon beds should, however, precede ion removal, for the adsorption of organic substances by activated carbon is greatly enhanced by the presence of calcium and magnesium ions. According to Weber et al. (1983), the adsorption of humic materials by activated carbon is pH-dependent and is influenced by the presence of inorganic ions in the solution. Calcium is slightly more effective than magnesium, and divalent ions are more influential than monovalent ions by an order of magnitude; potassium ions are slightly more effective than sodium ions. The salubrious effects of lower pHs on increasing adsorption had previously been remarked upon by other investigators (Schnitzer and Kodama, 1966).

A plausible explanation may derive from the Fuoss effect as discussed by Ong and Bisque (1966), and as advanced by Ghosh and Schnitzer (1979). The Fuoss effect states that large polymeric electrolytes, such as derive from humic acids, exist in solutions in a coiled configuration; as indeed do all polymers. Increasing ionic strengths increasingly promote the tightness of such coilings; polymeric molecules increasingly unwind and extend themselves in diluted solutions. The contractions of the humic acid molecules under the influence of higher ionic strengths has two adsorption-promoting consequences. The progressively coiled polymer molecules increasingly confine their hydrophilic moieties to become more hydrophobic, and the polymer molecular size decreases. The first effect furthers hydrophobic absorptions; the second increases the ease of interstice penetration. Thus the presence of ions such as hydronium, calcium, and magnesium increases both the capacity for adsorption and the rate. This is of significance because adsorption is rate-dependent.

Evidence that the adsorption upon active carbon surfaces of organic materials derived from humic substances is promoted by lower pHs was furnished by Weber et al. (1983) and by Schnitzer and Kodama (1966), and was stated also by Michaud (1988). Figure 7-16 (Weber et al., 1983) shows that the adsorption isotherm for humic acid on an activated carbon, while increased somewhat by going from pH 9.0 to 7.0, increases markedly when the pH is lowered to 3.5.

Lower temperatures favor adsorption if only because more elevated temperatures are more disruptive of the adsorptive bond. In aqueous solutions, however, higher temperatures reduce the solution viscosity. This promotes the probability of the species in question to diffuse to the adsorptive site. Overall, adsorption from aqueous solutions seems generally favored by higher temperatures. It results in a more rapid rate of adsorption to a lower degree or capacity.

It is possible to generalize regarding the adsorption of materials from aqueous media by viewing the adsorptive phenomenon as being in competition with the tendency of the material to remain in solution; the less water-soluble the material, the easier it is to remove it from solution by adsorption. By this measure, less ionized or nonpolar molecules are easier to adsorb, and hydrophobic adsorption is an important adsorption mechanism.

Nature of Adsorption

Adsorption is an interfacial occurrence in water contexts, usually between liquid and solid. It may, however, also involve gas/solid, gas/liquid, or liquid/liquid phenomena. The forces that result in absorptions can arise from charge-related considerations. The electrical attractions of valence that characterize ion exchanges are an example. Secondary valence effects or Van der Waals forces are another. Such secondary valence influences take place when the two electrons constituting the covalent bond are shared unequally by the two atoms involved. The valence bond is still in existence; this is not a case of ionization, of complete atomic separation, with one partner possessing both bonding electrons (anion) and the other none (cation). However, the unequal sharing of the bonding electrons renders the less possessive atom partially (or weakly) positively charged, and the electron-enriched atom partially negatively charged.

Adsorptions occur from the attractions between oppositely charged sites resident on the atoms of the adsorbent. (The species that is adsorbed is generally called the *adsorbate*; that which does the adsorbing is labeled the *adsorbent*). Distinctions are sometimes made among *absorption* (into), *adsorption* (onto), and even sorption (when both mechanisms are included or the distinction cannot be made); and between chemical and physical *sorptions*. Chemical absorption is seen to involve stronger forces, as between ions. Weaker attractions, and hence more easily disrupted into desorption, as in the case of Van der Waals bonding, are physical adsorptions.

Adsorption may also be independent of charge phenomena. Hydrophobic adsorption, where the driving mechanism is the minimization of the free energy of a system, involves a joining together of lyophilic (hydrophobic) areas or molecules when these are dispersed or dissolved in a hydrophilic (aqueous) medium. These organic molecules, usually nonpolar or only weakly polar (hence, lyophilic or hydrophobic) and, therefore, only reluctantly or sparingly soluble in water, prefer to adsorb to activated carbon surfaces, which are also only weakly charged at best. This is in preference to remaining dissolved or suspended in water with its strong polar character. The phenomena involved are a fulfillment of the alchemist's dictum that "like dissolves (or attracts) like." It is for this reason that adsorption can be thought of as being competitive with solution chemistry: The less soluble, the more easily adsorbed; and vice versa. The effects of molecular weight; molecular shape effects such as branching; polarity; and solubility upon adsorption by carbon were all detailed in the literature for a large number of organic compounds (Giusti et al., 1974; Bahrani and Martin, 1976). In general, surface area and pore size of the adsorbent along with the particle size and shape of the adsorbate are most important. Indeed, the rate of adsorption is seen as being governed inversely by the diameter of the adsorbate species.

Activated Carbon

Granular activated carbon, widely employed for its adsorptive qualities, comes from many sources. Each has its champion, whether on the basis of efficiency, cost, or perceived cost effectiveness. Activated carbons derived from coconut or pecan shells seem to be widely endorsed. They are harder and therefore more resistant to generating fines. The GAC can be prepared also from bituminous coal; and from numerous materials of cellulosic origins that can be converted to charcoal by being heated at about 450 °C (900 °F) in an atmosphere that is restricted in oxygen so that combustion does not take place. This destructive distillation of the original substance drives off whatever is volatile at that temperature, and the residue is termed charcoal. The ground-up charcoal is then activated by being roasted at 1,000 to 1,100 °C (about 1,900 to 2,000 °F). The mechanism of creation of the active sites and also their exact nature are known largely by conjecture. The sites, and the activity of the carbon, correlate with iodine numbers, a measure of unsaturation, and with the presence of some oxygenated groupings. Water treatment generally uses GACs having iodine numbers above 900. Whatever the nature of the activated sites, they are very effective in adsorbing a myriad of molecular species, whether by charge attraction, hydrogen bonding, hydrophobic attraction, or other adsorptive mechanisms. Higher iodine numbers are more conducive to TOC adsorption. Chlorine removal is relatively independent of that property.

The activated carbon granules are highly porous. Depending upon the carbon, the porous structure may be regular or highly irregular. GAC from bituminous coals is said to give more regular pores than nut shell carbons. They are useful in liquid applications; the other in gas phase usage. The adsorptive properties for specific molecules are believed to be governed by the pore sizes and shapes. Typical GACs used in water treatment have pore-size distributions from 5 to 10,000 angstroms. (Sodium ions may be a few angstroms in diameter; organic molecules may be several hundred.) The surface area of GAC is enormous, typically 1,000 square meters per gram. Michaud (1988) calculated that 1 cubic foot of GAC, about 25 pounds, has a surface area of nearly 5 square miles. It is this extensive surface that favors the adsorption phenomenon.

The water quality may be affected by the particular carbon used, and different waters seem to perform better with different carbons. The choices to be made are usually not too well directed by technical evaluations. It seems fair to say that

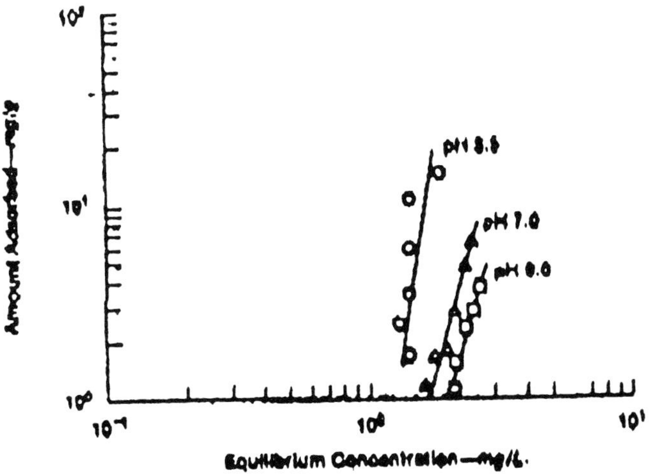

Figure 7-16. Adsorption isotherms for humic acid (A) on carbon (C); effect of pH.
Weber et al. (1983), Courtesy, American Water Works Association

which grade of carbon of what type is best for a given water requires appraisal by trial and error. However, the choice is perhaps too often made on the basis of price.

The carbon is treated in a furnace to render it into its activated form, into a structure amenable to being adsorptive. The carbon emerges from the hot furnace both activated and sterile. To ensure its retaining its relative freedom from organisms at the time of its loading into a carbon bed, at least one manufacturer gamma-irradiates the carbon, contained in 5-gallon plastic cans, just prior to its being loaded.

Granulated activated carbon yields extractables originating from the mineral ash resident in the charcoal. This gives rise to alkaline oxides such as magnesium oxide (MgO), calcium oxide (CaO), sodium oxide (Na_2O), and potassium oxide (K_2O). As water extractables, these oxides can raise the pH as much as 2 points, and can cause a hardness inimicable to RO operations. This makes for prolonged rinse-up times. Acid-washed grades of GAC are, therefore, made available. Acid washing will yield activated carbons that will produce cleaner effluents of lower pH. The acid washing can be performed in situ during the preconditioning soak cycle by adding about 0.5 liters of 35% hydrochloric acid (concentrated HCl) per foot of activated carbon in the bed. For critical operations, double or triple acid quantities may be employed. The overnight soaking is followed by backwashing to an acid-free effluent. Obviously, an acid-resistant vessel for housing the GAC must be used. Plastic constructions of PVC, of acrylonitrile-butadiene-styrene (ABS) polymer, or of most epoxides are suitable; mild steel, stainless steel, lead, copper, and galvanized iron are not. The acid-washed GAC is commercially available.

Acid treatment also removes aluminum, which might otherwise form difficult-to-solubilize aluminum silicates.

It is not possible to predict when the finite adsorptive capacity of carbon beds will be reached. That point in time must be assessed by measuring organic breakthrough levels, as by means of TOC analyzers. Regeneration of the carbon bed by alternating cycles of water and sodium hydroxide solutions of varying strengths serves to restore its adsorptive capacity, but only to a limited extent. Therefore, the bed's adsorptive capacity inevitably decreases progressively. In one case where activated carbon was being used to remove organic adsorbents, but primarily hydrogen sulfide (H_2S), regeneration with caustic restored the bed to an 80% to 85% capacity (Pope and Federici, 1989). More usually, such high degrees of bed recovery are not attained. Regeneration with sodium hydroxide is an onerous chore. It can easily take more than a day, especially in critical applications where a thorough removal of the caustic rinse is essential. In the instances cited above, Pope and Federici found that regeneration times of 5 to 15 days were required. Such a time interval would usually be excessive. However, rinsing the regenerated bed free of sodium hydroxide is not easily accomplished.

(See page 373). Where long rinse-up times are involved, continual use of the water system could necessitate another GAC bed in standby capacity.

Carbon Fines and Backwashing

The deep carbon beds are, in effect, depth-type filters. Thus they accumulate particulate matter and in time develop increasing pressure drops. This necessitates their being cleansed by backwashing. To enable this operation to be carried out, a freeboard of some 50% within the carbon bed shell is required. Backwashing is also required to rid the bed of carbon fines, which are generated by the abrasion of the carbon granules against one another as in steaming operations, in rebedding, and even in backwashing itself. The creation of fines is undesirable. For this reason harder (more abrasion-resistant) carbon types, such as from coconut shell, are advised.

Prior to bed reloading with new or pretreated carbon, it is better if the fines can be removed in a separate facility, perhaps by the carbon suppliers. Backwashing a new carbon bed to rid it of fines can be a messy job. Preflushed carbon commands a premium price, of course.

It is best for the carbon bed shell to be equipped with five valves. One, on the top, permits downward flow of the feedwater. The second, at the bottom, allows the treated water to flow from the bed. The third valve, also on the bottom of the bed shell, permits the backwash stream to enter. The fourth, on the top, allows the upflowing backwash waters to exit the tank or shell into the system via depth-type filters of about 10-μm nominal rating. The fifth valve, also on top, is to permit the backflow drainage to be dumped directly when the carbon fines being removed are especially plentiful. (This would spare the filters for more normal use.) The bottom distributor collector design for the bottom of the bed is important. One suitable type has slotted openings of about 10 μm in width to restrain the passage of the fines. The backwash rate is slower than for sand beds. The backwash rate should be less for smaller-sized carbon granules lest they be carried out of the bed. A commonly used carbon tolerates a backwash of 5 to 6 gpm/ft^2. Typically, the backwash rate does not exceed the service rate. Unlike deep-bed (multimedia) filters, backwashing of carbon beds seldom needs larger water lines. As will be seen, however, the backwashing of carbon is an irksome chore.

The need for backwashing is usually signaled by excessive pressure drops across the bed, although the practice may be automated to a timed cycle. The rates of backwash will vary with the mesh size of the GAC. Although backwashing will help to remove debris and particulate matter from the carbon beds, it will not rejuvenate them because it will essentially not remove the adsorbed material. Periodic backwashing serves also to correct the channeling to which all deep-beds constructions are liable.

The short life of activated carbon beds in the adsorption of organics is their chief limitation. Steamings, usually 10 to 30 minutes, serve to rejuvenate them somewhat by removing the more volatile adsorbents. Inevitably, repeated steamings become less efficacious. Carbon beds are usually replaced semi-annually or annually.

Sanitizing of Carbon Beds

The very act of chlorine removal renders water susceptible to organism invasion, perhaps from the carbon bed itself. As the top layers of the bed remove the chlorine from the water, the lower layers—moist, nutrient-rich, and unexposed to chlorine—are conducive to organism proliferation. Examples exist where carbon beds have served as sources of organism contamination and concomitant pyrogenicity.

The use of carbon beds requires, therefore, a means of sanitizing them. This poses no problem when the carbon container is made of stainless steel, rubber, or epoxy-coated carbon steel. Hard rubber liners that can endure 250 °F (121 °C) are available. These are known to yield extractables that are acceptable. A thin film, some few mils of epoxy coating, may prove less durable. However, less expensive installations may not withstand the corrosive action of sanitizing steam or of hot water. Therein lies the sanitizing problem.

The effective control of microorganism growth in carbon beds is otherwise difficult and expensive. At present there is no completely satisfactory way of controlling such organism growths.* Le Chavallier et al. (1984) found that organisms ensconsed on activated carbon particles, whether because sheltered in cracks and crevices or from adaptations making for their survival, exhibited a heightened ability to resist sanitizations. Counts coming out of the carbon beds can be 600 cfu/mL. The daily backwashing of carbon beds with chlorinated water can reduce counts from 10 to 80 cfu/mL. A 15-minute backwash followed by a 5-minute rinse is advocated.

Hot water or steam seem the best methods for sanitizing carbon beds. The use of hot water releases endotoxin from used activated carbon beds, according to Husted (1995). This should supply a desirable cleansing. The use is made of steam at atmospheric pressure, but this is more expensive than hot water. Furthermore, the steam, being a vapor, has a low viscosity. This may predispose it to avoid dense sections of the bed, and to find channels through it. Water, having the higher viscosity of a liquid, would have less of a tendency to channel. For this reason, hot water would seem to be the better sanitizer. For this reason too, "bumping" the carbon bed to eliminate channels is a recommended practice.

A Malaysian pharmaceutical company mixes steam and water in a suitable

*At least one facility expert has utilized hydrogen peroxide on his carbon beds to remove adsorbed organics as well as to sanitize. To the 150 to 200 gallons of water left in the bed was added 33% hydrogen peroxide. The reaction could be explosive. As a precaution, the manhole cover was removed from the carbon bed. The practice was found effective, but is too risky to be recommended.

mixer to attain water temperatures close to 100 °C. The heated water is fed concurrent and countercurrent for 40 minutes, mornings and evenings daily, to achieve carbon bed effluents containing as few as 10 cfu/mL.

Obviously, the liner of the shell containing the carbon must be capable of withstanding the steam. Brass or copper piping is suitable, but PVC piping, particularly prevalent in older installations, is not. Clean steam is required. Plant steam containing corrosion-inhibiting amines is not suitable for high-purity water systems.

Treatments with caustic rinses serve to sanitize carbon beds, because of their high pH. The caustic can require 24 hours and longer to be removed by aqueous rinsing, however, particularly if the water is cold. Caustic remnants may have deleterious effects upon downstream RO filters. (Indeed, it is stated anecdotally that a caustic treatment, of unspecified strength, resulted in the catastrophic breakup of carbon granules, of unspecified identity, with the devastating production of carbon fines throughout the system.)

Carbon beds are dry when first constructed. Heterotrophic organisms such as the pseudomonads common to aqueous habitats do not survive desiccation. Therefore, the dry carbon is relatively free of such vegetative microbes. If the water to be introduced into the new (dry) bed is first treated with UV before it encounters the carbon, this should serve to prolong its freedom from such organisms.

The large surface area of carbon beds provides ample space for biofilm formation and hence for pyrogen generation. Effluent waters from carbon beds were found to contain from 10 to 1,000 times more organisms than the incoming municipally treated waters (Fernandez et al., 1986). Geldreich et al. (1985) and Ridgway et al. (1981) put the proportion at 10 to 100 times higher than the incoming waters.

Collentro believed that carbon beds can effectively be sanitized by being heated to 80 °C. and then being allowed to cool; this should be done once every 1 to 4 weeks; the carbon should be replaced every 3 months (Collentro, 1985a and b).

Most important of all, the carbon bed should be kept under constant recirculation to discourage organism growth. The circulation rate can be slow, as low as 1 gpm/ft^2. Manfredi (1991) suggested the rate that results from a linear velocity of 5 ft/sec. through the water supply pipe. A low-horsepower pump could be dedicated to recirculation through an ultraviolet light.

Ultraviolet lamps are often used with carbon beds, to treat the exiting water. Continuous circulation in conjunction with UV lamps is even more desirable. Nominally rated filters, as of 3 to 10 μm, should be used downstream of the carbon beds to retain the carbon fines. Ultraviolet lamps should be employed downstream of these to control the organisms commonly emanating from the carbon beds.

Organism Control by pH Management

While each organism species has its own optimum pH range, bacteria are generally favored at pH neutral to slightly alkaline, and yeasts and molds favor neutral to slightly acidic. Most commonly encountered bacteria do not grow and may not survive at pHs below 4.6. Such pHs characterize waters emanating from cation-exchange beds. Haraguchi et at. (1987) suggested, therefore, the placement of the carbon bed between twin bed ion-exchangers to benefit from the bactericidal self-sanitizing effects of low pH. Nevertheless, such an arrangement, however beneficial to the carbon bed, would expose the cation-exchange resin to attack by the chlorine present in the water.

It is not an uncommon experience, however, for carbon beds, particularly when their design is compromised by the needs for economy, to be seen as troublesome in terms of organism control.

Successful Carbon Bed Operations

One example of a very successful carbon bed operation may serve to focus what can obviously be a diverse and sometimes contradictory experience. A pharmaceutical company has for some 2 decades now been utilizing a carbon bed downstream from sand beds and separated by filters from downstream ion-exchange beds. The carbon tank or shell is 6 feet high and 54 inches in diameter, and contains about 50% of freeboard. The normal effluent rate is about 120 gpm. The beds are backwashed twice daily, largely to cleanse them of iron deposits. The backwash is at the rate of 200 to 250 gpm. Microbial assays are performed on alternating days, thrice weekly. Microbial alert limits are set at 600 to 700 cfu/mL. The action limit is 1,000 cfu/mL for 3 consecutive days on the cold water system, ascertained as total heterotrophic plate counts. This action limit invokes hot (65 °C) water sanitization. The heated water is flushed into the bed and is then trickled to a total volume of 500 to 1,000 gallons in an overnight operation during a weekend. On one occasion, a bed required weekly sanitizing for a period of some 6 months before the bacterial burden was successfully maintained below 1,000 cfu/mL with only more occasional interventions. Carbon fines seem not to be a problem. Fines are removed from new beds by an upward flush (backwash), barely vigorous enough to overflow the fines to drain. This backflow fines-removal is done overnight. The successful operation of this carbon bed is ascribed to its continuous recirculative flow from its inception. The flow, through a 1- to 1/2-inch line capable of delivering about 30 gpm, is at a minimum of from 25 to 40 gpm (approximately 10 to 2 gpm/ft^2) regardless of whether water is being supplied to the downstream ion-exchange beds or not. The return loop to the carbon bed is by way of the preceding sand beds. In summary, the three elements of this carbon bed's maintenance are: continuous recirculation, twice-daily automated backwashes, and weekly sanitizing with 65 °C hot water.

At another pharmaceutical installation, the carbon beds are sanitized by the use of steam. Rebedding is performed every 3 years, and new carbon beds are initially given two steam sanitizations. The liner of the carbon shell is of an epoxy steam-resistant composition. The pressure differential across the carbon bed is 5 to 8 pounds per square inch gauge (psig). There is no pressure build-up over the use period. Each bed is steam-sanitized every 48 hours for 2 hours, and the temperature reached is at least 86 °C (180 °F). After each steaming, the carbon beds are backwashed to drain for 30 minutes at a flowrate of 84 gpm, somewhat more than the 70 gpm service flow. During the backwash the carbon bed is "bumped" to help loosen its compaction. The backwash is followed by a 6-minute forward rinse to help settle the bed. The effluent from the carbon bed is tested on alternate days. The bacterial counts are usually close to zero, though on occasion there are bacterial excursions. These are, however, rapidly corrected by the steam sanitizing.

Backwashing serves also to remove whatever particulate matter the carbon bed, as any other deep bed, accumulates in its action as a filter. Surprisingly, there are those who advise against backwashing. They believe the action may more widely scatter the trapped organisms. These are assumed to be retained within a finite zone presumably near the top of the bed. However, the purpose of backwashing is to float out retained particles, whether organisms or carbon fines, by flushing them out of the bed with a flowing stream. If this is not done, the pressure buildup within the bed could interfere with the proper water flow.

As a general rule, a daily backwash of carbon beds is recommended. A backwash is also indicated to remove the fines generated by steam sanitizing. Such sanitizing should be done long before the water exiting the carbon bed gives TNTC (too numerous to count) organism readings. Otherwise, RO membrane surfaces may become occluded and/or DI columns may become clogged. The use of filters downstream of the beds to retain the carbon fines, usually 3- to 10-μm-rated depth types, is suggested. At some pharmaceutical houses, microporous membrane filtration is utilized to more reliably retain microbes originating in deep-bed operations or in ion-exchange columns. The practice is, however, not widely emulated because of its cost.

It is commonly believed that carbon-bed sanitization using oxidizing re-agents, including the chlorine and free-chlorine reagents usually employed for such purposes, are ineffective because they react with and are destroyed by the carbon.

LeChevallier et al. (1984) found the organisms associated with carbon to be very resistant to chlorine. Presumably, these bacteria are protected by lodgment within cracks in the carbon, and are shielded by biofilm glycocalyx production.

It may be, however, that reaction rates and sanitizer deliveries can avail. At slow flowrates and diluted concentrations of sanitizers, destruction by carbon may predominate. At higher flowrates and concentrations, however, the competitive bactericidal reaction may occur (at least to some extent) at the more remote locales within the bed; these may ordinarily not be reached because slower flows of weaker doses are destroyed before they can get there. Thus, one pharmaceutical company sanitizes their carbon beds using 0.2 ppm of ozone in water periodically recirculated through the carbon beds. Organism counts are reduced, not eliminated. Presumably bacteria upon the carbon granule surfaces are destroyed. By means of this technique, the microbial growth within the carbon beds is kept under control. The ozone is destroyed, and carbon consumed, by interaction within the bed. The technique of using stronger concentrations of sanitizers more rapidly recirculated through the carbon beds, not yet widely practiced, is worthy of trial. Its price would be a more rapid consumption of the carbon bed.

The difficulties of sanitizing carbon beds has led many to eschew their use; and to manage organic removal instead by the use of macroreticulated anion-exchange resins, and chlorine removal by the chemical injection of sodium metabisulfite or of other reducing agents.

Chlorine Removal by Bisulfite

Chlorine can be eliminated by reduction reactions involving sulfites, bisulfites, or metabisulfites. The resulting sulfate ion can be removed by anion exchange. This action is often recommended as an avoidance of the problems associated with carbon beds, particularly their sanitization. It should be noted, however, that sulfite-digesting bacteria can contaminate the bisulfite solution being added to the water. The bisulfite units require sanitization. As an overview it can be stated that the installation of a carbon bed to remove chlorine requires an initial capital expenditure. The cost of a bisulfite addition system lies in its maintenance. About 30% of chlorine removal is presently accomplished using sodium bisulfite or one of its like-acting chemical relations.

Bisulfite in the form of an 8% solution is fed by a pulse-speed metering pump, as signaled by the feedback from a chlorine-residual meter. Unfortunately, the stoichiometric proportion is not that easily assured. Oxygen in the water serves to consume the bisulfite ion, and the chlorine content changes as it is destroyed.

A bisulfite concentration of 5 to 10 times the chlorine concentration of the feedwater is usually maintained (Sinha, 1990). Being a reducing agent, bisulfite is itself oxidized by the oxygen present in air and water. Therefore, bisulfite solutions deteriorate with time. Agitation of bisulfite solutions also promotes their contacts with oxygen and their deterioration.

Upon being oxidized by the chlorine (which thereby becomes destroyed by being reduced) the bisulfite ions become converted to sulfate ions; the chlorine forms chloride ions. Obviously sodium ions are added in the process.

There are those who consider it poor technique to introduce ions into a water system undergoing ultimate deionization. The use of bisulfite thus offends them.

Then, too, the use of chemical feeders may be of dubious reliability.

The chlorine is usually monitored randomly or on a maintenance schedule at best. On-line monitoring is infrequently employed. Where excess bisulfite is fed, the chlorine level is always zero. Therefore, chlorine monitors are of no use. Oxidation-Reduction Potential monitors should be used in their place. Their cost is about $1,500 (in 1994). When the intent is to permit the remaining presence, say of about 0.1 ppm chlorine, a chlorine monitor (about $2,000) is indicated.

The sodium sulfite, bisulfite, or metabisulfite are solids packaged in 90-pound bags. The bisulfite can also be obtained in the anion-exchange resin form (instead of the usual anion-exchange hydroxyl form.) The bisulfite anion-exchange resin, while used in the nuclear power generating industry, is expensive. Moreover, the resin regeneration kinetics are unfavorable. Where the regeneration of the anion-exchange hydroxide form requires 3 pounds of sodium hydroxide, the bisulfite form uses 14 pounds of sodium hydroxide.

Opinions differ on whether carbon or bisulfite is more suited to the removal of chlorine. The inclination is to avoid carbon and its fines upstream of an RO. To know exactly how much bisulfite to use, one should know the type of chlorine compound used, whether Cl_2 or chloramine, or other; and the adequacy of the contact time. Slower-reacting chlorine compounds require more time, translating to slower flow velocities, in order to be reduced and removed. Chlorine dioxide and the chloramines are among these. Too much bisulfite creates an unnecessary stress on the ion-exchange resins and/or RO units downstream. The bisulfite is generally automatically added by a pump activated by the chlorine level in the water. A failure to deliver the bisulfite adequately could result in the hydrolytic destruction of polyamide RO units. Indeed, in an exaggerated response to such possibilities, one installation was observed to rely upon both carbon beds and bisulfite addition.

Increasingly, chlorine is not removed from the water streams but is permitted to enter the deionizing resin beds. There it serves to sanitize against bacterial growth. The price is some degradative loss of the resin capacity. In one 60-gpm deionizing system, water treated with 0.3 to 0.5 ppm of chlorine is passed through twin deionizing resin beds followed by two mixed beds. The anion-exchange resin loses about 10% of its capacity over a 2-year period. The emerging water is free of chlorine and of chloride ions.

In one instance, the chlorine penetrated to the anion-exchange resin, causing by its degradative action the release of amines. By contrast, its consumption of the cation-exchange resin (the first encountered) presumably is spent largely on cross-link scission, as evinced by the high moisture uptake value of the altered resin. Where the chlorine is intentionally passed onto the DI resins, it would perhaps be best if the rate of flow confined its reaction to the cation-exchange bed.

Sinha (1990) in Figure 7-17 shows the effect of chlorine on the resistivity and the TOC levels for two primary mixed-beds in series after 2 hours of operation involving 0.3 ppm free chlorine. The feedwater resistivity, originally 17.9 megohm-cm, became 17.2 megohm-cm after the first bed. The original TOC value of 65 ppb changed to 80 ppb. All the chlorine was consumed. The water leaving the first mixed-bed and entering the second contained no free chlorine, and had a resistivity of 17.2 megohm-cm and a TOC content of 80 ppb. Upon exiting the second mixed bed the water had a resistivity of 17.8 megohm-cm and a TOC value of 68 ppb. The service flow was at 0.85 gal/ft^3

Indeed, the chlorine may be removed sacrificially in the softening process itself (while simultaneously acting as a sanitizer) by reacting with the cation-exchange resin doing the softening. This loss of resin can be accepted economically where the chlorine concentration is about 0.3 to 0.5 ppm.

The option to dispense with carbon beds is not available where chloramines are present. Bisulfite is not sufficiently efficacious in neutralizing these compounds.

Where reliance is upon chlorine neutralization by chemical injection, use should be made of an in-line continuous chlorine analyzer mounted in a bleed stream, and arranged to control a proportioning pump having variable speed to feed the sodium metabisulfite solution. This system can be alarmed against accidental exhaustion or interruption of the chlorine-reducing reagent. (Chlorine can also be analyzed for amperometrically, which is an accurate titration; whereas the colorimetric reaction more commonly used is quick but is not accurate. Ortho-toluidine, formerly used as a colorimetric indicator, is considered carcinogenic.) Use of the in-line analyzer and proportioning pump is to make certain that the life expectancy and usefulness of any thin-film composite RO unit downstream is not threatened. The economic justification of such an injection system to remove the chlorine by chemical neutralization becomes easier for larger systems where the costs of the volumes of carbon used are large enough to balance out the expenses of the chlorine analyzer, the injection pump, and their mutual servomechanism.

In summary, four functions are generally assigned the carbon beds: to lower the oxidative demand of the water by adsorbing organics; to decrease fouling damage to the DI resin by removal of humic acids, fulvic acids, and other organics; to remove residual chlorine; and to adsorb trihalomethanes (Nebel and Nebel, 1984).

Filters are used downstream of carbon beds to restrain the carbon fines that are inevitably sloughed into the flowing water. Traditionally, 3- to 10-μm-rated depth filters are used. Present practices include microporous membrane filters to restrain organisms. These must of course be maintained suitably, including sanitization. Filters are also used upstream of the ultraviolet units, since particles reduce the efficiency of these units.

FDA Observations Regarding Carbon Beds

An FDA inspector observed that, "The carbon filter is probably the weakest element in any DI system from the standpoint of microbial attack" (Farina). Standard operating procedures (SOPs) should be established and implemented to regularly backflush and/or periodically sanitize these beds—by steam, if their construction materials permit; otherwise by hot water, if possible. It is clear that carbon beds require periodic microbial monitoring. Monitoring schedules are not stipulated. They come to be developed on an historical basis derived initially from frequent testing, which eventually becomes less frequent. The FDA intends that the drug manufacturer have the written records to show that such monitoring is regularly scheduled and performed, and that any indicated corrections are instituted in timely fashion. Carbon beds can signal their need for cleaning or replacement by development of high pressure differentials. Such clogging, possibly the result of the organism proliferation, can then be attended to. Regrettably, the exhaustion of a carbon bed's capacity to remove organic materials does not manifest itself by an increase in the pressure drop. Although all too seldom practiced, the maintenance of the carbon bed under dynamic recirculative flow would serve to eliminate the organism proliferation characteristic of static systems.

To prevent stagnation in DI resin beds, a recirculation rate of 1.5 to 2.0 gpm/ft^2 of cross-sectional bed area (6.1 to 8.2 Lpm/cm^2) is recommended. Perhaps

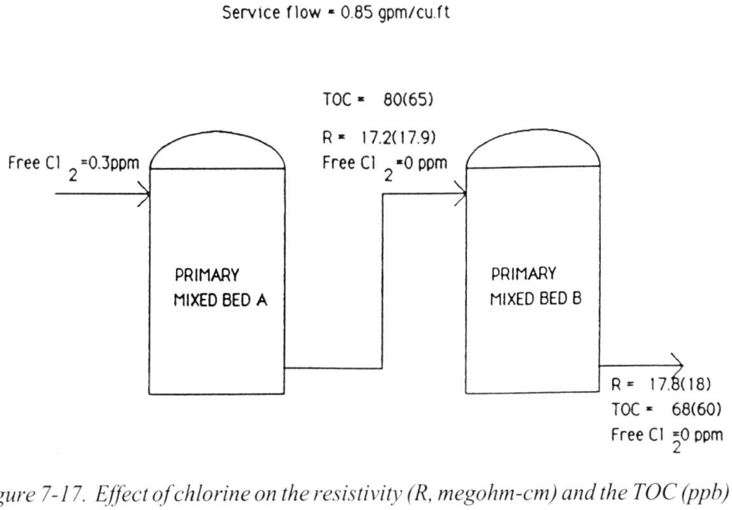

Figure 7-17. Effect of chlorine on the resistivity (R, megohm-cm) and the TOC (ppb) levels for the two primary mixed-beds, in series, after 2 hours of operation. Resistivities and TOC values before chlorine injection are shown inside the parentheses.

Sinha (1990); Courtesy, *Ultrapure Water* journal

such a recirculatory flowrate would serve also for carbon beds.

Hudack and Terribile (1989) recommended a 6- to 10-gpm/ft^2 recirculatory flow through twin beds, and a 20-gpm/ft^2 flow through mixed beds. Substantiating data were not given, nor was the method disclosed whereby these figures were produced. Perhaps such recirculatory flowrates would serve also for carbon beds.

Circulation of the water through the carbon bed may raise its temperature because of the pump action. To compensate for this, some of the heated water is sent to drain through a high temperature divert. The discarded water is replaced by colder chlorine-containing water that enters by way of the multimedia beds and the softener. This serves to replace some of the chlorine that is removed by the carbon. Some sanitizing benefit is sought thereby.

In an effort to secure adequate carbon bed capacity, even in standby, while maintaining a circulatory mode, the multimedia bed may be followed by two carbon beds in parallel operated simultaneously and continuously at, say, 70% of capacity. If one of the beds requires being shut down, the overall operation can still be continued.

In any given situation relating to any particular purification device or process, it is necessary to weigh the potential advantages proffered by the treatment against its shortcomings and limitations. In the case of carbon beds, if they begin to impose undue burdens by inserting high bacterial loads into the system, or by imposing the need for too-frequent sanitizing, then they can be avoided. Bisulfite or entrance into the ion-exchange resin beds, by a few tenths ppm per mL of chlorine, can be used to remove chlorine; and ion-exchange resins beds can be used to remove organics, which usually come to possess some ionic charges as a consequence of having undergone some degree of oxidation. It may not be possible to regenerate such resins totally, but they can gainfully be employed nonetheless. Also, ultrafiltration can be used to remove organic matter. However, there is a history of the successful use of carbon beds. They do require a proper maintenance. At least two companies, as previously detailed, have to good purpose long employed carbon beds, one for almost 3 decades.■

CHAPTER 8

ION EXCHANGE

There are three principal means whereby ionic components may be removed from aqueous solutions. Deionization, or demineralization, as some term it, by use of ion-exchange resins is one. Distillation is another. Reverse osmosis, whether pressure or electrically driven, is the third. Distillation is seen as being prodigal with energy costs. Reverse osmosis is higher than ion exchange in its capital costs, but lower in chemical costs. Reverse osmosis is also more demanding of feedwater pretreatment than is ion exchange.

The use of deionizing (DI) ion-exchange beds may well result in the bacterial contamination of their effluent waters. The beds are havens for the growth of organisms that enter with the feedwaters. Thus DI beds can also serve as sources of endotoxins derived from waterborne organisms. Ion-exchange therefore is not a USP- or FDA-approved method for preparing Water for Injection. It may, however, be used to prepare USP Purified Water. In pharmaceutical settings, all three principal purification methods, albeit in a proper sequence, may be used to prepare compendial water. In the semiconductor industry, use of ion exchange is widespread, usually in combination with RO and usually subsequent to it. Deionization by ion exchange is altogether a very important and widely used water purification method.

Deionization by Ion-Exchange Resins

Ion exchange is, with the possible exception of distillation, the oldest method used for the large-scale preparation of deionized water; and is referenced extensively in the literature (Anderson, 1979; Hill and Lorch, 1981; Owens, 1985; Applebaum, 1968; Calman and Simon, 1969; Strauss and Kunin, 1980; Kunin and Barrett, 1979; Kunin and McGarvey, 1955). It may be instructive to review the significance of some of the operational features of ion exchange; and to update our information on the relevant practices. Ion-exchange reactions are governed by equilibria and/or reaction kinetics.

Nomenclature

The pertinent functional group of the cation-exchange resin is its anion, and that of the anion-exchange resin is its cation: Ion exchangers are named not for what they are but rather for what they do. Thus the resin whose seat of activity is its anionic constituent is called a cation-exchange resin; the compound whose mode of action derives from its cationic moiety is called an anion-exchange resin. There are, unfortunately, examples in the literature where the cation-exchange resin has been called the cation resin or the cation component, while its anion-exchange counterpart is called the anion resin or the anion component. Such informal jargon is best avoided.

Strong and Weak Electrolyte Ion Exchangers

Both the acid and base ion-exchange resins exist in both strong and weak electrolyte forms (Figure 8-1). Strength is measured by the relative degree of ionic dissociation that characterizes the functional acidic or basic group that is substituent on the organic molecules forming the resin beads. The cross-linking of the organic moieties of these molecules serves to insolubilize them, thus rendering them nonmigrating, fixed in space on the resin bed. The ion species that are the same as the resin-anchored ions are called *co-ions*; their labile ionic companions of opposite charge are called *counterions*.

The strongly acidic type is almost always the polysulfonic acid derivative of polystyrene cross-linked through the agency of divinylbenzene. Electron resonance within the aromatic nucleus accounts for the strength of these acid groups. The sulfonic acid group substituent is highly dissociated in water. It has a strength equivalent to the first hydrogen ion* dissociation of aqueous sulfuric acid or even to that of hydrochloric acid:

$$H_2SO_4 <----> H^+ + HSO_4^- \qquad \text{Eq. 8-1}$$

The weakly acidic resins comprise cross-linked linear carboxylic acids in polymeric form, derivatives of acrylic and methacrylic acids:

$$R\text{-}COOH <----> RCOO^- + H^+ \qquad \text{Eq. 8-2}$$

Ion-exchange capacity, the ion-exchange equivalence per liter of resin, is greater for the weak acids because the functionality of their acidic groups is less diluted by the polyacrylate structure than is that of the stronger acids by the cross-linked polystyrene skeleton.

In aqueous media, the acidic ion-exchange molecules give rise to hydrogen ions, or more properly to hydronium ions:

$$R\text{-}SO_4H <----> RSO_4^- + H^+ \text{ (More } H^+\text{)} \qquad \text{Eq. 8-3}$$

$$R\text{-}COOH <----> RCOO^- + H^+ \text{ (Less } H^+\text{)} \qquad \text{Eq. 8-4}$$

$$H^+ + H_2O <----> H_3O^+ \qquad \text{Eq. 8-5}$$

The weakly acidic cation exchangers are not as fully ionized as their strongly acidic counterparts when used in their hydrogen form. Therefore they interchange with cations to a far more limited extent. When, however, alkalinity is present, as in the form of bicarbonate, carbonate, or hydroxide, the ionization of

*For convenience in representation, the hydrogen ion will be written as the proton, H^+, rather than in its more correct hydronium ion form, H_3O^+.

the weak acids is enhanced to the point where cation exchange may be significant. However, where divalent cation exchange does take place, it does so with great efficiency, because of the undissociated nature of the divalent cation weak-acid salt. Therefore weakly acidic cation exchange is used largely for the removal of water hardness. (Aranovitch and Ford, 1995).

The strongly basic ion exchangers are generally of two types; they owe their strengths, however, to the one structural feature they share. They are both quaternary ammonium bases. The chloromethylation of divinylbenzene cross-linked polystyrene, when followed by amination with trimethylamine, produces a polymeric benzyltrimethyl quaternary ammonium hydroxide, called Type I. When aminated instead by dimethylethanolamine, a different type of quaternary base, called Type II, is formed.

These two types of strongly basic ion exchangers differ chiefly in their propensities to exchange chloride and hydroxyl ions. Type I is somewhat more stable at higher temperatures. It can be regenerated at temperatures up to 50 or 60 °C (122 to 140 °F), as will shortly be discussed. The Type II is less stable thermally, but may be regenerated at up to 35 °C (95 °F). Actually, both types of resins undergo some decomposition even at room temperature. When first prepared, they have very high capacities. They lose some 5% to 10% of total capacity after a day or so. Thereafter, the Type I continues to lose capacity but

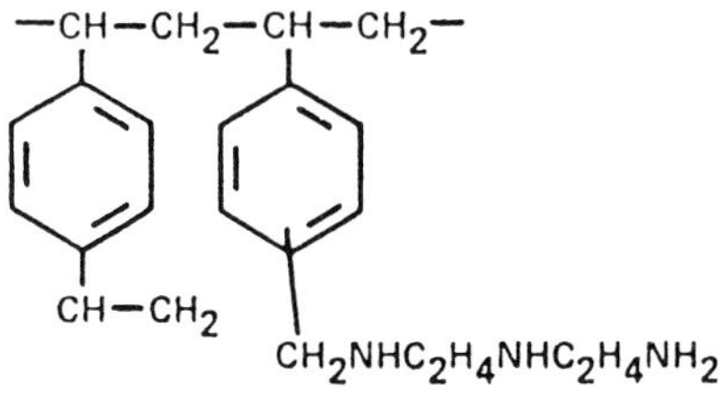

1. Weakly basic functionality

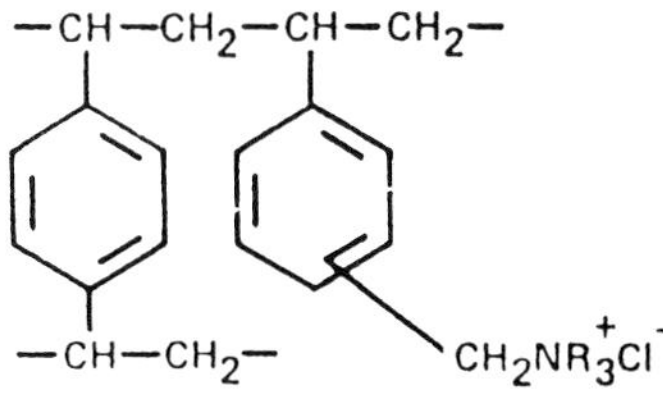

2. Strongly basic functionality

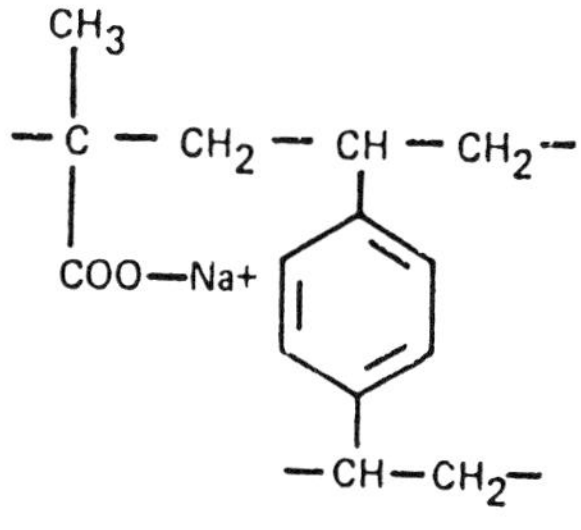

3. Weakly acidic functionality

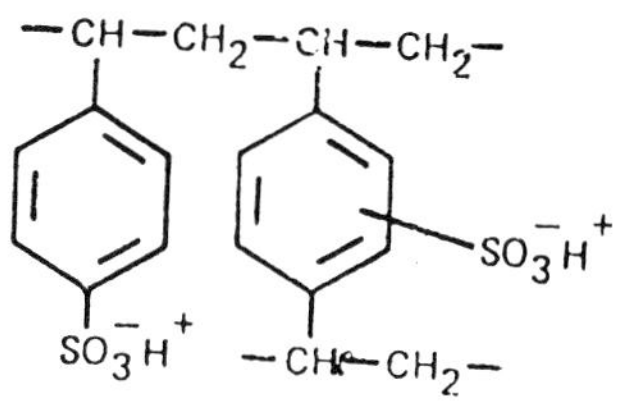

4. Strongly acidic functionality

Figure 8-1. Functional groups on anionic and cationic resins.
Kunin (1984); Courtesy, *Amber-Hi-Lites*

at a much slower constant rate. The Type II also levels off in a constant rate of capacity loss but at a somewhat higher rate. At room temperature, even with this constant diminution in capacity, the Type I can last for decades; the Type II can last for 5 years.

New Type I resins exude a fishy smell, caused by some few ppb of the trimethylamine that is one product of the Hofmann degradation to which these quaternary ammonium hydroxides are subject. Type II resins, on the other hand, give rise to minute quantities of acetaldehyde or ethanol, of a far less obnoxious odor. Because of the objectionable odor of Type I, it is the Type II resin that is often selected for use in perfumery and pharmaceutical settings. Both types are thermally stable, and hence free of odor, when they are in their salt forms. In addition to freedom from fishy odors, Type II strongly basic anion-exchange resin regenerates to a greater extent per pound of regenerant caustic used. At lower levels of regeneration, it is the more economical of the two resin types. When it does decompose thermally, it turns into a weakly basic tertiary amine resin. As a weakly basic resin, it will leak carbon dioxide and (soluble) silica. However, it will still be capable of removing chloride and sulfate ions. Regeneration of the Type II resin, it being more thermolabile than a Type I resin, should not be attempted at temperatures above 100 °F (38 °C). Type II resins are unsuited for polishing operations where the complete removal of weakly ionized materials is required.

Each type is fully dissociated ionically. They are both equivalent to sodium hydroxide in their basic strengths.

$$-CH_2-N^+(CH_3)_3OH^- \longleftrightarrow -CH_2-N^+(CH_3)_3 + OH^- \qquad \text{Eq. 8-6}$$

The weaker basic ion exchangers form a more diverse group of more complex structures. In essence, however, they are amine-like in character: for example, cross-linked polybenzyldimethylamine.

The weakly basic amine groups are not really ion exchangers. They pick up acids by forming onium-type addition compounds. The base strengths of the amine groups differ, depending upon the compositions of the amino-nitrogen substituents. There are also resins, intermediate in their strengths, based on their containing both amine groups and quaternary amine groups.

The economic penalty of deionization by ion-exchange resins derives from the character of the anion-exchange resins. They are more expensive, of lesser capacities, are less thermally stable, and cost more to regenerate.

The reason for the manufacture of both strong and weak resins is that the strong forms (highly dissociated into ions) are required to remove the ions of weak electrolytes (those that dissociate feebly), such as borates, soluble silica, and carbon dioxide. On the other hand, the weak electrolyte resins are preferred, when they can be used effectively, for the economics and ease of their regeneration.

Mechanisms Involved in Ion Exchange

The law of mass action. The ion-exchange resins responsible for deionization reactions are cross-linked polyelectrolytes immobilized by their organic structures. The avidity and completeness with which they exchange ions depend largely on two factors. The first of these is, for example as in the case of the cation-exchange resin, the concentration of the cations available for exchanging with the ionized hydrogen ion of the resin. The second is the concentration of hydrogen ions on the resin:

$$\begin{array}{c} R\text{-}SO_3\text{-}H \text{ <----> } RSO_3^- + H^+ \\ + \\ C^+ \text{ (cation)} \\ \downarrow\uparrow \\ RSO_3C + H^+ \end{array} \quad \text{Eq. 8-7}$$

According to the law of mass action, the greater the concentration of the exchanging cation, C^+, the greater the likelihood of its replacing H^+ from its association with the immobilized resin counterions, $R\text{-}SO_2\text{-}O^-$.

The law of mass action favors the ions with the greatest concentrations in their competition for pairing with the immobilized ion-exchange sites. The ion concentration, in turn, is dependent upon the temperature and the solvent polarity, as these influence the degree of ionization.

Some salts, the removal of whose ions is the object of the ion-exchange exercise, exist in aqueous solution in equilibrium form, however feeble their ionic dissociation may be:

$$AB \text{ <----> } A^+ + B^- \quad \text{Eq. 8-8}$$

On the other hand, many salts are completely dissociated even within the solid state of their crystal lattices:

$$Na^+Cl^- \text{ <----> } Na^+ + Cl^- \quad \text{Eq. 8-9}$$

When the aqueous solutions of such salts come into contact with the ion-exchange resins, the solution contains an ion mixture, for example, as of the following:

$$R\text{—}SO_3^- + H^+ + Ca^{2+} + SO_4^{2-} + Na^+ + Cl^- \quad \text{Eq. 8-10}$$

New equilibria can therefore become established:

$$(R\text{-}SO_3)_2Ca \text{ <----> } (R\text{-}SO_3)_2^{2-} + Ca^{2+} \quad \text{Eq. 8-11}$$

$$Na_2SO_4 \longleftrightarrow 2Na^+ + SO_4^{2-} \qquad \text{Eq. 8-12}$$

A similar circumstance involving ionic dissociation exists in the case of the basic ion-exchange resins. In this situation, the solution also contains a mixture of ions:

$$R\text{-}CH_2N^+R_3 + OH^- + Na^+ + Cl^- \qquad \text{Eq. 8-13}$$

However, all forms of the quaternary compounds, both the bases and the salts, are rather completely dissociated. The ion exchange is a statistical process based not only on the concentrations of the ions, but also on the selectivities that are an expression of the ionic charge densities that figure in the attractions, as well as the ionic radii that define the extent to which mutually attracted ions can approach one another.

The influence of Fajan's rule. The ease of ion replacement depends on such factors as ion concentration, temperature, and polarity or nonpolarity of the solvent; but it also depends largely on the charge densities of the competing ions and on the size of their radii. By charge density is meant the ratio of the charge to the ion size. The importance of radii size involves Fajan's rule.

The greater the charge density of a competing ion, the more likely its association with the ion exchanger, because the stronger the bonding attraction. How strong the ionic bonding is depends largely on the ionic radius, however. The smaller the ion, the closer it can approach the fixed opposite ion and the stronger the mutual attraction; and hence, the greater its selectivity.

The ionic radius of concern, however, is not that of the isolated ion, its crystallographic radius, but rather its radius as it exists in the aqueous solution surrounded by a shell of hydrating water molecules. The smaller the ion, the more closely it can approach water molecules, and the more avidly and plentifully it can be hydrated by them. The proton, the hydrogen ion, the smallest of all cations, may thus be surrounded by many water molecules. In its hydrated form, therefore, the smallest ion tends to become, conversely, the largest. Thus the proton is easily displaced from association with, say, cross-linked polystyrene sulfonic acid anions by the potassium ion, which, although crystallographically larger than the proton, has only five or six waters of hydration, and whose effective ionic radius in the hydrated state is therefore smaller. If alcohol is added to the aqueous salt solution, the degree of hydration is reduced, and the hydrogen ion or proton is less selectively replaced in ion-exchange reactions. Actually, ionic radii relate to the activity coefficients of the ions.

The degree of ion hydration follows Fajan's rule: The smaller the crystallographic ion radius, the greater the degree of hydration. Also, the greater the charge (or more properly, the charge density), and thus the ratio of charge to ion size, the greater the extent of hydration. In any case, the ion-exchange selectivity results in barium ions being preferred over strontium ions, which are preferred over calcium ions. The magnesium ion, being the smallest of the alkaline earth series, is the most hydrated. It therefore has the largest ionic radius in aqueous solutions; can approach the anion only at the greatest distance; and hence, has the least selectivity shown it. When monocharged ions are listed in decreasing order by the selectivity shown by their fixed anion, they are potassium, sodium, lithium, and hydrogen, in reverse of the crystallographic ion size and as a direct reflection of the hydrated ionic radius.

In the case of the anion-exchange resins, the hydroxyl ion also has a large ionic radius because, being relatively small in its crystallographic ion dimensions, it carries with it a large envelope of hydrating water molecules. Being strongly hydrated, the hydroxyl ion is therefore least preferred in ion-exchange reactions.

The effectiveness of the weak electrolyte ion-exchange resin depends strongly on pH, which of course influences the degree of protonization of the exchanger. Weakly basic anion-exchange resins therefore function best in acid media, below pH 7; while weakly acidic cation exchangers work best in basic media, above pH 7.

Ion selectivity. Selectivity has another facet wherein ion exchangers are concerned, one derived from the less-than-complete ionic dissociations of given molecular entities. Thus in weak acids the proton is selectively preferred by the fixed acid because its combination forms an undissociated covalent bond that drives the combining action to completion.

Metal ions such as copper (Cu^{2+}) often exhibit strong selectivities because they form chelates, or undissociated complexes whose undissociation tends to drive the ion exchange to completion.

The uptake of iodine by strongly basic anion exchange resin in the iodide form is another case in point. It is almost impossible to strip iodine from the resin without oxidizing it to the iodate. The bonding involves stable associative compound formation that is not of an ionic type (McGarvey, 1990).

$$RI + I_2 \longleftrightarrow RI_3 \qquad \text{Eq. 8-14}$$

It is therefore difficult to remove by attempted manipulations of ionic equilibria.

It is possible to give a ranking to the ion selectivities listed in Tables 8-1 and 8-2, as based upon the equilibrium constants of these ions relative to the resin-fixed ion-exchange counterions. These numbers find expression as the selectivity coefficients of the ions. They reflect the relative affinities of the ions for the appropriate ion-exchange groups.

When two or more ions are present (as is almost universally the case in practical situations), the equilibrium composition of the counterion, the fixed exchanger group in the resin, is a resultant of both the individual ion concentrations (mass action law) and the selectivity of the resin group for each ion. In effect, the selectivity coefficients mirror the relative competition of each ion for the counterion. It is this competition that determines which ion will break through the resin bed in any given situation. It has a major effect on the propensity of an ion-exchange bed to remove low concentrations of one ion in the presence of high concentrations of other ions. Thus the removal of sodium ions from ammoniated condensate water, or the removal of chloride ions from borated waters of high-pH reactor coolant in the power industry, are given by Frederick and Cartwright as examples where removal achieves only a few hundredths of a percent of the inherent ultimate capacity, due to the interfering presence of ions competing for the fixed exchange sites.

Competition among the ions for removal by the ion-exchange resins also explains the stratification of removed ions (exchanged) within the resin bed. (This is a matter of some importance in the utility of countercurrent regeneration,

Table 8-1
Relative Selectivity Coefficients of Various Cations

	X-4%	*X-8%*	*X-12%*	*X-16%*
Divalent Cations				
Barium (Ba)	6.15	8.7	11.6	16.5
Lead (Pb)	5.4	7.5	10.0	14.5
Mercury (Hg)	5.1	7.2	9.7	14.0
Strontium (Sr)	3.85	4.95	6.25	8.1
Calcium (Ca)	3.4	3.9	4.6	5.8
Nickel (Ni)	2.85	3.0	3.1	3.25
Cadmium (Cd)	2.8	2.95	3.3	3.95
Copper (Cu)	2.7	2.9	3.1	3.6
Cobalt (Co)	2.65	2.8	2.9	3.05
Zinc (Zn)	2.6	2.7	2.8	3.0
Iron (Fe)	2.4	2.55	2.7	2.9
Magnesium (Mg)	2.4	2.5	2.6	2.8
Manganese (Mn)	2.2	2.35	2.5	2.7
Monovalent Cations				
Silver (Ag)	6.0	7.6	12.0	17.0
Copper (Cu)	3.2	5.3	9.5	14.5
Cesium (Cs)	2.0	2.7	3.2	3.45
Rubidium (Rb)	1.9	2.6	3.1	3.4
Potassium (K)	1.75	2.5	3.05	3.35
Ammonium (NH_4^+)	1.6	1.95	2.3	2.5
Sodium (Na)	1.3	1.5	1.7	1.9
Hydrogen (H)*	1.0	1.0	1.0	1.0
Lithium (Li)	0.90	0.85	0.84	0.74

Courtesy, *Ultrapure Water* journal

as will be discussed.) As a mixture of, say, calcium and sodium ions flows through the cation-exchange bed, the calcium ions, of greater selectivity, are removed first. The exchanged sodium ions will form a band of sorts, an exchange layer, below that constituted by the calcium ions. If magnesium and potassium ions are also present, they will arrange themselves in strata, one above the other, between the calcium and sodium.

Regeneration. When regenerant acid is added at the top of the column, the hydrogen ions, present in high concentrations, replace the calcium in the topmost layer. Calcium ions in turn replace the magnesium, and so on in avalanche fashion. Since bed regenerations, for practical and economic reason, are seldom carried to their ultimate consummations, a heel of unregenerated resin usually remains in the resin bed. Upon the reinitiation of the service water flow, the first portion of the effluent water will reflect the ion-containing heel in its ionic content. As the ionic heel becomes removed by the hydrogen ions released in the exchange reaction, the water quality improves; eventually it becomes compromised again by ion breakthrough. See also page 396 regarding ion leakage.

Regeneration is by strong acids or bases where selectivity reversal is occasioned by the law of mass action. Conversion of the salt form of the immobilized sulfonic acid group to its acidic form will be favored by the addition of a massive concentration of H^+, such as from the resin's encounter with hydrochloric acid.

Regeneration occurs similarly, due to the law of mass action, when sodium hydroxide solution washes through the exhausted anion-exchange resin.

In the case of a weak base at high pH, above 7, the base that is formed is undissociated. Therefore the reversal is driven to completion:

Table 8-2
Relative Selectivity Coefficients of Various Anions

Ion	*Type I*	*Type II*	*Ion*	*Type I*	*Type II*
Benzenesulfonate	>500	75	Bisulfite	27	3
Salicylate	450	65	Bromate	27	3
Citrate	220	23	Nitrite	24	3
Iodide	175	17	Chloride	22	2.3
Phenate	110	27	Bicarbonate	6.0	1.2
Bisulfate	85	15	Iodate	5.5	0.5
Chlorate	74	12	Formate	4.6	0.5
Nitrate	65	8	Acetate	3.2	0.5
Bromide	50	6	Propionate	2.6	0.3
Cyanide	28	3	Fluoride	1.6	0.3
			Hydroxide*	1.0	1.0

Courtesy, *Ultrapure Water* journal

$$RNH_2 + H^+ + Cl^- \text{<---->} RNH_3^+ + Cl^- + Na^+ + OH^- \text{------>} RNH_2 + Na^+ + Cl^- + H_2O \quad \text{Eq. 8-15}$$

The acid/base interaction to form undissociated water also makes for an effective regeneration reaction. Therefore weakly basic anion-exchange resins are easily regenerated by base (just as weakly acidic resins are readily regenerated by acid).

The greater ease with which weak anion/cation exchange resins can be regenerated, coupled with their higher capacities and lower costs, is economically important.

Order of Ion Removal: Cation, then Anion

The individual cation-exchange resin bed is the first ion-exchange unit the water encounters. The cations, such as sodium and calcium, are removed by exchange with hydrogen ions from the resin. The emerging solution is consequently acidic.

Were the anions of the solution to be exchanged first, the emerging solution would contain hydroxyl ions, exchanged for its sulfate and chloride ions. It would therefore be basic. The alkaline pH in this case would cause the precipitation of the as-yet-unexchanged cations such as calcium, magnesium, iron, and aluminum. The eventual fouling of the ion-exchange bed would be considerable. This is why cation removal from the water by cation-exchange action is practiced first (Figure 8-2).

The ion-exchange reaction represents an equilibrium situation. It is effective only to approximately 60% because of the equilibrium position of the sulfonate salt dissociation into ions:

Table 8-3
Selectivity Equilibria

$$R^+\text{--}OH^- + Cl^- \text{<---->} R^+\text{--}Cl^- + OH^-$$

$$K_{OH}^{Cl} = \frac{[Cl]_R}{[OH]_R} \times \frac{[OH]_S}{[Cl]_S}$$

$[Cl]_R$ and $[OH]_R$ are concentrations in the resin
$[Cl]_S$ and $[OH]_S$ are concentrations in the solution
KClOH is called the Selectivity Coefficient

Hoffman (1985); Courtesy, Rohm and Haas Co.

$$R\text{-}SO_3H + Na^+ \quad \text{-- 60\% -->} \quad R\text{-}SO_3\text{-}Na + H^+ \qquad \text{Eq. 8-16}$$
$$\text{<-- 40\% --}$$

Of course, the degree of effectiveness depends on such factors as concentration, temperature, time, and the nature of the ions involved. When the solution containing the 40% of unexchanged cations encounters another section of cation-exchange resin, it loses another 60% of this 40% of cation quantity. By a progression of such encounters, the cation concentration can be reduced to desired levels. To accomplish this, however, the cation-exchange resin must be arranged in the form of column. The anion-exchange resins function in the same manner. By following the cation-exchange resin, however, they operate more effectively.

It is because of the acid/base (H^+ plus OH^-) interaction to form undissociated water that anionic exchange resins operate more effectively than the cationic. Their function gives rise to the hydroxyl ions, and because their use follows that of the cation-exchange resin where the H^+ are produced, undissociated water molecules are the end product. This drives the reaction to completion.

Cocurrent Twin-Bed Demineralization

This flow is called cocurrent separate-bed or two-bed demineralization or ion exchange. By co-current is meant that the service flow of the water being deionized is in the same direction of flow as will ultimately be assumed by the regeneration solutions. Cation-exchange resin is placed in the first column; anion-exchange resin in the second, separate column.

The columns are not filled to the top with resin. There is usually from 50%

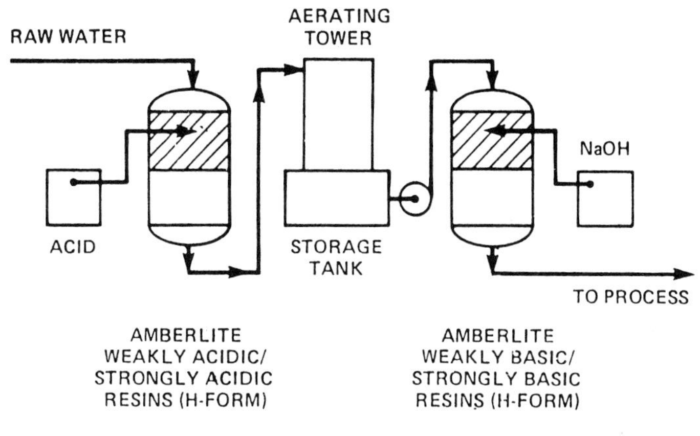

Figure 8-2. Cationic and anionic stratified beds with degasifier.
Hoffman (1985); Courtesy, Rohm and Haas Co.

to 100% freeboard allowed for backwashing. During their ion-exchange actions, the resin beds inevitably accumulate foreign particulate matter, for they also act as deep-bed, depth-type filters. The resin beads also undergo continual abrasion and alternate shrinkage and swelling as they go from their acidic or basic forms to those of combinations with ions, and then back again during their regeneration to the acid and base forms. This occasions osmotic contractions and swellings that gradually cause bead fragmentations. Even new resins may contain resin fines. Backwashing the resin beds to a condition of fluidity releases the fines and trapped particles, and floats them out of the column by means of a collector located at the top of the column. The backwashing water flow enters the column through jets located in a distributor at the bottom of the column. Failure to remove the resin fines and aggregated particles serves to densify the resin bed, endowing it with an increasing resistance to the flow of the service water, the water being demineralized. In fact, the newly loaded column is first backwashed and then is allowed to settle before use. Backwashing also relieves the compression of the bed. This serves to alleviate the pressure drop across the bed.

The water being treated is flowed into the cation-exchange column through the topmost collector/distributor. The treated water exits the first column by way of the bottom collector/distributor. The water leaving the cation-exchange column then enters the anion-exchange column to repeat a similar pattern of flow. It is essential that the inlet distributor evenly disperse the water over the entire expanse of the bed surface. Otherwise the water, descending and percolating only where it falls, will miss areas of the bed, and lead to wastage of the unused resin. The underdrain or collector functions as a header that keeps resin in but lets water out. Its apertures must therefore be correctly sized for the type of resin being used.

The flow of water through the resin bed should, in accord with the resin manufacturer's recommendations, allow sufficient contact time for the ion-exchange reaction to occur. The reaction is not immediate; a proper flowrate is required. The resin has, of course, a finite exchange capacity. When it is exhausted, Na^+, HCO_3^-, or $HSiO^-_3$, those least readily exchanged, will emerge first. The resin bed must then be regenerated. It is sometimes the practice in semiconductor operations to anticipate the breakthrough of ions and to initiate the regeneration step when some drop in the water resistivity has been signaled, as when water with a resistivity of 18-megohm-cm decreases to a reading of 15 megohm-cm (Figure 8-3).

Situated some few inches above the resin bed in each column is a regeneration header through which the regenerant chemicals are fed during the rejuvenating cycle. The regenerant solutions must be of the proper dilution (soon to be discussed), and must be allotted an adequate contact time to effect the conversion of the resin. This is done by way of proper flowrates. In regenerating the cation-exchange bed, acid is used. The renewal of the anion-exchange resin requires the use of strong base. The contact time for the acid regenerant may be 20 to 60 minutes. After the acid flow is turned off, a water rinse of greater volume follows. The correct volumes, flowrates, and concentrations are provided in the resin manuals furnished by the resin producers. Their recommendations should be followed. In the flushing by water following the treatment of the anion-exchange resin, decationated water should be used. Ordinary water may contain magnesium ions, which can interact with the alkali to give sparingly soluble, gelatinous magnesium hydroxide precipitates. Such precipitations should be avoided. The regeneration and washing free of regenerant solution in the case of the anion-exchange bed involves similar considerations of contact times and flowrates. A high-rate flush of demineralized water through both columns readies them for the next use (Figure 8-4).

Regenerant Solutions

Sulfuric or hydrochloric acid may be used to regenerate the cation-exchange resin. Sulfuric acid is not as efficient a regenerant as hydrochloric acid; however, it is cheaper and is free of the noxious fumes emanating from concentrated hydrochloric acid (36%). Sulfuric acid is therefore used in the power industry where costs are very important. Hydrochloric acid, under conditions of proper

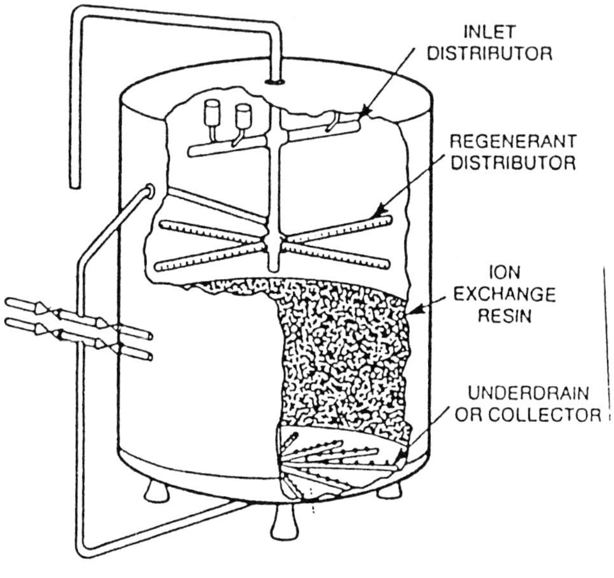

Figure 8-3. Cocurrentflow regeneration.
Courtesy, Rohm and Haas Co.

ventilation, is used most frequently when regenerations are performed only twice weekly or once every 10 days or so. It is more widely used in the pharmaceutical industry where smaller systems are involved.

An equal concentration of hydrochloric acid will more effectively regenerate a spent cation-exchange resin than will sulfuric acid. Hydrochloric acid, HCl, provides 1 mole of H^+ per 36.5 g or 1 mole of acid. One mole of sulfuric acid, 98 g, supplies 2 moles of H^+. On a comparative weight-efficiency basis, however, sulfuric acid furnishes 1 mole of H^+ per 49 g of acid. Moreover, the second H^+ formed by the dissociation of acid is not readily available:

$$H^+ + HSO_4^- \longleftrightarrow 2H^+ + SO_4^{2-} \qquad \text{Eq. 8-17}$$

Hydrochloric acid in its commercially concentrated form is at approximately 36% strength; it is essentially a 10-molar (M) solution. A 10-M sulfuric acid solution would be at a concentration of 98%. Dilution of so strong a sulfuric acid liberates a high heat of mixing that is a hazard and requires dissipation. The acid (which is heavier) should always be mixed into the water (which is lighter). The reverse can cause an explosive showering of steam and acid. A sulfuric-acid regeneration system should come equipped with an interlock of the acid pump or valve with a flow switch to moderate the dilution with water. Direct dilution of concentrated sulfuric acid of 66 Baumé (93%) to about 20% strength creates temperature transients that approach the boiling point. This strength of hot acid can be ruinous to PVC piping, among other things. The acid strength of the sulfuric or hydrochloric acid used for regeneration is usually around 4%.

When sulfuric acid is used, the concern is with the generation of insoluble calcium sulfate. This salt has some slight solubility (about 0.2%) in water, but its solutions can exist in a supersaturated state. In the regeneration profile for calcium, amounts as high as 27% are seen. This is explained as being caused by supersaturation. McGarvey (1990b) believed that the greater solubilities may be caused in part by calcium bisulfate. The sulfuric acid solutions used generally do not exceed 2% in strength. It is more advisable to initiate the cation-exchange regeneration using diluted sulfuric acid strengths and to progress stagewise to stronger concentrations, in order not to exceed the calcium sulfate solubility product at any point. A 1.5%, 2%, and then 4% sulfuric acid series, depending upon circumstances, would be preferable, to eliminate the peak calcium load without causing calcium sulfate deposition. This is coupled with high flowrates, perhaps 1 gallon per minute per cubic foot (gpm/ft^3) to begin with, and dropping to 0.7 gpm/ft^3 when the stronger acid feeds begin. The object is to get the band of calcium-form resin out of the column as soon as possible. Temperature is important. Calcium sulfate forms crystals very rapidly in hot water, calcium sulfate supersaturation being compromised by heat.

After forming in ion-exchange beds, the calcium sulfate normally redissolves, although large crystals could persist. Upon dissolving, however, the calcium, now in ionic form, releases sodium by successfully competing with it for the ion-exchange sites, and decreases the capacity of the resin. This ion-replacement phenomenon gives rise to a long, ragged rinse. For all these reasons, regeneration is better with hydrochloric acid, in 4% strength at regeneration rates of 0.5 gpm/ft^3; temperature concerns are absent. However, hydrogen chloride presents a corrosion problem. It corrodes stainless steel; Hastalloy or other special alloys are required for its handling. It is the greater corrosivity of hydrochloric acid that detracts most strongly from the wider use that its greater regeneration powers would warrant; although its storage requires venting for its hydrogen chloride fumes as well. Although less expensive, the use of sulfuric acid is hardly without comparable hazard.

Strong anionic-exchange resins are used to remove ionic silica from waters. Their regeneration is arduous and slow. The caustic used for this purpose is of 4% strength. It, the resin bed, and the rinsewater are heated to 50 °C (120 °F). The caustic solution is flowed at the rate of about 0.5 gpm/ft^3. When the silica content is high, the contact time should be at least 90 minutes. The use of a heated caustic regeneration of an extended duration is essential to the securing of low-silica waters. Caustic is often shipped in the form of 50% aqueous solution. This freezes at about 4.5 °C (40 °F), which interdicts its outside storage in some climates.

The hotter the regenerating caustic soda is, the better. The quaternary ammonium bases are relatively thermolabile, however, and can be decomposed by heat. The Hofmann degradation that ensues involves the rupture of a carbon-nitrogen bond, and partial or even total loss of ion-exchange capability will result. The regenerating practice is thus confined to temperatures below 50 °C (122 °F) for Type I strongly basic anion-exchange resins, and below 30 °C (86 °F) for Type II. Actually, thermal degradation occurs to some extent even at these temperatures, but the amount of functional loss is not judged excessive in terms of the resin service life. Heated caustic usually removes any silica that may have polymerized within the anion-exchange beads.

The regeneration of the strongly basic resin is difficult because the regenerating hydroxyl ions, aggrandized in their ionic size by their waters of hydration, find it difficult to approach the fixed cations and to displace competitively the salt-forming counterions.

The regeneration process stems from the effectiveness of the mass action law in upsetting the equilibrium of the ionic dissociation of the cation-exchange salt, removing (by replacement with H^+) its associated cation's counterions. In the case of the anion-exchange salt, the associated anionic counterion is replaced from the resin-salt formations that may be relatively undissociated, and hence practically irreversible. Heavy metal salts often form such entities. Such irreversible cation bonding would permanently reduce the resin's ion-exchange capacity.

The purity of the regenerating agents is thus of importance. One does not wish inadvertently to introduce heavy ion impurities. For instance, when sodium hydroxide is used, a particularly good grade, called Rayon-Grade, is often stipulated. Lesser grades contain chloride and/or ferric ion impurities. Naturally, purity has its economic price.

It is common to soften the water used in regenerations. This may seem unwise as the sodium-form cation exchange adds more sodium ions that are more difficult to remove. The practice serves, however, to prevent the formation of voluminous magnesium hydroxide precipitates.

Ion Leakage

There is a tendency to consider chemical reactions, such as those involved in DI resin regenerations, as leading to complete chemical transformations. Often, however, reaction proceeds to some equilibrium point; it does not attain a perfect conversion. Thus a resin bed may be totally exhausted by the passage of a brine solution; its fresh regeneration may reveal the bed to have a lower capacity that it should be capable of; then additional regenerations may boost the realized capacity to expected levels. The first regeneration (which achieved its proper equilibrium point, a less-than-complete conversion), was not necessarily faulty. The second regeneration increased the bed capacity because attainment of its equilibrium position resulted in a regenerative transformation of part of the exhausted fraction remaining from the first regeneration.

(Similarly, reverse osmosis purifications should not be thought of in terms of realizing absolute rejections. Such operations yield log reductions, not complete eliminations.)

Ion-exchange resins manifest a lower selectivity for monovalent ions because these exhibit a lower charge/charge interaction. The more highly charged multivalent ions, because of their higher charge densities, combine more avidly with the resin ion sites of opposite charges, the counterions. Thus accomplishing the removal of sodium ions to a level of less than 1 ppm is not easy. The attainment of this low concentration level is especially difficult if the sodium ion concentration exceeds 10 ppm to begin with. (This is not the case in counterflow operations.)

To the extent that sodium ion is present as the water issues from a cation-exchange column, it will become transformed by and emerge from the anion-exchange column as sodium hydroxide with strongly basic resins. The pH will be above 7. The specifications for Purified Water for pharmaceutical purposes call for a pH range of 5 to 7. This can be achieved using a two-bed system if weakly basic resins are used. Likewise, sodium-ion leakage from the cation-exchange bed is unacceptable for semiconductor or power industry needs. The leakage of chloride or silicate ions from anion-exchange beds is also undesirable. Soluble, ionizable silica, as will be discussed, may be difficult to remove because of its largely undissociated form. Chloride ions slip through the beds, as do sodium ions, because of their lower charge densities.

The resulting alkalinity emanating from twin-bed arrangements is sometimes erroneously ascribed to alkali that is residual from the regeneration process. It may also be disguised by the ubiquitous presence of carbon dioxide, which has acidic effects bacause of its feeble aqueous dissociation. The concentration of sodium ion must be reduced by ion exchange to a value of less than 1 ppm if this alkaline generation is to be avoided.

When high sodium-ion concentration arises from a preceding water-softening treatment, one approach to the problem is to limit the softening of the water to the 1-grain level. The treated water will be sufficiently softened so as not to produce scaling, and the sodium-ion loading will be minimized.

Sodium-ion leakage transcends the importance of the sodium ion itself. The sodium-ion effluent from the cation-exchange bed creates sodium hydroxide in the strongly basic anion-exchange bed. This has a regenerative effect that can

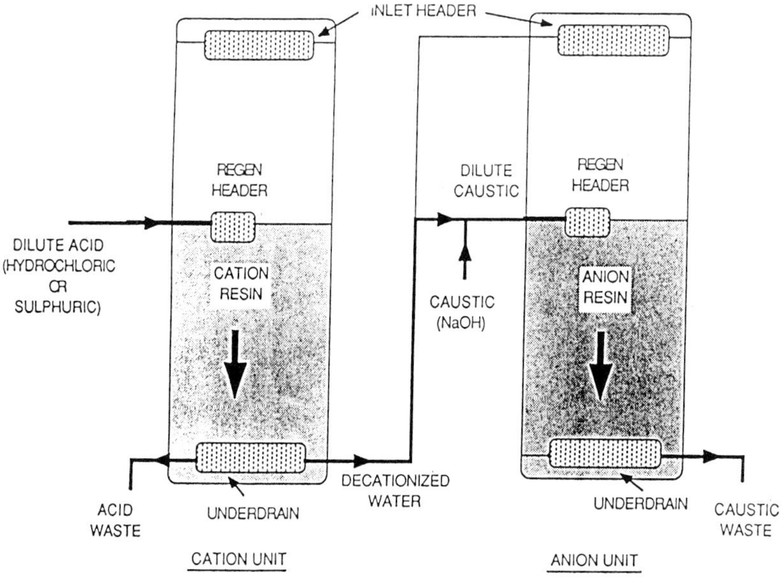

Figure 8-4. Cocurrent two-bed regeneration cycle.
Courtesy, *Ultrapure Water* journal

result in the release of silica from the latter bed. Silica breakthrough can occur, which may erroneously be attributed to an insufficiency in the anion-exchange bed. To avoid this incorrect diagnosis, sodium-ion leakage from the cation-exchange bed should be assessed directly, as by the use of sodium-ion electrodes (Foster, 1991).

The completeness of ion-exchange reactions is governed by the ratio of ion concentration in the water to the number of ion-exchange sites. This is the ratio that finds reflection in the probability of ions encountering the exchange sites. When the ratio is higher in ions, their removal is favored by the law of mass action. The ratio can be excessively high locally within the ion-exchange column, in which case the ion-exchange sites can be swamped by ions. Those ions uncaptured will permeate to the next downstream section of the bed, to be captured there. If the capacity of the bed becomes exhausted, however, the number of ions in excess of the member of exchange sites will exit the bed. This is sometimes called *ion slippage* or *ion leakage*. It can also be caused by so high a water velocity as not to provide adequate time for ion/ion-exchange encounter and reaction. According to Applebaum (1968, p 149), the final reduction to trace amounts usually requires a bed more than 24 inches deep. Since monovalent ions are exchanged least selectively, the phenomenon of ion slippage usually manifests itself as sodium leakage.

There are several ways in which ion leakage can be minimized. First, higher regeneration dosages can be used to accomplish more complete regenerations. Also, the ion-exchange bed can be made deeper, à la Applebaum; a third, cation-exchange, bed can be added to twin-bed arrangements; mixed-bed polishing may be employed; and the number of ion-exchange sites may be added to by the use of countercurrent or counterflow regeneration. A decrease in the ratio of ions to ion-exchange sites is sought by increasing the latter so that the desired exchange reactions will be favored by the mass action law, even for sparse ion concentrations, by the high incidence of ion-exchange sites. Increased ion-exchange efficiency would result.

Mixed-bed arrangements are often used after twin-bed installations in order to deal with sodium and silica leakage from the twin beds. As will be seen, twin beds followed by a third cation-exchange bed (or even another twin-bed installation) may be used to overcome the leakage problem.

Economics generally dictate what installations—two-bed, mixed-bed, or both—are used to effect deionization.

Hoffman (1985) stated that two-bed demineralizers typically produced a water marked by significant sodium leakage of 1 to 3 ppm, along with a silica leakage of 0.05 to 1.0 ppm. The effluent was generally alkaline with a resistivity of 0.1 to 0.5 megohm-cm. As the two-bed performance deteriorated with age, whether caused by anion-exchange resin degradation or by fouling, the leakage became worse. The passage of other inorganic ion species was seldom seen.

Mixed-bed ion-exchange units downstream from the twin beds were used to correct the situation so that very-high-resistivity water emerged.

Silica leakage management. Pate (1991b) offered a comparison of different purification methods meant to effect the removal of silica. A 4 ´ 2 array single-pass RO of cellulose acetate followed by a mixed-bed ion-exchange unit reduced a dissolved silica level of 25,000 ppb to 5 ppb. However, occasional excursions from incoming water variations, from mixed-bed exhaustions, and from RO rejection problems may cause short-term silica levels of 50 ppb. These in turn may briefly stress the polishing system and may potentially impact wafer manufacture.

The use of a two-pass RO system followed by a mixed-bed ion exchange is more effective in reducing the silica load on the mixed bed. Pate (1991) used cellulose acetate RO in a 4×2 array for the first pass, and a 4×2 array thin-film composite for the second RO. The need to regenerate the mixed-bed ion exchanger decreased from a frequency of once every 3 to 4 days, to once every 3 to 4 weeks. The risk of operating the mixed-bed unit to silica exhaustion followed by silica leakage was also minimized in this two-pass-RO-plus-mixed-bed arrangement.

According to Pate (1991b), the thin-film RO was superior to cellulose acetate RO in the rejection of silica by a comparison of 95% to 92%. However, the polyamide RO was more prone to fouling by hardness and by high SDIs. A double-pass RO wherein cellulose acetate was followed by thin-film poly-amide had very good resistance to fouling and rejected silica by 99%. The best percentage of silica removal, 99.9%, was attained using an anion-exchange column downstream from the single-pass RO but in advance of the mixed bed. The mixed bed was required in all these examples. Its presence helped to provide a very good dissolved-silica removal efficiency. The use of such three-staged water purification systems consistently furnished a high-quality water with a very low silica content. The more customary two-stage RO/DI arrangement usually achieved a product of like grade, but not consistently so.

Pate (1991b) used two mixed-bed deionizers in series to assure the polishing removal of silica to below 0.5 ppb. Over a 3-month period, when the water feeding into the dual polishing unit was at 5 ppb, the water exiting the first mixed bed reached 3 ppb, and 0.5 ppb emerging from the second mixed bed. The flow was then altered to enter the second bed first, and then to pass through the regenerated first bed. By an alternation of this flow pattern, the soluble silica count in the product water was kept from exceeding 5 ppb.

The best purification scheme utilized a single-pass RO based upon a 4×2 thin-film composite array, prior to twin beds and followed by a mixed bed. This purification system consistently yielded 1-ppb silica levels from source water with 50,000-ppb silica concentrations.

The Mixed Bed

Mixed-bed arrangements consist of an intimate mixture of anion-exchange and cation-exchange resin particles. They function as if they were a series of separate ion-exchange beds in which, because of the intimacy of the mix, the cations and anions are removed simultaneously (McGarvey, 1990a).

Mixed beds perform as if water molecules are the immediate product of their reaction. These are largely undissociated into ions. It is this that drives the ion-exchange equilibrium of mixed beds to so high a degree of complete ion exchange; hence the characterization of the mixed-bed operation as a polishing function.

The mixed bed usually contains equal exchange capacities of strong anionic and cationic resins. Because of volume capacity differences, this equates to about 60% anion and 40% cation exchanger in volume. If equal volumes of each were used, and particularly if difficult to remove carbon dioxide and silica were present, the system would generally be anion-exchange limited. Some redress to this situation would be supplied where the carbon dioxide is removed by degassing.

If, for instance, 100 ft^3 of strongly acidic cation-exchange resin had a capacity of 20 kilograins per cubic foot (kgr/ft^3) and an equal amount of strongly basic anion-exchange resin of capacity of 13 kgr/ft^3, then more anion-exchange resin

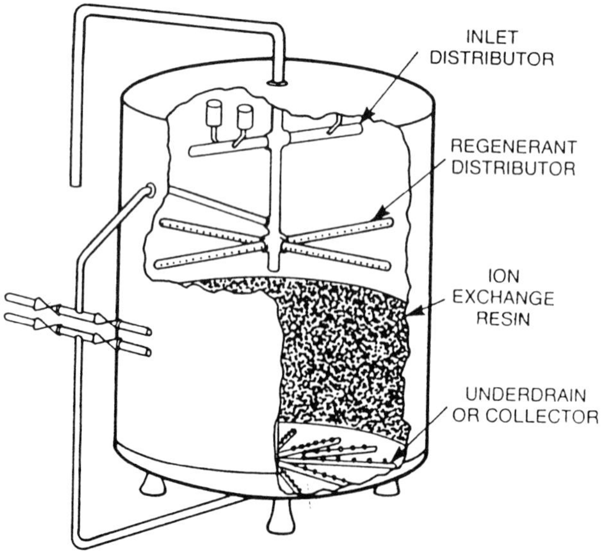

Figure 8-5. Typical commercial ion-exchange unit.
Courtesy, Dr. Robert Kunin

would be required to give a balanced system.

Typically, a 1-ft^2 column would contain 24 inches (18-inch minimum) of cationic resin, overlaid by 36 inches of anionic resin. A freeboard equal to the sum of these heights (5 ft) is allowed for easy separation of the resins in the regeneration stage. The 100% freeboard gives the typical mixed-bed unit a height of 8 to 10 feet. The open space above the resin beds is required to allow for their separation during backwashing. Both resins expand during this operation, the cationic (anion exchange) more so than the anionic (cation exchange).

The cation-exchange resin (also called the cation component or the cation resin) is loaded in first. Underlying it is the collector for spent regenerant. This collector is separated by a space from the bottom of the tank, where is located an arrangement that serves as an acid distributor, an air distributor, and a rinse and effluent collector. The bottom collector should be so positioned that no spent regenerant can be trapped below it. Nor may it be surrounded by resin, lest this serve to harbor traces of acid or even caustic (which would occasion a long rinse cycle). In order not to provide space for resin or spent regenerant, the tank bottom is sometimes cemented in around the distributor piping (Figures 8-5 and 8-6).

It may be advisable or even necessary to backwash the bed to remove fines and manufacturing debris. (On a few occasions this can take up to several hours.) This is done by way of a distributor at the bottom of the bed. The upwelling water and its burden of resin fines escapes the column through the top collector.

An intermediate distributor will eventually interface with the cation-exchange resin below and the anion-exchange resin above. This distributor's proper positioning relative to the height of the bed is very important, as it bears on the capacity of the regenerated mixed bed and its subsequent performance. As will be seen, a sharp demarcation between both resin types is required to optimize the regeneration of the exhausted resins. The interface collector should best be within 1 to 2 inches of the top of the cation-exchange resin layer when that layer is in its acid form, its most swollen manifestation. If the collector is too high

Table 8-4
General Shrink/Swell Characteristics of Ion Exchange Resins

Resin type	*Regenerated Form*	*Exhausted Form*	*Volume change*
Strongly acidic	H^+	Na^+	(-) 2 to 10%
Weakly acidic	H^+	Na^+	(+) 30 to 90%
Strongly basic	OH^-	Cl^-	(-) 10 to 25%
Weakly basic	Free base	Cl^-	(+) 15 to 40%

Courtesy, Brian J. Hoffman, Rohm and Haas Co.

above the bed, resin is added. (If cation-exchange resin in its sodium form is used to load the column, room must correctly be gauged and adjusted to allow for its expansion to that height upon regeneration.) If too much resin is present (that is, if its level is above the fixed interface collector), the excess is removed, as by siphoning through a garden hose, or else the backwash stream is allowed to remove that resin from the column. The location of the interface collector at 1 inch above the cation-exchange resin in its regenerated form allows for the redress of some shrinkage that may have occurred, and to permit a more exact adjustment following a more complete regeneration with acid flowed from the bottom distributor upward and out of the interface collector (Figures 8-7 and 8-8, Table 8-4).

The fixed interface collector having been correctly positioned by adjustment of the cation-exchange resin bed height, the anion-exchange resin beads are next loaded into the column (the mixed-bed shell), until the caustic distributor is about 5 to 6 inches above the top of the anion-exchange bed, following backwash of a few hours to remove fines and residuals. This allows sufficient room for the expansion of this resin during its regeneration to its base form. Care is taken not to place the distributor so close to the resin as to cause damage by compression as the bed undergoes swelling.

At the very top of the shell containing the mixed-bed resins is an influent distributor and backwash collector. The space between it and the caustic distributor is calculated to allow for a 100% volume expansion of the bed. This furnishes the headroom required to permit separation of the anion and cation resins just prior to their chemical regeneration. The disengagement of the two resins should take place in less than 5 minutes. If the bottom of the bed does not have room to expand, the anion-exchange beads will be forced out of the shell by way of the top distributor, and a long backwash will be required to achieve good separation.

The resins are placed into their mixed form by having air or nitrogen blown through the beds. The gas used should be free of oil, and of particles such as may become entrained by air compressors. In pharmaceutical usage, nitrogen gas generated from liquid nitrogen is employed. A gas pressure of 10 psig or somewhat higher is normally used. The usual gas flowrate is appoximately 5 to 10 ft^3 standard cubic foot per minute per square foot of tank area. Mixing time is about 15 minutes. Before the mixing is commenced, the water level above the beds is adjusted to about 3 to 40 inches to provide for good mixing. The exact depth of this layer, is, however, equipment-dependent. Too low a water level will permit the water to be blown out of the bed by the air pressure, and mixing would be impossible. Too high a water level will encourage a layer of the anion-exchange resin (less dense) to form on top of it, and this too should be avoided.

Service cycle. Following the removal of the resin fines the mixed bed is ready for use with the resins in their full acid and base forms (Figure 8-9). Mixed beds are appropriately used in the polishing mode to remove some few parts per million of impurities. The service water flow is rapid, to maximize the use of the large resin volume. The mixed-bed service flow is greater than 10 gpm/ft^2. The kinetics of the service cycle are, therefore, very important. This relates to film diffusion kinetics, which reflect the amount of resin surface area. Regeneration kinetics are a different story. Here one deals with a high concentration in the bulk phase, and with a much slower diffusion because one is working counter to the resin selectivity. Regeneration is invariably controlled by particle diffusion.

The service cycle is eventually terminated for any of several reasons: A high pressure drop manifests itself; there is high silica or sodium leakage; the effluent

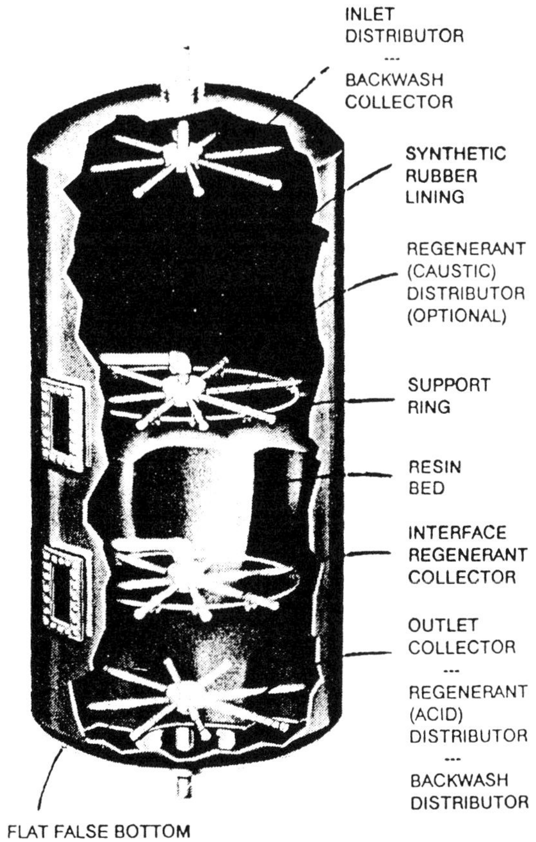

Figure 8-6. Cutaway view of a mixed-bed unit.
Coulter and Thomas (1987); Courtesy, *Ultrapure Water* journal

attains a high conductivity; or the total gallons of throughput so advise. Usually, the bed is used in the ion-exchange operation until some ionic breakthrough point is reached. The accepted breakthrough level depends upon the application and the purity of the water it demands. In some instances where a resistivity of 18 megohm-cm is required, a breakthrough has resulted in a precipitous drop in resistivity. Within 5 to 10 bed volumes of water the resistivity decreased to 10 megohm-cm. A mixed-bed operation, to provide margin, may be terminated when the resistivity decreases to 15 megohm-cm. The mixed bed is then regenerated (Figures 8-10 and 8-11).

Backwash cycle. Normally, the resin regeneration step involves a backwashing of the mixed resins to effect their separation into two layers, so positioned relative to the distributors and collectors in the column as to enable each to receive its appropriate treatment. The backwashing water flow serves also to release and wash out the suspended material collected by the bed during the service cycle.

The backwashing action can normally take 30 minutes, possibly less or even 45 minutes. Given that the service cycle of the ion-exchange bed can be 3 weeks or so, it would not seem critical to shorten the backwashing step or lengthen it by another 20 minutes.

Backwashing requires a freeboard of 100% to permit a proper agitation and disruptive mixing of the resin bed. If the freeboard is less, such an agitation may carry resin out of the column. If the turbulence is restrained in order to avoid this wasteful occurrence, the compacted resin layer at the bottom of the column may not be sufficiently disrupted. The disengagement of the two resins should take place in about 30 minutes. Poor separation presages lower exchange capacity and low-resistivity product water because of ion leakage. Ample room for bed separation provided by the space between the topmost backwash collector and the caustic distributor is therefore very important.

A staged backwash is required. The initial backwash rate is at a linear velocity of about 6 gpm/ft^2. This will serve to disrupt the bed. The water velocity is then reduced to about 4 gpm/ft^2 in order to avoid blowing resin out of the bed. However, the operator searching for the interface of the resins in the sight glass (halfway up the column) may be confused by the currents caused by the positioned distributor and support structures in the column. The flow is then reduced to about 2 gpm/ft^2, at which rate the formation of the resin interface becomes evident.

Some columns are built with an additional sight glass near the bottom, in order to make possible the viewing of the bottom compacted resin layer to make sure it is sufficiently disrupted. The bottom window feature is not too common. Its insertion into the column must be performed correctly lest it compromise the integrity of the bottom of the column and result in a violation of the vessel fabrication code.

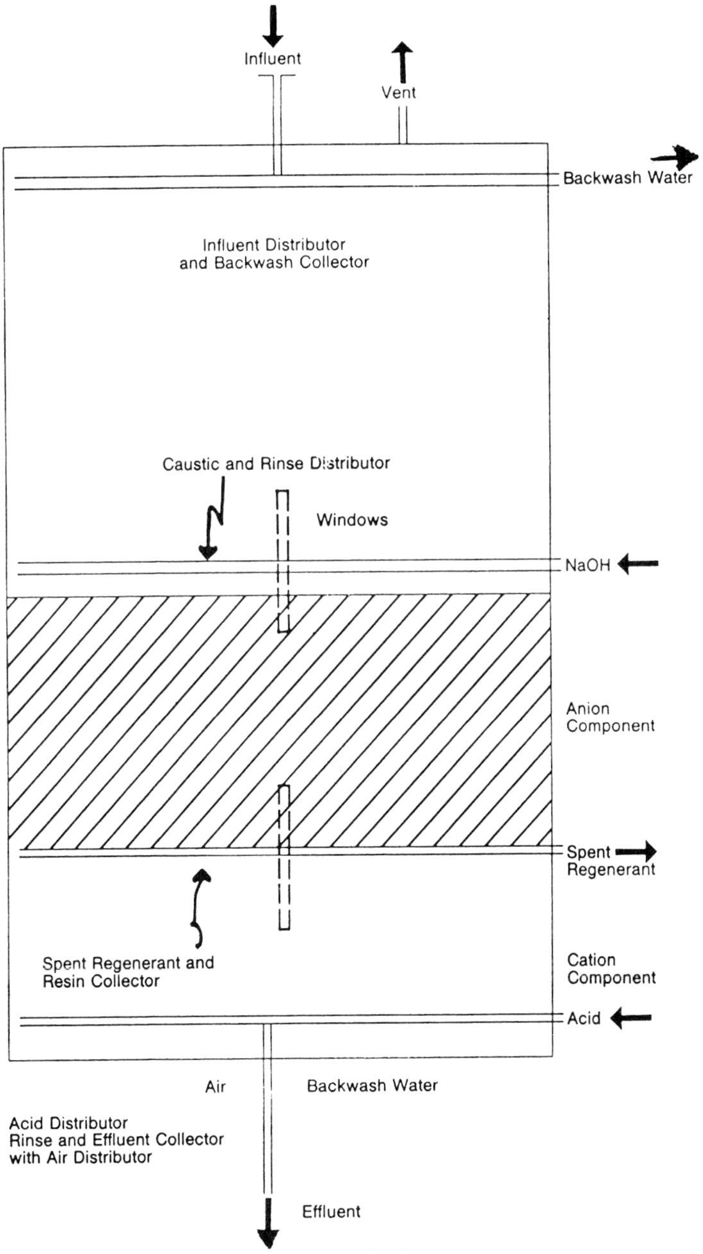

Figure 8-7. Illustrative diagram of a mixed bed.
McGarvey (1990a); Courtesy, Semiconductor Pure Water Conference

Regeneration cycle. The distribution and collection system should provide uniform contact of resin and regeneration throughout the bed, and should thus prevent regenerant hideout.

In the regeneration, alkali is flowed down through the upper separated resin layer, while water is flowed upward through the bottom layer to form a blocking layer. The two flows are regulated to meet at the interface of the two resin layers, to be removed by the header positioned at the interface. Regeneration of the cation-exchange resin (the bottom layer) is by acid flow up from the bottom of the containing tank, while the blocking flow of water is from the top down; the flows are balanced so that their joined stream is carried off by the interface header. Alternatively, the rejuvenating acid flow can be downward from the pipe at the interface, to be carried off at the bottom. The appropriate regenerants may be flowed simultaneously to exit the interface collector. Indeed, this is the common mode, for it saves regeneration time. It must be performed adroitly, however, lest it lead to complications caused by calcium sulfate depositions and by silica gel formation.

With the use of fixed headers it becomes important to cause the positioning of the resin layer interface at just that level in the column. Otherwise, some of one resin layer or the other will wastefully be denied its proper regeneration. Even worse, cross-contamination of the resins will result. The proper degree of expansive resin swelling, a consequence of the water temperature used, may govern the position of the layer interface.

There are various ways in which mixed-bed regenerations can be performed (Chapman et al., 1983b).

Following the attainment of an adequate regeneration as shown by restoration

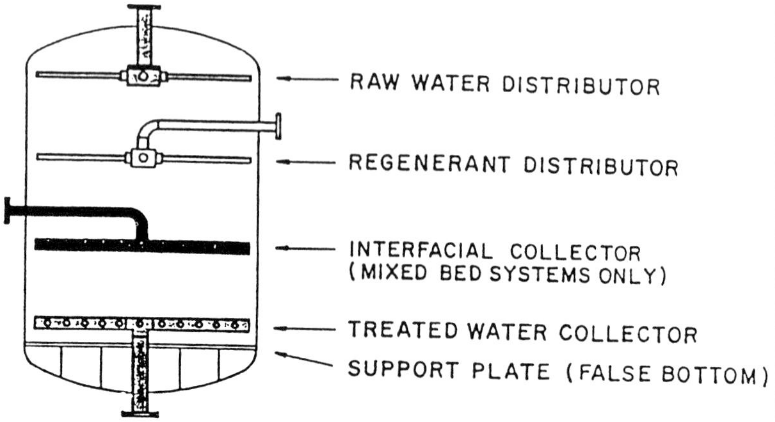

Figure 8-8. Ion exchange internals.
Courtesy, Brian J. Hoffman, Rohm and Haas Co.

of acceptable water quality, displacement of the regenerant by way of a slow rinse is instituted. This is followed by a fast rinse, essentially part of the service cycle except that the water is diverted to drain.

The regenerated resins can now be restored by air mixing to their mixed-bed arrangement ready for the service cycle. The rate of air flow used is from 5 to 10 SCFM (standard cubic feet per minute)/ft^2 of tank area.

The removal of the remnants of the regenerating acid, especially when hydrochloric acid is used, is particularly important where the deionized water is to be employed as feedwater for a still. Chloride ions will lead to the stress cracking of the stainless steel stills. The results can be catastrophic. This is to be guarded against particularly in the regeneration of mixed-bed resins. When twin-bed DI systems are used, hydrochloric acid unremoved from the cation-exchange bed will be neutralized and the chloride ion will be removed in the

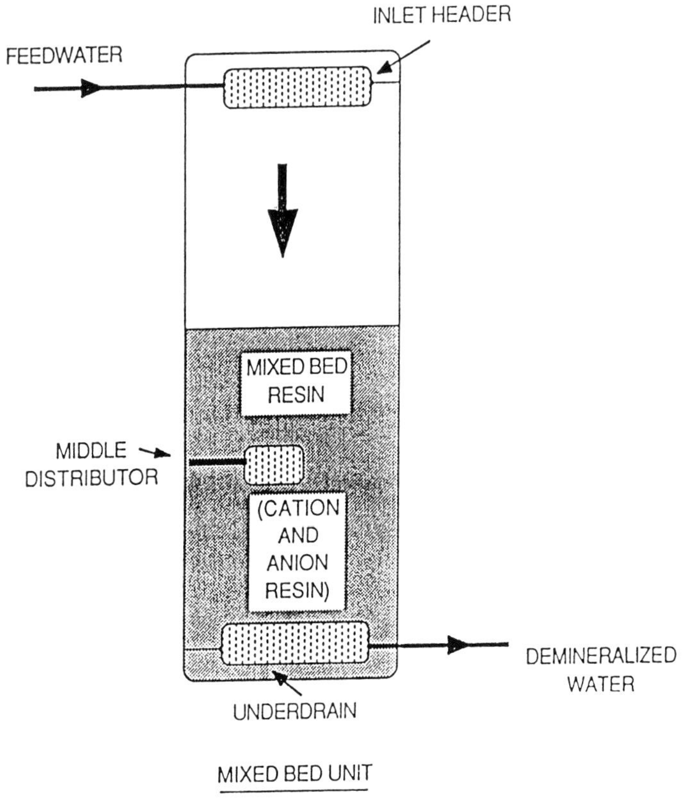

Figure 8-9. Mixed bed, service cycle.
Courtesy, *Ultrapure Water* journal

anion-exchange bed. That option is absent in the mixed-bed regeneration operation.

Resin separation. Backwashing of the exhausted mixed bed permits stratification of the two constituting resins on the basis of their relative densities. The particle size ranges are also important. The particle size distribution of the cation-exchange resin ought not include too many small particles. Its density will be about 1.3. The particle size distribution of the anion-exchange resin ought not to contain too many large particles. Its density will be about 1.07. Therefore the two resin types can be separated on the basis of Stokes' law, the lower-density anion exchange resin forming the upper layer.*

Resin bead size. The size of the resin beads is generally between 16 and 50 mesh, though 20 to 40 mesh is often preferred. Smaller beads, packing closer, would give better ion-exchange kinetics. Having greater surface-to-volume ratios, they

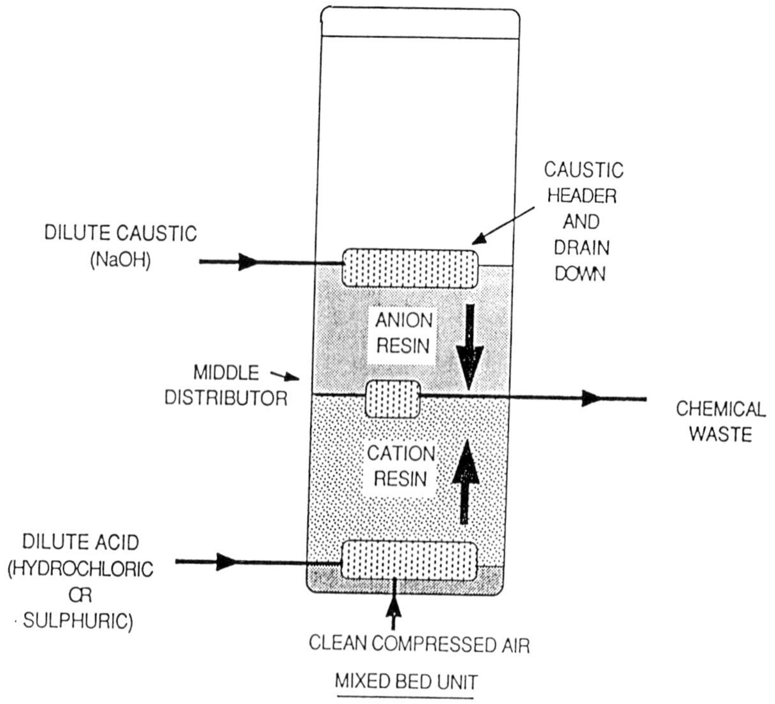

Figure 8-10. Mixed bed, regeneration cycle.
Courtesy, *Ultrapure Water* journal

regenerate faster. Some benefit derives. More important, however, is that the regeneration is diffusion-limited. That is why it is performed slowly. If the regeneration step is carried out at rates of 0.3 to 0.5 gpm/ft^3 in a well-designed column, resins will normally attain their regeneration status. Faster regeneration rates should not be used. The closer packing of smaller beads causes higher pressure drop. This is reflected directly in higher pumping costs, and in the additional sturdiness required of pipes, containers, and similar components. The pressure drops across the resin in ion-exchange beds are usually small, about 3 or 5 psig per foot of bed. Another consideration weighs against finer bead sizes. The ion-exchange beds often accumulate suspended matter from the water. This is periodically removed by backwashing the beds. If the resin beads are fine enough, they can be lost to excessive extents in the backwash operation as the suspended matter is dislodged and removed. The 16- to 50-mesh beads that are commonly used are coarse enough not to be lost during normal backwash operations. Cutler (1987) stated that a difference in harmonic mean size (HMS) of up to 200 micrometers should be selected for good remixing capabilities. With tighter uniformity coefficients, smaller HMS become acceptable. (Harmonic mean sizes are calculated using particle counters or screen analyses.)

The completeness of separation of the resins constituting a mixed bed depends upon maximization of their density differences, however, and this requires that the ion-exchange capacity of each resin be exhausted. Brine, brine and caustic solution, or even caustic itself (as in semiconductor operations) are used for this purpose. The exhausted resins can now be better separated into two layers (the anion-exchange on top) for the individual regenerations. The use of a "brine kill" will indeed maximize the density differences caused by the creation of the anion-exchange resin in its chloride form. Abrams (1991) pointed out, however, the severe economic penalty involved. The chloride form is far more difficult to regenerate into its hydroxylic counterpart and therefore necessitates the use of far more alkali to achieve it. This entails a severe economic penalty.

There are also commercially available resins that are sufficiently different in their densities even when they are only partly exhausted. These are more expensive than standard resins, but can often be an excellent choice for mixed-bed operations. They avoid the need for an exhaustion of the resins by the use of brine to facilitate their separation. They find application in semiconductor usage where resin regenerations are performed when the water resistivity declines to 15 from 18 megohm-cm.

The particle density of the cation-exchanger in the hydrogen form is 1.18 to 1.22. In the hydroxyl form it is 1.06. Therefore, it ought to be possible to separate the two resins in their regenerated forms. However, a tendency towards clumping exists. (See page 436). A loss of water into the bulk phase from

*Settling, according to Stokes' law, is directly proportional to both particle size and particle density. Both these factors are, however, independent of one another. True density is a fundamental property of materials.

hydrogen-form and hydroxyl-form groups may be responsible. Substituting sodium ions for at least some of the hydroxyl ions reduces clumping from this source. In going from the hydrogen to sodium form the density increased from 1.18 or 1.22 to 1.25 or 1.30. This helps the separation. If chloride is substituted for hydroxyl the increase in density is negligible; from 1.06 to 1.08. Furthermore, multiple regenerations may be required to remove the chloride sufficiently, as measured by ion chromatography, although chloride leakage on the next cycle may be brought low enough to escape detection by conductivity measurements. Therefore, a sodium hydroxide but not a brine kill should be used when resin exhaustion is undertaken, despite the fact that the chloride form has less tendency to clump than the hydroxyl form.

Allen's law concerning resin bead separations. According to Stoke's law, given particles of equal density, the larger ones settle out first. In the case of particles of equal size, the more dense ones have greater settling velocities; they settle out sooner.

Knowing the resin bead particle size distribution and the bead densities, calculations can be made to plot the settling velocities of the different resin beads. The plotting of the settling velocities versus the particle size of the resin beads allows one to see whether the settling velocity curves of the anion-exchange beads and the cation-exchange beads overlap. If they do, the conclusion is usually reached that the beads cannot be separated. This conclusion is, however, too simplistic. It assumes the free settling velocities the respective beads would have in water, the suspending medium.

Allen's law points out that free settling velocities do not describe the actual situation. The beads undergo a hindered settling imposed by the complexity of the suspending medium that is not water but rather a suspension of resin beads in water; furthermore its density changes progressively from the top to the bottom of the column. The hindered settling picture is a far more complex model than the free settling velocity peculiar to the density of water.

In actuality, anion and cation beads may permit separations even when their free settling curves overlap. The denser medium of resin-beads-cum-water gives a boost to the likelihood of separations. Thus, in the separation of the resins of a mixed-bed, the denser cation-exchange beads in their settling out tend to squeeze the anion-exchange beads up and out; a better separation results.

Removing the bigger anion-exchange beads and the smaller cation-exchange beads helps effect the separation even more.

With conventionally sized beads, a mixture of small-size cation beads and large-size anion beads exists at the interface region. Ion-exchange capacity may be lost because of the inadequate regeneration of this interfacial zone. However, there is a restricted ability to increase the size of the cation beads or to use anionic beads of a smaller size. Decreasing the anion bead size increases the pressure drop across the bed. Increasing the size of the cation beads decreases their kinetic performance. It is difficult therefore to minimize the mixed zone by these means. However, the use of optimally sized resin beads can avoid this situation, to the betterment of more usable bed capacity, a diminution of ion leakage, and less cross-contamination.

Given the use of ordinary resins in the mixed-bed operations, perfect separations of the resin type are seldom attained. Some small percentage of each resin may erroneously be either above or below the line of the regenerant distributor. Instead of becoming regenerated, the resin portion is rendered totally exhausted by the wrong application of regenerant chemicals. Contributing to this small amount of cross-contamination is the lack of perfection in distributor design. The cross-contamination results in the acid regenerant converting the anion-exchange resin to its chloride or sulfate salt form, and the cation-exchange resin being converted to or maintained in its sodium salt form. If a mixed-bed demineralizer takes several hours to rinse up, it is generally indicative of a poor resin separation. The effective loss of 10% or so of the resin is not the worst part; that is in the increase in the rinse-up time.

A reduction in the criticality of a sharp interface can be achieved through the introduction of a third resin, of intermediate density and without functional beads. Actually, it is the combination of particle size and particle density that is important to the hydraulic settling characteristics that govern the resin separations. In any case, the use of such a mediating resin serves to reduce the extent of cation-exchange intermingling. These special non-charge-bearing, or inert resins are different in color, which helps to define the interfacing layer they provide. They are expensive. Presumably, however, they provide value in terms of better regeneration and higher product water quality (Figure 8-12). This is of significance where the mixed bed is being applied in a polishing mode in more demanding applications. Otherwise, with a less well-defined interface, some higher quantities of sodium and chloride leakage would result.

The mode of regeneration of the separated beds follows the protocol of the two-bed regeneration: a slow regeneration using the appropriate reagents at proper concentrations, followed by a slow rinse to encourage the diffusive removal of the regenerants, succeeded by a fast rinse to remove traces adsorbed to surfaces. In good regenerations involving good resin separations, the final rinse can usually give water with a resistivity of 1 megohm-cm within 10 to 15 minutes. It is fair to say, however, that the regeneration of mixed beds can offer problems. Mixed beds that require frequent regeneration, as in a system composed just of a carbon bed and a mixed bed, are not too popular with plant operators.

Three-Bed Systems

The complexities of mixed-bed regenerations lead to the advocacy that cation leakage (usually sodium) from twin-bed operations be countered by the downstream installation of additional single beds. Thus Applebaum (1968) referenced the use of "multibed" plants, where a primary two-bed demineralizer was followed by a secondary two-bed demineralizer. Abrams (1990) advised the use of mixed beds for polishing operations, and the use of separate beds for makeup water. Sodium leakage from two-bed demineralizers would be contained by the addition of a third cation-exchange bed to remove the leaked cations.

Kunin (1984) saw two-bed demineralization followed by cation-exchange polishing as minimizing the use of acid regenerant, decreasing the quantity of regenerant waste, and improving the quality of the product water. Though twin-bed systems may exhibit sodium leakage, the presence of small quantities of such leaked ions in the product water need not always be objectionable. They might be tolerated in *USP* Purified Water contexts used if it were not for the fact that the sodium ion manifests itself in conjunction with hydroxyl ions. Thus the pH of the product water is in the range of 8 to 9, above the neutral level specified by *USP*. (This alkalinity is sometimes incorrectly attributed to residues of the caustic employed in the anion-exchange regeneration.) The cation-exchange polishing bed has a very high capacity relative to the sodium ion level. Therefore the polishing bed may be operated at high flowrates (up to 25 gpm/ft^2). Its size may be significantly smaller than that of twin beds, and it can be regenerated effectively with low acid dosage, usually about 3 pounds per cubic foot (lb/ft^3) compared to 6 lb/ft^3 for normal cation-bed operations (Bernatowicz and Collins, 1986).

The most popular *USP* Purified Water system is a two-bed ion-exchange unit

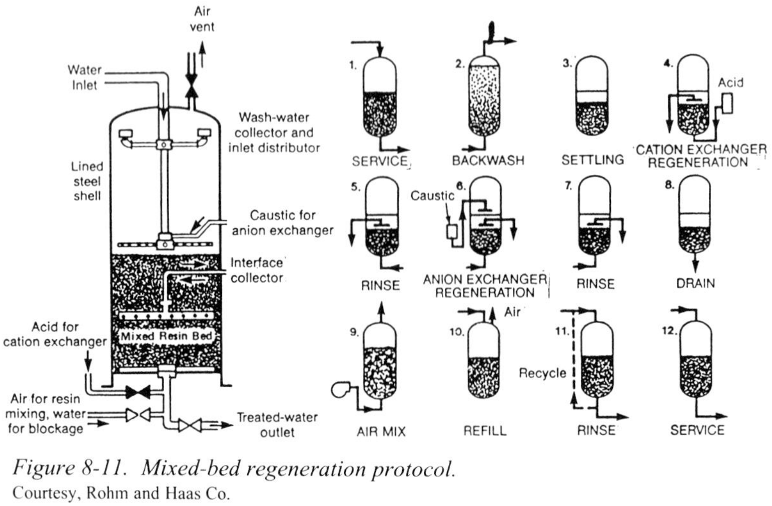

Figure 8-11. Mixed-bed regeneration protocol.
Courtesy, Rohm and Haas Co.

followed by a mixed bed; the latter unit is to contain sodium ion leakage and thus assure the required pH 7 level. But the same result can be had from a three-bed unit at a less than half the cost and with a less-demanding operation. However, as Abrams (1990) points out, two-bed units operated countercurrent also offer advantages.

Bernatowicz and Collins (1986) described two such systems used to produce *USP* Purified Water. The first of these consisted of well water fed to a carbon filter prior to a two-bed deionizer utilizing upflow countercurrent design, followed by a cation-exchange polishing unit, a 1-μm-rated cartridge filter, and an in-line UV sterilizer device. The well water had a TDS level of 310 ppm. The two-bed unit initially produced water of with a resistivity of 8 megohm-cm and a pH of 7.5. The cation-exchange polisher brought the water to a specific resistance of 12 to 14 megohm-cm and a pH of 7. After processing 15,000 gallons, the water effluent from the two beds had a resistivity of 1 to 2 megohm-cm, and after the polisher it was 6 to 8 megohm-cm at a pH of 6.5.

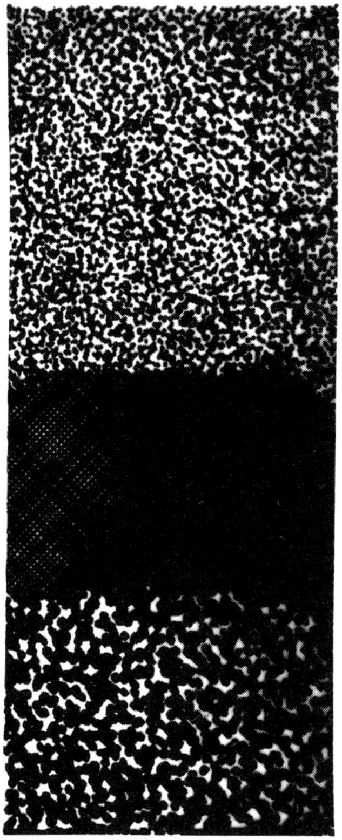

Figure 8-12. Use of inert resin to aid separation.
Courtesy, Rohm and Haas Co,

The second trifold system described by Bernatowicz and Collins (1986) was comprised of depth filtration, carbon filtration, cocurrent two-bed demineralizers, cation-exchange polishing, a 3-μm-rated filter, and an in-line UV installation. This was an on-demand system wherein the product water was recirculated during low-flow periods. Initially, the water produced by the two-bed unit had a resistivity of 400,000 to 600,000 ohms-cm and an 8.5 pH. Polishing brought this to 7 or 8 megohm-cm and pH of 6.9. The ion leakage from the two beds unfortunately increased with time, as did also the pH. Amelioration of the situation by the cation-exchange polisher brought the pH to 6.1 (because of the presence of weakly ionized anions), and the resistivity to 3.5 megohm-cm.

Cutler (1987) pointed out that the appropriate resin functionality depends primarily upon the design of the system. For example, a strongly acidic exchanger followed by a weakly basic exchanger (SA-WB) will leave silica levels unchanged, but will give water typically 10 to 30 μs/cm in conductivity. A strongly acidic exchanger followed by strongly basic (SA-SB) reduces silica to 0.02 to 0.10 ppm. The water will have conductances of 5 to 15 μs/cm. The arrangement of weakly acidic, strongly acidic, weakly basic, strongly basic (WA-SA-WB-SB) can reduce silica to 0.02 ppm and give waters having conductivities of 5 to 15 μs/cm. A strongly acidic, strongly basic couple reinforced by another similar pair (SA-SB-SA-SB) will yield the same low silica levels, 0.02 ppm, but with a product-water conductivity of less than 1 μs/cm. The four-bed arrangement of strongly acidic followed by a weakly basic succeeded by strongly acidic and strongly basic (SA-WB-SA-SB), while giving conductivity values of under 1 μs/cm, may lead, perhaps surprisingly, to somewhat lower silica readings, namely, 0.01 to 0.02 ppm. The same values should eventuate from waters from mixed beds. (It will be recalled that conductivity, measured in microsiemens/centimeter, previously in micromhos/cm, is the reciprocal of resistivity measured in megohm-cm.)

The mixed-bed system is best in terms of effluent quality, but not in terms of regenerant utilization. However, using a mixed bed following a two-bed deionizer will mean less frequent need to regenerate the mixed bed. This may encourage organism growth. To avoid this, short cycling becomes important. Short cycling will, as intended, mean more frequent regeneration, and the sanitization derived therefrom.

Table 8-5 compares the waters prepared by co-current two-bed systems and by a mixed-bed arrangement. In terms of total dissolved solids, the two-bed

Table 8-5
Deionizer Comparison

	Co-current Two Bed	*Mixed Bed*
Effluent (TDS)	1-10 ppm	0-0.5 ppm
Effulent (resistivity)	50,000-400,000 ohm-cm	1,000,000-18,300,000 ohm-cm
pH	4-10	7
Relative chemical efficiency	1.2-4	1
Ease of operation	Easier	More difficult

Courtesy, *Ultrapure Water* journal

yields from 1 to 10 ppm, and the mixed-bed approaches 0 to 0.5 ppm. The corresponding resistivities are 50,000 to 400,000 ohm-cm and 1 to 18.3 megohm-cm, respectively. Resistivity readings are always temperature-corrected to 25 °C. Usually this is internally compensated for within the resistivity meter itself. As regards pH, the water effluent from a two-bed system can be from 4 to 10; while that flowing from a mixed-bed should have a value of 7. The mixed-bed is not as chemically efficient as the separate beds because of the resin separation problem at the interface distributor. With regard to the removal of ions from a water, no other ion-exchange arrangement or any RO system can match the performance of a mixed bed, except in power generation condensate polishing where the influent impurities are in low ppb concentrations. This is more difficult to operate than other deionization units, however.

Countercurrent Regeneration

The construction and flow operations of ion-exchange beds were originally modeled after those of deep-bed filters, as of sand with which there has been much experience. The sand layer usually rests upon a gravel support layer that is, in turn, kept in position by a sustaining screen or grating through which the filtered water can exit. The water flows downward through the sand bed, and its force compresses the sand against the bottom restraints. This confers cohesion upon the deep bed. Indeed, the water flow can be so small as not to provide sufficient sand compaction, in which case channeling can occur. To effect desired bed compactions, the same downward flow principles are utilized in ion-exchange operations.

Periodically, sand beds are rid of their accumulated debris by being flushed. The most efficient flushing is by backwashing. The bed, having no physical restraints on top, is able to be brought to a quicksand consistency conducive to foreign-particle release. An accompaniment of the deep-bed disruption is the floating away as well of less-dense sand particles. In the case of sand this loss is generally unimportant. It would be of economic significance, however, if the loss were of ion-exchange resin. Therefore, in ion-exchange bed regenerations the chemical flows were initially (and in the United States still largely are) in the same direction as the service water flow: downward against the physical restraints whose presence preserves the bed compaction. *Co-current*, more correctly, *coflow*, describes this situation where the service flow and the regeneration flow are in the same direction.

For ion-exchange bed applications, there are advantages to countercurrent flows of water and regenerant. This arrangement is called a *counterflow* or *countercurrent* operation. There is a fundamental difference in the technology and performance between the coflow and counterflow practices. Counterflow or countercurrent operations are to be preferred. They result in ion-leakages that are of a magnitude less while saving on chemicals and reducing wastewater. Many ion-exchange experts consider cocurrent operations an improper way to apply ion-exchange despite the widespread usage in the United States. They decry the larger quantities of chemical regenerants consumed and of wastewaters produced in coflow operations as consequences of a perverted technology; wastefully excessive to the requirements of correct ion-exchange practices, namely, counterflow operations.

In the operation of an ion-exchange column, the ion-exchange resin becomes exhausted from the top down. The ion-exchange sites further upstream are the first to be utilized. The completeness of their conversion is assured by the initial high ratio of ions to ion-exchange sites. The ion-exchange sites lower down the bed are less depleted, and toward the bottom of the column may remain unspent altogether. To prevent sodium ion leakage, the ion-exchange operation is best left with a margin of safety. The ion-exchange operation is therefore not conducted to complete exhaustion. The beds are operated to a breakthrough point, to a percentage of total exhaustion. In semiconductor usage, the bed operation may be halted before the effluent waters decrease in quality to 15 megohm-cm resistivity.

Consider the regeneration of the cation-exchange column. As it is carried out in co-current fashion, the incoming hydrogen ions (or hydronium ions, H_3O^+) preferentially displace the sodium ions, then the magnesium, then the calcium ions, in accordance with the more tenacious hold of the multivalent elements. Also, as the multivalent elements are released, they in turn displace the monocharged ions downstream in a continuing progression. As a result, there may come to be a broad band of resin in the hydrogen form on top of the column, with narrower bands of resin combined with magnesium and calcium below that, and yet another band in the sodium form beneath that. If the regeneration proceeds to a sufficient extent, the sodium band may be eluted by the downflowing calcium ions released by displacement by the regenerating hydrogen ion. There will, in any case, be a heel of some unregenerated resin left at the end of the regeneration cycle because it is not economically feasible to completely convert the resin to the hydrogen form. (The unregenerated zone is perhaps 3 to 6 inches deep.) This co-current regeneration is limited by the law of diminishing returns. More and more acidic regenerant is required to obtain progressively less and less added conversions. Furthermore, it increases the problem of acid disposal. Even the dumping of water can be expensive, (in 1994), costing as high as $8 per 1.000 gallons. (Figures 8-13 and 8-14)

When ion exchange is again resumed, the water first issuing from the column will contain ions eluted from the unconverted heel; sodium (and possibly other ion) leakage will be evident. Eventually, the water quality will improve until, as the bed nears exhaustion, its breakthrough will be reached. If, however, the exhausted bed were to be subject to countercurrent regeneration, the broad band of hydrogen-form resin would become situated at the bottom of the column with overlays of resin in calcium, magnesium, and sodium forms. The resumption of ion-exchange operations would then not occasion any sodium leakage into the descending and exiting waters until the column reached its breakthrough point.

For the counterflow of regenerant chemical solutions to be in an upflow configuration, some form of restraint must be imposed on the top of the resin column to maintain its proper degree of compaction in order to prevent the physical movement, the disturbance, of the ion-exchange wave front. This may be managed in any of several ways; by blocking the flow of water, or by an imposition of air pressure, or the hindrance of physical restraints that are porous to permit the passage of regenerant solution but that will not become clogged by resin beads. Among the physical restraints is a layer of inert plastic beads restrained by screens. In co-current regeneration, more acid is used to minimize sodium leakage; therefore countercurrent regeneration may lead to savings on

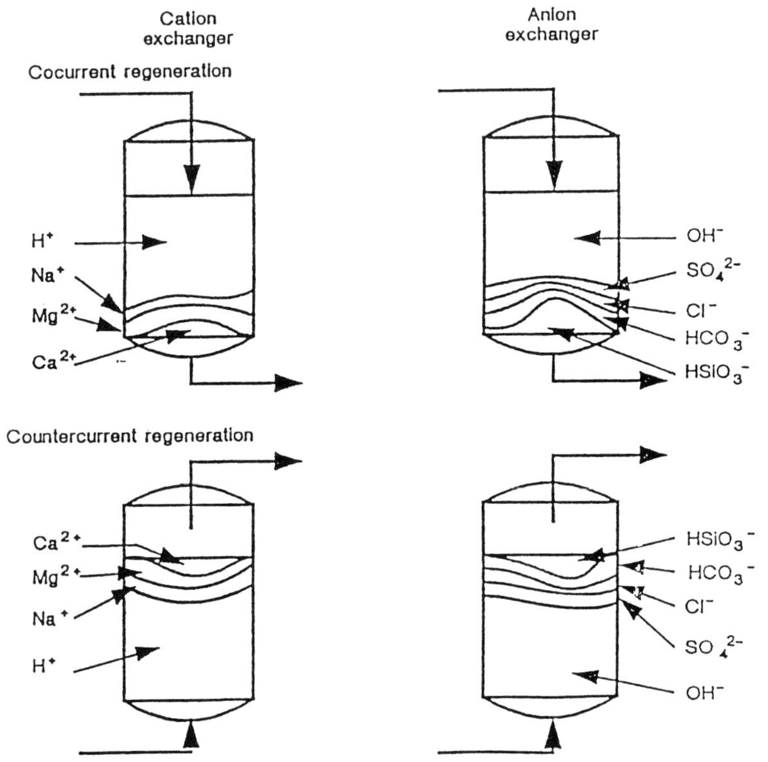

Figure 8-13. Cocurrent and countercurrent egeneration of ion-exchange beds..
Courtesy, Rohm and Haas Co,

regeneration chemicals. Where 4 pounds of sulfuric acid may be needed in co-current operations, 2 pounds may suffice in a counterflow practice. About 5% to 20% more regenerant is needed than the stoichometric amount in a countercurrent regeneration. The product water effluent from a co-current regenerated bed can attain 5 to 10 μS (100,000 to 200,000 ohm-cm, 0.1 to 0.2 meghom-cm).

Countercurrent procedures wherein the service water flow is upward (instead of the almost universally used downwards) and the regeneration flow is downwards ought to be best because upward flow would tend automatically to stratify the finer resin beads at the top of the column, making for a higher packing density that would offer its greater efficiency to the exchange of the diminishing ion concentration at the (upward) end of the column. Additionally, the bed would remain compacted during the downward flow of the regenerants. This would avoid inefficiencies in the regeneration that would lead to ion leakages in the next cycle.

The layer of inert polymeric granules against which the resin beads are compacted permits the passage of the service water along with suspended solids and resin fines. Normal size beads are retained. In those countercurrent installations in which the service flow is downward, the counterflow of regenerant is at a rate so sufficiently high as to maintain compaction against the low-density, inert plastic granules positioned at the top collector/distributor.

Kemp (1984) described the operation of such a countercurrent system utilizing service water upflow. Bed compaction was provided by a layer of rigid, inert, low-density plastic granules above the resin beads. The resin formed a compact layer against the layer of inert material at linear flow velocities of 4 gpm/ft^2. Below this layer a fluidized zone was formed. (The zone proportions were controlled by the flow velocities and the resin density.) The fluidized zone offered the advantage of intimate contact between the resin beads and the water whose ions were being exchanged.

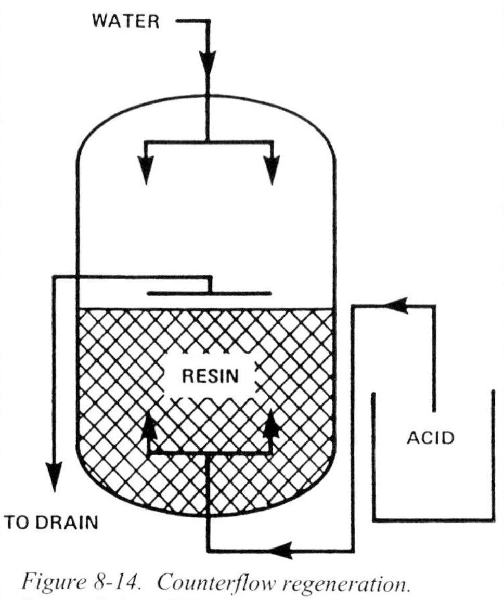

Figure 8-14. Counterflow regeneration.
Courtesy, Rohm and Haas Co,

In the co-current operations, as is the practice with sand beds, backwashing of the bed is practiced following the regeneration step. In the case of counterflow practices, backwashing is inadvisable because the layer of hydrogen-form ion-exchange should be kept in as stable a position as possible. Backwashing is disruptive. In countercurrent operations, backwashing is thus practical only once every ten cycles or so, instead of every cycle. Even so, it may take a couple of cycles or even double or triple regenerations for the hydrogen-form resin zone to settle down properly. To enable backwashing to be performed only every quarter or every year, in order to minimize disruption of the hydrogen-form resin layer, the service water requires being filtered to reduce or eliminate its particle load. Backwashing is done on differential pressure countercurrent.

The formation of $CaSO_4$ could be different in countercurrent regenerations. There, the sulfuric acid first regenerates sodium from the lowest band of cation-containing resin. The sodium sulfate thus generated may have a more sensitive effect than does sulfuric acid upon calcium sulfate.

Despite the advantages inherent in countercurrent regeneration, its logic has not proved to be compelling. Upward flows must be designed and managed for rather constant flowrates lest bed disruptions result. Their control is not that easily attained. In general, co-current operations are less sensitive. Countercurrent equipment is perhaps 15% to 25% more expensive than co-current equipment, and requires a somewhat greater expertise in operations to realize its inherent promises.

Countercurrent two-beds dominate the European scene to the extent of almost 90%; in the United States, only about 15% to 20% of the separate beds being built are countercurrent. It is easy to produce water with a resistivity of 1-megohm-cm using countercurrent two-bed systems. Producing water superior to co-current in quality, countercurrent operations save considerably on regenerants. At the same level of chemical usage, counterflow units can produce water with a resistivity of 2 to 3 megohm-cm (Zoccolante, 1990). In a co-current two-bed, the amount of chemical used is 3 or 4 times that actually required for regeneration. The excess chemicals require neutralization before being disposed of. In the countercurrent regeneration, only about 5% to 10% of excess quantities are involved. Some utilities with makeup water systems of several hundred gpm do use separate-bed countercurrent regeneration for the saved cost of regenerant chemicals.

According to Zoccolante (1995), the effluent quality for separate bed deionizers is normally in the range of 1 to 10 ppm total dissolved solids using cocurrent regeneration. Countercurrent regeneration yields waters having one-tenth that quantity TDS. The resistivity range for waters is 0.05 to 0.5 megohms-cm using the cocurrent technique; but from 0.5 to 10 megohms-cm for countercurrent regeneration. The pH range is wide; from 3 to 11, and can shift from alkaline to acid during the service cycle.

Mixed-bed effluent qualities are normally in the range of 0 to 0.5 ppm TDS, and their resistivities normally lie in the range of 1 to 18.3 megohms-cm. At high resistivity levels the pH of the product water is very close to 7.0; otherwise it is normally from 6.8 to 7.2.

Some Equipment Considerations

Some operators prefer an eductor to a positive displacement pump for the delivery of regenerative chemicals. Eductors, which operate on the venturi principle, require no moving parts; have less tendency to leak under pressure; and cannot be overpressurized and are thus safer. In contrast, positive displacement pumps deliver full strokes, but if the vacuum side is blocked, the stroke will be empty. This last fact notwithstanding, positive displacement pumps are consistent in their delivery of regenerant chemicals, which is a critical consideration where proper flowrates and precise dilution proportions are required. Eductors have the disadvantage of a delivery rate that is a function of the water pressure. It is true that regulators can be utilized to standardize the water pressure. Nevertheless, the eductor output is governed by back-pressure effects. For the delivery of ion-exchange regeneration reagents, positive displacement pumps are preferred for their relative reliability. Chemical pumps are used more frequently for larger units, and eductors for smaller units.

The introduction of oil by way of the airstream or the water backwash can have serious consequences. Oil entrainment onto the resin bead surfaces can effectively block and eliminate the ion-exchange sites from further participatory actions. Where oily impurities have been introduced, their removal can be accomplished by detergent washing. Unwanted microorganisms may also be introduced by way of the airstream used to remix the resins. It is best that air filtered through 0.2-μm-rated membranes be used for the remix.

Equipment such as PVC piping, pressure gauges, and diaphragms should be sturdy enough to withstand the inevitable water hammers. Diaphragm valves, although expensive, are recommended as being reliable against leaking (as of backwash water). The resin columns should be equipped with manholes, particularly near the distributors, to permit easy access and safe entry. They should also be equipped with a removal port at the bottom of the column. Proper water and regenerant solution distribution is very important. Circular distributors may not be suitable in wide-diameter columns because of the spaces at the perimeter between the spokes. Lateral distributors are preferable because they can be added as needed to cover the area of the resins. (See Figures 8-15 and 8-16).

The ease of water penetration into the racks is a function of its surface tension. This is much influenced by temperature and by the organic content of the water.

Removal of Carbon Dioxide

Carbon dioxide in water yields an acidic reaction, through the dissociation of carbonic acid, whose acid anhydride is CO_2, into hydrogen ions and bicarbonate ions. Complete conversion of bicarbonate to CO_2 gives water of about pH 5 (see page 353).

$$H_2O + CO_2 <----> H_2CO_3 <----> H^+ + HCO_3^- \qquad \text{Eq. 8-18}$$

The elimination of the carbon dioxide and of its low-pH-causing activities can be accomplished using ion-exchange resins in one of two ways. In either case, the aqueous solution containing, say, sodium chloride and calcium bicarbonate, is first reacted with a cation-exchange resin.

The generation of hydrogen ion by the cation-exchange reaction serves to shift the carbonic acid dissociation point toward its un-ionized form, in favor of water and carbon dioxide release.

Air free of carbon dioxide can then be used to sweep the solution free of the CO_2 before it is subjected to anion-exchange action. (See Chapter 7, page 356). Mechanical removal of the dissolved carbon dioxide serves to save on the strongly basic anion-exchange resin that would otherwise be required to remove it, a genuine economic consideration. Removal of the CO_2 by strongly basic anion-exchange resin is through the agency of bicarbonate ion removal:

$$CO_2 + H_2O <----> H_2CO_3 <----> H^+ + HCO_3^- \qquad \text{Eq. 8-19}$$
$$CH_2NR_3OH <----> OH^- + NR_3^+ + H^+ + HCO_3^-$$
$$\uparrow\downarrow$$
$$H_2O + CH_2NR_3HCO_3$$

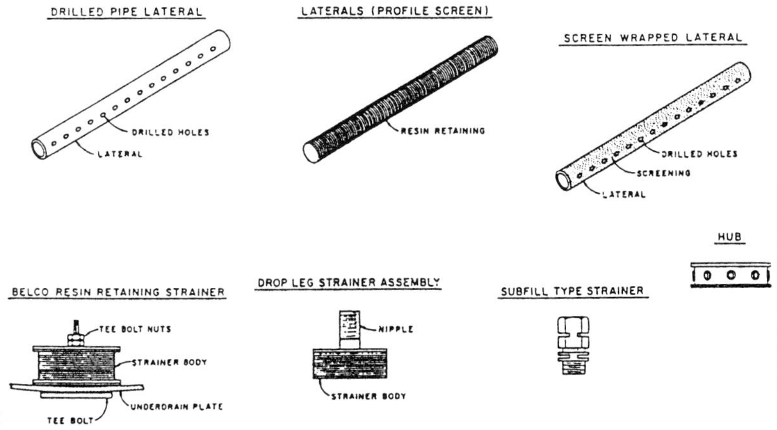

Figure 8-15. Internal components.

Brian J. Hoffman (1985); Courtesy: Hohm and Haas Co.

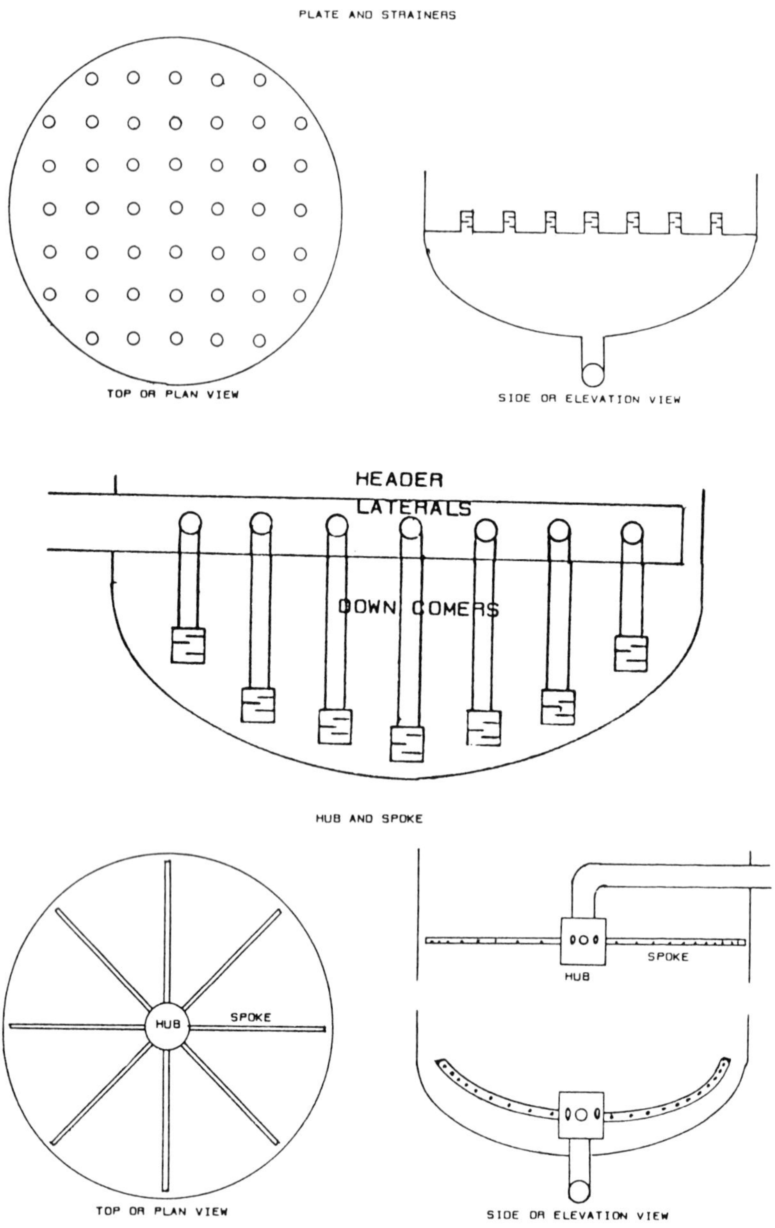

Figure 8-16. Various distributor arrangements.
Owens (1985); Courtesy, Tall Oaks Publishing Inc.

The technique of sweeping away the CO_2 necessitates the cost of a second pump. There exists a rule of thumb, the 50/50 rule, to give guidance in choosing between these two alternatives. When the water flow exceeds 50 gallons per minute (190 liters per minute) and its carbon dioxide content is over 50 ppm, the technique involving the expenditure for a second pump is economically justified. Otherwise, the carbon dioxide is removed in the form of the bicarbonate ion at the expense of the anion-exchange resin. The guidance of the 50/50 rule must be used with discretion. The use of degasifiers, as already discussed, threatens the introduction of organisms into the water system. Where the presence of organisms is of overriding concern, as in pharmaceuticals, the use of degasifiers is largely eschewed, and the 50/50 rule is ignored. In practice, the removal of carbon dioxide by degassing leaves about 5 to 10 ppm of CO_2 in the water (Figure 8-17).

The equilibration of water with carbon dioxide causes a lowering of the resistivity of the water. The effect is not constant. It reflects the degree of equilibration that takes place, and it is a function of time and of the partial pressure of the carbon dioxide. Water with a resistivity of 18 megohm-cm can decrease to 2 megohm-cm in the presence of carbon dioxide if its flow is stopped long enough for full equilibration to occur. The corresponding water conductivity is 0.5/μS-cm.

The Resin Bead Form

Gel type. The first-developed types of resin beads, those consisting of a polymeric hydrocarbonaceous cross-linked molecular network to which are periodically appended functional ion-exchange groups, were of the gel form. They are prepared by the vinyl polymerization of a solution of divinylbenzene (DVB) in styrene suspended in water. The size of the suspended organic droplets is regulated by the vigor with which the mixture is agitated. They are caused to undergo vinyl polymerization by the free radicals generated by a peroxidic initiation. By the termination of the polymerization, the suspended liquid droplets have become converted into gel-type spheres of cross-linked polystyrene, later to be converted chemically to functional-group-bearing resins (Owens, 1985, Chapter 4).

The ionic groups hydrate in contact with water. As a result the resin swells. The degree of cross-linking supplied by the divinylbenzene limits the extent of swelling. The cross-linking confers mechanical strength upon the resin bead. Within certain limits, however, the restraint on the degree of swelling, reciprocal to the increase in tensile and compressive strengths, circumscribes the resin's capacity for ion exchange. Untrammeled swelling predisposes to a more generous degree of ion exchange, but also makes for a weaker resin bead. The styrene/DVB formulation is the archetypal structure of such resin beads. They can be and are prepared by the vinyl polymerization of other molecular systems as well. Ethyl acrylate and methyl methacrylate are among other monomers that may be used. The same principles apply to other polymeric systems as well.

Organic extractables in gel-type resins. There are important consequences that arise from the gel structure of the resin. The total organic carbon (TOC) of importance in new resins is in the form of sulfonates. In addition, there is inevitably a portion of unconverted styrene monomer (along with low-molecular-weight polystyrene homopolymers, and accompanied by unreacted portions of DVB) that in any case contains a good proportion of non-DVB material. This material, along with other extraneous molecules both organic and inorganic, remains within the gel in bead form as well as upon its surface. Despite copious washing of the resin beads, a portion of this material (soluble sulfonates and amines included) remains to leach subsequently as TOC into waters being treated.

The unwanted impurities are removed from the interior of the bead by washing or leaching processes that are diffusion-limited. Diffusive removal is heavily time- and temperature-dependent. It is impeded by the viscosity of the gel. Ultimately, impurity removal is fastest from the surface of the bead. However, the ratio of surface to volume is smallest for spherical shapes.

The resins may be steamed and washed to reduce their leachables. When installed, these resins may be washed again for a very long time in very pure water. The leaching of TOC by water is a diffusion-limited phenomenon driven

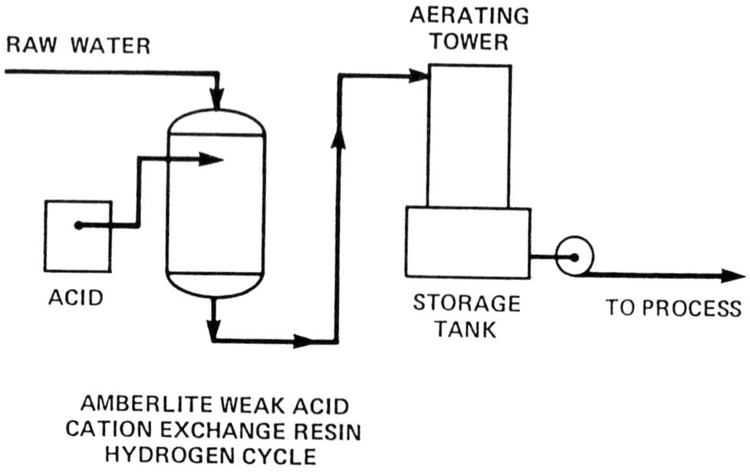

Figure 8-17. Elimination of water hardness and of carbon dioxide.
Courtesy, Rohm and Haas Co.

by the concentration gradient between the TOC in the resin and the TOC in the watery extract. The use of a TOC destruction device in a recirculating loop can be helpful in avoiding the leveling of the TOC gradient, and in saving water.

Ammerer (1989) used ultraviolet light in conjunction with titanium dioxide catalyst in a recirculating loop to destroy TOC. One way or another, TOC levels of around 100 ppb (or even as high as 200 to 500 ppb) emanating from resin beds initially may be flushed down at least to 20 ppb or less (Ammerer, 1989), or even to as little as 5 ppb.

It is questionable, given the diffusion-impeding viscosity of the gel and the polymeric nature of some of the TOC, whether complete TOC extraction is at all possible. However, its rate of leaching can be so low as to add very little TOC to a volume of water per unit time. Indeed, the faster the rate of water flow, the lower the TOC level may be for this very reason. Extraction by the flowing water of TOC from the resin beads is diffusion-limited, reflecting principally the influences of temperature and of time. If a given volume of water flows slowly through a given quantity of resin (i.e., over a given surface area), there is a greater opportunity for its picking up TOC than if the water flowed more rapidly, thereby minimizing resin-surface-to-water interfacing. The faster flow would yield lower TOC concentrations.

This same problem is involved in the fouling of the resin beads by TOC, soon to be discussed. It is also an aspect of TOC removal by ion exchange, also soon to be considered.

The problems posed by the slow rate of diffusion in and out of gels was appreciated by ion-exchange resin users even before current concerns regarding TOC asserted themselves. Organic matter in the water being treated (often arising from vegetative origins whose hydrolytic and oxidative degradation generated humic, fulvic, and other acid types) fouled the resin beads, especially the anion-exchange resins. These foulants could usually be cleaned from the accessible resin bead surfaces. Allowed to diffuse into the gel interiors of the beads over extended periods of bed operations, they were difficult to remove. Diffusive entrance and removal both take a long time, while the period dedicated to resin regeneration is relatively short. Under conditions of TOC fouling and long durations between bed regenerations, an inevitable loss of resin capacity results.

Macroreticular resins. Macroreticular resins are, in effect, openly porous types. Their polymeric matrix is the familiar gel. Its sections within the bead are thinner, however, and more accessible to diffusion because the bead is honeycombed with open pores.

The internal pores result from the inclusion of extractable material in the polymerization formula. This material does not participate in the vinyl polymerization. After the bead is formed, the extractable material is appropriately removed, as by solvent, to leave a porous structure.

Polystyrene, prepolymerized and therefore not subject to vinyl cross-linking with DVB, is such a material. It can be removed from the bead by solvent. Cross-linked polystyrene is insoluble, however, because of the three-dimensional molecular network established by cross-linking. Another way of introducing porosity in the beads is to include a polar material such as tertiary butyl alcohol in the polymerization reaction. This serves to precipitate the copolymer before it is completely gelled. It emerges with a macroreticular structure, a polymeric mass riddled with pores and passageways. It therefore has more surface; it is more openly porous than the polymeric gel. In consequence, diffusion into and out of its interior is more rapid, and more of its adsorptive sequestration is of the more easily removed surface type; albeit the surfaces are those of pore channels.

There is another virtue to the macroreticular resin beads. They are more generously cross-linked than the gel type. They contain some 20% of DVB in their polymerization recipes. If the gel types were as heavily cross-linked they would be so restrained in their degree of ion transport as to be limited in their ion-

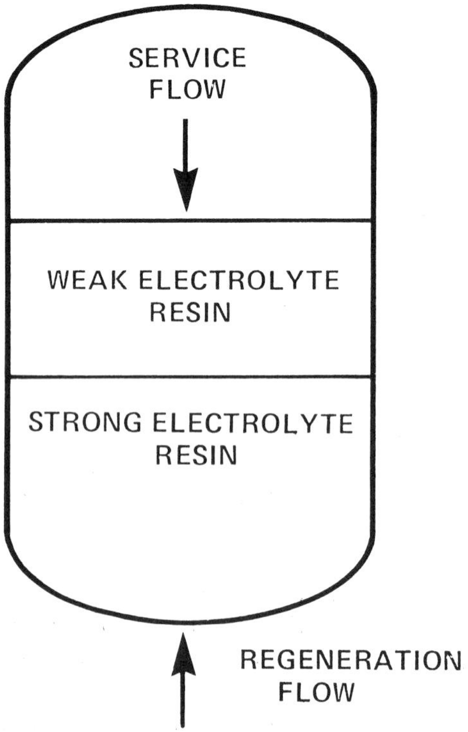

Figure 8-18. A layered bed construction.
Courtesy, Dr. Robert Kunin

exchange capacities. The open porosity of the macroreticular types makes their more extensive surface, more readily accessible and keeps their capacities from being unduly compromised. Higher degrees of cross-linking confer greater mechanical strength. The alternate swelling and shrinking of the beads, in addition to their being subject to constant abrasion, causes bead fragmentation and wear. Some claim the gel types fragment more, often breaking into halves and quarters; this is possibly a response to inner strains in a more compact structure. Abrams (1976) found such generalizations misleading. By way of a pump-based impact test, he found that gel-type beads may actually be superior, but the matter remains in dispute.

The larger spaces within the macroreticular resin beads come at the expense of some capacity. The higher cross-linking of the macroreticular resins gives them a higher selectivity, but does make them more difficult to regenerate. Their greater physical stability is an advantage, although gel-type resins are adequately strong for innumerable applications.

The higher cross-linked densities of the macroreticular-type resins provide additional stability against oxidative degradation, such as is occasioned by chlorine being permitted to enter the resin beds. This is an increasingly frequent occurrence that finesses the use of carbon beds or of bisulfite to remove the chlorine. Its entering the ion-exchange beds may serve to some extent also to sanitize them against organisms.

Gel versus macroreticular beads. Abrams (1976) listed the following advantages for condensate polishing of gel-type resins over the macroporous or macroreticular types of resins: higher capacities, more favorable regeneration efficiencies, lower cost, and a lower tendency to produce colloidal particles.

The greater the degree of cross-linking, the higher the mechanical strength of the bead, but also the more restrained its degree of swelling. Limitations to the swelling find expression, however, in the ion-exchange selectivities of the resins. The selectivity ratios for the Na/H ions and the Cl/OH ions increase with the styrene/divinylbenzene cross-linking. The situation as presented by Abrams (1976) is as follows:

	Degree of Cross-Linking	
Ion	*8%*	*16%*
H^+	1.0	1.0
Na^+	1.5	1.9
NH_4^+	1.95	2.5

The gel types are usually cross-linked to an 8% extent. The amount of cross-linking for macroporous types is higher, possibly to about 20%. Therefore the latter have higher Na/H selectivities.

The effect has been discussed of the greater degrees of cross-linking (necessary to macroreticular bead integrity) upon the increase in ion selectivity. The more accessible structure of the open bead type means that more ions and foulants are surface-deposited and/or are diffused a relatively small distance into the gel material constituting the bead's polymeric matrix. By contrast, the gel-type bead has relatively little surface; and its adsorbing action requires a deeper penetration by adsorbents into the polymeric mass. Therefore the diffusion-limited removal of the adsorbents, whether ions or foulants, requires more time with the gel-type bead.

Gel-type resins perform their ion-exchange functions well. The periods between resin replacements as necessitated by irreversible fouling can be prolonged even when the water being treated does contain organic foulants. A maintenance program can be helpful. The resins should be soaked in a brine/caustic solution for a minimum of 4 hours (the longer the better) every 3 months to remove the adsorbed TOC. It is helpful but not essential to use a warm soak solution. By means of such treatments, resin replacements on account of TOC fouling can be postponed, perhaps for a 50% increase in life. Resin life is highly application-dependent.

Not surprisingly, the strongly basic anion-exchange resins foul more avidly than the weak. It is easier to rid the weakly resins of their TOC. The weakly resins swell more, to a 20% or 30% extent, and shrink more upon regeneration. This exaggerated osmotic effect, with its concomitant greater cycles of resin expansions and contractions, serves to better eliminate the imprisoned organic matter. Thus layered constructions of weakly basic resins atop of strongly basic resins are used to prolong the life of the latter against TOC fouling. Indeed, the weakly basic resin can be regenerated more efficiently. The strongly basic resin should be used only when it is required to remove such weak acids as carbon dioxide (the anhydride of carbonic acid), and the silicic acids (silica). About 6 pounds of caustic are required to regenerate a cubic foot of strongly basic resin, but 4 pounds or less of caustic to regenerate a cubic foot of weakly basic resin. For a large installation, the difference in chemical costs can be appreciable (Figure 8-18).

The weakly basic resins have amine functionalities. The unshared electrons of the amino nitrogen atom participate in onium-type addition-compound formation, and combine with mineral acids to form amine salts. In regeneration, this acid is removed by the rejuvenating caustic, which is competitively stronger than the amine. The regeneration is not really an ion-exchange action but rather a straightforward neutralization, easily and efficiently accomplished.

The resin beads can also be protected against organic fouling by the prefilter action of ultrafiltration membranes or reverse osmosis units. In their prefilter roles, these serve sacrificially to prolong the life of the ion-exchange beds. It needs perhaps to be mentioned, and will subsequently be detailed, that cleaning such prefilters of the organic foulants they collect in the process shortens their own service lives. In this regard, ultrafilters (usually composed of polysulfones) better endure the rigors of cleaning than do RO membranes. Especially in electronics applications, RO is placed upstream of DI units. It is questionable whether without this arrangement the ion-exchange units could furnish water with 18-megohm-cm resistivity for extended periods of time.

Resin Fouling

Ion-exchange performance, particularly the mixed bed, is governed by the attainment of equilibria that characterize the separation and regeneration chemistry. Departures from the optimum levels of the equilibria may lead to ions slipping through the beds, to ion leakage. Ion leakage may also derive from kinetic causes. If the rate of ion-exchange becomes retarded, ions may come to pass through the beds before they are removed. In the service cycle, the water is run at high rates, the impurity level being low. The ion removal depends upon film diffusion kinetics. The ions must reach the bead surfaces to become exchanged. Therefore, the surface or film diffusion kinetics are the rate-controlling step. Fouling of the resin surfaces can, therefore, dramatically affect the ion-exchange rate kinetics. The water flow through the column may be slowed to have a more favorable effect upon the diffusion of the ion through the fouling film. However, if the rate is reduced much below 9 or 10 gpm/ft^2, the laminar boundary water film itself serves to impede the diffusive access of ions to the bead exchange-sites. Care should be taken to avoid fouling of the resin surfaces.

To begin with, being deep beds, ion-exchange columns serve as filters for particulate matter. They, therefore, require particulate removal protection to at least some degree. A large variety of fouling may arise in connection with ion-exchange resins. It may be helpful to summarize the approaches to solving certain of these problems.

Fouling by oil, which may originate from the exhaust vapors of compressors and pumps, is a particularly irksome occurrence. The resin may be cleansed by use of a heated solution of a nonfoaming surfactant, typically used in concentrations of 0.05% to 0.1%. (Recommendations for specific brands of surfactants may be obtained by contacting a manufacturer or supplier of ion exchange resins.) In cases of severe oil fouling, 1% caustic may be added to the heated surfactant solution.

The principal cause of premature resin failure may well be that occasioned by organic fouling, often permitted to proceed to irreversible extents. The foulants allowed to diffuse into the gel structure of the beads may prove very difficult to remove. Light surface fouling sometimes shows itself by an early sulfate-ion breakthrough when high flowrates are used in mixed-bed operations.

Sulfate ions, being divalent, are not difficult to remove by anion exchange. Enough fouling may occur, however, to deny the ready presence of two adjacent charged sites needed for sulfate-ion removal. Although charge capacity may still exist in the resin, sulfate ion may nevertheless slip through. This occurrence, sulfate leakage, is of real concern in the power industry. It should be noted that following cation exchange, the monovalent bisulfate is the ion of consequence. (Figure 8-19).

The problem of organic fouling requires treating the resin with a 10% brine solution (10 pounds of salt per cubic foot of resin), or with a preparation of 1 pound of caustic and 7 to 8 pounds of salt per cubic foot of resin in more recalcitrant cases. In either instance, the solution should be heated to 50 to 60°C (120 to 140 °F). Some believe it efficacious to add surfactant to the brine or brine/caustic mix. However, the use of anionic surfactants in conjunction with anion-exchange resins is to be strongly avoided in order to avoid fouling.

Anion-exchange resin fouling in single beds is generally caused by the adsorption of high-molecular-weight organic acids (TOC). Its prevention, as by prepositioned RO, is easier than its cure. Anion-exchange resin fouling also results from the accumulation of TOC originating in the cation-exchange resins. The reduction in extractables from the cation-exchange resins minimizes this source of TOC. Cation-exchange resins may exhaust in mixed-bed operations from the thermal degradation products emanating from anion-exchange resins exposed to excessive temperature. One such product may be trimethylamine. It combines with the cation-exchange groups but is easily removed upon resin regeneration. Such degradations are the product of time and temperature (Cutler,

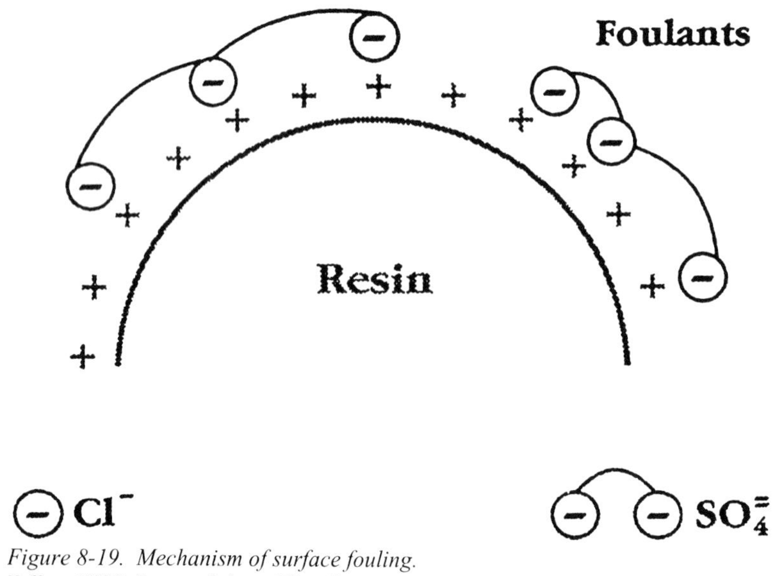

Figure 8-19. Mechanism of surface fouling.
Hoffman (1985); Courtesy, Rohm and Haas Co.

1987).

Organic fouling of the resins manifests itself as a reluctance to rinse up. It may necessitate a resin replacement. To minimize such situations, McGarvey (1990) advised a brine treatment every 6 months or so. The disposal of the brine may be a problem. Periodic examinations of the resins should be made as a forecast of fouling.

Silica-fouling removal from anion-exchange resin calls for a minimum 4-hour treatment of the resin with a 10% brine solution (10 pounds of salt per cubic foot of resin) containing 4% to 5% of caustic soda at 60 °C (140 °F). Brine itself will not remove polymeric silica, the usual form of silica fouling. A triple regeneration is advised, followed by a very thorough backwash to remove the resin fines that form. Where mixed beds are involved, alkali treatment is postponed until all magnesium has been removed from the bed. This is necessary to avoid the formation of magnesium hydroxide precipitation.

Magnesium hydroxide fouling of anion resins may follow the exhaustion of cation-exchange beds. The previously described solution of brine and caustic should be used on separated anion-exchange beds. If magnesium fouling occurs in mixed beds, brine should be used without the caustic.

Fouling by iron and/or manganese can be set right by a soaking in hydrochloric acid.

The fouling of ion-exchange beds by accumulated particulate matter, a cause of decrease in flowrates, requires the ministrations of backwashing. This should be done with caution. If air pressure is used, too vigorous an application can dislodge the laterals and distributors. It can be helpful in the backwashing to add 0.05% to 0.1% of a nonfoaming, nonionic surfactant.

The use of sulfuric acid in regeneration of the cation exchanger may lead to the fouling of the ion-exchange resins by calcium sulfate precipitation. Hydrochloric acid solutions of 5% strength can be used over a period of 2 hours at 50 to 60 °C (120 to 140 °F) to remove calcium sulfate deposits. Obviously, such treatments are to be avoided where stainless steel is present in screens or other articles, lest corrosive stress cracking occur.

Silica Fouling

Silica chemistry is unusual and complex. The solubility of silica is limited, and is both pH- and temperature-sensitive. Its more concentrated solutions may lead to its polymerization and precipitation. Silica is removed by strongly basic anion-exchange resins. It penetrates into the resin, however, where the amount of water available is restricted. Its concentration builds in this area of restricted and competitive hydration to the point where the individual silica structures begin to complex with themselves to produce silica polymers that are obstructive to removal. The trick is to prevent the silica within the bead from reaching high levels.

It is easy to overload the resins with silica. New or highly regenerated resins have a lot of capacity. After several cycles, wherein the system is run to a silica end point, silica polymerization begins to build, and regenerations are less effective. Eventually, the system runs at a higher level of silica leakage because the silica polymer begins to redissolve. One must, therefore, be cognizant of the silica levels in the water and of the amount being loaded into the ion-exchange resin. Unfortunately, numerical limits are difficult to recommend, given variables such as pH and temperatures. Thus, in two-bed systems where there is sodium leakage from the cation-exchange bed, the higher-pH waters entering the anion-exchange beds may serve to minimize silica polymerization, the polymer being more solubilized at higher pHs. In a very cold climate, silica polymerization may be reduced; however, higher-baseline silica leakage may obtain. If, as one is running to a silica end point, the level begins to build in the effluent water, the silica content of the water collected in a large storage tank may still be very acceptable. However, silica loading in the resin may become excessive. In cases where a mixed bed follows a two-bed arrangement, the ultimate reliance for silica removal should not be imposed upon the mixed-bed lest the anion-exchange column of the two-bed arrangement became overloaded. If silica polymer becomes released from the anion-exchange bed it would escape capture by the mixed bed. It could be reconverted to ionic silica in a boiler, its presence a puzzlement to all concerned since silica analysis would not have indicated its presence below the anion-exchange bed. Overloading or overrunning the bed with silica should be avoided. A conservative silica removal program should be practiced.

Silica and Silica Removal

The difference between a strong- and a weak-electrolyte ion-exchange resin is the degree of dissociation. The stronger resin dissociates more, furnishing more resin-anchored ionic sites for exchange. This is important where the sequestration of ions from weakly dissociated molecules is desired. Thus the strongly basic anion-exchange resins are required for carbon dioxide or soluble silica removal.

Silica can exist in water in the soluble form of essentially undissociated silicic acid, the exact chemistry of which is obscurely complex (See Chapter 6). Highly undissociated, its presence is not detectable by conductivity measurements. It dissociates even less than does boric acid or carbonic acid. Its presence in solution may be depicted as follows:

$$H_2O \cdot SiO_2 \text{ <----> } H^+ + HSiO_3^- \qquad \text{Eq. 8-20}$$

To capture the minuscule quantity of silicate ion, a very avid anion-exchange group is necessary, one that will supply as large a complement of cations as possible for salt formation. This means a strongly basic resin, the aromatic quaternary ammonium hydroxide type. The weaker polyamine types will not suffice.

$$
\begin{array}{c}
H_2SiO_3 \;<\text{----}>\; H^+ + HSiO_2^- \\
+ \\
2R\text{—}CH_2NR_3OH \;<\text{----}>\; 2OH^- + 2R\text{-}CH_2\text{—}N^+R_3 \\
\downarrow\uparrow \\
H_2O + (R\text{—}CH_2\text{—}NR_3)_2SiO_2
\end{array}
\qquad \text{Eq. 8-21}
$$

Ongoing salt formation between the quaternary ammonium ion and the silicate ion continuously upsets the undissociated silicic acid/silicate ion equilibrium, causing even more silicic acid to dissociate into ions. This results in the eventual removal from solution of the undissociated silicic acid.

Soluble silica can be removed through anion exchange using strongly basic quaternary ammonium hydroxide exchange media. The means of applying this method are also amenable to variation, as dictated by economic considerations, so that the strongly basic anion-exchange resin is not unnecessarily consumed. Thus if the water, purified of its cations as it emerges from the cation exchanger, is led into a bed or column of weakly basic anion-exchange resin first, then most of the anions (but not silica or carbon dioxide, too feebly dissociated) will be removed. Silica can then be eliminated in a subsequent treatment involving a strongly basic anion-exchange resin. With the use of a three-bed system, most of the anion-exchange activity takes place on the more easily regenerated, weaker anion-exchange resin. The strongly basic anion-exchange final bed is preserved largely for silica (and carbon dioxide) removal. It will also arrest iron and aluminum when these are constituents of negatively charged colloids (Figure 8-20).

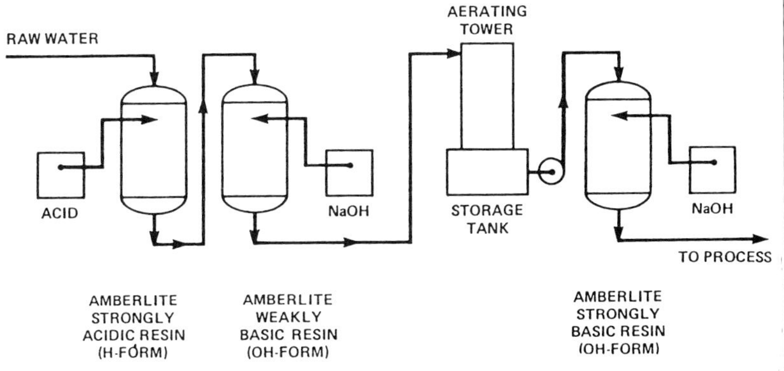

Figure 8-20. Three-bed system deionization with weakly and strongly basic anion exchangers.
Courtesy, Dr. Robert Kunin

The weakly basic column in a three-bed system adds to regeneration efficiency. It is sometimes possible to regenerate the weak base with the spent regeneration solution from the strongly basic column. In essence, the weakly basic regeneration is then for free. Thus, to regenerate the anion-exchange resins, sodium hydroxide is pumped countercurrent, first through the strongly basic resin, and then through the weakly basic resin. This order provides the strong regenerative reaction of concentrated sodium hydroxide where it is most needed, at the strongly basic anion-exchange resin bed. The rejuvenating caustic soda does become diluted as it flows through the first bed. Its strength, however, suffices for the renewal of the weakly basic anion-exchange resin in the second bed.

High-Purity Resins

In the semiconductor industry, organic substances are considered far more undesirable than they usually are in most drug manufacturing. In addition to the contributions of organics forthcoming from vegetative, farm, and industrial sources, there is concern for that leached or extracted from filters, from the activated carbon, and from the DI resins themselves.

These impurities can be unconverted monomers or low-molecular-weight polymers. They may be nonfunctional or even ion-containing substitution compounds. Decomposition products and oxidative and hydrolytic products of the organic resins may time-dependently contribute organic impurities.

Normal, typical commercial ion-exchange resins do contain leachables. In particular, long-chain sulfonic acid leachables can foul anion-exchange resins. New resin should be regenerated and rinsed a few times before being put in use. After such treatment and some period of use, leachables will become almost undetectable. Idle ion-exchange units after several months or even weeks should be recycled to help remove leachables. It is fair to say that it is unusual to find less than 1 ppb of organic matter in ion-exchange resin-treated waters.

Virgin resins are used in order to protect against cross contamination from usages by others. Such resins have not been exposed to a sodium cycle. These resins, their exchange sites not preempted by sodium, have a capacity 25% to 30% greater than ordinary DI resins in the sodium form even after a second regeneration to remove sodium. Actually, sodium is easy to remove if enough acid is used. Additionally, these resins are very low in metallic extractables, never having been used in ion exchange.

Certain grades of resins are referred to as nuclear-grade resins. They may indeed have specifications set by nuclear plant users, with different specifications variously set by different plants, usually with regard to particular metals. The stipulated properties may or may not confer benefits upon other users or applications, and can be unnecessarily costly. The implication that nuclear-grade means higher standards of purity or more desirable purity may be misleading. Virgin resins of equal purity and regeneration are available.

The significance of the "nuclear grade" is that it is manufactured to conform with stipulated standards, of whatever general significance, and that it passes a defined test confirming an ability to undergo a specified high degree of regeneration. In other words, it is produced to some user specifications. It has a discipline in addition to that of the manufacturer imposed upon its preparation.

Efforts to manufacture low-TOC ion-exchange resins were described by Borgquist and Brodie (1989).

Cutler (1987) discussed the considerations involved in the correct selection of ion-exchange resins. She discussed temperature effects on resin fouling in terms of thermal stability; pointed out that smaller resin beads are less susceptible to breakage as caused by osmotic shock than are larger beads; indicated the degradative effects of dissolved oxygen (especially at elevated temperatures and as prompted by heavy-metal catalysts) on the resin cross-links and upon the resulting organic fouling of downstream resins; and emphasized the importance of resin bead size in providing for their separation in mixed-bed regenerations and in avoiding excessive pressure drops.

Resin Life Expectancy

The resin life expectancy is dependent upon the criticality of the application. In normal industrial ion-exchange context, such as water softening, cation-exchange resins may last for 4 to 7 years, while 3 to 6 years of use may be had of anion-exchange resins. If, however, one wishes to reduce TOC in the effluent water to a few parts per billion, as in high-performance applications, the arduous demand would foreshorten those time periods.

Normal resin bead attrition is about 5% per year. This mostly physical attrition is minimized by soft pump start-ups.

Resin Bead Examination

Among the qualifying tests that resin manufacturers perform on their products are examinations for capacity and moisture content. The latter is very important in that it offers a measure of the degradation a resin bead undergoes with time. The cross-link density of the resin restricts the extent of swelling by its uptake of moisture. As will be seen, the oxidative degradation of the resin molecules by hypochlorite, chlorine, ozone, and even the aging caused by oxygen over time cuts these cross links. This permits a less restrained moisture uptake and a larger concomitant swelling. The increase in moisture content is thus a measure of the resin's decrepitude. Resin beads are also measured for their ability to withstand crushing. The whole-bead content is assessed by microscopic analysis and/or by inclined plane testing wherein only whole beads roll to the bottom of the plane. The measurement of bead size is also very important. A range of 16 to 50 mesh is usual; a range of 20 to 40 mesh is often preferred.

A user should periodically (perhaps yearly) reexamine the resins, or have them examined, for cleanliness, freedom from oil, moisture content, capacity, and ability to be regenerated. Test columns are constructed and operated to assess the actual capacity and ease of regeneration. Long rinse-up times, short operational cycles, and poor product water quality are possible indications of the need for resin replacement.

At shutdowns, resins should be stored in brine to discourage microbial growth and to prevent freezing. Such storage also helps to prevent organic fouling. The subject of periodic resin examination and analysis was discussed by Fisher and Otten (1985).

Resin Bead Clustering or Clumping

The regeneration of mixed beds requires that the cation-exchange and anion-exchange resins be separated so that each may receive its separate and opposite treatment: the former, an exposure to acid; the latter, to base. If the two types of resins are not completely separated, portions of one or the other or of both will, if exposed to the inappropriate regenerant, not become regenerated.

Mixed-bed regeneration sometimes does not achieve its proper level. This can be traced to a clustering of cation beads with anion beads. The clusters are not separated during the backwashing operation. Therefore, the affected beads are incompletely regenerated. This results in cross contamination, thereby increasing the ion leakage and reduced capacity of the mixed bed.

Sometimes several regenerations are required to attain the proper level of regeneration. According to the electrostatic theory, clustering takes place among oppositely charged resin beads, principally involving the small unexhausted portions of these always left at the end of an ion-exchange operation. (Much larger proportions of unexhausted resin are left in certain semiconductor operations wherein the mixed beds are regenerated as soon as the water quality drops to around 15-megohm-cm resistivity. To minimize presumed charge-related clumping, mixed beds are fully exhausted by a caustic wash before the resin separation commences. McGarvey (1990) believed it significant that air bubbles are often present where resin clumping occurs. Wetting effects are, therefore, believed to be part of the phenomenon. The beads would seem to be hydrophobic. Also, resins having the same charge sometimes cluster—particularly the weakly acidic types, but also the weakly basic varieties. Effects other than charge-related are therefore suspected. Hydrophobicity imparted by trace organic residuals used in the manufacture of the beads possibly seems implicated.

Indeed, one theory is that the clustering is caused by hydrophobic adsorptions operating among hydrophobic spots or areas on the resin beads. Actually, cross-linked polystyrene is a hydrophobic material except as this property becomes relieved in the molecular areas of the polymeric chains where ionic functional groups are present. The presence of hydrophobic spots also helps to explain the association of clumping with the presence of air bubbles. Rinsing the beads with detergent solutions helps. A sulfonated alkylated aromatic surfactant (or indeed most other surfactants) would adsorb its nonpolar moieties onto hydrophobic surfaces, leaving the polar, ionic groups extended into the water. Such a coating on resin beads would serve to militate against hydrophobic clustering, with the polar groups on the different resin particles repelling one another. This, in fact, is the classic effect of better wetting as caused by surfactants. In any case, treatment with detergent is often as effective as caustic washes. Such washes are sometimes employed prophylactically in a repetitive routine in the hope of preventing the poorer regeneration that results from clumping.

The cause of resin clustering is still in dispute, however. There may be more than one cause. Some resins, perhaps notably those prepared from ethyl acrylate, are inherently sticky. This can also be said to a degree for the resins constituted of polystyrene cross-linked by divinylbenzene. Those prepared from ethyl methacrylate seem not to be so tacky. Mechanical adhesions may therefore be involved.

New resins may clump in mixed beds for quite a few cycles when high-purity water is being polished. As the resin bed becomes used more and more, clumping diminishes. Some degree of irreversible organic fouling may come to modify the surface properties and may insulate the resin surfaces from one another. Perhaps in imitation of this effect, some resin manufactures have added small portions of bentonite or even of the oppositely charged resin fines (perhaps 25 to 50 grams per 50 ft^3 of resin) to their resin preparations, to coat the surfaces to prevent the resin clumping.

Mixed beds that achieve very low loadings, essentially zero utilization, function poorly because of clumping of the anionic and cationic components. This can be troublesome in the early cycles before the clumping disappears (McGarvey and Tamaki, 1989).

Chu (1989a and 1989b) found that after anion-exchange resin beads were exposed to trihalomethanes, they tended to clump, and adhered tenaciously to glass surfaces. Cation-exchange beads were not similarly affected.

Cutler (1987) said that to eliminate clumping, resins need to undergo some degree of fouling. Thus clumping effects are observed when resins are first put into service. The declumping of macroreticulated resins is ascribed to the adhering to their surfaces of colloids set free by backwashing or air scouring. These particles, it is believed, intersperse between the resin beads to forestall their agglomeration.

Cutler (1987) reported that the tendency for resins constituting a mixed bed to clump, manifest when the resins were separately regenerated, disappeared when the resins were exhausted and regenerated in their mixed forms. Presumably molecular entities responsible for clumping are mutually removed from each resin by the other when they are in intimate contact.

Because resin clumping becomes manifest usually as poor regeneration that necessitates an additional regeneration, efforts are sometimes made to forestall its appearance by routinely doing multiple regenerations before remixing the resins. As part of this effort, the mixed bed is first exhausted with caustic, or it is washed with a detergent solution. There is at present no standard, single way of dealing with the situation.

Organism Growth in DI Beds

It is well recognized that ion-exchange beds are potential sources of organism contamination (Chapman et al., 1983). Their dark, dank interiors; large surface areas; favorable ambient temperatures; and apparently sufficient nutrients favor organism growth, whether of microbes originally present in the water or of those adventitiously introduced into the process thereafter. The strongly basic anion-exchange resin, the quaternary ammonium base, is a bactericide.

Single beds have fewer bacterial problems, possibly because of the pH differences encountered. The pH in the cation-exchange bed is low. In the anion-exchange bed it is high. Neither of these pH environments is conducive to organism growth. Mixed beds more generally exhibit microbial problems, because of their pH-neutral effluents.

The risk of organism contamination increases with the removal of chlorine from the water being processed. Although chlorine degrades the resin, increasingly it is permitted to pass into the beds to sanitize them and to avoid the troublesome use of carbon. Chlorine concentrations of 0.2 or 0.3 ppm are used. However, chlorine concentrations of 2 or 3 ppm could be much too harmful to the resins. The 0.3-ppm chlorine concentrations do give rise to TOC, but in amounts that are (presently) tolerable in pharmaceutical water systems. However, the same quantities of TOC could be ruinous in high-performance semiconductor applications. The suitability of the practice depends, therefore, upon the application.

There is no known way of completely preventing organism growth in DI beds. The belief is widely and firmly held that the recirculation of water through an ion-exchange bed is effective in reducing its bacterial growth. There are those who question this belief; they see no rationale to it. Usually recirculatory flow is made through an ultraviolet light unit. The UV irradiation itself would have salubrious effects. It is pointed out, however, that bacteria are firmly attached to the resins by charge considerations and that their attachments, even as biofilm, are too firm to be disrupted by the recirculatory flow. Typical recirculatory flowrates are essentially at service flowrates or a bit lower, 1.5 to 2.0 gpm/ft^3 (6.1 to 8.2 L/min·cm^3).

The experimental work of Fleming (1988) has already been referenced (page 97) as showing no difference in bacteria levels between two ion-exchange columns, one maintained in static conditions, the other in continous recirculative flow. Flemming conclude that the recirculative flow confers no benefits with regard to discouraging organism proliferation. (See Figure 2-7).

Higher flowrates will the more soon exhaust the resins, however, necessitating their more frequent regeneration, which helps considerably to minimize bacterial growth.

Service flows of usually about 2 gpm/ft^3 give about 3 to 3.5 minutes of contact time. Flows can be much higher, however, depending upon circumstances. For example, in a semiconductor installation dealing with a water of low dissolved solids concentration, the flows can be 5 to 10 gpm/ft^3. In general, however, the flows are based upon the hydraulic character of the distribution system in the beds. Plant operations cannot tolerate wide variations in the service flow. Thus, if the flow customarily set at 5 gpm/ft^3 is reduced to 1 gpm/ft^3, the collector and distributors built into the equipment may malfunction; they may not prime or distribute well. Bed channeling leading to short cycles may result. This problem is resolved by including a water recycling system so that when the bed's full output is not on demand, the excess is recycled. The exigencies for recycling to discourage bacterial growth need therefore not usually be designed for. It will result from the recycling intended to insure proper bed functioning at various rates of flow. The recycle system usually includes an ultraviolet light installation to reduce bacterial counts (and TOC).

Organism growths do flourish in stagnant ion-exchange beds; those removed from use for longer time periods. In the case of DI beds, organism growth can be prevented by storing the cation-exchange bed under regenerating acid, and by filling the anion-exchange column with sodium hydroxide. The harshness of these regenerant chemicals will serve to sanitize. The beds will also be in a state of readiness for regeneration. In the case of mixed beds, long-term storage under sodium hydroxide is advised to eliminate organism growths. The price will have to be paid in the (cation-exchanger) regeneration cost (Hoffman 1994).

Not all ion-exchange beds are equally hospitable to organisms. In twin-bed arrangements the water generated in the cation-exchanger resins is acidic, an environment unconducive to microbial growth. Particularly if sodium leakage is taking place, the anion-exchange bed may be of an elevated pH unfavorable to organisms. The more pH neutral surroundings within a mixed- bed are more receptive to microbial presences.

Sanitizing of DI Beds

--by regeneration. A microbe count of 100 colony-forming units per 100 mL downstream from mixed DI beds is generally considered acceptable. When bacteriological monitoring discloses a trend towards higher numbers, sanitization is performed. Mittelman (1987) suggested that mixed beds in particular, being on-line for extended periods of time, should be regenerated (as a means of sanitization) on the basis of significant bacterial numbers rather than on the less frequent need for ion-exchange renewal. Ordinarily, regeneration is delayed in order to minimize the expenditures and the handling of the regenerant chemicals. Indeed, the need to handle the regenerant reagents is considered by some a sufficient hazard to avoid the use of ion-exchange demineralizations, as by substituting CDI, continuous deionization (See page 517). In pharmaceuticals, however, the efficiency of the chemical usage is secondary to control of the organism. It is usual in such usages to perform frequent regenerations. Unfortunately, the sanitizing regenerant chemicals do not reach the tank surfaces above the resin layers. These may, therefore, remain unsanitized.

Deionizing resin beds become sanitized upon contact with the acids and bases that are their regenerating agents. Frequent regeneration is the sovereign means of avoiding organism contamination of and from ion-exchange resin beds. This is why ion-exchange planning tends toward the use of downsized parallel systems. Downsizing forces the discipline of frequent DI bed regeneration (sanitization), with one set of beds being regenerated while the other is undergoing use.

Regeneration, automated or otherwise, is usually considered nevertheless to be an unwelcome chore. Views differ regarding a frequency of regeneration that should be tolerable. Many believe, however, that a frequency of as often as once per 24 hours is not excessive. The effluents from many DI systems may yield close to zero within such a period, even though the bioburden on the resin particles themselves may be very high. Generally, bacterial counts of some hundred colony-forming units per 100 mL are considered tolerable. To stretch the time intervals between sanitizations by regenerations, chemical sanitizations may be resorted to.

The release of organims from DI beds is not a phenomenon to be ignored. Many USP Purified Water systems rely upon ion-exchange to remove the chemical impurities followed by filtration to remove the microbes. However, the reliability of the filtrative action is promoted (or its compromise is less threatened), the lower the organism level. Considering the risk posed by the likelihood of adventitious organisms eventuating in the finished water, it would be wise to sanitize as frequently as possible, to minimize the microbial load on the filters. To further the practicality of such an operation, ion-exchange planning trends towards the downsizing of ion-exchange beds,to compel their more frequent regeneration. An FDA letter to the pharmaceutical industry warns that the proliferation of organism into the effluent water and not ion breakthrough should be the signal for resin bed regeneration (Michels 1981). This warning letter was occasioned by the presence of *P. Cepacia* found in Povidone Iodine solutions prepared from ion-exchange treated waters. Parallel sets of DI beds may be utilized, one being in stand-by condition while the other is being utilized.

A more recent practice makes use of shallow (typically 6 inch deep) fully packed beds of fine mesh ion-exchange resins, some 1/4 the usual bead diameter, at high flow rates, and regenerated automatically in counter-current fashion. The cycle times are very short; approximately 30 minutes in water treatment applications (Fletcher and Pace 1995, Brown and Fletcher 1986). The utilization of fine resin beads necessitates that the feedwater be pretreatment with a high quality, multimedia filter specifically selected and graded for this usage. This type demineralization system has been applied to boiler makeup water. The extention of its short cycle, frequent regeneration characteristics to the preparation of pharmaceutical waters is indicated.

Increasingly, also, efforts are made to protect DI beds against organism invasions. Membrane devices such as tangential flow units, RO systems, or ultrafiltration units are thus placed upstream of the DI beds to arrest organisms filtratively. U.V lamps are also used to kill organisms. Also, UV light systems, RO, or ultrafiltration units are placed downstream of the DI beds to counter organism presences that might emerge from the deionizing system.

--by chemical sanitizers. Chemical sanitizations of DI resin beds are limited by the same concerns that accompany the sanitization of other surfaces, membranes, and other devices. Most sanitizers are oxidants (e.g., active chlorine compounds and peroxides). These threaten the chemical integrity of resins, impairing their functionality.

Sanitizing of resin beds can be accomplished using sodium hypochlorite solutions of strengths in keeping with the recommendations of the manufacturer of the specific resin. Contact time should be less than 1 hour. Such a treatment should follow rinsing of the DI beds with a 10% brine solution (9 pounds of salt per cubic foot of resin) (Chapman et al., 1983c). The reason it is necessary to use the brine treatment prior to the sodium hypochlorite is that the quaternary ammonium hydroxide form is far more susceptible to oxidative degradations and to thermal decompositions than is the corresponding salt form. Inevitably, the active chlorine will cause some resin degradation and will result in some TOC generation. Also, the sodium ions will help to deplete the cation-exchange resin. Actually, one resin manufacturer adds a portion of hypochlorite before he sends the resin out in order to stabilize it against bacterial growth. Obviously, repetitive treatments with active chlorine compounds or with chlorine will continue to degrade the resin. Concentrations of 0.1 to 0.4 ppm are generally considered safe; not that such quantities do not cause degradations of the resin—they do, but an acceptable trade-off is seen in terms of sanitization. An increasing practice is to sanitize the resins and to remove chlorine from chlorinated waters by permitting the chlorine to enter the resin beds. (See page 377).

Chloramine in unspecified concentrations and contact times has been recommended for resin bed sanitizations.

--by peracetic acid. Zoccolante (1990) advised the use of hydrogen peroxide stabilized peracetic acid as a sanitizing agent, claiming that while it will exhaust resin it will not degrade it. Ganzi and Paresi (1990) stated that peracetic acid is difficult to rinse from resin beds. They advised the use of 1% sodium percarbonate solution, prepared by the action of hydrogen peroxide on sodium carbonate solutions. No particular use of this compound has been noticed, however.
At least one resin manufacturer advises resin sanitizations using 2% peracetic acid in a two bed volume over a thirty minute period followed by a one hour soak.. The peracetic acid is then removed by flushing; its complete removal being checked by pH measurements.

--by formaldehyde. Formaldehyde, an effective sanitizing agent, has been implicated as a probable carcinogen. It is free of oxidizing potential and will therefore not harm the DI resins. However, not only its handling entails risks but the disposal of its rinsewaters requires proper protocols to accord with EPA concerns. Nevertheless, formaldehyde is used as a DI resin sanitizing agent.

The Occupational Safety and Health Administration (OSHA) has set limits of 0.75 ppm (reduced from 1 ppm) averaged over an 8-hour period as the exposure limit for formaldehyde. (If this exposure level causes significant eye, nose, and throat irritations, based on a physician's professional judgment, the individual is to be removed for a period of up to 6 months to an area of at least 25% less formaldehyde exposure than that causing the irritations).

The maximum discharge wash-water concentration permitted by EPA reflects a concern for the sewage processing system, specifically for the organisms involved in its organic digestive process. This may vary locally, depending upon the particular publicly owned treatment works (usually the appropriate municipal sewage plant). To learn the acceptable maximum discharge level permitted in a given locale, inquiries should be directed to the regional or state EPA office relative to their regional pretreatment program involving formaldehyde. The same considerations apply to the discharge of sulfuric acid, caustic soda, or other chemicals resulting from ion-exchange regenerations and other processes.

Formaldehyde solutions of 0.25% to 0.4% prepared from formalin (40% formaldehyde) are left in contact with the resin bed at room temperature for from 30 to 60 minutes. The formaldehyde must then be thoroughly washed from the resin beds as evidenced by a control test (involving, for example, Formalert test kits); and the wash waters then properly disposed of.

Abrams (1991) stated that a rinse of 10 to 15 gal/ft^3 of resin should suffice. Longer rinses have also been recorded. In any case, the salinity of the rinsewater should be low in order not to consume the capacity of the sanitized bed (Chapman et al., 1983c).

--by hot water sanitization. There is a trend to the use of hot-water sanitization.

The water is circulated through the resin beds while gradually being raised in temperature. The circulating water is then cooled slowly. The problem with this technique is with the thermal instability of the strong anion-exchange resins. The Type I quaternary ammonium benzyltrimethylamine can be kept at around 82 °C (180°F) for 1/2 to 4 hours or so without compromising its service life unduly, provided the resin is in its salt form. Otherwise, in its base form, it would lose one-half its capacity in a single 4-hour treatment. The Type II quaternary ammonium dimethylethanolamine has a maximum operating temperature of 40 °C (104 °F). Similarly treated, its life in high-purity applications could be foreshortened to 3 months or so. Other strongly-basic anion exchange resins may have greater stabilities. However, none is impervious to thermal degradation. It may be argued, in given cases, that the amount of resin degradation will not significantly diminish the bed's ion-exchange capacity by the time its scheduled replacement is due. In such instances, the generation of TOC, the organic degradation compounds, requires consideration. In polishing contexts, their presence may be objectionable. Yet some advise sanitization by heating to 160 °F (71 °C) periodically for a few hours. The resin is replaced after 3 to 6 months. Some resins can endure this type of treatment over a 1-year period.

The use of thermal sanitizations of ion-exchange beds is especially attractive for mixed-bed operations where the sanitizations derive from resin regeneration, a relatively onerous chore. Husted and Rutkowski (1991), using both total count and epifluorescence microbiological assay techniques, studied the effects of temperatures from 60 to 72 °C upon the sanitization of mixed beds. The mixed beds were contained in PVDF-coated stainless steel vessels. The heated high-purity water of 18.2-megohm-cm resistivity was measured for temperature and for organism content as it flowed into and out of the beds on its way to discard.

Intriguingly, Husted and Rutkowski (1991) found that large quantities of TOC, particles, and organisms were shed by the resins undergoing the hot-water treatment. Apparently, the binding affinities of the resins decrease at higher temperatures. This alone should commend the use of elevated water treatments.

Additionally, Husted and Rutkowski (1991) found that large numbers of microbes were killed by exposure to the heated water, beginning near 45 °C. Where single mixed beds were investigated (as distinct from two in series, as also studied) no viable cells were discovered in samples of several liters once 45 °C was measured at the bed outlet. Furthermore, the effluent waters remained significantly lower in colony-forming-unit counts for 14 days following the thermal treatment. However, short exposures to 60 °C did not produce sterile waters; not all cell types present were sufficiently susceptible to the heat. Interestingly, large numbers of particles, organisms, and TOC were released by the mixed beds as they were being heated.

Husted and Rutkowski (1991) suggested that DI bed colonization may derive from the inlet piping biofilm, but that most organism population diversity can be eliminated by low-temperature heating and that this ought to retard subsequent bed recolonization and effluent cell rebound. On the basis of these findings, the Husted and Rutkowski hot-water technique for sanitizing ion-exchange beds, particularly of the mixed-bed variety, merits a wider application than it has thus far been accorded.

The Michels Letter

The Michels letter (1981) was occasioned by the finding that *P. cepacia* were growing in and being passed out of the ion-exchange beds. However, its advocacy of more frequent ion-exchange bed regenerations (sanitizations) as a means of controlling microbial growth, while well advised, lacks the practicality of quantitative guidance. Microbial levels downstream from such beds are usually high; 200 cfu/mL are commonplace, although hot water sanitizations can minimize the counts. One can utilize a prophylactic practice; (e.g weekly regenerations). Otherwise, the trend of organism release should be plotted, and sanitization (bed regeneration) should be instituted when a significant release of microbes becomes evident. Husted and Rutkowski (1991) advise that such releases are sharp occurrences, possibly caused by the displacement of the weakly held (weakly ionic) organisms by the descending sodium ion front, itself forced down the ion-exchange column by more strongly held competing ions. In any case, Michel's letter nonwithstanding, pseudomonads can be expected to be released from the ion-exchange beds in an ongoing fashion. In practice, downstream filtration is relied upon to control the release of organisms from the DI beds.

FDA Observations Regarding DI Resin Beds

Farina, an FDA inspector at the Brooklyn, N.Y., district office, pointed out that the need for DI bed regeneration is normally monitored by either resistivity meters or by "recharge" lights. The latter are in use particularly when the DI resin facility is arranged for on a service basis. Neither signal indicating the need for regeneration of the DI resins is at all indicative of the resin bed's microbiological status. That requires being assessed by direct microbiological assays conducted on water samples drawn preferably both before and after the bed in question, at a frequency shown by a testing history (as initially developed by rather frequent tests) to be sensitive to the disclosure of the water quality trends.

To validate the correlation between a desired end-product quality and the acceptable microbiological levels of the water used in compounding, the FDA may require a daily validation over the production of a month's duration, to be followed by weekly and then monthly validations over the period of a year. Actually, to sustain a trend-revealing water quality program, all types of water systems should be tested at least weekly at test ports both before and after each purification unit. Observations by FDA inspectors strongly advise the use of DI resin beds in conjunction with following UV light treatment units in a dynamic flow mode, that is, under constant recirculation to minimize the promotive effects of stagnation on organism growth. Typical flows of 1.5 to 2.0 gpm/ft^2 of cross-sectional bed area (6.1 to 8.2 gpm/cm^2) are used.

The microbe proliferation concerns regarding nonflowing DI systems also extend, in FDA thinking, to newly regenerated DI resin beds available under wet conditions. Such storage conditions should be investigated with the service supplier. If the new tanks contain wet resins, tantamount to stagnant flows, then the units require sanitizing before being placed in service. The use of sanitizing agents, except for formaldehyde, consume some of the resin's capacity for ion exchange, and require being flushed out with deionized water to avoid further capacity loss. Hot-water sanitization may offer advantages for standby units.

Service DI Resin

The regeneration of DI resin beds, and particularly of mixed beds, is perhaps the most onerous chore in all of water system maintenance. The regeneration of mixed beds requires the separation of the cationic and anionic exchangers. A line dividing the resins is required to enable a separate treatment for each resin. This line should be visible through a sight window built into the column containing the resin; but the degree of swelling of the resins may cause the line to change positions. As a result, each resin phase may receive less than optimal regeneration.

The degradation of the cation exchanger caused by dissolved oxygen, chlorine, or certain sanitizers may break down the polystyrene's cross-linkages. This boosts the degree of swelling caused by water imbibition; the resin then exhibits an excessive moisture uptake that shifts the resin interface, creating difficulties where a fixed header (interface collector/distributor) is involved. The anion-exchange resins may lose their functional groups, the seat of water imbibition, and may therefore shrink.

To avoid these problems, as well as the risks to personnel associated with the handling of the strong acids and bases needed for regeneration, the work is sometimes contracted out on a service basis. This also finesses the problems associated with chemical discharges.

The problem for pharmaceutical waters is the validation of such service. How is one assured that some other company's resins are not returned in place of one's own; and how to guard against receipt of a resin previously used in electroplating applications wherein heavy metal ions abound, possibly detrimental if leached in pharmaceutical contexts? At a price, a company can, first of all, obtain and have retained for its services its own resin tanks. Second, the resin returned for regeneration can be segregated as to usage. That is, it will be pooled only with resins received from other water purification operations. It would be segregated from resins employed in industries considered hazardous to pharmaceutical applications. The resins returned in regenerated form would therefore be innocuous.

All this the service company should corroborate by written records made available for the drug manufacturer's records. The records should also be available for on-site inspection and FDA perusal. Finally, but at a substantial cost, a company can have made available to them a dedicated resin supply, regenerated and resupplied strictly for its own purposes.

In-place regenerable deionizers entail a higher capital cost, but lower operating expenses than do off-site regenerated ion-exchangers. However, while they involve chemical handling and disposal, something the off-site regeneration obviates, they permit more direct control over the process and its water quality. Non-regenerable new resin deionizers, often used in polishing loops, cost the highest amount to operate, but enable the greatest quality control. Their use should include resin supplier batch QC documentation.

Oxidative Attack upon Ion-Exchange Resins

The free-radical chain reaction that characterizes an attack by oxidizers such as chlorine, ozone, hydrogen peroxide, or UV radiation (or any combination thereof) ultimately results in the chain scission of the polymeric carbon-to-carbon backbone. It may also directly attack the functional group responsible for ion exchange. In the latter case, the resin capacity for ion exchange will decrease. Such loss is irreversible. The oxidative fragmentation of the cross-linked carbon-to-carbon structure may also produce organic entities that may foul the resins. The TOC thus produced that contains ionic charges such as carboxylic acids (commonly products of oxidative degradations) may foul anion-exchange groups; whether this is reversible or permanent depends upon the exact nature of the foulant. Not all TOC generated by oxidative degradation is acidic in nature. In general, TOC can be absorbed hydrophobically to most resin bead surfaces, including ion-exchange functional groups, thus interfering with their performance. Particularly noxious as TOC foulants are the longer-chain fragments set free from the resin polymer and the polymeric fragments generated by the oxidative degradation. These are difficult to remove from the resin beads.

Both the cation-exchange and the anion-exchange carbon-to-carbon cross-linked networks undergo chain scission. However, the quaternary ammonium carbon-to-nitrogen bond of the anion exchanger is far more labile under oxidative attack than is the carbon-to-sulfur bond of the sulfonic acid group present on the cation exchanger. The loss of anion-exchange capacity under oxidative attack thus becomes evident early on. This does not mean, however, that cross-link scission in the anion-exchange molecule does not take place. These linkages gain no exemption against oxidative attack just because a carbon-to-nitrogen bond exists elsewhere in the molecule. This disruption is secondary as far as functional diminution is concerned, but, as in the case of the cation-exchange degradation, it too creates TOC. The TOC generated by the disruption of the carbon-to-nitrogen linkage of the anion exchanger yields trimethylamine or methanol. Neither will specifically foul the functional groups of the cation-exchange resin. They do, however, constitute TOC, and as such they are potential foulants of resin bead surfaces.

Where fouling causes diminution in capacity, it may be restored by regeneration. It is comprehended that the oxidative alterations give rise to polymeric fragments bearing carboxylic acids. These would be taken up by the strongly basic anion-exchange groups of the anion resins. They would not be expected to enter exchanges with cation-exchange resins. Where anion-exchange resin undergoes loss of its positively charged quaternary ammonium group, that will be taken up by the cation-exchange group. It is conceivable, additionally, that some fouling of any resin beads may be caused by the deposition, perhaps involving hydrophobic adsorptions, of the generated TOC upon the extensive surfaces offered by such beads.

The chain scission that occurs in the polymeric molecules as a result of the oxidative free-radical attacks would take place regardless of whether the polymers supported cation-exchange or anion-exchange functional group substituents. The degree of cross-linking would, however, be important. Cross-linking creates three-dimensional polymers whose breakdown into soluble, detectable TOC would require enough chain scission to set free two-dimensional fragments. Three-dimensional networks inherently tend towards molecular complexities that are not soluble. The more cross-linking, therefore, the more degradation a polymer may endure until it is destroyed as an entity by the chain-scission reactions. Such chain scission, progressively weakening three-dimensional restraints against swelling, are measurable by the moisture-holding capacity of the resin where functional groups exist to imbibe water.

In work with 0.1-ppm ozone concentrations on mixed-bed resin combinations, Yarnell et al. (1989) found that cation-exchange capacity better withstood the oxidative attack than did the anionic-exchange capacity. The carbon/sulfonic acid bond was stable under the conditions studied. The resin combinations performed reasonably well up to 200 hours of exposure. Hoffman et al. (1987) studied the effects of chlorine allowed to enter mixed-bed resins. The conclusions drawn by Hoffman and his associates in both these studies differed somewhat in certain particulars. The general findings, however, were that regardless of the resin, chain scission did take place, better resisted by more cross-linking; that this occurrence was not adequately signaled by the resin's moisture-holding capacity; that the TOC generated did foul its accompanying resin counterpart in mixed-bed operations; that capacity losses caused by fouling could be retrieved by regeneration; but that continued exposure to the oxidant, on a time-concentration basis, progressively led to irremediable degradation. Significant resin degradation manifested itself as resin fines that were found in the downstream filters following backwashing.

As Hoffman et al. (1987) saw it, chlorine exists in its aqueous solutions as the hypochlorite ion. Being an ion, the hypochlorite radical, OCl^-, is attracted to and inside the anion-exchange resin. There it readily cleaves the carbon-carbon cross-link bonds. The rsulting polymer fragments, probably including amine functions, serve to foul the carbon-nitrogen bonds of the anion- exchange resin, but this is of lesser importance. When the resin cross-link level is greater, the resin structure is more resistant to the effects of oxidation. Concomitantly, the cation-exchange resin also undergoes decross-linking. The stronger carbon-sulfur-bond representing its cation-exchange function is not affected. However its sulfonic acid-bearing polymeric fragments may foul the anion-exchange resin so badly as to reduce its kinetic performance markedly. The fouling of the resins by the organic entities (particularly polymeric) generated by the oxidative degradations leads to kinetic failures in the mixed beds. In twin beds, the effects of the foulants may be less noticeable.

Ozone is a far stronger oxidant than chlorine. Unlike the chlorite ion (chlorine in solution), ozone is not directed specifically to the anion-exchange resin. Overall, then, ozone, unlike chlorine, primarily degrades the cation-exchange resin. Where the chain scission results in sulfonated polymeric fragments that foul the anion-exchange resin, restitution of normal ion-exchange kinetics is almost beyond the ability of the regeneration process. This mode of attack by ozone on mixed beds was confirmed by the work of Yarnell et al. (1989).

The investigations of Hoffman et al. (1987) indicate that chlorine, and to a much lesser extent ozone, may be permitted entrance into ion-exchange beds only in applications relatively insensitive to TOC fouling and to the loss of exchange capacity. The practice becomes even more restricted where mixed-bed arrangements are involved. Moreover, the introduction of oxidants into ion-exchange beds devoted to high-performance applications is totally inappropriate.

Emery et al. (1988) studied the chemical constituents in TOC forthcoming from ion-exchange resins subjected to degradations resulting from conditions meant to reflect industrial usage. Parr bomb oxidations of ion-exchange resins for 24-hour periods with oxygen at 100, 150, and 200 °C were used to simulate the oxidative molecular alterations. High-pressure liquid chromatography (HPLC) was utilized to compare and identify the decomposition products. Tetramethylammonium hydroxide was identified as a compound originating from the anion-exchange resin. This would be expected as a result of the Hofmann degradation typical of quaternary compounds at elevated temperatures. Hydroquinone, quinone, phenol, and toluene were other compounds identified after the Parr bomb oxidations.

Ion-exchange resin manufacturers offer beads having some resistivity to chlorine, which is more than occasionally allowed to enter the DI beds.

Traps for Organic Foulants

Ion-exchange beds may be fouled by organic matter. This occurrence, usually confined to surface waters, results in long rinse-up times, decreased capacities, shorter throughputs, and silica leakage. It makes necessary the replacement of the resin, commonly the anion exchanger, after only a couple of years or less.

To protect the beds, organic traps consisting of anion-exchange resin can be placed upstream of the ion-exchange beds. The organic matter, whether naturally or in consequence of its having become partially oxidized, bears carboxylic acid groups, and so is removed by an anion exchanger. The ion-exchange resin used is usually of a macroreticular type, although gel types are also used. The flowrates at which these organic traps are used should not exceed 3 gpm/ft^3 of resin for 5-ppm organics. A lower rate of 2 gpm/ft^3 should be used for organic concentrations of 5 to 20 ppm.

At least one resin exhibits an uptake of 30 gm of organic material (expressed as potassium permanganate consumed) per liter of resin (Applebaum, 1969). Optimum regeneration utilizes 1 pound of caustic soda mixed with 7 to 8 pounds of salt per cubic foot of resin. However, treatment with 10 pounds of salt per cubic foot of resin suffices and is generally used. The regenerant solutions are best used at 49 to 60 °C (120 to 140 °F). Such resins also remove sulfite and bicarbonate ions, exchanging them for chlorides.

Where the removal of organic acids is by anion exchange, it may be best to use a linear-acrylic weakly basic anion exchanger for its nonselectivity so that its regeneration can be accomplished expeditiously. Also, macroreticular resins should be used to maximize the bead surface presented for interaction. Acrylic resins, both strong and weak, resist fouling because they more readily desorb foulants. The anion-exchange resins must be regenerated frequently. Otherwise, the humic and/or fulvic acids, initially surface depositions on the resin beads, will diffuse into the interior of the reticulated beads. Then their removal, diffusion-limited, will be very slow. The first indication of a humic/fulvic acid problem is an interference with soluble silica removal by the strongly basic anion-exchange resin. A second symptom of the condition is the emergence of an acidic water, even after mixed-bed treatment. Frequent anion-exchange regeneration is prescribed. A third symptom is a longer rinse time. One wishes, of course, to avoid chemical hideout such as can be caused by a poor distributor design. The anion-exchange resin rinse should be at the rate of 30 to 50 g/ft^3 (the literature says 75 g/ft^3), but with the age of the resin this can be increased to 150 g/ft^3.

To free anion-exchange beds of organic materials that may have settled therein, periodic flushings with strong brine solutions of some 10% concentration should be made. The frequency of such treatments, whether weekly or monthly, must be based on experience. The organic matter will thereby desorb, turning the brine into a murky yellow or brown fluid. The chloride ions of the brine solution replace the organic complex more efficiently than do hydroxyl ions. Therefore, brine is more efficacious than is sodium hydroxide solution in the desorption from the resin beads of the organic matter, presumably held as acidic complexes.

Carbon beds are often advocated for the removal of organic foulants. For this purpose, unlike for their removal of chlorine, they require very slow flowrates; too slow, usually, to be practical (see Chapter 7, page 363).

Traps for Resin Fines

In the water purification field, a device may be named after the service it is intended to perform, rather than for its form or design. Thus, the term "resin trap" can refer to a 10-µm filter or to any plumbing device that contains within it a screen for restraining resin finds sloughed from the DI resin beds. Such devices can be made from PVC or stainless steel; the latter is more common in pharmaceutical usage. The restraining screens within these devices are described in mesh sizes rather than in terms of micron pore sizes. The screens are usually 100 mesh; the fines being retained are from 15 to 60 mesh sizes. (The larger the mesh size of a screen, the smaller the spatial openings between the constituting wires or fibers).

The abrasions normal to the osmotic expansions and contractions of the beads in their ion-exchanging and regeneration cycles result in the production of resin fines. This too is the normal consequence of whatever oxidative degradation the resins undergo, rendering the cation-exchange resin beads less cross-linked and hence more gelatinous.

Resin fines, on a time-dependent basis, are inevitably, if slowly, formed in the resin beds, to be carried out of the column by the flowing stream. It is therefore common practice to position a prefilter, usually of about 5- to 10-µm rating, downstream from the beds to act as a scavenger for resin particles.

Removal of Organics

Traditionally, organic molecules are removed from high-purity waters by the restraining actions of reverse osmosis membranes. However, RO impediments to the passage of lower-molecular-weight organics are reduced. Generally, molecular weights lower than about 200 are not expected to be restrained from passing the RO membrane. The molecular shape seems also to be a factor. Therefore, the removal of volatile organics (VOC) by reverse osmosis is not dependable. It is possible, however, for 185 (184.9) nm ultraviolet light to generate hydroxyl free radicals in high-purity water. These degrade most organic materials. Chain scission occurs to yield progressively smaller molecular-weight entities. Theoretically and eventually, carbon dioxide and water are the end products of this oxidative degradation of organic matter (Francis, 1989). Long before these ultimate products are formed, however, relatively stable carboxylic acids are formed through precursors less stable to free-radical attack.

These include alcohols, aldehydes, and ketones. The practical purposes of organic removal are served by irradiating the water with 185-nm UV and removing the carboxylic acids formed by the use of anion-exchange resins. Some organic matter will incidentally be removed by adsorption onto the resin bead surfaces (as also upon activated carbon) regardless of whether they be cation- or anion-exchange in nature, and independent of charge considerations. Trace organics are removed following reverse osmosis by the use of anion-exchange resins in polishing modes even though they themselves may leach organics.

Pretreatment of Ion-Exchange Feedwaters

As stated, the ion-exchange beds can act as deep-bed filters. To avoid their progressive blockage by suspended particles, these should be removed by the use of multimedia filters or cartridge filters. The deposition of iron or manganese precipitates should be avoided by using greensand (zeolite) beds. Oxidative degradation of the resins by chloride can be escaped by removal of same using activated carbon beds or by the injection of sodium bisulfite. Organic scavengers can serve to remove surface-fouling TOC. Bacterial fouling can be controlled or reduced by the use of ultraviolet radiation.■

CHAPTER 9

REVERSE OSMOSIS, ULTRAFILTRATION, AND ELECTRICALLY DRIVEN DEMINERALIZATIONS

Reverse osmosis offers a means of removing ionic components from their aqueous solutions. It also serves to remove most soluble organic compounds; and to restrain the passage of insoluble particles, both viable and otherwise. The process is widely utilized for these purposes in the preparation of high-purity rinsewaters in the electronics industry. Increasingly, RO is employed in the power industry in the preparation of makeup water, to replace that consumed in use or lost as steam. In the pharmaceutical industry, RO is designated by the USP as one of the two methods permissible in the preparation of Water for Injection; distillation is the other. The FDA, however, will permit its use for this purpose only when two-pass product-staged RO is involved; this is a recognition that RO membranes are not always of such perfect reliability as to ensure sterile effluent.

The two chief alternatives to RO for preparing high-purity water are distillation and ion exchange. Reverse osmosis requires a lower expenditure of energy than distillation; but is generally (although not universally) more sensitive to the pretreatment of feedwaters than is ion exchange. A surface water with a very high organic load could be purified using RO without undue fouling, by manipulation of the amount of RO recovery. However, even macroreticular resins might become irreversibly fouled thereby. Nevertheless, RO seems more sensitive to abuse by operators than is ion exchange.

Reverse osmosis membranes are thin microporous polymeric (usually) films. As explained in Chapter 5, which deals with polymeric membranes, the RO pores derive from the interstitial spaces present in all solid matter. They are not the artificially enlarged pores common to the microporous filters of commerce. The dimensions of the pores of RO membranes are on the order of 25 to 100 angstroms. Such small orifices severely restrict the permeation of water. A practical permeation rate therefore necessitates an aggrandizement of surface-to-liquid area interfacing, along with an enhanced thinness of the polymeric barrier. Both of these techniques have been developed for RO devices.

Not all polymers exhibit the same intersegmental spacing. It was discovered that certain polymers, when disposed as films and confronted with salt water, could, under pressure, be permeated by the water while discriminating against passage of the salt (Beasley, 1977). Certain of these polymers, notably those composed of cellulose acetates, of certain aromatic polyamides, and of polysulfonated polysulfones, are offered for achieving the desalination of saline waters.

The Principles of Osmosis and Reverse Osmosis

Osmosis occurs when a semipermeable membrane, one permeable to water but not to salts or organic molecules in solution, separates water or a dilute solution from a more concentrated solution. Water molecules have a stronger tendency to escape from water than from a solution. Water flows through the membrane from the dilute to the concentrated side in an effort to equalize the osmotic pressures of the two solutions. If the juxtaposition of the two solutions is made in the two arms of a U-tube, with the semipermeable barrier in the horizontal section between them, the water rises in the more concentrated arm and diminishes in the arm containing the dilute solution (or pure water). The relative heights of the solutions at equilibrium are a measure of their osmotic pressure differences.

The process of osmosis can be reversed. Pressure could be impressed upon a dilute solution confronting such a semipermeable membrane. Water would be forced through the membrane barrier to yield pure, or purer, water on the far side; and a proportionately more concentrated solution on the near side. Since the liberation of the pure water from its solutions is caused by the reversal of the osmotic pressure, the operation is termed reverse osmosis. In practical contexts, it serves to prepare pure water from aqueous solutions by the imposition of pressure in conjunction with semipermeable RO membranes. As an alternative to ion exchange, RO avoids the costs of chemical regenerants, the risks associated with their use, and the need to train personnel to avoid those risks. The decision points on when to use RO and when to employ ion exchange will be addressed.

Mechanisms of Reverse Osmosis

Some five different mechanisms have been advanced to rationalize the RO phenomenon. The differences among these may, at least to some extent, be semantic. One hypothesis that explains the process adequately holds that water molecules wet the polymer surface by hydrogen bonding to its polar groups. By this means, under the impetus of the applied pressure, the water negotiates the pore passageways, the interstitial polymeric spacings. The hydrophilic nature of the polymer is a factor. The more hydrophilic the polymer, the greater the density of its polar substituents; and therefore the less pressure may be required to intrude water, as into the pores of hydrophobic filters. The water molecules thus permeate the RO membrane. However, the hydrated ions are too large to pass through the RO membrane pores.

The ions contained in the water are of different sizes. Because of their electrical charges they acquire skirts of water molecules, shells of hydration. According to Fajan's rule, the smaller the crystallographic ion size, the larger its envelope of hydration; and the larger its hydrated or actual size. Charge density is important here. The greater the ion's electrical charge and the smaller the ion's crystallographic size, the more water molecules it binds into its hydration shell, and the larger its actual overall dimension. Therefore, a sulfate ion of atomic weight 96 with two charges is larger in its overall hydrated size than the hydrated chloride ion of atomic weight 35.5 with one charge. The sizes of hydrated ions militate against their permeating the interstitial spaces (pores) of the RO membranes, and the sulfate ion is more easily excluded than is the chloride ion.

More than size exclusion is involved in the RO function. A solubility influence, as defined by cohesive energy density, plays a part. When the cohesive energy densities of the polymer and organic compound are sufficiently similar, they will form a (solid) solution. This permits the passage of one through the other. Thus certain organic molecules, such as phenol, formaldehyde, and acetic acid, are passed preferentially by cellulose acetate membranes. Additionally (probably based on considerations of size), organic compounds having molecular weights lower than 100 or 200 are not rejected by RO membranes, depending upon the molecular characteristics of the RO polymer.

Whatever the spatial limitation responsible for salt rejection, it is related to the dimensions of the spaces present in the polymer film or membrane. It is obvious that such small apertures would also prevent the passage of particulate matter such as organisms, and even of such molecules in true solution as proteins, or the lipopolysaccharides that are a cause of pyrogenicity. It is for this reason that RO membranes find utility in Water for Injection production.

Operational Considerations

The pressure imposed upon a feedwater in an RO operation has two components: that required to overcome the osmotic pressure of the solution to liberate the pure water; and that required to overcome the resistance to flow posed by the membrane. As regards the second consideration, there is a straight-line relationship between the driving pressure and the rate of water permeation through the same semipermeable membrane. A salt-containing water can have an osmotic pressure of 350 to 500 psig. If one wishes a water flow as occasioned by, say, 300-psig pressure, then the total pump pressure required would be some 650 to

800 psig. Many RO systems operate on municipally treated waters. These generally have osmotic pressures of about 1 psig per 100 ppm of total dissolved solids. A feedwater of 200 ppm of TDS would require only 2 psig of pressure to overcome its osmotic pressure; the remainder of the applied pump pressure would drive the water flow and determine its rate of permeation.

In most actual plant operations, the applied pump pressure serves virtually to drive the water; the osmotic pressure restraints are negligible. Pump pressures used are typically from 200 to 400 psig. Cellulose acetate RO units may require as high as 500 to 550 psig; thin-film composite RO devices usually are operated at 200 to 250 psig. The feedwater entering an RO unit emerges in two sections: the permeate stream and the reject stream. The term *concentrate* is often preferred to the term r*eject stream*.

Recovery

The term *recovery* refers to the percentage of the feedwater flow that becomes product water. (See Figure 9-1). Typically for large systems it is about 75%. The 25% of the feedwater, previously processed by pretreatments, that is discarded is the single greatest negative feature of RO operations. It is a costly waste. In comparison, if the TDS of the feedwater is below 20 to 50 ppm, the ion-exchange demineralizers may require only 2% to 5% of the feedwater for regenerations. (Above about 50 ppm of TDS, possibly at 200 ppm, the regenerations may consume 10% or higher.) It may well be, however, that with water being used to effect other processes such as resin separations and rinse-ups, the consumption is much higher. In any case, the remainder becomes product water. The more concentrated the feedwater, the greater the percentage that it is necessary to waste. If the TDS of a particular feedwater is 4 times that of an average

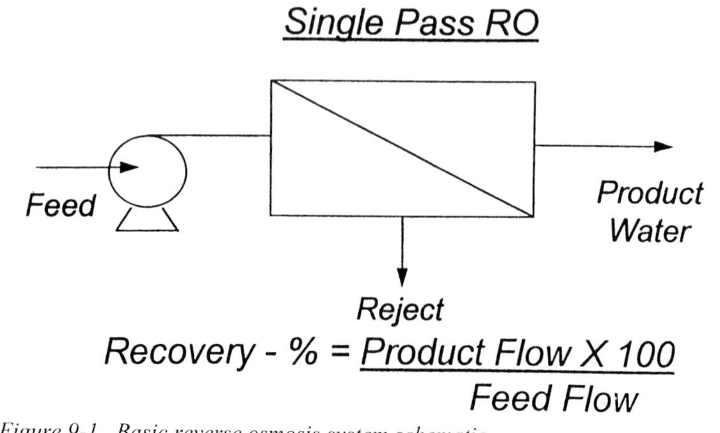

Figure 9-1. Basic reverse osmosis system schematic.
Courtesy; Gary Zoccolante, U.S. Filter Co.

municipally treated water, the amount sent to waste can well exceed 25%. It is good economics somehow to utilize the reject stream. Usually its purity permits its use in makeup for cooling towers, for compressor cooling, and even for watering the grass. The reject stream comes off from the RO unit under pressure. Therefore, the costs of storage and repumping can be avoided. Discharging water to the sewer can be expensive, as much as $8 per 1,000 gallons (as of 1994). In contrast, ion-exchange operations can consume as little as 1% to 10% in the regeneration step.

In common with the operation of other purification units, circulation of water through the RO is advised to minimize microbial growth (planktonic organisms) when the unit is not in service. This entails a consumption of water. If the conservation of water is a prime consideration, the RO unit should be shut down when not in use. Post shutdown, the unit should be flushed with product water. This is seldom done.

Limit to Recovery

Since the major cost of RO operations is that of the unrecovered water, usually expensively pretreated, that is sent to waste, its volume is best minimized. Yet there are limits to RO recoveries. Recovery in any given situation can vary widely, from 30% to 90% or so. Recovery influences the rejection. As the percentage recovery is increased, the water product quality decreases.

The osmotic pressure of the water itself imposes limitations. As the treated water becomes more concentrated, its osmotic pressure climbs. It is not the osmotic pressure of the original feedwater but the average osmotic pressure of the waters fed succeeding membranes in the RO device that is the consideration. This is very important where brackish water or seawater is being desalinated. Where municipally treated waters are involved, the osmotic pressure of the water is normally not of real concern.

The concentration of sparingly soluble salts in the reject waters being treated by the next membrane in an RO device is important. If 75% of the water is being recovered, the concentrations of such sparingly soluble salts as calcium sulfate and calcium carbonate will have increased fourfold in the reject stream. This concentration is likely to cause precipitation of these salts by exceeding their solubility product. (*Solubility product* and *supersaturation* are discussed below). An 80% recovery increases the impurities fivefold. If the feedwaters were to contain 0.5 ppm of barium ions, their fourfold increase to 2 ppm would lead to the precipitation of barium sulfate. Cleaning this especially insoluble deposit from the RO membrane surface would be very difficult. Such fouling is best avoided.

In most cases this is not a large factor, however, as RO operations are generally preceded by an acid feed or by a water-softening pretreatment that substantially reduces the initial divalent cation content of the RO feedwater. Even at a fourfold increase in reject stream concentrations, such wastewater is not a scaling solution, which commends the use of such reject streams for cooling purposes.

Chloride ions are among the more difficult to reject, and in pharmaceutical waters their maximum concentration is stipulated by regulations. If feedwaters were high in their chloride content, and if a single-pass RO unit were being used, the product waters could end up with an excessive amount of chloride ions. This is an example of too high a recovery influencing the product water quality.

Rejection

The percentage of the ions and soluble organics rejected by RO units depends upon the RO membrane type. The older cellulose acetate (CA) types reject about 90% over a fair period of time. The newer "blend" CA polymers give 97% to 98% salt rejections (Comb, 1991). The common perception is that the thin-film composite polyamide (PA) polymer membranes reject even better. Higher rejection percentages are in any case attained at lower recovery rates. (Precise performance data are not easily obtained and compared. They are sometimes obscured by the conflicting claims of competitive marketing; each claim is based upon particular interpretations of data and conditions.) Leakage, not failure to reject, may be involved in the limitation of 98% or 99% rejection that is reached. Salt impurities may inevitable intrude to some small extent.

The water being treated in an RO unit flows through a succession of membranes, becoming progressively more concentrated in its passage. The 98% values mentioned above reflect the relatively low concentration of the feedwater seen by the first membrane. The last membrane may confront a water stream concentrated at least fourfold over the original feed stream. The few percentages of ions not rejected represent a sizable amount, however, when the impurity level is many times that of the original feedwater. The permeate is removed from each vessel separately. That from the last vessel is a very small portion of the total, because of both the smaller volumes and the higher osmotic pressures of its feed.

Overall, then, an RO unit will generally not attain the high 98% rejection rating characteristic of a single RO membrane operating on diluted feedwater. Curiously, some units may achieve their high advertised rejections only because the reject level for the single membrane may have been (for whatever reason) characterized too modestly, the RO membrane being actually better than rated.

Regarding the rejection of organics, sunny ratings of 99% are sometimes advertised. These figures may derive from the rejection of human albumin. The fulvic and humic acids more commonly encountered as organic contaminants may not give such high rejection percentages. If the organic concentration is 1 ppm going in, it will not be 10 ppb coming out. The actual amount of rejection will depend upon the size and shape of the organic molecule. Reverse osmosis rejection of naturally occurring water color constituents and of humic acids may be very satisfactory. The point being made, however, is that advertised claims are once in a while exaggerated. Generally, TOC reductions of a high order are effected by RO.

Reverse osmosis devices reject organics rather well if these organics are larger than 200 in molecular weight going to the cellulose acetate membranes, and over 100 to the thin-film composite membranes.

There is a belief, logical if unconfirmed, that waters treated by RO are less hospitable to organisms because the nutritional medium for the microbes, the water's organic content, is reduced. Whatever the actual case, in pharmaceutical settings the CA devices are preferred over the PA despite their lower rejections because they pass dissolved chlorine, which tends to keep the permeated waters bactericidal. Very high ion rejections are unnecessary in most pharmaceutical water applications, but the concern with the organism content is paramount.

In some RO units, part of the reject or concentrate stream is pumped back to join the feed stream. This is done to maintain the turbulent flow necessary to minimize fouling, and overall it minimizes the volume of reject water. In small units without recirculation, recovery can run as low as 30%.

Ion Rejection

Not all ions are equally rejected by RO membranes. The mechanism of RO rejection is imperfectly understood. In contrast, the response of ion exchange to the Law of Mass Action and to the influence of charge densities in accordance with Fajan's rule is relatively straightforward. In RO rejection, divalent ions are generally rejected to upward of 99% by polyamide, the monovalent ions upward of about 97%. For this reason, sodium and chloride ions, being comparatively difficult to reject, are used in test concentrations of 1,000 to 2,000 ppm of sodium chloride to characterize RO membrane rejection qualities. Sourirajan (1963, 1964) showed that for cellulose acetate membranes, anions could be arranged in the following decreasing order of rejection: citrate, tartrate, sulfate, acetate, chloride, bromide, nitrate, iodide, and thiocyanide; and cations in a like order: magnesium, barium, strontium, calcium, lithium, sodium, and potassium. Rejection is a direct function of the valence of the ion, but of other unknown influences as well. The hydrated ion size exerts an effect.

pH Considerations

For reasons relating to their hydrolytic stability, as will be discussed, cellulose acetate RO membranes are normally operated in the pH range of 4 to 7.5. This usually requires an acid feed. Actually, CA can be operated at a pH 10, at the expense of considerably shortening life by accelerated hydrolysis. The thin-film composite polyamide RO membranes can be utilized over a much wider pH range. With the correct protection against mineral scaling, they can perform at a pH above 10. At pH 8.5, polyamide can reject bicarbonate ions, a matter of potential importance. The pH of the feedwater does not contribute importantly to the RO performance as regards sodium chloride, but it does affect bicarbonate and carbon dioxide.

The use of charged RO membranes has shown a rejection that was a function of pH and of the ion concentration (Kamiyama et al., 1990). Positively charged RO membrane showed a preference for chloride ion permeation over sodium ions. The results reflect the difficulty for an ion to permeate a membrane of like charge. Moreover, at a 10-ppm concentration, transport of the sodium ion through the positively charged membrane was fivefold, for a 97% rejection, compared with 99.4% at the 1-ppm concentration. This concentration effect mirrors the common reaction of charged membranes to concentrations of like-charged entities. At higher concentrations, the repelling charges on the membrane become swamped. At lower challenge densities, their repulsion of like charges is more efficient.

As expected, pH influenced the rejection qualities of the charged membranes (Kamiyama et al., 1990). Depending upon the particular membrane, there was a reversal of sodium ion and chloride ion rejection once a given pH value was attained. At pHs above its pK_a, the acidic groups of a given membrane assumed their negative charges. These facilitated the passage of sodium ions and interfered with the permeation of chloride ions. In principle, the positively charged membrane had its amine sites largely in an ionized condition below pH 10, whereupon it preferentially passed chloride ions.

Pressure

Water flux through RO membrane varies directly with the transmembrane pressure. This relationship is normal to the permeation of all microporous materials. In the case of RO membranes, higher pressures may also engage flows through pores that were too small to be involved at lower pressures. At the higher pressures, the water tension at the smaller pores becomes broken, bringing them into production (Comb, 1991). Above 30 psig there is no practical effect on the rejection of the ions per se. Since higher pressures cause a greater water permeation, however, the overall effect in diluting the ions not rejected is tantamount to higher rejections, the product water being less concentrated. Reverse osmosis operations are usually performed at 200 to 400 psig. The higher rejection possible at 1,000 psig is an impractical attainment.

Cellulose acetate units give unacceptable rejections at very low pressures. For these units, good rejections can be had at 150 psig, and better rejections at 300 psig. The higher the pressure, the better the overall rejection. Rejections by thin-film RO are less affected by pressures as low as 30 psig.

A certain minimum pressure is required in any RO operation to impart such a velocity to the reject stream as to keep it turbulent in order to enable it, by its tangential flow, to sweep the membrane surface free of polarizing contaminants.

Temperature
There is actually a slight loss of ion rejection with rise in temperature, but the relationship is close to linear. Temperature, as also pressure, is therefore used in RO operational design work. The membrane area determines, along with the feedwater quality, how much water can be processed. Using temperature or pressure decides how this volume is to be attained. Many RO units contain preheaters that raise the water temperature to about 21 to 25 °C (70 to 77 °F). The increase in temperature reduces the water viscosity. This boosts productivity by allowing for an easier passage of the water through the membranes.

By convention, RO membranes are rated for their performance at 25° C (77 °F). This leads to a popular misconception that RO operations are to be performed at that specific temperature. Reverse osmosis practices may be and are carried out at any temperature. At feedwater temperatures above 10 °C (50 °F) RO operations become practical. Rejection itself does not alter much in the usual temperature range of 10 to 26.6 °C (50 to 80 °F). However, the flux rating changes markedly with an increase in temperature. Overall, the effluent is diluted. This equates with an enhanced rejection. Instead of operating a cellulose acetate RO at 300 psig on room-temperature water, one can employ 150-psig pressure on water at an elevated temperature to get the same results. The flux for a typical thin-film composite at 25 °C (77 °F) is twice that at 9 °C (48 °F).

Heating chlorinated feedwaters diminishes their chlorine content, that reagent being a volatile gas. It is customary, therefore, to pass the chlorinated feedwater through the sand or multimedia bed before heating it by way of a heat exchanger in order for the higher chlorine concentration to be more discouraging to organism growth in the filter. Alternatively, the cold, chlorinated water can be heated by mixing it with heated potable water. The mixing valve is less expensive than a heat exchanger. However, the mixed water entering the deep bed filter will then have a lower chlorine content. More frequent sanitizations of the filter may be necessitated. More to the point, the incoming water during sudden cold weather occurrences, albeit set for heating by mixing, may still not be at 25 °C (77 °F). This could mean that water permeation would be dimished, perhaps to too low a level.

To overcome this possibility, a larger (more expensive) pump may be needed, or a larger (more expensive) RO unit may be utilized. Any of these approaches is acceptable technically. The choice is made chiefly on an economic basis.

It is generally more economical to pay for pumping energy, however, than for heating energy. If well water at 13 °C (55 °F) is being subjected to RO purification, it is usually operationally less expensive to use higher pressures or larger-size RO units to obtain given flows than to heat the water from 13 °C (55 °F) to 21 °C (70 °F) or higher. On the other hand, heat is often used because it may permit lower outlays for capital costs. Keeping these low in a water purification operation is a common concern; expenses in the actual operation are apparently more easily tolerated. If waste heat is available, its utilization to heat the feedwater makes good economic sense.

Perhaps the most important effect of temperature on RO operations is its influence on carbon dioxide solubility. The higher the water temperature, the lesser the amount of dissolved carbon dioxide, and the lower the resulting conductivity of the water.

RO Membrane Compaction

Higher temperatures dispose cellulose acetate RO membranes especially to greater degrees of compaction because these membranes are thermoplastic polymers. They soften with heat. This in turn results in lower flux. In general, the perception is that higher temperatures compromise the membrane service life. However, the effect upon membrane life is a minor item. Higher RO operating temperatures may also overcome the tendency towards supersaturation, as of calcium sulfate, thus promoting mineral scale deposition upon the membrane.

Compaction of the membrane leads to losses in the permeation rate. For cellulose acetate RO membranes, these losses have been estimated to be 10%, 15%, and 20% for 1, 2, and 3 years service, respectively, at about 350 to 450 psig (1,378 to 1,723 kPa) driving pressure. In the case of polyamide RO membranes, the losses have been seen as being lower, namely 8%, 13%, and 18% over the same service durations (Paulson and Bertelson, 1990). These authors cautioned, however, that these compaction values, productive of membrane densification with concomitant loss in void volume and permeation rate, were obtained when "pure water" was presumed to be used in the compaction tests. They cited Rudie et al. (1985), who purified the test water by using ultrafilters of 20,000 daltons as prefilters immediately ahead of the RO test cells. Rudie et al. (1985) actually observed less compaction at 600 psig (4,130 kPa) for cellulose acetate after 1,000 hours, as measured by flux reduction, than is generally expected to occur at 400 psig (2,760 kPa). The implication was that a portion of the flux decline normally attributed to membrane compaction was actually the product of fouling caused by the use of "pure water."

Rudie et al. (1985) compared the flux declines of an RO membrane operating at 25 °C and at zero permeate pressure, and variously protected by ultrafilters characterized by different dalton ratings and operating at 35, 100, and 800 pounds per square inch differential (psid). The UF-protected RO showed no flux decline at any of the tested differential pressures, which would be an indication of freedom from compaction (Figure 9-2).

Comparing RO Polymers

Historically, cellulose acetate and cellulose acetate blends were the polymers from which the earliest RO devices were prepared. The polyamide RO membranes, usually in the form of thin-film composites (polyamide, PA), are of more recent

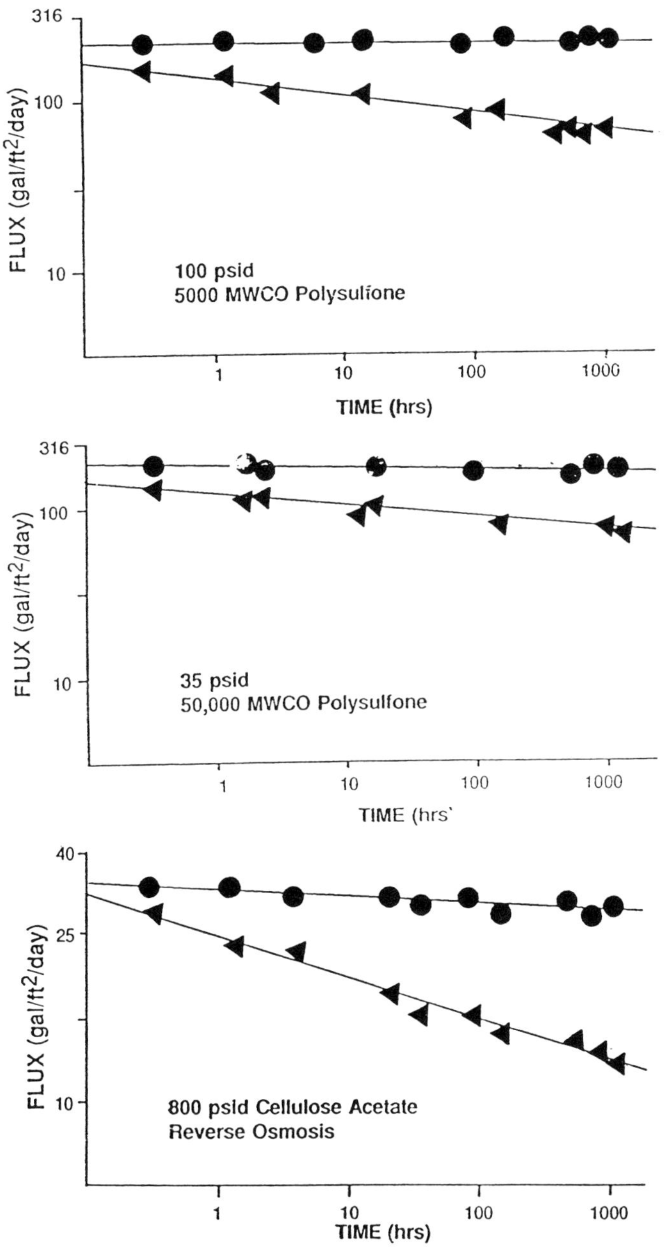

Figure 9-2. Flux reduction: compaction or fouling?
Rudie et al. (1985); Courtesy, American Chemical Society

manufacture.* The present consensus is that the PA units perform better in rejections and yield higher fluxes. They compact less than the cellulose acetate membranes, and therefore tend to retain their initial high flowrates. In consequence, PA units are lower in their electrical pumping energy demand, particularly as they operate at lower pressures. Moreover, they are hydrolytically stable over a more extensive pH range; and are not degraded by cellulose-digesting organisms. Accordingly, claims of long service lives are made for PA units.

The single greatest detriment to PA units is their ruinous susceptibility to oxidative decrepitude, especially as caused by chlorine. An index of the damage caused to PA membranes by chlorine is a decrease in their rejection rate, as measured in thousandths of ppm. The polymeric structure of the polyamide contains residual diamines. It is these residual linkages that cause its sensitivity to chlorine. Not surprisingly, the thin-film composite ROs have been widely used because of their superior performances, their susceptibility to chlorine (and other oxidizers) notwithstanding (Gupta, 1986a). Indeed, the superior rejection qualities of thin-film composite ROs have led a New England company to control a high bacterial load with ozone, and to destroy the ozone with 185-nm UV just prior to the water entering the RO. The high rejection rate of the PA membrane is sought despite the risk of the strong oxidizing powers of ozone to the RO.

Cellulosic membranes do cost less than the PA. However, the polymer undergoes some finite hydrolysis at all pHs, but minimally at pHs from 4.5 to 5 (Vos et al., 1966). Albeit RO practices utilizing CA membranes are preferentially conducted at pH 5 to 7.5, CA inevitably hydrolyzes; its rejection decreases with time. That of PA membranes remains flat. Reverse osmosis units of PA thus compare more favorably with CA over longer service durations.

The typical end-of-life for a CA membrane is signaled by a reduced salt rejection, to the low 90 percentiles. The end-of-life failure for the PA membrane is marked by a reduction in flow. The typical operating pressure of a cellulose acetate/RO is about 400 psig; for the PA, about 225 psig. The nanofilters, the more open constructions of these RO membranes (See page 188) utilize lower pressures, about 200 psig for the CA type, and 150 psig for the PA variety (Comb 1994).

The CA membranes have a normal salt rejection of 97.5%; 70% for the corresponding nanofilters (NF). The salt rejection normal to the PA membrane is 98 to 99%; for the NF constituted of polyamide it is also about 70%. These rejection levels reflect single ion measurements. (Comb 1994).

The CA units can be expected to last from 2 to 5 years, mostly 2. Reduction

*There is some ambiguity in the use of the term *polyamide*. Most thin-film composites are composed of a functional polyamide skin overlaying a porous polysulfone support structure. DuPont's hollow-fiber Permasep units are composed of aromatic polyamide. Some use the term *polyamide* only for the hollow-fiber devices. Here, the term polyamide refers to the polymer type, regardless of the form in which it is arranged. The abbreviation TFC is often used for *thin-film composite*. This is not appropriate, as TFC is an actual trademark of one type of PA thin-film composite. To avoid this usage, the acronym PA is used here to indicate thin-film composites of polyamide membranes.

in service life down to 1 to 1.5 years may be occasioned by operations at higher or lower pHs. The PA units can last from 3 to 5 years, mostly 3; but they are essentially not chlorine tolerant. Since the production of the polyamide thin-film composite involves a two step process, its cost is about double that of the CA unit (Comb 1994).

The pH range of 4.5 to 5 is not used for reverse osmosis, for many reasons. Cellulose acetate rejects best, as measured on mixed ions, at pH 6. (Polyamide rejects best at pH 7.5 to 8.) Additionally, for those who fear overshooting to the pH levels ruinous to CA membrane, pH 5.5 to 6 provides a safety margin. Moreover, pH represents a logarithmic function. A 10-times increase in the amount of acid is needed to increase the pH from 4.5 to 5.5. Also, the cost of neutralizing this acid prior to disposing of the reject stream is a real consideration. Acid addition is demanding in operational accuracy, as is also its neutralization. These require the added expenses of a mixing tank, an acid proportioning pump, and a pH monitor and cell. Regulations by OSHA about waste disposal are also a factor.

Acidification creates free carbon dioxide in equilibrium with bicarbonate ion, and can be removed by vacuum degasification or by sweeping the water with a purging airstream. Such decarbonation is not mandatory. If carbon dioxide is present, however, it will permeate the RO units. Its equilibration with water yields, at about 5 ppm, resistivities of about 250,000 ohms-cm. Carbon dioxide can be removed from its aqueous solutions by the use of strongly basic anion-exchange resins—at significant cost, however, if the volume is substantial.

Carbon dioxide permeates all RO membranes. Its creation is avoided by the use of PA membranes at pHs of 8 to 8.5, which enables the rejection of bicarbonate ion, thus obviating the use of acid and the problem of carbon dioxide removal. At these pHs, however, other means of scale control (e.g., softening) are required. The removal of carbon dioxide, as bicarbonate, eliminating its presence from the permeate, improves the conductivity of the product water.

Figure 7-9 gives the percent passage of carbon dioxide through polyamide RO membranes as a function of pH. Below pH 6, about 80% of CO_2 exists as such. Beginning at about pH 6.3 its conversion to bicarbonate takes place rapidly, and its passage to CO_2 diminishes precipitously. Above pH 8.3, all the carbon dioxide is in the form of carbonate ion; no dissolved CO_2 gas exists to pass the RO membrane.

$$CO_2 + H_2O \text{ ----> } H_2CO_3$$
$$H_2CO_3 \text{ ----> } H^+ + HCO_3^- \qquad pKa = 6.38$$
$$HCO_3^- \text{ ----> } H^+ + CO_3^{2-} \qquad pKa = 10.37$$

Intriguingly, CA membranes are said to have been devoured by waterborne cellulose-digesting organisms over relatively short time periods. Reports allude to such incidents taking place over long weekends in stagnant (nonflowing) systems. The answer to the problem is the maintenance of a chlorine residue or of a continuous recirculation. Usually, recirculation is used for thin-film PA membranes, which do not tolerate chlorine. Actually, enzymatic digestions may not be involved. Changes in pH, occasioned by the organisms, may cause hydrolytic decompositions.

Cellulose acetate is relatively resistant to oxidizing agents like hypochlorite. The ability of CA to endure chlorine and to be permeated by chlorine is a great advantage. Hango (1989), from long experience, judged that cellulose acetate RO produces the best quality water while requiring the least maintenance. Performing at 75% to 80% recovery, Hango's cellulose acetate RO operations required cleanings only every 2 to 5 years. The presence of 0.1 ppm of chlorine downstream of the RO unit served to sanitize the entire line into the DI resin beds, whose consequent degradation seemed negligible. Temporary hardness was handled by acid addition, followed by carbon dioxide removal by a degasifier utilizing an airstream treated with a HEPA filter. The continuing presence of chlorine helped to safeguard against microbial recontamination. Indeed, the chlorine residual upstream of the ion-exchange beds (wherein it was removed) conferred such a bacteriostatic disposition to the water as to continue to influence its quality downstream of the beds. The flux through the cellulose acetate RO was only about 60% or so of that of a PA unit, but its cost was also about 60% of that of an equivalent PA. On a cost-per-gallon basis, Hango believed, cellulose acetate RO was superior.

Nevertheless, new cellulose acetate installations seem to be in decline, and very little new research and development is being expended on CA reverse osmosis possibilities.

Polyamide RO membranes are resistant to hydrolysis between the pHs of 4 and 11. At pH 8, these RO filters exhibit a high rejection of bicarbonate ion. Therefore it has been possible to remove the carbon dioxide in the form of bicarbonate ion using polyamide RO membrane at pH 8 (Kraft, 1985). Depending upon the calcium ion concentration in the water, however, calcium carbonate scale formation on the membrane surface is a possibility at this pH. The probability can be ascertained by determining the Langelier saturation index of the water. The most economical method of controlling calcium carbonate scale formation is by acid dosing. Unfortunately, the polyamide RO membrane suffers a reduction in its bicarbonate ion rejection below pH 8. Softening is of value here. The sodium ion from the cation exchanger that substitutes for the bivalent ions that are removed in the softening are more difficult for the RO to reject. This is offset by the reduction in scaling. An alternative is to utilize additives such as sodium hexametaphosphate, 20 mg/L in the RO feedwater (Kraft, 1985).

The polyamide polymer contains free carboxylic acid groups, functional group components normally present as chain endings. These groups, dissociated in the form of negative ions, strongly adsorb cationic surfactants and just as irreversibly combine with polymeric cationic flocculants. Flux reductions of as much as 35% have been reported.

There are those who believe that metals such as copper, aluminum, or 1 ppm of barium or strontium also combine irreversibly with the aberrant carboxylic acid groups of the polyamide membranes. Concentrations of 0.4 ppm of aluminum, as from excessive alum treatments, can shut down PA membranes in weeks or even days. According to this theory, users of potable waters prepared using alum coagulation and flocculation should therefore use polyamide RO membranes with due caution.

Others strongly disagree. They believe that flux decline is the result of barium sulfate being precipitated under conditions where improper prefiltration and inadequate crossflow turbulence are used.

A new RO type consists of polysulfonated polysulfone. The polysulfone polymer bears sulfonic acid groups. It is popularly referred to as a *polysulfone RO*, which is an unfortunate nomenclature as it does not indicate the presence of the sulfonic acid radicals that distinguish it. Its mode of action differs from that of the conventional RO membranes. The sulfonated polysulfone works on the Donnan exclusion principle. Anions bearing like negative charges are repelled by the sulfonic acid groups; thus they fail to permeate the RO. In order to maintain electrical neutrality, their cationic counterions are compelled not to traverse the RO barrier. Therefore all ions are rejected by the sulfonated RO membrane. The sulfonic acid groups screen a spatial area, as it were. As such, they can be swamped by a flood of cations. The rejection efficiency of this new RO thus reflects an inverse relationship to the rate of fluid flow, as influenced by differential pressure. The degree of water softening is important in the minimization of divalent ions that can neutralize the ionized sulfonic acid groups, by combining with them into relatively undissociated forms. Decreasing the anion population is important in avoiding the swamping effect, the overwhelming of the sulfonic acid group defenses against anion passage. Like most water purification units, the purer the water it confronts, the better the polysulfonated polysulfone works. It resembles cellulose triacetate RO in its higher operating pressure, and in its somewhat lower rejections.

Rejecting on the basis of ionic charges, the polysulfonated polysulfone RO has a poor rejection of TOC and of nonreactive (nonionic) silica.

The chlorine resistance of the sulfonated polysulfone RO module is remarkable. It has been demonstrated to withstand 100 ppm of chlorine at pHs of 5.5 to 6.0 for at least 400 hours without significant decrease in flux or rejection. After 1,100 hours at 200 psig of feed pressure and 20% recovery at 20 °C, a salt discrimination loss of 6% to 7.2% was detected. Because of its permeability to and inertness to chlorine, RO units using this module can be sanitized and freed of foulants by the use of sodium hypochlorite of 100 ppm of active chlorine equivalent at pHs of 5.5 to 10. At pHs of 5.5 to 7.0, 50% of chlorine will permeate at 200 psig. The wide pH stability range of these units permits cleaning with hydrochloric acid at pH 2, or with sodium hydroxide at pH 12, just as is possible for more familiar RO membranes. It is, however, their inertness to active chlorine compounds that is noteworthy. The polysulfonated polysulfone can be "shocked" with 100 ppm of chlorine; cellulose acetate will endure 5 ppm or so, the polyamides virtually none. The appended sulfonic acid groups explain the influence of pH on this membrane, as well as its susceptibility to fouling by divalent cations capable of forming undissociated (insoluble) sulfonate salts. The use of this RO type requires thorough water softening Parise at al. (1987),

Kamiyama et al. (1990) listed a number of less usually encountered RO membrane types, including aromatic/aliphatic polyureas, heterocyclic/aromatic polyamides, and fully aromatic polyamides.

Reverse osmosis membranes cannot be depended upon to furnish sterile water. In one RO installation, for example, the final 0.1-μm-rated microporous filters downstream became blocked with annoying frequency. These filters responded to sanitization by sodium hypochlorite, a sign that the filter blockage was occasioned by bacterial growth. Eventually, replacement of the RO units with new RO devices resulted in a freedom from clogging of the final membranes. The underlying causality in the above experience was seen as being the nonsterilizing qualities of the original RO set. Given the large quantities of RO membrane manufactured, it is not surprising that such filters on occasion depart from perfection in organism retention. Their overall ionic rejection remains unimpaired, however.

There is also a contrary view, which says that RO membranes are integral but that their downstream surfaces become colonized by organisms from below. Be that as it may, tests performed at the U.S. Public Health Service Bureau of Epidemiology some 15 years ago concluded that all RO membranes experience the grow-through of organisms under certain conditions.

Summary of RO Membrane Polymers

The most popular RO types are the thin-film composites. These are usually run at 200 to 250 psig, or around 300 psig for a cold-water supply, and give very high rejections, even of bicarbonate and silica (98% rejection of silica). If run at below 100 psig, and certainly at below 30 psig, as from a need to reduce productions or because the RO unit is oversized, the rejection could diminish to 95% or 96%. Productivity changes more drastically with pressure than does rejection. Despite the chlorine rating given by manufacturers to PA membranes, their resistance to oxidants in general and to chlorine in particular is very poor. Using dechlorinated waters, polyamide RO units can achieve long service lives. Polyamide polymer is resistant to degradation by organisms, and offers the highest flux of any RO membrane.

Cellulose acetate RO is generally the lowest in rejection, and its flux is only low to medium. However, it involves the lowest capital cost. Where low bacteria counts are the overriding consideration, as in pharmaceuticals, the inertness of CA units to chlorine may make them the RO polymer of choice.

Sulfonated polysulfone rejects better than CA membranes but not so well as those of PA. It requires operating pressures in the same ranges as required by the CA units. Despite their expense, where the aim is to chlorinate without acidification, these membranes may be the best choice. Experience with these membranes is not yet sufficient to indicate reliably the length of their service lives. (See Table 9-1).

Membrane degradations may result, as from catastrophic oxidative alterations in the molecular structures and properties of polyamides by chlorine or other oxidants; by the slower and therefore more subtle degradations of cellulose acetate by the same agents; by the hydrolysis of CA membranes; and by the actual bacterial digestion of cellulose acetate under certain conditions. Degradation of the RO membrane, of whatever type by whatever agency, results in the loss of its reverse osmotic purifying functionality, so that the RO unit becomes ruined and must be replaced.

Kremen and Knappe (1994) challened the common belief that cellulose acetate RO membranes are digestively degraded by microorganisms (the phenomenon is sometimes referred to as *head-end* loss); on occasion, it is anecdotally alleged, even to the point of almost total obliteration. These investigators ascribe the observed degradations as being cauded by the oxidative decrepitude induced by the presence of sodium hypochlorite catalyzed by trace quantities of ferric oxide and "other ubiquitous particulates." Indeed, they stated that organisms rarely attack cellulose membranes even when present in large numbers. The possibility of pH-related effects has already been mentioned.

Kremen and Knappe (1994) asserted that head-end deterioration, characterized by a decrease in salt rejection and an increase in water permeation, arises from the chlorine present in the feedwaters. It has been observed when the chlorine content is from 0.5 to 1 mg/mL, and when the oxidation-catalyzing

Table 9-1
Reverse Osmosis Membrane Operating Parameters

	Cellulose acetate	*Polyamide*	*Thin-film composite*	*Sulfone composite*
pH	4-7	4-11	2-11	2-12
Chlorine tolerance	Good	Poor	Poor	Excellent
Resistance to bacteria	Poor	Good	Good	Good
Temperature limit (°C)	35	38	50	70
Rejection (%)	90-98	90-95	98	95-98

particulates are present. The decline in RO performance first affects the lead end of the head-end elements, and, unless halted, progresses on a patterned basis with respect to the element position.

Removal of chlorine, as by any of the conventional means, arrests (or prevents) the degradation. Of course, the biocidal protection of the chlorine is canceled forthwith as well. Kremen and Knappe (1994) advocated instead the addition of a slight excess of ammonia to the system. This lowers the redox potential to the point where oxidation of the cellulose can no longer take place. Advantageously, the chloramide formed by interaction of the chlorine and ammonia serves to keep the waters in a disinfected condition.

RO Membrane Design

While RO membranes do restrain the passage of ions and permit permeation of water, their flux (the volume of water passed per unit area of membrane per unit time) are low. (Flux is described in terms of liters per square meter per hour, or as gallons per square foot per day [GFD], for instance.) Overcoming this problem has occasioned three approaches: the devising of asymmetric membranes, the maximizing of the membrane surface/water interchange of the RO unit, and the application of tangential flow. The success of these approaches has led to the practicality of RO devices (Gupta, 1986b).

Asymmetric Membranes

Loeb and Sourirajan (1962) devised the membrane casting technique whereby a thin, dense, functional layer of polymer comes to overlay a much thicker, much more open support layer of the same polymer to compose an asymmetric structure, so called because of its side-to-side differences in morphology.

Subsequently, very thin films of aromatic polyamides were devised by the interaction, for instance, between a hexane solution of a dicarboxylic acylhalide or acid with one of, for example, metaphenylenediamine. The resulting thin polyamide film then is constructed as an overlay upon an open, porous polysulfone membrane. These constructions are known as thin-film composites.

By either of the techniques and their variations, asymmetric RO membranes are manufactured.

The asymmetric membrane rejects the passage of ions, such as salts, but permits an acceptable rate of permeation by water. The denseness of the thin skin establishes the membrane's discriminatory qualities. Its thinness serves to limit the resistance that this density imposes on the flux of permeating molecules. The thicker but less dense porous understructure acts merely as a mechanical support for the metering skin.

Tangential Flow

In any population of particles there is a particle-size distribution. In most particulate distributions there are more small particles than large (Johnston, 1990). The finer the pores in a filter, the more particles it will retain and the earlier it will clog. As explained in Chapter 5, "Particulate Removal by Filtration," the dead-ended mode of filtration commonly practiced for microporous filters is inappropriate for reverse osmosis or ultrafilters. Crossflow filtration wherein the tangential sweep of the liquid is across the filter surface is necessitated. This serves to remove or at least reduce the polarized layer of particles whose filtrative accretion would otherwise prematurely abbreviate the useful service life of the RO device.

Inevitably a fouling layer of some thickness forms. The thickness is a resultant of several factors, including the velocity and turbulence of the liquid stream, the roughness of the filter surface, and the surface interaction with the particles by way of adsorptive forces. However formed, and of whatever dimensions, this deposition, usually a thin filter cake, reduces the permeate flux. Attempts have been made to predict the steady-state permeate flux as a function of the operating conditions (Korin, 1990). Advantage is taken to utilize the action of the bulk flow tangent to the membrane to limit the accumulation of the immobile cake layer (Blatt et al., 1970).

Crossflow velocity is the average of the feed and concentrate or reject flows, $Q_{ave} = (Q_f + O_c) \div 2$. Its practical measure may be made in terms of the feed flow, however. The economic considerations of tangential flow filtration were investigated by Korin (1990).

The design factors involved in the devising of tangential flow systems, particularly for biotechnology applications, were detailed by Dosmar and Wolber (1991). Considerations regarding piping, valves, pumps, and instrumentation were discussed.

Concentration Polarization

An inevitable consequence of the retention by the RO membrane of ions, other solutes, and particulates is the buildup in the concentration of these entities in the neighborhood of the membrane. This concentration polarization, although minimized by the sweeping action of tangential flow, and corrected for by concentration-gradient back diffusion, always occurs in any membrane process. Hydraulic resistance by the concentration polarization layer is negligible, except as higher applied differential pressures may compact particulates. The flux losses occasioned by concentration polarization are therefore of osmotic pressure origins. The concentration polarization effect can become stabilized in an RO operation. A steady state results from achieving such an equilibrium. For this reason, the phenomenon of concentration polarization should not be considered to be fouling (Paulson, 1987). However, concentration polarization may lead to the exceeding of a substance's solubility product. A deposition may then result that can foul the membrane.

The consequences of concentration polarization resulting from an accumulation of particulate matter are self-evident: Blockage of the filter surface occurs, resulting in a diminution of effective filtration area. Concentration polarization of solute and ions will also occur. As the water leaves the solution side of the RO membrane to permeate the intersegmental spaces within the polymer, it deposits its dissolved ions and solute molecules in close propinquity to the membrane. The ionic concentrations increase in this boundary layer. This creates an osmotic back-pressure demand that renders progressively more difficult further reverse osmotic demineralization. This can be countered by the use of higher applied pressures. It is best dealt with by employing a more vigorous sweep of the tangential flow.

In dead-end filtration where the flowrate decay is rather steep, the filtration cost is reckoned in terms of the membrane cost. In the rapid stream velocities of the crossflow or tangential filtration mode, the flow decay is much more gradual. The cost is made in terms of pumping expense rather than of membrane. In devising their various RO modules, most manufacturers try to achieve a compromise position between the extremes.

If a plot is made of rate of filtration versus average transmembrane pressure, a straight-line relationship will usually result for clean water. Here, the resistance of the filter alone dictates the flow. Departures from linearity constitute evidence that a deposited layer or a concentration polarization layer has formed on the upstream side of the membrane. In such cases, increasing the pressure does not proportionally increase the flowrate. Even in the tangential flow mode, some concentration polarization is always present, and pressure increases may not be efficacious. In effect, the polarization layer can become the rate-limiting filter. Added pressure may serve only to waste the added pumping costs and to cause compaction of the polarized layer.

The consequences of concentration polarization can be overcome by encouraging rediffusion or removal of the polarized material back into the bulk solution. The purpose of tangential flow is to accomplish this removal by the sweeping action of a liquid flow. This crossflow sweep must be strong enough to minimize, by shearing away, the polarized layer overlying the filter surfaces. The material involved in the concentration polarization, thus removed, is recirculated for further treatment. (See Figure 9-3).

Figure 9-4 shows a schematic for a tangential flow system consisting of a liquid reservoir, a pump, a tangential flow filtration module, and utilizing concentrate recirculation and permeate collection. Figure 9-5 is a photograph of an actual system designed for concentrating cells in the laboratory.

The velocity of the recirculating liquid on the upstream side of the membrane is regulated by means of the pump and two valves, with the inlet valve admitting the solution to the filter module and the outlet valve governing its exit. The greater the disparity in the extents of openness of these valves, the greater the velocity of flow. Throttling the outlet valve for any setting of the inlet valve serves to diminish the velocity of the circulating stream and increase the transmembrane pressure.

A third or permeate valve on the downstream side of the membrane regulates the permeate flow through it and thus serves to define the filtrate pressure. The applied differential pressure across the membranes, the average transmembrane pressure, is the average of the inlet and outlet recirculating pressures, less the permeate pressure. As in all filtrations, the average differential pressure governs the rate of a filtration unit until such time as filter-cake formation or fouling of the membrane supersede.

Because, as in any filtration, the rate of filtration is desired to be as high as possible, the object in a tangential flow is to restrict the permeate flow as little as possible. The permeate pressure is normally kept at zero; the permeate valve is wide open. If, however, polarization effects become manifest, the filtration rate can be scaled back to minimize the rate of concentration polarization.

The concentration polarization of ions tends to become progressively worse as an RO operation continues. As the effective filtration area decreases because of carbonate, sulfate, or other scaling, the water flux decreases and there is a

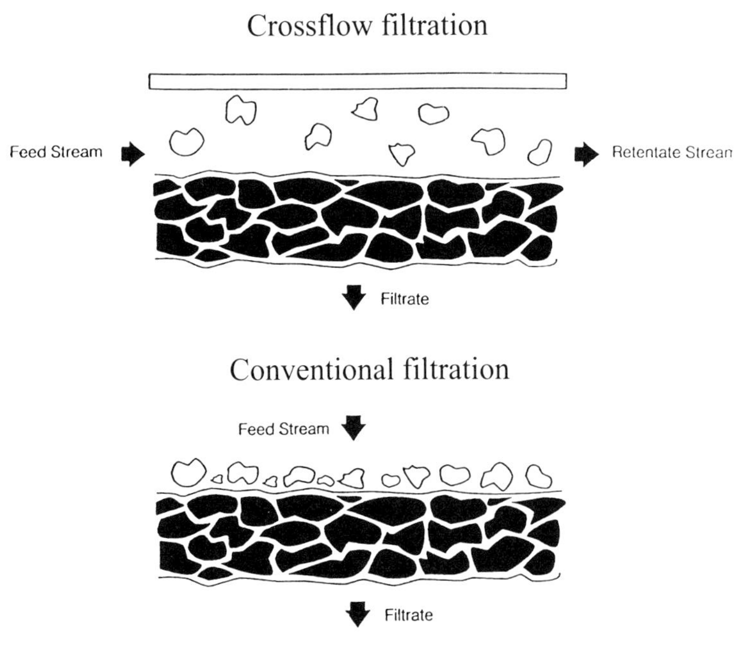

Figure 9-3. Crossflow filtration conventionalfFiltration.
Courtesy, Millipore Corp.

decrease as well in ion rejection by the membrane; the permeate increases in ionic content. This decrease in permeate rejection should be taken as evidence of ionic concentration polarization. It occurs because ion rejection by the membrane is not absolute. Like ion exchange, it is a percentage, about 95%, of the confronting ion concentration. In some cases, a 3% to 4% drop in rejection occurs for a 10% drop in permeation. Some use a 1% drop as indicating a need to clean the RO membrane. In many cases, however, a drop in permeate quality (in overall rejection) signals the onset of fouling even before a drop in permeate rate manifests itself. Concentration polarization arises from the depletion of solvent molecules, with a corresponding increase in solute concentration. This is a result of the pressure-driven permeation. The condition comes to characterize the boundary layers of membranes wherein water passes while particles (whether colloidal or otherwise) and/or ions are retained. This is typical of reverse osmosis and ultrafilter operations, and even of microporous filtrations, although with less severe consequences in the latter case. Minimization of concentration polariza-

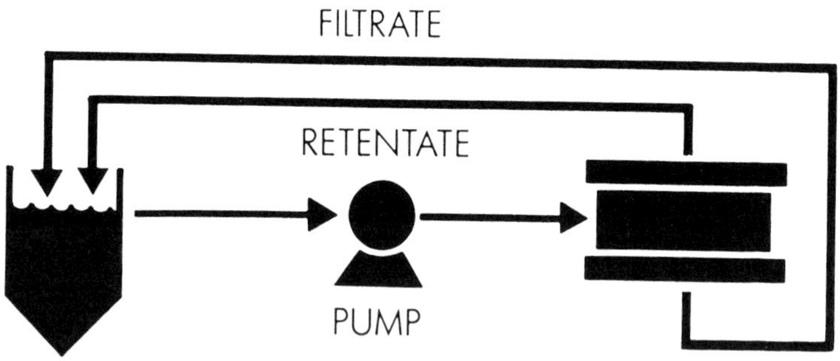

Figure 9-4. Total recycle, tangential flow system.
Courtesy, Millipore Corp.

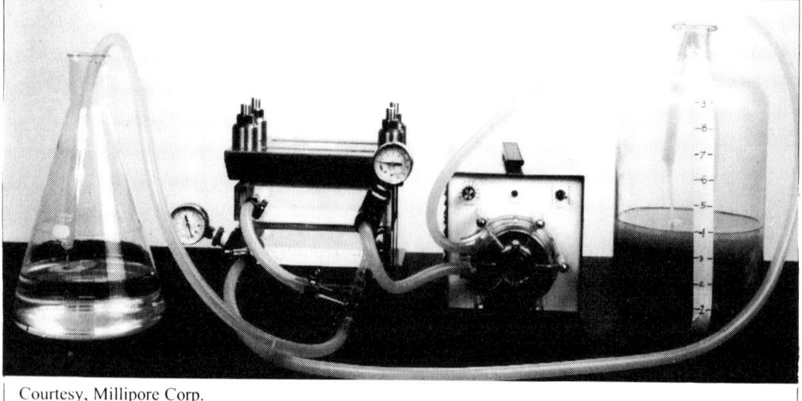

Courtesy, Millipore Corp.

tion beyond the inevitable few-angstrom boundary layer necessitates use of the crossflow, or tangential cycling mode. The velocity of the crossflow must be above a Reynolds number of 3,000 or 4,000 (as variously advocated): enough to create turbulent flow.

A Reynolds number, also referred to as N_{RE}, is any of several dimensionless quantities of the form LV p/u that are all proportional to the ratio of the internal force versus viscous force in a flow system. L is the characteristic linear dimension of the flow channel (in feet), V is the velocity (ft/sec), p is the fluid density (lb/ft^3), and u is the fluid velocity (lb/ft·sec). The critical Reynolds number corresponds to the transition from turbulent to laminar flow as the velocity is reduced (Perry and Chilton, 1973; Chapman et al., 1983a).

Membrane Element Configurations

The modes of maximizing membrane surface to liquid volume that are used in RO construction, as described below, are also used in the devising of ultrafiltration units. Practical application of the RO concept necessitates a compact disposition, one offering a high productivity of treated water per unit volume occupied by the device. This problem has been approached by each of four different arrangements: plate and frame, hollow fibers, tubes, and spiral-wound membranes.

Pohland (1981) has gathered into tabular form a comparison of the various RO modes with their attendant area of membrane surface per unit volume (Table 9-2).

Plate-and-frame mode. In the first arrangement, RO membrane sheets are used in a plate-and-frame mode (Böddeker et al., 1978). This choice has the advantage of permitting the selection of RO and UF membranes as the particular circumstances require. Also, it has a low sensitivity to feedwater conditions. It is not noteworthy for its optimization of membrane area; and it is not, perhaps for this reason, much used. Its square footage costs are simply too high. It finds application largely in research-and-development settings and in processing and waste treatment applications.

Table 9-2
RO Membrane Configurations

Module	*Membrane Area* *(m^2/m^3)*	*Device Volume* *(ft^2/ft^3)*
Plate and frame	165	50
Hollow tube	335	100
Spiral wound	1,000	300
Hollow fiber	16,500	5,000

Pohland (1981); Courtesy, McGraw-Hill.

Hollow fibers. In a noteworthy development, the DuPont Company introduced hollow fibers of an aromatic polyamide composition having small diameters of approximately 42 μm. Subsequently, Dow introduced a hollow-fiber device made of cellulose triacetate. Laterally arranged into cylindrical bundles containing a very large number of fibers and with a very large total surface area, the hollow-fiber modules constitute the most compact RO membrane disposition commercially available.

The hollow fibers would plug all too easily were feedwaters led into them. The arrangement is for feedwater to be flowed among but outside them, under the impetus of pressure contained by the shell. The hollow-fiber device, where the spaces among the fibers are on the order of 25 mm, is usually preceded by 5- to 10-μm-rated prefilters, designed to remove particulate matter. The permeate water issuing from within the fibers is collected. Although the hollow-fiber walls are thin, the outside diameter of some fibers attains about 95 mm, about twice the diameter of the lumen (inner diameter), some 42 mm. The fibers are therefore strong enough not to collapse under the high applied differential pressures used, 28 bar (400 psig) (Figure 9-6).

The problem with hollow fibers relates to their fragility. They may be tested successfully at one pressure, yet may fail in actual use at lower pressures. Apparently, a wave phenomenon serves to flex them excessively in actual flow. Their use is therefore often confined to pressures of 30 to 35 psig. At these pressures, the liquid flow through them remains in the laminar region. When, as for the Permasep devices, the flow is from the outside in, the flow is not really tangential but is essentially dead-ended.

The high packing densities of hollow-fiber devices compensate for their lower permeation rates. The systems are very sensitive to feedwater particulates. Their high pressure drop limits the driving pressure available to them. Additionally, the DuPont and Toyabo hollow-fiber elements cannot be operated at turbulent flows.

The devising of a hollow fiber constituted an impressive technological accomplishment. However, the resulting devices require excessive pretreatment to prevent their fouling. They are prone to faster blockage by scale formation, and the turbulence necessary to prevent clogging by sediment is difficult to achieve due to the fragility of the fibers.

Hollow-fiber RO devices are still used in seawater desalinations, although they have a low recovery. Otherwise, they seem to be utilized mostly in retrofit contexts, and in ultrafiltration work.

Tubes. Tubular RO devices are also available. Such tubes can be produced with the dense rejecting layer of the asymmetric structure on either the inside or the outside. The tubular arrangement serves to maximize the membrane area / device volume relationship, although hardly to the extent of the hollow fibers.

Most tubular arrangements are of 1/2-inch diameters. An advantage of the tubes is that the inner diameters are too large to be plugged by the suspended sediments and other large particulates present in feedwaters. By the same token, they lend themselves to easy cleaning.

Tubular modules have a relatively small membrane area per unit volume, however, and thus a low packing density. To minimize concentration polarization and particle buildup adjacent to the membrane surface, turbulent flow is required. To achieve this, high fluid velocities of 3 to 4 ft/sec are required in such tubes. The long tubular flow paths and turbulence result in high pressure drops and in higher energy costs.

Tubular units have fluxes of 10 to 25 gal/day/ft^2 at 400 to 600 psig (40 to 100 liters/day 929 cm^2 at 28 to 40 bar).

Tubular units are very inefficient, and are not much used in water purification applications. In addition, their installation requires room, a consideration not often easily available. In general, thin-film configurations, such as are forthcoming from spiral-wound modules, are seen to be more attractive economically (Short, 1990). They require far less membrane surface to interface adequately with feedwater volume.

There are some small-diameter tubes, possibly of 100-mil inner diameters, that, although they are often referred to as hollow fibers, do not suffer the same deficiencies. These tubes can withstand high enough differential pressures to

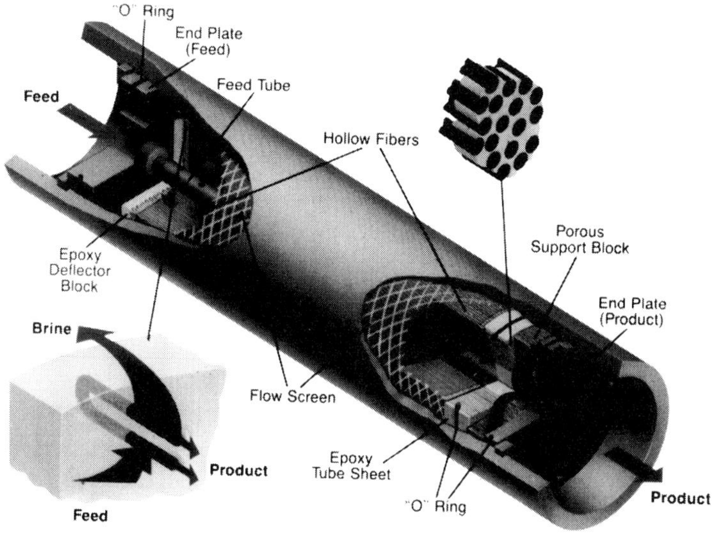

Figure 9-6. DuPont hollow fine fiber "Permasep" permeator.
Courtesy, DuPont de Nemours

impart turbulence to the liquids they carry; it is hoped, enough to minimize concentration polarization. Such small-diameter tubes are little used, however.

Spiral-wound modules. Spiral-wound modules have been amply described in the literature (Truby and Sleigh, 1974; Pohland, 1981). They are, in essence, jelly-roll formations of RO membranes sandwiching fabric spacers, and sealed* on three sides. The fourth, open side is sealed around the perforations of a center core, usually of PVC. The water that permeates the membranes from the outside is directed by the sandwiched spacer to flow into the openings of the central pipe (Figure 9-7).

Additional spacers, in turn, separate these sandwiches and direct the feedwater to the outsides of the membranes of which they are composed. One side of each membrane faces feedwater; the other side interfaces the treated permeate. The spacers are of a mesh construction designed to create turbulence in the flowing feedwater stream. One problem with these spacers is that they may cause a hang-up of particles by what has been called the snow fence phenomenon.

The entire membrane assemblage is spirally wound around the central core or pipe. Each such packet is called a leaf. From three to five leaves are normally spirally wound around a core. The feedwater enters one end of the tube that surrounds the core with its spirally wound leaves, and concentrate exits the other. The permeating water emerges as RO-treated effluent from the central pipe.

The optimization of membrane surface derives from using two membrane

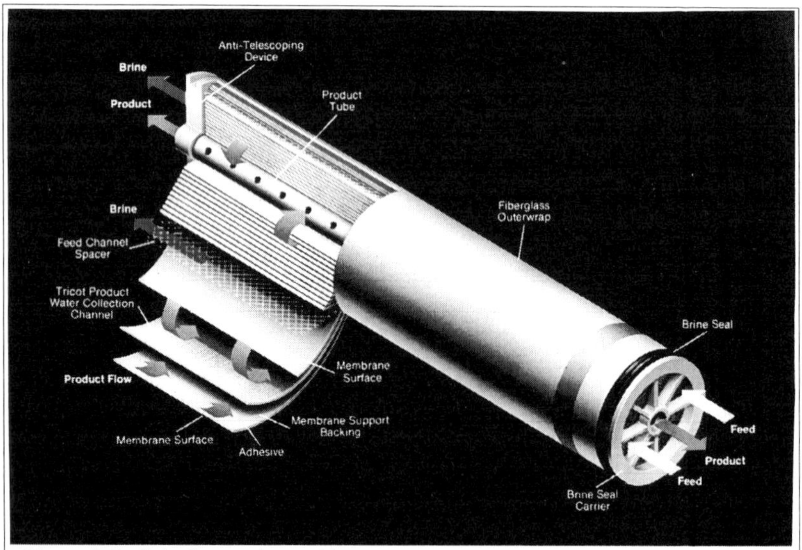

Figure 9-7. Spiral-wound cartridge.
Courtesy, DuPont de Nemours

areas per single permeate spacer, and from the disposition of the whole in cylindrical form. Spiral-wound units (and also the other RO modes) come in modular form and can be additively assembled to form units of whatever capacity is required.

Spiral-wound modules have the advantage of short feed flowpaths. Hence they exhibit low pressure losses. A key to the success of the spiral-wound configuration is the mesh spacer used, which causes turbulent flows at low velocities, thus reducing concentration polarization possibilities. The attainment of high packing densities is not difficult to achieve using spiral-wound modules. With feedwaters containing very fine solids, however, moderate to serious fouling problems may result (Truby and Sleigh, 1974). Most RO devices, perhaps 90%, are of the spiral-wound variety.

Spiral-wound arrangements perform best on waters with a silt density index less than 3 to 5. Hollow fibers require cleaner waters as regards total suspended solids. It may be that the higher packing densities of hollow-fiber devices militate against them when high-SDI waters are fed into their cores for permeation through the fiber walls and collection within the hollow-fiber bundle. Not enough turbulence can be created for practical processing rates, given the low flux of the membrane material. If, however, such waters are fed into the fibers to permeate into the core or shell of the device, the high TDS material tends directly to clog the lumina of the hollow fibers.

As spiral-wound RO units become progressively fouled, their permeation rates may fall off before the loss of discrimination against ions becomes evident. It is usual to clean spiral-wound RO arrangements when their salt rejection has decreased by a 1% or 2%, when they exhibit a 25% increase in differential feed to waste pressures, or when they have suffered a 10% reduction in the rate of permeate flow. Usually, rejection diminishes before permeation decreases.

The colloid level in an RO feedstream is usually limited to 1.0 nephelometric turbidity units (NTU) or less of turbidity, and to an SDI of no more than 4 to 5. However roughly estimated, these levels serve widely as guidelines in RO operations (Bates et al., 1988).

Jackson (1990) stated, "A spiral module is a dynamic, non-linear system in function. Therefore, what is known about a system is empirical." He added, "Even when general information already exists, the tendency has been to keep it confidential." It must be evident, therefore, that under the present conditions not too much can be gleaned concerning design details from the literature forthcoming from a proprietarily oriented manufacturer. Jackson (1990) listed the following as the factors to be considered in designing spiral-wound modules: cost, reliability of performance, component availability, potential market, interchangeability, and system size/complexity.

*See LeFave (1990) for the design, formulation, and testing of adhesives for RO constructions.

ring failure should be tested for to avoid needless RO element replacements.

As regards O-rings, Hango (1990) had this to say:

> "One disadvantage of the spiral-wound systems is the large number of O-ring seals and brine seals. Periodic conductivity profiles are needed to detect leaks. In order to prevent premature membrane seal failure, the following steps are recommended:
>
> a. Install new membranes with the factory representative on site. The small additional cost protects a large investment.
>
> b. Minimize start-stop operation of the RO systems by providing adequate permeate storage.
>
> c. Provide slow-acting feedwater valves to ramp membrane pressure gradually. The pump should start with the valves closed. Open gradually over a 20-second period. This will reduce membrane movement and seal failure.
>
> d. Install spacers with care to eliminate end play.
>
> e. Keep the RO system full of water to prevent air pockets and sudden pressure changes. Instrument sample lines can drain the system if not properly designed."

Considerations of Physical Space Availability

In designing an RO unit, the first considerations are the feedwater quality and the desired flowrate capacity, especially the latter. The unit diameter is then decided upon: 8, 4, or 2 1/2 inch. For 50 gpm or larger, an 8-inch diameter is usually the least expensive when a once-through water flow is used. When reject recycling is used, however, 8-inch units can be used for flows approaching 30 gpm (Zoccolante, 1991). Using 4-inch units provides four times as many elements, providing more possibilities for staging, but is more expensive.

Units 8 inches in diameter and 40 inches long constitute about 75% of the market. Longer units are not desired; such distances may prove too long to permit the flush-removal of particulates. Units of 16-inch-diameters had been constructed, but they proved too heavy and cumbersome to be useful.

For product flows of 2 or 3 gpm, diameters of 2-1/2 inches are enough, provided the desired RO polymer is constructed in that size. The 4-inch diameters fills the range in between. The chief design point is the maintenance of the required exit velocity from every membrane. However, as a rule of thumb, 4-inch units are used to produce up to 20 gpm; 8-inch units are for larger quantities.

However, staging considerations are also involved. A 20-gpm unit could be built around a single 8-inch element.* However, no staging advantages with their higher recoveries would be forthcoming. A 20-gpm RO could also be constructed around 24 4-inch elements. The fluxs of the membranes permit either arrangement. The decision involves how many membranes per vessel and how to stage the vessels. In whatever diameter, 40-inch-long elements require 4 feet of space at each end so that operators may get membranes in and out of the pressure vessels to replace them. Reverse osmosis units require adequate space, and the space available for the unit now enters the picture.

If eighteen elements of any diameter are required, and the biggest pressure vessel holds six elements, then three vessels in total would suffice. These can be arranged in a single array, with all the vessels in parallel, or as a 2:1 array. The latter would be preferred for reasons of recovery. Either arrangement would yield 70 gpm as required. The single array would need 40 inches plus twice 4 feet, about 12 feet. The 2:1 array need not require double the length of space available. The piping could be adjusted in the 2:1 array so that all three vessels are parallel, in line with one another. Either arrangement would yield 70 gpm as required.

Sometimes customers are forced to purchase more expensive ROs with three or four membranes per vessel, rather than longer vessels containing five or six membranes, in order to accommodate the space they have available. When pressure vessels are added with no increase in flow, the cost increases considerably. Two vessels to hold three membranes each are almost twice as expensive as one vessel to hold six. Another cost consideration is the added expense of employing more manifolding.

The rate of flow determines the number of membranes that are needed. The goal is the least expensive device that will furnish the required volume flow. Since both temperature and pressure determine the output of the RO, a choice can be exercised. A heat exchanger can precede the RO. Hotter water permeates the RO at a higher rate. Alternatively, higher pump pressures may be employed to secure more rapid flows. Temperatures in excess of 38 °C (100°F) shorten the service life of the membrane. Higher pumping pressures entail their own costs. Generally, however, the less expensive alternative is to utilize higher pressures. (See page 461).

Configuration Design of the RO Unit

The supplier of the RO membrane will supply data sheets setting forth the limitations on water recovery to be expected from each membrane. Typically this will be in the 10% to 20% range. Unless the reject stream is recirculated, a one-membrane RO limits the recovery to that amount. To reach a total recovery of 75% to 80%, enough membranes are required to treat progressively the processed streams, increasingly more concentrated, from the previous membranes. Usually RO units of 10- to 15-gpm capacity can allow 75% to 85% recoveries, except on unusually concentrated feedwaters. Smaller-capacity ROs will give

*Comb (1991) advised that an 8-inch element should not be run at more than 5 to 6 gpm.

lower recoveries.

Considerations of permeate quality also limit the amount of water recovered from RO systems. Product quality decreases as the waters being processed come to have higher salt concentrations. This is so because the amount of salt rejected is a percentage of that confronting the membrane, and the final stages of the RO are challenged by the more concentrated reject streams of the earlier stages. This is less important where the RO operation is followed by ion exchange, as in a polishing activity. Where ion exchange is being avoided, whether through an effort to eliminate the handling of regenerant chemicals, or the desire to prepare pharmaceutical waters solely by use of single- or double-pass RO, concerns of permeate quality may limit the amount of RO recovery. In such instances, sending more water to waste, decreasing the percentage recovery, will benefit the quality of the recovered water.

Only a few RO unit manufacturers produce their own membrane. In any case, RO membrane manufacturers supply data sheets detailing operational requirements for their membranes. Test conditions are given for specific test solutions in terms of factors such as gallons per day, pressure, temperature (both minimum and maximum), limits on pH, and maximum influx flowrates. The RO device manufacturer should guarantee that his unit conforms to the membrane manufacturer's stipulations.

Waste-Staged Design

Within the pressure vessels, the membranes connect with one another in a series/parallel arrangement designed to maintain high flow through the membranes. Typically, only about 10% to 15% of the feedwater is converted to product by each membrane. The resulting high rate of flow promotes turbulence and keeps the rejected contaminants from settling out. The water emerging from one pressure vessel is fed in a series arrangement into a second. Since some of the water is removed as product water, the maintenance of a water velocity that is both high and constant necessitates a decreasing number of pressure vessels in the second stage in series, and even fewer in the succeeding third stage.

The following scheme summarizes a simplified RO: A prefilter precedes the pump that supplies feedwater in parallel to each of four pressure vessels of a first stage. The product water is collected. The reject water, now more concentrated, emerges from the four vessels to be fed in parallel to the three pressure vessels of the second stage, in series with the first. This reject water, yet more concentrated, is fed in parallel to the next two pressure vessels of a third stage. Such an RO arrangement is called a 4:3:2 array. The reject stream (effluent) from the third stage is typically 25% of the original feedwater flowrate. The RO system recovery is 75%. It will be recalled that the feedwaters to the succeeding stages increase progressively in their total dissolved solids. The ionic contents emerging from the succeeding stages are also progressively greater, although the percentage of rejection remains the same. The overall percentage of rejection is a weighted average of that of the three stages. The purpose of the reject-staged design is to minimize water discard and to increase the recovery.

The reject-staged arrangement is also made use of in the disposition of two separate RO units. The wastewater from one unit is fed into a second RO unit in order to minimize the overall discard of water. The permeate from the first unit is purer, that unit having been operated using a more dilute feedwater. The product waters from both RO units may then be blended. Unfortunately, the blending will diminish the purity of the first product water.

Alternatively, the product water from the second RO, where still of fairly high TDS, too high to give an acceptable blend, can be used as feedwater to the first RO unit to give an improved product water, say at 75% recovery, from the first unit (Zoccolante, 1991).

Product staging, to be considered subsequently, uses the product water from the first stage as feedwater to the second. Also called double-pass RO, its purpose is to improve the quality of the ultimate product water. It is this arrangement of double-pass RO that the FDA intends to be used in the preparation of Water for Injection (WFI), as will be discussed.

RO/DI Arrangements

Whittet (1981) pointed out that reverse osmosis characteristically reduced the TDS contents of water by some 95%, and pharmaceutical waters may contain no more than 10 mg/L of total dissolved solids. He concluded that the use of RO to prepare such waters from ordinary waters must additionally involve mixed-bed resin polishing deionization, either before or after the reverse osmosis step. A single-pass RO will most probably not prepare water of purified water (PW) quality. However, followed by an ion-exchange unit, PW quality can be assured.

Of course, the use of ion exchange after RO could not be made for WFI applications. Ion exchange need not be used at all. Two-pass RO can be employed. In any case, since 1981, RO membranes have improved markedly in their rejection qualities.

Various arrangements of ion exchange and RO units are used on different waters in accordance with particular purification intentions. Some utilize ion exchange before RO, others reverse the order. Ion exchange before RO is rarer by far. It is, however, used by some Japanese chip manufacturers who consider the ion-exchange unit an ideal pretreatment for the RO, one that renders the RO operation more dependable.

Ion exchange is sometimes used in advance of the RO in order to reduce or prevent fouling of the membrane, first by reduction of the organic load, and second to avoid scale formation. An example is where the feedwaters are high in silica content, as in the Southwest where water recovery from RO operations must also be high. Typically, where silica in the waste stream exceeds 120 ppm, there is a great potential for RO fouling. If the feedwaters contain 80 ppm of silica, and if feedwater recovery is only 50% or so (and often it may be crucial to recover 90% to 95%), the reject water may contain about 160 ppm of silica. In such situations, particularly where high water recovery is required, the prior intervention of ion exchange to reduce the silica burden may be indicated. Silica values above about 100 ppm in reject streams may cause flux reductions of even over 75% over a 48-hour period. The RO can be used after the DI resins to eliminate colloids, bacteria, and organics. Some believe that ion-exchange resins are more easily fouled by silica than is RO. The form of the silica probably governs. However, the use of a weakly acidic cation-exchange resin before RO removes the divalent ions and prevents the deposition of alkaline earth sulfates upon the RO membrane.

It must be pointed out, however, that the use of strongly basic anion-exchange resin to process waters containing 120 ppm of silica would be very expensive.

The installation of RO units after ion-exchange beds, in effect the use of RO for point-of-use filtration, was utilized by Lewis et al. (1990) to reduce both particle counts and TOC levels in the rinsewaters for semiconductors. Utilization of this arrangement resulted in an immediate reduction in TOC and achieved a steady state after 216 hours. A continuing slow rise in TOC rejection brought the ultimate TOC elimination to 79.6%. Particle reduction to an asymptotic level was slower, but reached the 75% to 80% range after 288 hours. Another 244 hours lowered the particle count to a high of 98.3%, and the count finally settled to an overall level of 96.5%. The RO unit employed by Lewis et al. (1990) was a spiral-wound polyamide thin-film composite. The unit design was a 3:2:1 array using fiberglass pressure vessels. The feed piping was polished stainless steel; the product piping, PVDF. Clearly, in the cited work, the use of RO for point-of-use filtration achieved its objectives in lowering the TOC content and the particle counts in the product water.

Quinn (1989) believed that a computer-designed RO/ion-exchange program could lead to the rapid optimization of the RO/ion-exchange system, including the selection of the RO membrane from among the types available. If the feedwater contains high levels of foulants, a spiral-wound configuration would be selected. Where high pressure and rejection membranes (more costly) are used, ion-exchange capital and operating costs are minimized by the use of a simple mixed-bed deionizer. In effect, the RO serves a polishing function.

In the power industry, the more usual arrangement is for the RO unit to precede the ion exchange. The focus is on colloid removal. Reverse osmosis membranes accomplish this, albeit at the expense of becoming fouled in consequence. If the DI resins were first in line, it is feared that the colloids, usually constituted of organics, silica, and inorganics, exhibiting only low conductivities overall, would not be captured by the ion exchange. They would penetrate the DI beds, eventually to become destabilized (possibly by the subsequent RO action itself), with the result that their ionic and inorganic components would then be liberated. If, on the other hand, the RO treatment came first, even if it resulted in colloidal destabilization and ionic release, harm would be prevented by the subsequent ion-exchange action. Moreover, RO is more tolerant to organics than is ion exchange. In all applications, the primary motivation in preceding the ion exchange with RO is to minimize the frequency of the DI resin regeneration, with attendant reduction in regeneration chemical consumption.

The RO process tends to destabilize colloids because the increasing salt content of the reject stream serves to decrease the thickness of the double layer stabilizing the colloidal particles. However, the ultimate salt concentration reached is determined by the percentage of the water rejected, and the rate of makeup water fed to the system. These can be regulated. Sodium ion softening by ion exchange serves to increase the electrical charge on the colloid and to increase its double layer by removal of its di- and trivalent cations, thus effecting such stabilization.

In pharmaceutical contexts, the choice of RO to substitute for twin-bed deionizers finds at least partial justification in the resulting freedom from the bother, risks, and costs of regenerating the DI resin beds. It is a continuation of this logic to utilize the mixed DI beds after the RO operation in order, by sparing the DI resins, to minimize the need for their regenerations.

The placement of the RO before the ion exchange helps to protect the resin beds from needless accumulations such as particles, organisms, and organic matter. McAfee and McCormack (1988) stated that the placement of an RO before ion-exchange beds increased the service life of the latter twentyfold, and paid back the investment in the RO within 4 years. If the DI beds require sanitizations that are not otherwise performed, however, they may have to undergo regeneration for that purpose, their unconsumed capacity notwithstanding. In that case, the savings in regeneration chemicals cannot be realized. A large majority of RO and DI combinations utilize the RO in front of the DI bed, perhaps mostly to spare the ion-exchange unit. About 20% of deionization systems rely upon two-pass RO.

An Example of RO Preceding DI

It has been reported (Sullivan, 1982) that Eli Lilly Co. in Indianapolis used reverse osmosis to remove a "relatively high concentration of organic substances" from Indianapolis metropolitan water, derived principally from surface sources. The water thus treated removed 90% of the dissolved solids as well as the organic matter. As a consequence, the deionizers that followed the RO treatment were spared heavy ionic loadings as well as organic fouling (of the cation-exchange resins.)

Initially, chlorine removal, zeolite softening, and prefiltration were used to protect polyamide RO units. The prefiltration consisted of polyelectrolyte coagulation plus mixed-media pressure filters (not otherwise defined). Eventually, better results in terms of RO unit life were secured using cellulose triacetate RO membranes. This permitted the use of chlorination to reduce the bacterial content of the system. Carbon beds to remove the original municipal chlorination served to render these beds as breeding grounds for bacteria. However, chlorine removal by sodium bisulfite caused little improvement. It was found that the PVC piping being used seemed to encourage organism growth. Another action taken was the substitution of stainless steel piping for the PVC, a move that reduced the bacterial growth. To reduce the stored water to a bacterial content of less than 1,000 organisms per 100 mL necessitated heating the water to 120 °F (40 °C).

Some unusual findings resulted from the Lilly study. For instance, the RO units removed pyrogens but were ineffectual at bacterial removal. The mixed-bed deionizers were not "bacterial breeders." Regenerated frequently, they reduced both the bacteria and pyrogen levels. The deionized water thus prepared usually had close to zero organism counts per milliliter, had no detectable pyrogens, and had a resistivity consistently in excess of 10 MΩ.

Placement of the reverse osmosis unit before the DI bed is intended to spare the ion-exchanger and to decrease the frequency of its regeneration. The disadvantage is the common finding that organisms grow in the resin beds and populate the effluent waters. Therefore, the arrangement of RO before DI is less popular in pharmaceutical water settings.

Another example in the making of Purified Water utilizing this purification mode is given by Boireau (1993). A municipally treated feedwater was tempered to 25 °C. It was subjected to multimedia filtration before being pumped from its storage tank through an activated carbon bed for the removal of TOC. The water was then led through a 20-μm cartridge filter into a UV unit, to be succeeded by a cation-exchange softening treatment. It was next filtered through a 5-μm cartridge filter preparatory to its undergoing RO action. The RO permeate was flowed through another UV unit before entering a mixed-bed deionizer. The emerging water was again led through a UV treatment, finally to be filtered through a 0.2-μm-rated microporous membrane.

The prepared Purified Water was stored in a 7,000-gal tank of 316-L electropolished stainless steel fitted with a 0.2-μm-rated vent filter. The distribution piping was of electropolished, orbital-welded 316-L stainless. The water temperature was maintained at 25-30 °C by an in-line heat exchanger. Water recirculation was continuous within the loop, which contained a UV unit after the pump. Thirty-four points of use, sanitized weekly by 1-hour flushes of hot water (80 to 90 °C) are used to distribute the Purified Water for cell culture needs, for buffer and media preparation, and for equipment washing.

The Purified Water produced by the system was expected to have a 99% pass-rate at a bioburden level of no more than 100 cfu/100 mL; a pass-rate greater than 99.9% for the bacterial endotoxin standard of no more than 10 EU/mL; and a pass-rate of 100% for the USP chemistry. These standards, it should be noted, are tighter than those usually required for USP Purified Water.

RO and Organics

Clearly, when reverse osmosis is used to remove organics from waters, the retained material will, in its accumulation, serve as a foulant and will eventually have to be removed to restore the effective filtration area to the RO process.

Generally speaking, RO membranes do not reject organic molecules having molecular weights lower than 200 for CA and 100 for PA. In fact, they preferentially pass phenol, alcohols, and acetic and formic acids. However, suitably larger organic molecules are restrained from passage by RO membranes.

Particularly in semiconductor operations, it is not enough to produce water with a resistivity of 18 megohm-cm. The water must also be free of colloids and of TOC. It is understood that waters may be of 18-megohm-cm resistivity but may nevertheless contain TOC. Reverse osmosis membrane processes are often utilized for the TOC removal.

Tables 9-3 to 9-5 from McGarvey and Tamaki (1989) present the compositions of three different waters. The first (A) was characterized by a high solids content (TDS), the second (B) had a high organic content, and the third (C) had a high degree of hardness. The first water was similar to a well water in an arid region, with a TDS of 450 ppm. It was high in chlorides but low in silica and in organics. The second, having a low TDS, 50 ppm, but being high in organics, was characteristic of the surface waters encountered in northern Europe and Canada, and in parts of the United States. The third water, high in silica and in hardness,

Table 9-3
Deionization of High-Solids Water A

Components	*Two-Bed DI*	*RO* Plus Two-Bed DI*
Total cations, ppm as $CaCO_3$	450	18
% Sodium	67	83
% Magnesium	11	6
% Calcium	22	11
% Silica	2.2	6
% Chlorides	56	51
% Sulfates	22	14
% Alkalinity	22	29**
Total anions, ppm as $CaCO_3$	460	34.5

*It is assumed that the RO membrane has a rejection rate of 98% for divalent and 95% for monovalent cation (except for silica, 80% rejected; and carbon dioxide, 90% rejected).
**Assumes that alkalinity is largely free carbon dioxide from the neutralization to avoid precipitation in the concentrate.
McGarvey and Tamaki, (1989); Courtesy, *Ultrapure Water* journal

represented waters found in the southern United States, where silica can reach 100 ppm.

All three of these waters could easily be purified to a resistivity of 18 megohm-cm. To accomplish this, Water A would ordinarily be subjected to a two-bed demineralization followed by a mixed-bed polishing. The absence of significant hardness, silica, and organics would require very little pretreatment.

Both Waters B and C would ordinarily be treated with some type of coagulation and would be subjected to a carbon treatment to effect TOC removal (reduction) before being demineralized. The use of RO to achieve the removal of the higher-molecular-weight organics would be proper. In conjunction with ion exchange, it would yield water with a resistivity of 18 megohm-cm and less than 50 ppb of organics (once the resins were conditioned [i.e., rinsed free of their TOC content]) (McGarvey and Tamaki, 1989). Because of the high organic content of Water B, it would be advantageous to position the RO in advance of the ion-exchange beds, to protect the DI from fouling, it being easier to clean the RO membrane surfaces. In addition, control of the suspended solids of Water B would call for its pretreatment, as by coagulation and/or prefiltration. Polishing of the product water by a mixed-bed treatment would be required despite the low TDS.

The RO treatment of Water C prior to two-bed demineralization would serve to reduce both the TDS and silica content before exposure to the ion-exchange actions. Even ultrafiltration can be of help to the ion-exchange operation because, although it will not remove ions, it will restrain colloids, and will trap organic matter in excess of 750 daltons in size (molecular weight), thus sparing the DI beds.

When RO fouling is excessive, as when cleaning of the membrane requires

Table 9-4
Deionization of High-Organic Water B

Components	*Two-Bed DI*	*RO* Plus Two-Bed DI*
Total cations, ppm as $CaCO_3$	50	1.75
% Sodium	50	71
% Magnesium	30	18
% Calcium	20	11
% Silica	10	22
% Chlorides	36	34
% Sulfates	36	22
% Alkalinity	18	22**
Total anions, ppm as $CaCO_3$	55	4.5

*It is assumed that the RO membrane has a rejection rate of 98% for divalent and 95% for monovalent cation (except for silica, 80% rejected; and carbon dioxide, 90% rejected).
**Assumes that alkalinity is largely free carbon dioxide from the neutralization to avoid precipitation in the concentrate.
McGarvey and Tamaki (1989); Courtesy, *Ultrapure Water* journal

being performed every 4 or 8 weeks. an organic scavenger ion-exchange resin should be employed as an RO pretreatment. This should reduce TOC by about 85%.

RO in General Pharmaceutical Use

Reverse osmosis is used to prepare WFI by some pharmaceutical processors, but increasingly for the manufacture of Purified Water. The pharmaceutical water systems are small; most are 10 to 15 gpm (37.5 to 56.78 Lpm) in capacity. A 300 gpm (1,135-Lpm) system, such as is used by a large-volume parenteral manufacturer, is big for a pharmaceutical RO system. Primarily RO is used in small compounding areas where low volume and low capacities are required, about or below 5 gpm or so. Cost considerations and the unavailability of small stills govern here. Convenience and logistics may also be a factor. Thus RO is used by the Army in the field to constitute drugs from dry powders. It is also used by medical device manufacturers, as in tubing rinse operations. Additionally, it finds utilization in total parenteral nutritional care in home contexts. Two-pass RO in product-staging mode is an approved procedure for preparing WFI. The predominant method is, however, by distillation.

The most common usage of RO in pharmaceutical settings consists of a chlorinated water feed led through depth filters, through a carbon bed, and through a PA reverse osmosis unit by way of water softener into a storage tank. This type of makeup system is sized for the gpd volume required, as produced over a 16- to 18-hour period.

As for all other water systems, the feedwater analysis is the basis for the system design. The pretreatment portion in particular is built in response to the feedwater analysis. Thus, the multimedia beds are designed to remove particles

Table 9-5
Deionization of High-Hardness Water C

Components	*Two-Bed DI*	*RO* Plus Two-Bed DI*
Total cations, ppm as $CaCO_3$	330	9.6
% Sodium	30	52
% Magnesium	25	17
% Calcium	45	31
% Silica	11	20
% Chlorides	22	29
% Sulfates	27	13
% Alkalinity	40	38**
Total anions, ppm as $CaCO_3$	370	39.5

*It is assumed that the RO membrane has a rejection rate of 98% for divalent and 95% for monovalent cation (except for silica, 80% rejected; and carbon dioxide, 90% rejected).
**Assumes that alkalinity is largely free carbon dioxide from the neutralization to avoid precipitation in the concentrate.
McGarvey and Tamaki (1989); Courtesy, *Ultrapure Water* journal

down to 10 um in size. The softeners are designed to permit higher recoveries to be made by the RO units. Recoveries are usually at the 75 to 85% level. Greater recoveries can introduce problems by increasing the salt concentrations in the reject streams to the point where precipitation and scaling commences. Typically, strong anion-exchange resins are used in their sodium form in the water softeners to remove the scaling elements, although the dissolved solids level remains the same. Countercurrent regeneration of these resins reduces the use of regenerating salt and the frequency of backwashing. Cartridge filtration is relied upon to remove the resin fines. Carbon is relied upon for TOC removal. The RO feedwaters are kept at 77 °F (25 °C). The productivity in terms of the water volume produced is reduced at lower temperatures. During periods when the water is not being used, it is kept circulating through the carbon bed. Its temperature increase caused by the pump action is moderated by the use of a high temperature diversion, with cooler water replacing the heated water that is sent to drain (Comb, 1994).

The stored, RO-treated water is fed to a mixed-bed deionizer, then successively through a resin trap and ultraviolet light sterilizer, and finally through a 0.2-µm-rated sterilizing-grade microporous membrane filter, after which the water is recirculated to the storage tank. The sterilizing filter should have a long service life, the RO unit having removed colloids.

The pump used to distribute and recirculate the water is sized to do so at linear velocities of greater than 5 ft/sec (5 to 10 ft/sec) in order to discourage biofilm development by organisms on surfaces encountering the water. The mixed-bed deionizers are usually regenerated by off-site services, in keeping with the logic attending the choice of RO in the first place, namely, a desire to avoid the chemical handling and the labor of DI bed regenerations. The carbon bed should be backwashed daily and should be sanitized on a scheduled basis, as indicated by need.

Test ports should be present before and after each major piece of purification equipment, to enable appraisal of its operational status. A test port should definitely be installed beyond the last point of use, at the furthest reach of the pipe system, to enable weekly (if not daily) analyses to be made of the water's SDI, TOC, TDS, and (especially) microbial contents. In pharmaceutical usage, system sanitization, which can easily consume an entire day, should be performed weekly. The proper schedule for sanitizations should be established on a historical basis of need.

To obtain the low organism counts expected of such water purification systems, the successive purification units in the overall train should have a cascading effect. The overall effect mirrors the purity of the starting water quality as it influences and is modified by a carbon bed or a water softener. The brine could create TNTC (too numerous to count) organism growth for the water softener. The same could be the case for the carbon bed. There is not one right number for a given component. The water leaving the carbon bed, in essence the prefilter to the RO, probably has the highest organism count in the system: typically about 10^2 colony-forming units per milliliter. Exiting the two-bed deionizer, if such were next present, the count could be 10^1 cfu/mL; and the same count after a mixed bed. Emerging from the RO unit, the water could have a count of 10 cfu/100 mL; and after the ultraviolet unit it could be reduced to 1 cfu/100 mL. The point being made is that the organism removal efficiencies of RO units, of UV light installations, and even of sterilizing filters, are not absolutes. The cleaner the water going into the unit, the cleaner the water coming out. A superior operation therefore involves the optimization of each and every component in the purification train.

The RO unit is perhaps best run in a recirculation mode to minimize bacterial endotoxin and organism levels. Otherwise, the inoperative RO unit should be stored containing sanitizer.

Imperfections in RO Membranes

At least from a theoretical point of view, the structure of RO membranes precludes the passage of organisms or pyrogens. Yet from time to time, even careful RO operations do result in downstream contamination by organisms. How to reconcile the theoretical with the actual? Rationalization is made that the membranes are not to be impugned, but that the O-ring boundaries and mechanical brine seals separating the feedwaters from the permeate may be less than perfect, so that occasional cross-contamination may result.

As Zoccolante (1995) sees it, most spiral wound reverse osmosis membranes incorporate a brine seal at the leading end of the reverse osmosis element. This seal is designed to expand between the membrane and the pressure vessel which contains the RO membrane. The purpose of the seal is to prevent passage of water between the membrane and the pressure vessel and to divert the flow of water across the RO membrane surface. The brine seal can cause bacterial problems since a stagnant water condition is inherently created by the presence of the seal. Some membranes are produced today without a brine seal on the leading end. These membranes are commonly referred to as loose wrap or full fit and are configured in several different ways with the same goal of allowing modest controlled flow between the reverse osmosis membrane and the pressure vessel. This type of membrane is superior for use in pharmaceutical reverse osmosis units as bacterial contamination is minimized. This type of membrane also allows the sanitizing solution to reach the outer surface of the membrane near the pressure vessel which is also difficult to accomplish with conventional brine seal RO elements.

However, it is known that even with regard to the salt rejection for which they were originally intended, RO membranes are "leaky." Carter (1976) stated that solutes pass through RO membranes because of the solubility/diffusion phenomenon, whereby salts dissolve in the membrane at high pressure and diffuse through to reappear on the low-pressure side. He also hypothesized concerning the presence of large pores and/or "pinholes."

Those familiar with the problems of manufacturing large expanses of membranes will hardly reject as unlikely the occasional occurrence of flaws, or be surprised by their inability to be detected on the statistical basis of a practical number of quality control samples. In any case, at least at present, RO devices are manufactured to standards significant to desalination operations rather than to Water for Injection production. The two applications are hardly identical. Desalination can tolerate some degree of membrane imperfection. The bulk flow of salt will not be of significance, given the total volume of salt-free water flow. In the WFI situation, however, the passage of some few organisms through a membrane imperfection can have an impact of real significance.

Whatever the likelihood of flawed membranes, there is also reason to believe that organisms invade RO systems from downstream directions in response to chemotactic stimuli (Husted, 1993).

It seems fair to say that the possibilities of having flawed membranes or broken fibers in devices make RO an uncertain method of achieving sterility. This is the view of the FDA, based on the extensive observations made by their inspectors in their examination of pharmaceutical industry practices. Therefore, the FDA advises that WFI system validation is far more likely to be achieved using dual-pass, product-staged RO units. Manufacturers are free to attempt WFI production by the use of single-stage RO. In the FDA experience, such efforts are far more difficult to validate. Therefore, the FDA will examine such data very critically. (Repetitive filtrations in critical operations such as filtrative sterilizations have long enjoyed serious endorsements.)

Organisms Downstream of RO

Bacterial growth downstream of RO membranes poses problems. Heat sanitizations may be precluded, necessitating organism control by chemicals. Zoccolante (1993) held that a mixture of peracetic acid and hydrogen peroxide is best for this purpose, particularly where thin-film polyamide membranes are involved. In this regard, cellulose triacetate membranes have the advantage of passing dissolved bactericidal chlorine.

Two-Pass Product-Staged Design

The FDA requires that Water for Injection being prepared by the use of reverse osmosis be the result of two-pass product-staged units. The product water effluent from the first stage is used as the feed stream for the second stage. In such arrangements there is almost never a need to clean the second stage. (See Table 9-6). Therefore, it can be smaller. If it is of the same size it can, when necessary, be used independently as a single stage. In two-pass product-staged systems the first stage recovery is usually set at 75%; the second stage at 90%. A two-pass RO system will yield water that will pass the USP chlorides limits test even on a high chloride content water. The water that is effluent may exceed 1 megohm-cm in resistivity.

Double-Pass Pumping; Product Staged

(The term *double-pass* as used here is synonymous with two-pass, and with product-staged RO.)

The double-pass RO system can be arranged in different ways. A single outsized pump can be used ahead of the system, large enough to drive the water through both RO units. This generally would require 400 to 500 psig of pressure even for low-pressure membranes. Polyamide types and cellulose acetate ROs would require higher pressures. A second way would be to use a smaller and hence less costly pump to move the water through the first RO. The product water would then be repressurized using a second, interstage pump to pass it through the second RO stage.

An outsized pump, although more expensive than a smaller one, need not be markedly so. A single pump, say of 400-gpm capacity, is less expensive than two 200-gpm pumps. The size of a single pump may be limited, however, by the ability of the first RO stage to withstand its pressure. To reduce the size of the single pump to conform to the first-stage pressure rating may require the use of heated water. The energy costs of heating water are more expensive than pumping costs. If necessary, two pumps are bought at a higher capital outlay, and cold water is used. Depending upon the quantity of water being processed, the cost for the extra pump may easily be recovered by the savings in heating energy.

The energy required to run a single pump is about the same as for the total of two pumps, one for each stage. This is so because the energy required is defined by the number of membrane elements being serviced. There are disadvantages to a single pump. Exerting high back pressure in the first RO permeate requires the high-pressure strength of stainless steel piping. This is costly. The use of two

Table 9-6
Reverse Osmosis Rejection*

	Single stage RO	*Double stage RO*
Dissolved inorganics	90-98	>99
Dissolved organics	>99	>99.99
Pyrogens	>99	>99.99
Bacteria	>99	>99.99

* Rejection is the percent of a contaminant group removed from the feed stream.

pumps permits the independent operation of each unit. This is useful where sampling ports and clean-in-place connections are used to permit independent RO unit upkeep. More important, independent RO unit operations (two pumps) do not necessitate a continuous operation. The first unit may be shut down while the dynamic operation of the second stage is maintained. This saves on water to the drain. The use of two separate RO units in series offers the greater versatility of two independent units.

Where small RO units are involved, say of 4-gpm productivity, a single feed pump would be cheaper. However, the water would require being heated to 24 to 27 °C (75 to 80 °F) to minimize the pressure requirements to practical limits. If the quantity of water being prepared is about 40 gpm, the use of an interstage pump allows a greater leeway of water temperatures and pump pressures. For example, the feedwater temperature could be 10 to 13 °C (50 to 55 °F), and the pressure required could range from 250 to 320 psig. The quality of the product waters produced would be the same either way, as long as the driving pressure is sufficient.

One of the costs of an RO operation is the discard of the reject stream. The amount of water discarded in double-pass RO operations is almost the same as in single-pass; however, the overall recovery is about the same. The second RO unit utilizes RO product water. Almost every potential for scaling and fouling has been eliminated. The second RO stage can thus be operated at significantly higher fluxs and recoveries. The second-stage wastewater exceeds the quality of the original feedwater. For example, if the original feedwater had a TDS of 200 ppm, the wastewater from the second stage could be about 30 ppm. The reject stream from the second stage is therefore sent back to the first-stage RO. A single-stage recovery would run at about 75%, a double stage at about 73% overall, the second stage operating at about 90%. A two-pass RO system will yield water that will pass the USP chlorides limits test even on a high chloride content water. The water that is effluent may exceed 1 megohm-cm in resistivity.

Various Two-Pass Systems

A more general treatment of dual-pass operations was presented by Comb and Schneekloth (1989) in a study based upon combinations of cellulose acetate and polyamide RO units, namely two PA units, two CA units, and an arrangement consisting of CA followed by PA. Also considered were the advantages of using one pump overall; or two pumps, one for each stage.

The arrangements involving paired polyamide RO devices reflected the advantages resulting from the higher rejections exhibited by the RO polymer. The limitations of PA/PA couples derived from polyamide's susceptibility to decomposition by chlorine. Removal of chlorine from the water by activated carbon exposed the membranes to the accumulation of bacteria sloughed from the carbon beds. Moreover, the water being bereft of biocidal chlorine, the final permeate product could become microbiologically contaminated from organisms downstream of the second RO. The alternative removal of chlorine by bisulfite, and the pyrogenic consequences of bacterial contamination has already been discussed. (See page 376.)

The advantage of a two-pass CA/CA arrangement was that the cellulose acetate polymer was relatively resistant to chlorine. Moreover, it passed chlorine, to provide a biocidal content to the permeate product. However, for this system optimally to resist microbiological recontamination, some level of continuous bacteriostatic feed was recommended, and it was imperative that at least the second-stage RO be operated continuously.

A static system, whether RO unit, carbon bed, or ion-exchange bed, encourages organism growth. Dynamic, continuously flowing systems minimize such organism proliferations. Because of its greater control of organisms because of its permeation by chlorine, a CA/CA two-pass RO system is generally preferred in pharmaceutical contexts.

Comb and Schneekloth (1990) demonstrated that the use of a CA/PA dual-pass RO pair provided the level of silica rejection that is the concern of the electronics industry. Cellulosic RO, operating on chlorinated waters, kept biological recontamination under control both up and downstream. The purer downstream water kept the microbiological contamination of the second (polyamide) RO unit to a minimum despite the absence of chlorine. Chlorine was removed from the product water of the first stage before it entered the second RO unit. Bisulfite addition was relied upon to achieve this end; both the bisulfite ion and the sulfate ion (the oxidation product of chlorine removal) were well rejected by the polyamide second-pass RO.

Table 9-7 shows the comparative RO performances of the PA/PA, CA/CA, and CA/PA systems. In any case, the tolerance of cellulose acetate RO membrane to chlorine suggests its greater suitability for the preparation of pharmaceutical waters where organisms are of greatest concern. Overall, the application of a dual-pass CA/PA pair permits the second unit to manifest its rejection properties while operating in a microbiologically clean environment. Product water exiting a dual-pass RO system provides very clean water to

Table 9-7
Comparison of Different Water Supplies

City Water	*Irvine, Cal.*	*Boston, Mass.*	*Syracuse, N.Y.*	*Santa Barbara, Cal.*
System design	PA/PA	PA/PA	CA/CA*	CA/PA
Feedwater	806 µS	75 µS	95 µS	1,160 µS
Product water	0.5 µS	1.0 megohm-cm	7 µS	4.4 µS

*Low-pressure CA design
µS - microsiemens
Comb and Schneekloth (1989); Courtesy, *Ultrapure Water* journal

subsequent mixed-bed polishers, proportionately reducing their loads. The Comb and Schneekloth teaching was elaborated upon by Comb and Fulford (1991).

More recently, Weitnauer and Comb (1995) investigated the subject of recoveries from two-pass RO systems, both passes of PA, relative to the rejection rates resulting from such recoveries. They concluded that a system designed to recover 75% in the first RO unit followed by only 70% in the second gives product waters having conductivities better able to meet the conductivity requirements of *USP 23* than do a 75% recovery for the second unit (Figures 9-8a, 9-8b). The lower recoveries in the second RO wasted very little product water as the reject stream is pure enough to mix with feedwater for the first unit. These investigators doubted, however, that the use of CA units in place of either of the two PA reverse osmosis arrangements could effect rejections sufficient to meet the USP 23 conductivity requirements.

Polyamide Two-Pass RO

The FDA insistence upon double-pass, product-staged RO for the production of WFI not based upon distillation is predicated upon the probability that single-pass RO systems will not yield microbial counts conducive to the low pyrogenicity levels required. It is a predilection independent of economic considerations. The use of double-pass RO may be advanced upon economic grounds as well, however. It has been stated that the cost of equipment required for a double-pass RO system would be just about twice that for a single system.

The lower power requirements of the thin-film composite RO units, however, along with their higher permeation rates as occasioned by the thinness of the membrane discrimination layer, were stated by Pittner et al. (1986) to result in an overall savings over the use of a single-pass cellulose triacetate system. These investigators stated that a PA membrane can produce the same flow of treated water as a CA membrane at approximately half the applied differential pressure. Alternatively, operating at the same feedwater pressure, the cost of operating a PA double-pass RO system that yields greatly reduced ionic contents will be about the same as for a single-pass CA arrangement. In economic terms, Pittner et al. (1986) characterized the advantages of double-pass PA RO systems by stating that "twice as much separation can be obtained at the same energy cost."

In this mode of operation, two-pass RO does more than fulfill its customary role of reducing the ion load (typically by 90% to 95%), preparatory to the water's being polished by a succeeding ion-exchange treatment. In the more usual role, RO may not remove as high a proportion of the dissolved solids as a two-bed ion-exchange unit. In the double-pass arrangement, the water may become demineralized enough not to require ion-exchange polishing. Pittner et al. (1986) found that the water exiting a two-pass PA RO unit was generally in the resistivity range of 3 to 4 megohm-cm. Mixed-bed ion-exchange polishing

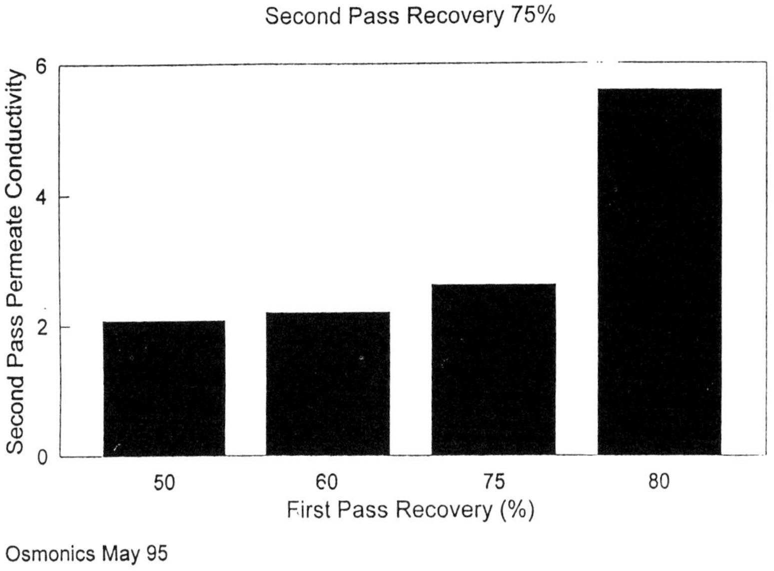

Figure 9-8a. Second-pass conductivity versus first-pass recovery.

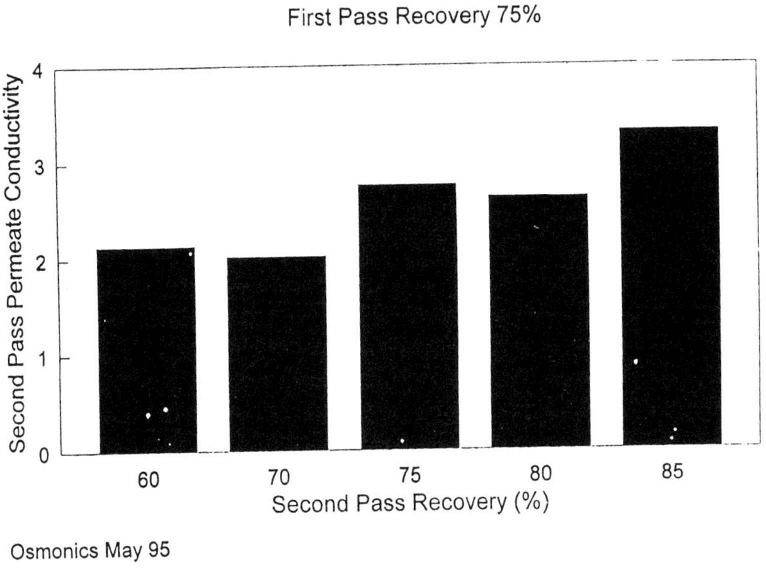

Figure 9-8b . Second-pass conductivity versus second-pass recovery.
Weitnauer and Comb (1995); Courtesy, *Medical Techsources*

improved this water to 18-megohm-cm resistivity. A similar ion-exchange polishing on a single-pass RO produced water of 10- to 15-megohm-cm resistivity. Based upon these data, thin-film double-pass RO offers a standalone makeup water system in the resistivity range of 3 to 4 megohm-cm, and capable of being polished by ion-exchange to the 18-megohm-cm resistivity required in semiconductor usage. The two-pass RO serves essentially to replace the RO and ion-exchange treatment that more usually precede mixed-bed polishing.

In the system advocated by Pittner et al., (1986), the feedwater was raised to a pressure of 400 to 500 psig, sufficient to drive the water through both RO units in series. To motivate the product water through the second of the two RO units, the discharge pressure from the first RO device had to be at 200 to 250 psig. Permeate backflow at this pressure would have destroyed the integrity of the upstream RO. This was guarded against by use of a spring-loaded check valve and a bleed valve between the two RO arrays. Municipal water was softened by a sodium-form ion exchange operating at 12 gpm at 13 °C (55 °F). The water was dechlorinated chemically and the pH was adjusted to 8.0 to 10.0.

Under 400 psig supplied by a 15-horsepower multistage pump, the water was fed into the first polyamide RO unit. The concentrate flow at 230 psig was 12 gpm. The permeate then entered the second RO array, from which concentrate issued at 4 gpm. The permeate, its resistivity at about 1 megohm-cm, was stored. Prior to use it was treated in a mixed ion-exchange facility. The deionized water was passed through a UV light unit, and finally through a 0.2-μm-rated membrane filter.

Interestingly, the ionic removal by each RO unit is not the same, largely because of a pH effect resulting from the first RO unit's rejecting some ions better than others. To bring the ion rejection of the second pass up to the level of the first requires pH adjustment. The water becomes more acidic as it passes through through the RO because the membrane fails to remove ever-present carbon dioxide. This pH adjustment between the two passes greatly increases the resistivity of the product water. (Another approach is to put storage, either atmospheric or pressurized, in between the units to accommodate variable flows.)

Silica removal. Ammerer and Dahmen (1990) reported on a double-pass RO system utilizing two spiral-wound PA/PA membranes addressed primarily to the removal of a high silica content. Previously, a single-pass RO system had been used. In both cases, mixed-bed polishing post-RO served further to treat the effluent waters. The results (see Table 9-8) clearly showed the advantages of two-pass RO over the single pass. Moreover, the two-pass system was utilized to eliminate the previously included water-softening pretreatment.

Reverse osmosis can usefully be employed in silica removal for total rejection of suspended and colloidal forms, and for partial rejection of the soluble type, with 60% to 90+% of soluble silica being rejected. Various RO membrane compositions reject silica differently. According to FilmTec (1988), "After 10 days in field operating conditions ranging from 200 to 500 psig at ambient temperatures, single-pass silica rejection varies for different types of RO membranes, averaging 84% for cellulose acetate blend membranes, 89% for cellulose triacetate membranes, and 98.2% for advanced thin-film composite membranes using polyamide compounds in the membrane surface construction."

Subsequent ion-exchange treatment, twin beds followed by mixed bed, or mixed bed alone, serves further to reduce the silica levels. However, the complexities of silica chemistry are such that mixed-bed demineralizations are reported to produce low-molecular-weight silica compounds not amenable to further removal by ion exchange. Also, the formation of silica oligomers, 20 to 30 angstroms in size, have been described. Their removal by the use of strongly basic anion exchange (desilicization) prior to the mixed-bed encounters has been recommended (Hoffman, 1985). Nonionic dissolved silica, if there is any, is imperfectly rejected by RO. (See pages 296 and 399.)

As Ammerer and Dahmen (1990) described, the pretreatment consisted of dual multimedia filters, chemical addition, degasification, and cartridge filtration. Softeners were not used. Thus the bicarbonate present in the water had to be reduced to avoid scaling of the RO membranes. Through the chemical injection of acid, the majority of the bicarbonate was converted into carbon dioxide. Antiscalant polymer addition controlled the scaling tendencies of trace heavy metals and any remaining bicarbonate. This combined effect minimized scaling problems with the RO membrane. The forced-draft degasifier was positioned ahead of the double-pass RO to remove the vast majority of the carbon dioxide formed by the earlier feedwater reaction of acid and bicarbonate. Following decarbonation, the repressurization and filtration took place; and the trace carbon dioxide remaining from feedwater degasification passed through the first-pass membrane of the double-pass RO. The pH to the second stage was

Table 9-8
Silica Profiles (ppm)

Sample Point	*Single-Pass RO*	*Double-Pass RO*
Incoming feedwater	25.8	28.7
Pre-RO	27.9	29.2
Interstage RO	—	3.2
Post-RO	7.7	0.147
Pre mixed bed	1.77	0.147
Post mixed bed	0.009	0.005
Distribution loop inlet	0.010	0.007

Ammerer and Dahmen (1990); Courtesy, *Ultrapure Water* journal adjusted using caustic injection, converting the trace carbon dioxide to sodium bicarbonate, which was rejected by the spiral-wound PA membrane. The concentrate flow from the second pass was directed back and combined with the feed to the first stage of the RO system. The pH adjustment to second-stage RO membrane further enhanced the excellent rejection characteristics for both silica and organic compounds.

> Particulates and TOC introduced during forced-draft degasification are no longer present in the water processed through the double-pass RO unit, and final product water resistivity is greatly improved over conventional single-pass RO results. Mixed-bed polishers are positioned downstream from the double-pass RO to further reduce silica levels, prior to DI water storage and distribution to the fab. (Ammerer and Dahmen, 1990)

Interestingly, the use of two polyamide membrane units on the double-pass RO system would have permitted the removal of bicarbonate at pH 8 to 8.5 (Kraft, 1986). However, softening to prevent calcium carbonate formation would be necessary. The need for the initial acidification for the degasifier, and for the subsequent pH adjustment between the RO stages would have been obviated. Ammerer and Dahmen (1990) claimed, however, that the pH adjustments used in conjunction with their double-pass RO usage yielded not only the better silica and TOC removals reported, but produced as well an overall superior total ionic content reduction than would result from the double-pass operation at an all-alkaline pH. Be that as it may, pH adjustment between the two stages of dual-pass ROs is an operating arrangement covered by patent (Pittner, 1986). Even better bicarbonate rejection would result from raising the pH after the decarbonator and before the first RO unit (Cartwright, 1991).

A cautionary note should be sounded relative to the use of dual RO units of different polymeric compositions, such as CA/PA. The removal of foulants from RO membranes is often accomplished using cleansers of different pH, and dependent at times upon their oxidative actions. In such instances, what may suit cellulose acetate RO may be incompatible with polyamide structures. For example, PA is stable over a broad pH spectrum, CA is not; PA cannot withstand active chlorine compounds, CA can. Therefore, each RO unit must be cleaned individually, and the solution exiting one must be kept from entering the other. An egress to drain between the two RO units is required.

According to Benedek and Johnston (1988), the quality of water produced by a two-bed DI system from a 300-ppm TDS feedwater is approximately 2 to 4 ppm of TDS. These investigators believed that, using the same feedwater, single-pass RO would yield a permeate of 8 to 9 ppm of TDS, and two-pass product-staged RO would give 0.3 to 0.5 ppm of TDS. In addition, the RO system would reduce (and possibly remove) bacteria, particles, and organic matter. If thin-film polyamide RO accomplishes 98% rejections, 300 ppm of TDS should yield 6 ppm. However, using the figure of 9 ppm, it can be seen that single-pass RO would suffice where the application need not have waters of less than 9 ppm of TDS.

For semiconductor applications where water quality is the determinant, two system choices are possible: either single-pass RO followed by primary and secondary mixed-bed polishing, or double-pass RO with service-exchanged mixed-bed polishing. The higher costs of the two-pass RO system may be offset by the benefits derived from its better quality water, namely, higher product yields. Benedek and Johnston (1988) also believed that either single-pass RO or twin-bed ion exchange is adequate to provide the feedwater for the distillation operations usually relied upon in pharmaceutical contexts for high-purity water preparation. Although the stills generally perform better on lower-TDS waters, and although ion-exchange treatment gives lower TDS values than does single-pass RO, these investigators favored the single-pass RO as being more economical while furnishing a water quality adequate for distillation needs.

Effect of Dual-Pass RO on DI Usage

Growing usage of dual-pass RO will cause the use of two-bed ion exchange to dwindle. Twin beds are needed most of the time when single-pass RO is used, but they may be dispensed with where double-pass RO is employed. The twin-bed arrangement is environmentally inefficient, using 3 to 4 times its amount in the chemicals employed for their regeneration. The mixed beds will always be needed where single-pass RO is used. They supply a polishing function. Single-pass RO is therefore coupled with mixed DI beds. Double-pass RO could obviate some mixed-bed applications. Mixed beds cost more, and are more difficult to operate. However, they confer high quality to the water. A single-train twin-bed deionizer is the cheapest installation. However, a dependable 24-hour operation makes necessary a standby unit. Where high-resistivity waters are desired, as in the semiconductor field, a choice exists between a twin-bed DI resin unit followed by a mixed bed, and an RO unit followed by a mixed bed. The choice ineluctably leads to pretreatment considerations, to the user's views regarding regeneration in place or off-site (service contract), and to the use of cold DI resin regeneration (if on-site) or to heating the water to 25 °C (77 °F) to optimize the RO operation.

Double-pass product-staged waters should exhibit resistivities from 750,000 to 1 or 2 megohm-cm. A two-bed ion-exchange system should provide water with about 100,000- to 500,000-ohm-cm resistivity. Conductivity is the reciprocal of resistivity. Thus 20,000-ohm-cm resistivity water has a conductivity of 50 microsiemens, μS. Interestingly, 1 ppm of total dissolved solids, depending upon the specific salts present, has a conductivity of about 2 micromhos or microsiemens.

According to Yabe et al. (1989), a one-stage RO, useful in reducing the ionic content of a water to 5% to 10% of its original value, can be product-staged to yield water with resistivities of 1 to 3 megohm-cm on a continuous basis. This is so because the second stage, in its 99% to 95% reduction of ions, renders negligible the product quality variations forthcoming from the first stage.

The resulting product waters usually have a resistivity of several megohm-cm. For 18-megohm-cm resistivity, ion-exchange treatment is required. The product-staged double-pass RO water is suitable for USP Purified Water, and for bioengineering applications.

Gagnon et al. (1991) stated that RO with polishing mixed-bed deionization is most cost-effective when the feedwater TDS levels are 300 ppm or greater; between 150 and 300 ppm, either RO or two-bed ion-exchange may gainfully be employed; below 150 ppm of TDS, two-bed ion-exchange followed by a polishing mixed bed is most appropriate. The usefulness of this advice depends, however, upon the intended water application. In semiconductor applications, the water will most likely be treated by RO in any case because of a concern with particles and with TOC. Data from Whipple (1987) at Dow suggested that 75 ppm of TDS, not 300 ppm, constituted the crossover point between RO and ion exchange. Data from Dow suggested that RO preceding DI is always more cost-effective for less than 150 ppm of TDS.

Ultrafilters

The formation of RO membranes from their casting solutions was previously described. It was stated that the ultimate bulk density of a polymer is not necessarily realized. Variations of this density, reflective of the interstitial spaces or "pores" in the membrane, can be shaded to give a more open porosity. To quote from Chapter 5, page 198:

> By the preparative manipulations of the polymer casting formulas it is thus possible to manufacture a spectrum of 'solid' polymeric membranes characterized by differing intersegmental space dimensions. It is these more open film forms that are used in the practices of ultrafiltration. These differences in spacings translate to "cutoff" values, usually defined in terms of the ability of the ultrafilter to retain protein molecules of different sizes as related to molecular weights. The shape of the protein molecules also exerts its influence.
>
> The implication of the cutoff ratings of the ultrafilters is that they retain larger molecules while permitting the passage of smaller ones. They would seem suitable, therefore, for the separation of different size of protein molecules.

Actually, neither the rating systems, usually described by the dalton unit rather than by molecular-weight cutoffs, nor the UF membrane interstitial spacings permit exact separations. The UF separations that are possible are of a magnitudinal difference. A ultrafilter can be utilized, perhaps, to separate a 20,000-molecular-weight protein from one of 50,000. It will probably not differentiate between proteins of 15,000 and 30,000 molecular weight. Also complicating the picture is the lack of uniform rating standards among UF membrane manufacturers.

Ultrafiltration membranes are prepared from a variety of polymers (among them polysulfone and PVDF) in a number of different modes. These filters offer a porosity between that of the microporous membranes and that of the reverse osmosis membranes. By far, UF hollow fibers dominate the market today. Yet UF is also available in spiral-wound formats and in flat-sheet forms, variants of early plate-and-frame configurations. The units typically utilize tangential flow patterns. The hollow-fiber configuration flows water from the inside out, the reverse of the RO configuration.* As a result, higher velocities with their greater turbulences are realized; therefore, the fibers clog less readily. However, recoveries made from these UF units may average about 95%, so that the high turbulent flows at the beginning of the fiber have decreased markedly by the end. Fouling depositions build at the trailing end of the unit. Reversing the flow periodically serves to clean out this debris. This is particularly useful in highly fouling waters. In such applications, hollow-fiber UF units can save the expense of nonrenewable microporous cartridge filters, because they are backwashable, a rare quality for membranes.

Ultrafilters are often applied in polishing operations, even after RO treatments, to make certain that colloids, organisms, endotoxin, and larger TOC entities are removed before the points of use. In such settings the impurity burdens are minimal. This permits dead-end filtration to be applied without unduly shortening the service life of the UF unit. The use of tangential flow in such cases would result, at 95% recovery, in a waste of 5% of processed water that already probably cost $10 to $20 per thousand gallons to purify. Thus in biotechnical applications the water purification train may include RO, ion exchange, and UF, but the UF may utilize dead-end filtration. In the dead-end filtration mode, the concentration valve is typically opened for short periods to periodically flush out the membrane device.

Sharpe (1985) discussed the successful application of ultrafilter units to the removal of colloidal silica and of colloidal humic and fulvic acids from the feedwaters of two power generating plants. He attempted to determine the more appropriate positioning for the ultrafiltration unit, whether pre- or post-demineralizer. Its placement before the demineralizer would (proportionate to how burdened the feedwater is with colloidal matter) occasion more frequent cleaning of the UF, but would better protect the demineralizer against fouling. Down-

* The DuPont Permasep hollow-fiber RO units intended for seawater desalination were fed from the inside out.

stream from the demineralizer, an ultrafilter would still perform its function of arresting the passage of colloidal particles, but would be spared frequent cleanings by the sacrificial interpositioning of the demineralizer unit, which would assume part of the colloidal load. Sharpe (1985) held that the post-demineralizer position is the better. It permits a high permeation rate for the UF with a reasonably cost-effective cleaning cycle productive of a long service life. His experience suggested a twofold penalty on flux, and a sevenfold penalty on chemical cleaning or pretreatment, versus post-DI applications.

A concern has been expressed that the lower water velocities imposed by UF filters may increase the incubation of organisms in a system (Henley, 1991). Be that as it may, some 13 Japanese power generating operations have utilized hollow-fiber UF in their condensate polishing, and 19 employed them for rad waste processing (D'Angelo, 1991).

Ultrafiltration application to raw waters could be an uncertain practice, given the TSS of the feedwater. The UF, being a tight filter, would be highly retentive, and its use could necessitate too frequent cleanings. Like RO, UF retains endotoxin, organisms, colloids, and larger organic entities. Use is made of ultrafiltration in the power industry to remove silica in its colloidal form (Sharpe, 1985). However, being more open than an RO, its flux is higher. It may require 25 psig of driving pressure, whereas RO may need 300 psig or so. Ultrafilters can thus be used advantageously for the above removal purposes.

The distinction between RO and UF is blurred. From the 0.1-μm rating of microporous membranes to the 10,000 daltons of ultrafilters, organics can be removed, but not ions. Below the 10,000-dalton ratings is the province of the RO membranes. They discriminate against organics, but only against the larger hydrated ions. The divalent ions, having higher charge densities, carry more extensive skirts of hydration and are, therefore, more easily excluded on the basis of size. Thus, the sulfate ion exists in the decahydrate form. Accordingly, it does not permeate even the nanofilters.

UF as Prefilters for RO and Stills

Suspended solids carried into the RO module by the feedwaters tend physically to obstruct the membrane. This occurrence should be avoided by pretreatments involving sedimentation and settling. Colloids should be removed by coagulation and settling, or by deep-bed filtration. The tangential mode of flow by which all RO modules operate serves well here to sweep away such suspended solid accumulations before they become excessively troublesome. In addition, the RO units are protected by prefilters. Usually, depth-type prefilters are used, although there is a tendency towards tighter filters that are more retentive of smaller particles. If the water flows were found to be penalized unduly thereby, more-open filters would be substituted. As in most filtrations, the filter rating choice is in the direction of accomplishing the required objective, namely, the restraint of particles. The rate of flow is usually the secondary consideration. It can be addressed by recourse to larger filter areas, if need be.

The pecuniary blandishments of string-wound depth-type filters for this application are considerable. They may also be insidious. The less expensive, more open depth-type filters are often secured by knife-edge seals. These seldom ensure against bypass by particles smaller than 1 μm or so. In one case where such depth filters were used, grow-through manifested itself after only 4 hours.

Although undefined, a correlation should exist among the SDI of a feedwater, the frequency of RO cleaning it would occasion, and the tightness of the prefilter required to minimize both.

Ultrafilters are currently being retrofitted in front of stills to remove bacterial endotoxins. Concerns have been expressed by the FDA regarding the hesitancy of some still manufacturers to guarantee more than 4 logs reduction of endotoxin. The possibility of sudden releases of bacterial endotoxins in large quantities from preceding ion-exchange beds are the concerns. Ultrafilters, usually of the 100,000 daltons character, are used to remove the bacterial endotoxins from the feedwater entering the stills. (See page 69 and 538). Ultrafilters give better apparent endotoxin removals than do RO units because their flows are greater at any given pressure.

Ultrafilters are also used as prefilters for RO units. These are expensive filters whose utilization requires justification. Placed upstream of RO, the ultrafilters, having dalton ratings of 100,000 or less, will remove the colloids, thus sparing the RO membranes. The ultrafilters are usually composed of polysulfone polymer. This polymer is relatively resistant to the cleansing and sanitizing agents needed periodically to remove accumulated colloidal and other fouling substances. They can withstand long exposures to 10% hydrogen peroxide or to 200 ppm of sodium hypochlorite. Zahka and Vakhshoori (1990) referenced a PVDF ultrafilter resistant to ozone. The service life of these prefilters is not unduly abbreviated by usage as prefilters to RO. The RO membranes' polymers are not so robust, enduring such cleaning not nearly so well as the polysulfone. The use of the chemically resistant polysulfone prefilters to remove colloids exempts the RO units from cleaning ordeals that they cannot well sustain. The relatively expensive ultrafilter may be justified in this application if it sufficiently prolongs the service life of the RO unit.

In one instance, a UF prefilter to a thin-film composite RO reduced the SDI_{15}* of a 50-gpm feedwater from 2 to 0.63. No other treatment was involved. A similar treatment for a 50-gpm feedwater of SDI_{15} of 5.95 reduced its value of SDI_{15} of 0.61. Two 100-gpm systems having SDI_{15} values of 620 and 1,010, respectively, were reduced correspondingly to SDI_{15} of 1.20 and 1.60. The SDI_{15} 1,010 water utilized a 10-μm filter upstream from the ultrafilter. The efficacy of

*It will be recalled that the SDI is a measure of the total suspended solids of a water. Hence, it is related to filter plugging tendencies. SDI_{15} is the SDI measured after a 15-minute flow interval. See pages 284 and 530.

ultrafiltration prefiltration for ROs was thus demonstrated.

A hollow-fiber ultrafiltration system of two parallel arrangements, each capable of providing 125 gpm of permeate, was used by Burns and Booth (1988) as prefilter for an RO unit at the Millstone nuclear facility. Typical conversion rates for the UF feedwater were 86%, while 20 gpm were rejected and 20 gpm were recycled. The UF system consisted of two parallel module racks of 100 hollow-fiber cartridges per rack. Each module rack consisted of two sets of upper and lower racks, containing 25 hollow-fiber cartridges each.

The skid-mounted RO unit in a 3:2:1 array was served by a multistage centrifugal pump. Each vessel contained six spiral-wound, 40-inch-long, 8-inch-diameter RO membranes composed of a cellulose acetate/cellulose triacetate blend. Recovery values were 66% to 70%, the net flow being 210 gpm. Operations of the UF/RO system were limited by a daily 2-hour period for cleaning of the ultrafilter.

The compositions of the feedwater and permeate water, as well as of the reject stream, are shown in Table 9-9. The permeate product water achieved 5–μS/cm conductivity, containing 8.5 TDS, down from 51.8 TDS. Use of the ultrafilter followed by RO required the addition of an acid pump and tank to control the pH to avoid calcium carbonate scaling of the RO membranes.

The wisdom of the above arrangement can be questioned. Daily cleaning was needed. Usually, such a cleaning frequency would be considered intolerable, as an RO unit may operate for months between cleanings. Ultrafilters foul more readily than RO systems because, being more open, they process more water at a given differential pressure. Ultrafilters thus tend to have higher recoveries per element and per system than RO. The general situation may be a 90% recovery for UF compared to 75% for RO, and with worse staging for the UF. A faster loading results for the UF. If the 15% difference in recoveries were used as blowdown for the RO, the cleanings required would diminish significantly without any UF protection. Zoccolante (1991) pointed out that the use of UF at 90% or so of recovery could deposit so much material per element and per system as to require cleanings at an impractical rate. It seemed far wiser and more economical to Zoccolante to obtain the same effect at realistic rates of cleaning by operating the RO itself at lower recovery levels without the use of UF.

As Ridgway (1987) pointed out, the use of ultrafilters as prefilters for RO units of questionable economic benefit in larger systems where flux losses are important. It all depends upon the fouling characteristics of the feedwater, with higher TSS and organism levels predisposing to more rapid ultrafilter blockage. Too frequently occasioned cleaning of ultrafilters tends to cancel out the advantages of their use. For such waters, alum treatment or additional prefiltration is indicated. The TSS level is simply too high to warrant UF or RO confrontation.

In the actual event, it is difficult to persuade the use of ultrafilters that can cost significantly more than depth filters, even through the employment of filters having nominal ratings of 5 to 25 mm are obviously less apt to retain microorganisms adequately.

Yabe et al. (1989) found that the UF membranes they tested shed particles when tapped. Accordingly, vibrations were used to rid these filters of particles. Vibrations having a frequency of 5 to 10 kilohertz (kHz) and an acceleration force of 1 to 2 g (gravitation constant) were used on UF filters. A monitoring of the water permeate following such treatment showed the treated filters to be free of further particle shedding. Previously they had released 2,000 to 3,000 particles per milliliter. Such UF units would serve suitably for final polishing filters even where vibrations are possible. The data supportive of the Yabe et al. (1989) findings are presented in Tables 9-10 and 9-11 and in Figure 9-9.

Electrically Driven Demineralizations

New techniques and advances in the old characterize continuing efforts at improving the means of accomplishing deionizations. These often hold great promise and should not be ignored. On occasion, some are furnished by single-source manufacturers. The literature, often in support of marketing endeavors, comes to reflect their singular points of view. These are no doubt honestly and competently presented. They may, however, lack a self-critical zeal. The limitations of such devices may on occasion not be asserted with objective clarity, and their practical applications may not yet be broad enough to supply it. This holds true even for the more established processes. For example, not all polyamide membranes offered for RO operations are equivalent. Yet by

Table 9-9
Millstone RO Feedwater, Concentrate, and Permeate*

	Feedwater	*Concentrate*	*Permeate*
Calcium	4.0	14.8	0
Magnesium	1.2	4.2	0
Sodium	8.6	35.0	1.6
Potassium	1.5	3.0	1.0
Hydroxide	0	0	0
Carbonate	0	0	0
Bicarbonate	11.6	21.5	2.4
Chloride	9.5	30.2	1.5
Nitrate	0.4	1.8	0.9
Sulfate	12.0	70.0	0
Silica	3.0	7.0	1.0
Conductivity	78 μmhos	210 μmhos	5 μmhos
TDS	51.8	188.0	8.5

*All values in mg/L unless otherwise indicated.
Burns and Booth (1988); Courtesy, *Ultrapure Water* journal

invoking the term PA, a given RO manufacturer may seek to associate his RO device with the superior performance of a better grade of PA unit. Here, however, competition imposes a policing action that is absent where single-source devices are being dealt with. The literature relating to innovative and valuable single-source processes requires being evaluated differently.

Electrodialysis. Electrodialysis (ED) as a demineralization process has been providing drinking water from brackish water for half a century. One notably successful application is in operation at Buckeye, Arizona. Electrodialysis is generally considered more cost-effective than reverse osmosis for waters in the salinity range of a few hundred to a few thousand ppm. Its application to pharmaceutical waters is of more recent origin, but, unlike RO, is limited by its inability to remove organism and endotoxins. The chief drawback to ED is that RO is generally considered a more economical method for accomplishing the same purpose. Yet there are ED installations that are operated on the grounds that they are less costly than RO. Electrodialysis does offer certain operating advantages. It is said to be able to operate at up to 200% of calcium sulfate saturation with zero chemical feeds and with no deleterious consequences to performance (Elyanow et al., 1981). Electrodialysis generally requires less pretreatment, as compared to RO. Presoftening, pH adjustments, or the use of

Table 9-10
Particle Release From Final Polisher Components After Tapping 10 Times

Component	*Particle Counts Downstream of Elements (particles/mL, >0.2 μm)*
Blank 1-10	
Cartridge polisher	1,180
UF module:	
Hollow fiber A	3,970
Hollow fiber B	1,460
PVC piping:	
Straight pipe	50
Joint: Elbow	65
Tee	73
Flange	30
Diaphragm valve	100
PVDF piping:	
Straight pipe	60
Joint: Elbow	38
Tee	30
Flange	13

Yabe et al. (1989); Courtesy, *Microcontamination*

sequestrants are usually not needed. The ED-treated water emerges with a neutral pH. It is thus not corrosive to stills, for which it is ultimately intended. Perhaps most intriguing of all is the longevity of the membranes involved. Useful life spans of 10 years have been reported.

Although commercial ED units are multicell units, it is convenient to explain electrodialysis on the basis of a single cell having three compartments (see Figure 9-10). Within the left compartment is a cathode. This compartment is separated from its neighbor by a cation-permeable membrane, which can be constituted of polysulfonated cross-linked polystyrene. The immobilized sulfonic acid groups, being negatively charged, permit the passage of cations, their oppositely charged counterions. However, they repel and hence forbid the passage of similarly charged anions.

The compartment on the right contains an anode and is bounded by an anion-permeable membrane, one constituted of quaternarized* amine groups immobilized by substitution on, for instance, cross-linked polystyrene. This membrane permits the passage of oppositely charged anions, the mobile counterions to the styrene-bound, positively charged, ionized quaternary radical. It repels, and thus interdicts, the passage of like-charged mobile cations.

The central compartment is bounded on its cathode side by the cation-permeable polysulfonated membrane, and on its anode side by the anion-permeable polyquaternerized membrane. When a direct current is passed through the cell, the cations migrate from the center compartment through the cation-permeable membrane to the cathode. The cations of the cathodic cell (left portion of Figure 9-10) do likewise. However, the cations of the anodic cell (right portion of Figure 9-10), drawn to the cathode, are enjoined from entering the central compartment by the anion-permeable membrane that forbids passage to like-charged cations. Simultaneously, the anions migrate from the center compartment through the anion-permeable quaternarized membrane on their way to the anode. This same membrane, however, frustrates the passage of cations, under the attraction of the cathode, from the anodic compartment into the central compartment. The anions in the cathodic compartment are kept from entering the central compartment by the barrier action of the polysulfonated membrane against like-charged ions The central compartment thus becomes deprived of both its anions and cations without the possibility of acquiring new ones.

The result of this direct current passage is that the central compartment becomes deionized or demineralized. Assemblies of hundreds of such cells results in an arrangement, a membrane sandwich bounded by electrodes at either end, capable of producing large flows of deionized water (Schmauss and Aiken,

*Quaternarization is the reaction of an amine, usually but not necessarily a tertiary amine, with (usually) an alkyl halide. In the process, the nitrogen atom of the amine moiety comes to share its generally unshared electron pair with the alkyl radical. In consequence, it acquires a positive charge to become cationic. The halide atom becomes an anion, its negative counterion.

1984).

To be sure, the concentration changes effected in the electrode compartments, depending on the constituents of the water, may cause precipitations, as of calcium carbonate, calcium sulfate, and barium sulfate. Water-softening pretreatments may be indicated. These and other electrochemical side reactions can detract from the efficiency of the ED process. Suitable manipulations and procedures are available to maximize its success, however. The periodic reversal of the current, of the polarity, is one such. It prevents the precipitation of salts having limited solubilities. Electrodialysis cannot operate above calcium saturation levels without chemical addition. (Electrodialysis reversal, the use of periodic current reversals, can operate above saturation levels.) For tap feeds, precipitation of calcium carbonate is more prevalent than that of calcium sulfate.

The ionic strength of carbon dioxide is too low to permit its removal by electrodialysis. To do so, the dissolved carbon dioxide needs to be converted by alkali into bicarbonate ions. Similarly, the handling of high TDS waters to avoid scale formation can be managed by use of hydrogen cation-exchange softening. Silica removal using ED can also be performed by a simple tailoring of the feedwaters by the addition of alkali, which results in an increase in the form of ionized silica removable by the anion membrane (Pasqua and Dvorin, 1988).

A cell pair consists of an anion-permeable membrane, a concentrate-stream spacer, a cation-permeable membrane, and a dilute-stream spacer. Fifty percent of the ions can be removed per cell pair. Above 50%, precipitates form from concentration polarization. The use of five stages can give a greater than 90% removal. The use of two or three stages in a pretreatment mode can yield a 75% to 80% removal of ions.

Electrodialysis will not remove organisms, pyrogens, soluble silica, or other

Table 9-11
Particle Contamination of Membrane Modules*

	Classification		
Location	*Hollow-Fiber UF (A)*	*Hollow-Fiber UF (B)*	*Spiral RO*
Permeable side of membrane	5.3×10^{11}	1.2×10^{13}	8.4×10^{11}
Permeable side of spacer net	1.3×10^{11}	3.4×10^{10}	3.0×10^{11}
Vessel inside	8.1×10^{10}	1.1×10^{10}	NA
Permeable side, total	7.4×10^{11}	1.2×10^{11}	1.1×10^{12}

*In particles per module greater than 0.05 μm
NA: Not applicable
Yabe et al. (1989); Courtesy, *Microcontamination*

nonionic entities. However, the equipment is reputed to be rugged, capable of long-term operations at temperatures as high as 45 °C and at pHs of from 1 to 10.

Electrodialysis is advocated as a roughing deionization method for producing water suitable for mixed deionizing resin-bed treatment, prolonging the operation of such beds. But the frequent regeneration of DI beds is sought as a means of sanitizing them. The chief potential application of ED to pharmaceutical needs is seen as an alternative to RO. Its advocates advise that an operating cost analysis based on an 85% water recovery shows about an 11% to 12% advantage over RO; while at the recovery level of 90%, it amounts to $0.26 per thousand gallons of product water (Larson and Walker, 1984). The combined initial capital and installation costs of an ED system may be higher by 10% to 15% than those of RO. The economic advantage of ED over RO is said to become evident when operating and maintenance costs are factored in. On this basis, ED provides an alternative to RO in the deionization of water intended for distillation.

Electrodialysis reversal. Electrodialysis itself is often limited by poor recoveries, 50% to 60%, and by a susceptibility to scaling. A major process improvement, electrodialysis reversal (EDR), minimizes scaling and brings recoveries to a range of 80% to 90%. This enhanced efficiency and its considerable reduction in need for pretreatments positions EDR to be an alternative to ion exchange for the demineralization of high TDS waters; and as a pretreatment of multibed ion exchangers, to reduce capital and operating costs.

Electrodialysis reversal features programmed periodic electrical polarity reversal to maintain a nonscaling condition on the membrane surface. This necessitates periods of discontinuous flow for 0.5 to 1.5 minutes at 15- to 45-minute intervals. A continuous brine stream carries product water impurities to

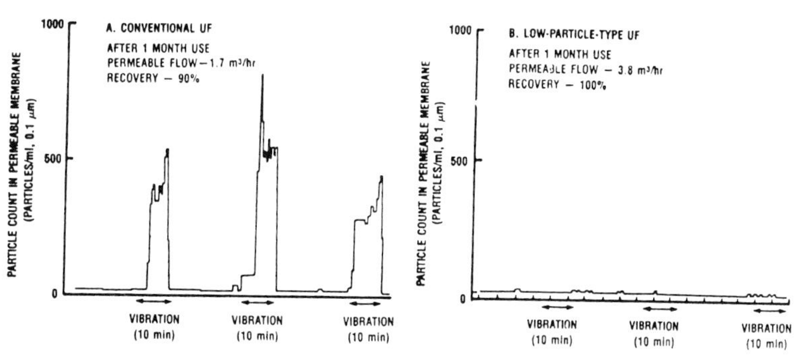

Figure 9-9. Particle generation from UF elements caused by vibration application
Yabe et al. (1989); Courtesy, *Microcontamination*

waste. Product water flow can be from 75% to 80% of the feed. Total organic carbon removals of 25% to 50% have been noted.

The electric power required for EDR is a function of the dissolved solids. Lower TDS requires less power. The major power cost is for pumping, as for ion exchange, not for the electrodialysis itself. Pressure drop is usually 50 psig through the system.

Cell pairs are composed of an anion and a cation membrane separated by a spacer to form a flowpath. Hundreds of cells are assembled to form a stack. Stacks are hydraulically connected to form stages. Each stage removes approximately 40% to 50% of ionized impurities. Elevated temperatures increase ionic mobility and, hence, impurities removal.

Katz and Clay (1986) described a systems approach to water purification designed to operate on waters of up to 1,000 ppm of TDS, regardless of seasonal water-source variations at operational temperatures of 4.5 °C to 32 °C (40 °F to 90 °F). It was made up of a polysulfone spiral-wound ultrafilter of 50,000 daltons. The spiral-wound format avoided the problem of bypass caused by hollow-fiber breakage. The polysulfone composition permitted hypochlorite sterilizations, and provided a very low SDI water of reduced organics, particulates, and organisms.

This was followed by a primary demineralization utilizing an EDR technique. This action produced approximately a 90% reduction in TDS along with TOC to the amounts of 15% to 80%, depending upon the organics' molecular weight and electrical charge. Electrodialysis reversal was selected for its ability to accept a

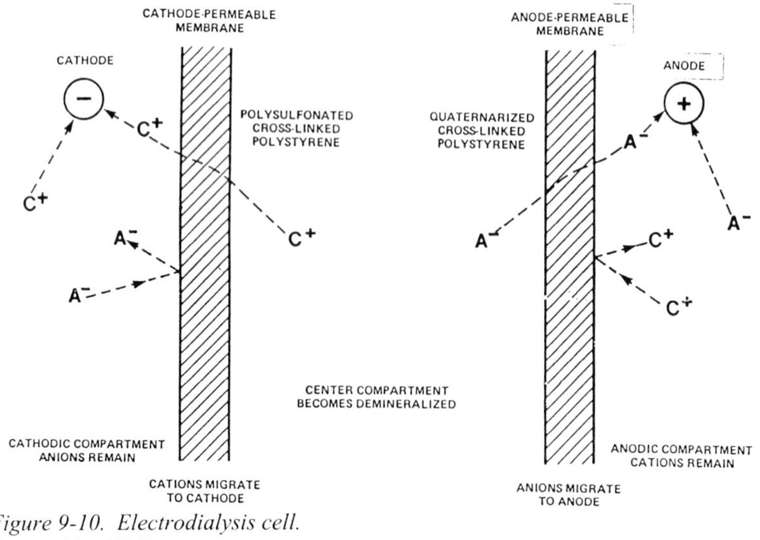

Figure 9-10. Electrodialysis cell.
Courtesy, Marcel Dekker

wide range of source waters without requiring chemical feeds or pH adjustments. This system component was amenable to continuous exposures to chlorine residuals at strengths up to 0.5 ppm.

The third element in the Katz and Clay (1986) system was a cellulose acetate hollow-fiber RO unit, selected for its compatibility with free chlorine. This was productive of organism control. The normal tendency of hollow-fiber RO devices to plug was said not to be a problem because of the prior ultrafilter and electrodialysis treatments. Also obviated was the need for scale control. Some 90% of the remaining minerals were removed by the RO, along with silica, and organics of 300 molecular weight or over.

The RO was followed by a polishing step consisting of constant recirculation through mixed-bed ion exchange and ultraviolet light installations. Water so treated was typically characterized by a conductivity of 0.5 to 15 μS/cm.

Its advocates see EDR as being economical for treating waters with a high TDS. By contrast, mixed-beds require low TDS values. Electrodialysis reversal removes 90% of silica, although mixed beds do better. An EDR treatment prior to mixed beds is suggested, using the hydroxyl form of the resin for the silica removal.

One advantage of the EDR method is that its membranes are impervious to fouling by the particulate and colloidal matter causative of high SDIs. Its diluting and concentrating compartments are fully reversible. Reversing the direction of the direct current several times an hour interchanges the demineralizing and concentrating streams, and purges particulates and sparingly soluble salts from the membranes. So operated, EDR in essence automatically and periodically, electrically and hydraulically backwashes its membranes (Katz and Clay, 1988).

Electrodialysis reversal has been applied to waters from the Canadian River having SDI_5 of 19.4 at peak loads, using a 200-gpm unit.

Electrodeionization. A variation on the electrodialysis method, called *electrodeionization*, can be achieved by the addition of mixed DI resins to the control or pure water compartment of the electrodialysis cell (Ganzi et al., 1987). The advantage of this modification is that the presence of the ion-exchange resins confers upon the pure water a degree of ionic conductivity it would otherwise lack. This maximizes electrical current transfers, minimal in high-purity waters themselves, and serves to insure the practical rate of the ion transfers. The arrangement also promotes the performance of the mixed-bed resins.

As in the case of electrodialysis, the electrodeionization equipment consists of alternating cation- and anion-permeable membranes and spacers that form compartments. Alternate compartments are filled with mixed ion-exchange resins. The result is a repeating element called a cell pair, as shown in Figure 9-11. Feedwater enters all the compartments in parallel. The imposition of a direct electrical current (DC) serves to motivate ions to move from the compartments containing the resins into the adjoining sections. The charge-selective displacement of ions by the transverse DC electric field depletes them from the ion-exchange-containing compartments, which become diluting regions. The transfer of ions across the appropriately charged boundary membranes into neighboring compartments transforms these compartments into concentrating sections.

The process operates in two different regimens. In conditions of high salinity the ion-exchange resins in their salt forms enhance the electrical conductivity in the ion-depleting compartments. This is in contrast to electrodeionization where, in the absence of ion-exchange resin at low conductivities, the remaining ions are not sufficiently electrically motivated to migrate. Under conditions of low salinity, as the ionic strength in the diluting stream decreases, the relative increase in mass transfer resistance in the thin water layer bounding the resin bead surfaces causes the development of high-voltage gradients at the water/resin interfaces. This can result in the lysing of water molecules into hydrogen and hydroxyl ions. These serve continuously to regenerate the mixed resin beds. The dissociation of water into its constituting ions depends not only upon the water purity, but also upon its flow velocity and upon the applied voltage.

In high-purity water, ion-exchange resins are typically more conductive than water by 2 or 3 magnitudes. Ion transfer within the diluting compartments is thus by way of the resins, not through the water. Water does not flow through the membranes. It is the ions that make this passage, directionally motivated by the direct current (White et al., 1989).

The water flowing through the concentrating compartments flushes the ions from the system to drain. The water moving through the diluting regions becomes product water.

As Griffin et al. (1991) describe it:

> Under the conditions of electroregeneration, the concentration of ions in the diluting chamber is very low. Here relatively high voltage gradients develop, creating currents at which the ion concentration at the resin surface approaches zero. When this voltage gradient exceeds a certain voltage potential, and the resin surface meets certain catalytic requirements, the water at the resin surface will spontaneously decompose to its hydrogen and hydroxide ionic components.
>
> This creation of hydrogen and hydroxide ions has important consequences. First, it allows the resins to remain highly conductive by placing resin in the hydrogen and hydroxide forms. Secondly, the resins in the regenerated forms can react with weakly ionized species, allowing transfer of species that would not otherwise occur.

As will shortly be seen, the generation of hydrogen and hydroxyl ions fleetingly localized into regions of extreme pH is hypothesized as causing cidal effects upon bacteria.

Among the reported successful applications of the electrodeionization device was a 10-gpm unit dedicated to boiler feedwater, which operated on well water that was pretreated to remove colloidal iron and to effect softening, and irradiated with UV light to reduce organism contamination. Following these steps were an activated carbon bed succeeded by a strongly basic anion scavenger, both dedicated to organic removal. This was capped by a 1 μm-rated prefilter prior to confronting the electrodeionizer. The system reduced the TDS from a range of 150 to 200 μS/cm, to less than 10 mS/cm (White et al., 1989). Applications of the system have also been made to semiconductor usage, and to general industrial purposes. As is evident from the pretreatment regimens employed, electrodeionization systems require protection against organic foulants. Relying upon ion-exchange resins and electrodialysis, albeit with advantages, electrodeionization reflects the general operational limitations of these techniques.

In another application, an electrodeionization device operated 21 hours per day over a 2-year period, converting feedwaters having conductivities of from 93 to 70 μS/cm into product waters of 1 μS/cm (Ganzi et al., 1987).

Continuous deionization (CDI) is a manufacturer's term for their particular electrodeionization device. A paper by Parise et al. (1990) described the use of a CDI system to provide water of the quality of pharmaceutical Water for Injection and of suitability to semiconductor rinsewater purposes. Parise et al. (1990) employed a module with the flow capacity of a typical full-scale commercial pharmaceutical application. Unfortunately, the achievement of Water for Injection quality is not alone sufficient to permit a device to be used to prepare WFI. The requirements in pharmaceutical applications have previously been discussed. They involve in the validation exercise a demonstrated consistency of performance along with an operational definition of the duration over which the performance can be depended upon. What requires being validated is not a small-scale device, however faithfully modeled, but an operational apparatus large enough to remove the engineering uncertainties inevitably associated with scaleups. This makes it difficult for promising new techniques such as electrodeionization to find their applicational niches in the pharmaceutical industry. Nevertheless, CDI installations have been validated for USP Purified Water manufacture in at least ten pharmaceutical houses. An ophthalmic drug producer uses one device of 20-gpm capacity. Other pharmaceutical producers utilize CDI installations of from 5 to 120 gpm. One large Midwestern drug house achieves a high USP Purified Water production by employing two modularized units, each of 50- to 64-gpm capacity.

Ganzi and Parise (1990) advocated a system based upon RO followed by electrodeionization to prepare water having the quality of Water for Injection. They demonstrated (by way of a laboratory-size installation of 5-gpm capacity operating on Bedford, Massachusetts, city water) that the RO effluent waters contained fewer than 10 cfu/100 mL of bacteria (95% confidence limits), and that the water exiting the electrodeionization unit contained less than 27 cfu/mL (95% confidence limits). The system terminated in a 0.22 μm-rated membrane filter. It was not entirely clear whether organism samples were taken before or after this sterilizing filter. In any case, the FDA-suggested guideline of fewer than 10 cfu/100 mL was achieved with only an 80% probability. What is more important, however, is that the USP stipulation of not more than 0.25 endotoxin units/mL was consistently met over the 4,000-hours (over 5 months) test duration (Cooper, February 1991). This performance has justified the use of electrodialysis for the successful preparation of USP Purified Water in a number of validated systems.

The RO is required to eliminate the hardness elements and TOC. The feedwater to the CDI portion of the assembly should have a TDS of less than 0.5 ppm, thereby reducing fouling. Because an RO unit is really integral with the CDI, if the RO imposes restrictions on the flowrate, the CDI undergoes the same restraints.

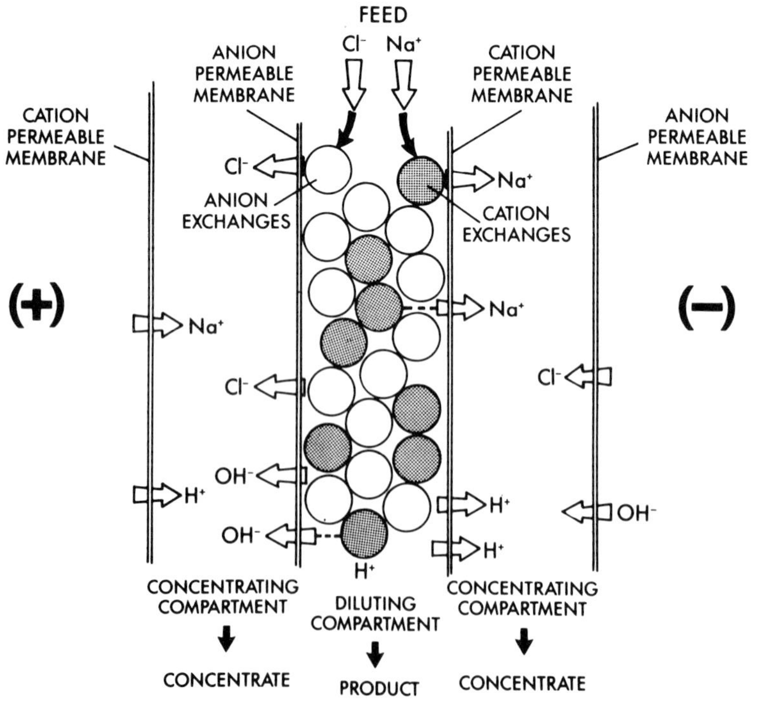

Figure 9-11. Principle of continuous deionization, an electrodeionization device.
Ganzi et al. (1987); Courtesy, *Ultrapure Water* journal

As regards the applicability of CDI to semiconductor pure water operations, Hango and White (1990) pronounced it a success. These investigators concluded that CDI has the potential to eliminate expensive and disruptive resin replacements, and to permit lower levels of ionic impurities than do conventional mixed-bed polishers. In comparative testing, Hango and White (1990) concluded that CDI produces water of as good quality as is derived from new mixed-bed polishers. The use of mixed-beds is still the accepted procedure for polishing operations.

A notable limitation to the electrically driven deionizations is the tendency of the membranes to become fouled by hard-water constituents. Because of their requirements for softened, pretreated waters, CDI devices are coupled with upstream RO units and downstream sterilizing membranes. It is this entire arrangement whose salubrious effects are being measured, not just those of the electrodeionization device.

Ganzi and Parise (1990) stated, "The removal of bacteria and bacterial endotoxins by RO are well documented and, because of their size, are unlikely to be removed by CDI." There is an obvious and stated concern with the organisms that can get through the RO or that may come to colonize its downstream side. But the RO is sanitized exhaustively to eliminate these very possibilities. It would seem there is no justification for ascribing to the electrodeionization unit the very actions the RO unit is known to be capable of conferring. The RO, if properly maintained, should reduce the organism counts to acceptable levels, and would eliminate endotoxin without any input from electrodeionization. Surprisingly, Tanaka et al. (1984) stated that the water dissociation that occurs in electrodialysis serves to kill *E. coli*. These investigators reported that increased current densities and decreased pH exerted a germicidal effect upon $10^8/cm^3$ suspensions of *E. coli* at 20 °C, particularly at current densities greater than the limiting current density of 0.8 A/cm^2 where "neutral disturbances" occur. The germicidal action was rationalized as being due to the localized production of H^+ and OH^-, inimicable to organisms, although at the macro level the water remains neutral.

Dunleavy (1991) found a similar germicidal effect operative in continuous deionization processes. He too rationalized its existence as being caused by localized neutrality disturbances. In the electrodialysis experience, Tanaka et al. (1984) employed ion-exchange membranes and electric current (i.e., electrodialysis). Dunleavy (1991) utilized electrodeionization that involved the use of ion-exchange resin as well. The use of the ion-exchange resin gave rise to the lysis of water into H^+ and OH^-, within the lower regions of the cells when few ions remained for carrying out the electric current. It was hypothesized that locally, at the micro level, bacteria-killing regions of high and low pH occurred, and that overall, the water maintained its neutrality through the mixing of the flowing water stream. Others ascribe the germicidal properties of CDI to the buildup of magnetic fields. Whatever the causes, waters exiting CDI units are said to be in bacterial balance with those entering. Sterilizing properties are not claimed. The CDI does require periodic sanitizations. Peracetic acid in concentrations of about 0.5% are useful at the same frequency as required by the RO unit. A rinse of less than 1 hour suffices. More strongly oxidizing sanitizers, destructive of the resin capacity, should not be used lest the oxidative degradation of the ion-exchange resin comes to compromise the "continual" feature of the CDI function.

That the electrically driven deionization processes are productive of organism reductions by effecting their destruction is a very significant advantage. Ganzi and Parise (1990) demonstrated that a system consisting of pretreatment, RO, CDI, and then a sterilizing filter also commendably reduced organic content and TDS. The CDI by itself offers a poor rejection of TOC and silica. Griffin et al. (1991) advocated the application of CDI to condensate polishing. Dunleavy (1991) discussed its application to the power generation industry in general.

Electrodeionization offers the demineralizing equivalence of mixed-bed resins without requiring the rigors of mixed-bed regenerations. Applications of electrodialysis in pharmaceuticals have been made in order to avoid the use of regenerant chemicals for ion-exchange resins, and to eliminate the costs of their disposal as necessitated by the EPA and environmental concerns. The use of the combination of RO, CDI, and filter is being directed to the preparation of waters being prepared for distillation to WFI. In any case, the availability and suitability of electrodeionization to the preparation of high-purity water offers another tool for the attainment of this objective.

Some users prefer the electrodeionization method to ion exchange. The sodium chloride used to regenerate anion-exchange water softeners is less expensive than the sulfuric acid used to regenerate cation-exchange resins (even more so than hydrochloric acid used for the same purpose), and is far less costly than the sodium hydroxide required for the anion-exchange regeneration. Additionally, with the use of electrodeionization, the handling of these chemicals is obviated as is also the disposal of their wastes.

Continuous deionization can give rejections of 99.9% under optimum conditions. It is a capital-intensive operation capable of yielding good process control.

Water for Bulk Pharmaceutical Chemicals

Waters used in the preparation of bulk pharmaceutical chemicals (BPC) will be affected by concerns about endotoxin limits where the ultimate preparations will be injectables and where the FDA will have interest in the bioburden (FDA, March 1991). Water for Injection need not be used for such purposes.

Restraint of the endotoxin content to 0.25 EU/mL limits the Gram-negative organism population as well. The storage of water intended for BPC purposes in recirculatory loops at 65 to 85 °C should ensure against increase in the attained endotoxin level, and ought to obviate concerns about the attendant bioburden. Purified Water does not, at present, carry an endotoxin specification. (For a fuller discussion of water for bulk pharmaceutical chemicals, see Chapter 14.

Membrane Fouling

Fouling is a condition wherein a membrane undergoes plugging or coating in such a manner that its flux, permeation, or output is reduced. Membrane fouling is, in this sense, a surface phenomenon. Fouling that results from a generalized surface deposition and blockage was shown by Probstein et al. (1981) to involve (at least in the case of a cellulose acetate membrane fouled by colloidal ferric hydroxide) the low activation energies characteristic of physical adsorption rather than of chemical bonding.

Nonspecific, arbitrary surface depositions and blockage can also occur in carbon beds, on ion-exchange resin beads, and in deep-bed filters in general. In carbon beds the adsorptive sites may become preempted, and on resin beads the ion-exchange groups may become involved as a consequence of their specific functionality. This is also considered fouling in that the function of the active site was not intended for the foulant. Thus in the fouling of ion-exchange resin sites, partly oxidized organics (weakly ionized) may usurp by ion exchange the sites intended for, say, chloride ion removal.

There is some ambiguity to the use of the term *fouling*. Some speak of mineral scales such as of calcium carbonate, calcium sulfate, barium sulfate, or calcium fluoride. They reserve the term *foulant* for deposits of biofilms (organisms), metallic oxides, silica, and various colloids (Amjad, 1987). Fouling is seen as the depletion of solids already present in the water (e.g., colloids or other suspended solids, including organisms that may then proliferate into biofilms that adhere to surfaces, whether membrane or other). Scaling is seen in this definition as a deposition of materials that have their genesis in the RO process. Each definition of *fouling* has its adherents; no usage is universal. (Bates et al., 1988).

Paulson (1987) defined membrane fouling as the condition wherein substances such as particulates, precipitates, and colloids accumulate on the membrane surface because of changes in the physical and/or chemical character of the feedwater. Fouling can be measured in terms of flux reduction; by the mass, volume, or density of the foulant; or by an increase in the feed-channel pressure drop. The latter is mirrored by the resistance to hydraulic flow, a decrease in flux that results from a blockage of the filter, and a diminution of the effective filtration area. In membrane fouling, a steady state is rarely obtained. The fouling and its effects usually continue to increase with time.

Fouling results from bacteria, organic substances, iron, manganese, silt, and/or silica. These are impurities that may be present in the feedwaters and that can therefore come to be deposited upon the RO membrane to reduce its effective filtration area. A reduction in the permeation rate results. A loss of RO rejection capabilities is also possible, (Zeiher et al., 1991).

Scaling or precipitation also result in a blockage of the RO membrane surface. It is caused by the RO operation rather than from a condition already present in the raw feedwaters. Thus, a calcium sulfate in the feedwaters in soluble quantities can come to exceed its solubility product, at about 2,000 ppm, during the RO operation. Its precipitation upon the membrane may result.

Fouling results in larger osmotic pressures and in the formation of gels. This must be compensated for by higher operational costs. To overcome the limitations of lower fluxes, larger membrane areas may be supplied at a cost. The cleaning of foulant from the membranes is also an economic tax, as is the downtime involved. Moreover, a chemical degradation of the membranes with a foreshortened service life may result from the foulants themselves, or from the reagents employed to clean the membranes.

The fouling of ultrafilters is similar to that of RO filters except that the minimization of osmotic pressure developments emphasizes the complication of gel deposition. This is caused by near-colloid-size macromolecular solute concentrations at the membrane surface. Microorganisms are encouraged to proliferate by the nutrients thus provided. Sanitizations, even independent of flux-restoring UF membrane cleaning, may be indicated.

Specific terms have sometimes been employed to describe particular types of fouling occurrences (Paulson, 1987). *Gel layer* describes the fouling of a membrane by gel-forming proteins. The term should not be broadened to reference fouling in general. Similarly, fouling can result in the dynamic formation of a foulant layer upon (usually) a more permeable membrane. The result is a better retention of smaller particles, albeit at a reduced rate of flux. Thus the term *dynamic membrane* usually has positive connotations, at variance with the negative implications that the term *fouling* generally conveys. However, dynamically formed membranes are not necessarily helpful, and higher sweep velocities need not give poorer retentions. Paulson (1987) cited higher rejections of dextran by an ultrafilter at a flow velocity of 8 meters per second than at 2 meters per second. High velocities apparently involve unelucidated complexities. Paulson (1987) referenced work directed towards differentiating more precisely between concentration polarization and fouling, between osmotic pressure effects and gel-layer influences.

Biofilm formation (see Chapter 2, page 90) is not without effect on flux decline. According to Characklis (1973), a biofilm of 0.8 to 1.6 mm (1/32 to 1/16 inch) caused a 12% reduction in flow through a 42-inch water main. A reduction by 55% of the flow through a 50-mile-long, 24-inch pipe was occasioned by a 0.6-mm (25-mil) thick biofilm.

Fluid Dynamics

The more vigorous the crossflow and the greater the turbulence of the flowing stream, the more mixing and the less fouling there will be at the membrane surface. Turbulence is seen to provide a scouring action that is antithetical to the layering of fouling deposits. In tubular and thin-channel configurations, flows of 2 meters per second are considered optimum flowrates. However, in spiral-wound arrangements (which means the great majority of cases), the usual rate is only about 20% that amount for water purifications. In ultrafiltrations where high fouling is involved, the rate may be up to 30% of the 2 meters per second considered optimum. The higher flowrates obtainable in the tubular models have often proved to be impractically expensive. Paulson (1987) points out furthermore that different types of foulants require different fluid managements. Thus hard, discrete particles may respond better to less rigorous flowrates than do soft particles or emulsified materials.

A comprehensive review of the sources of foulants and contaminants and of the pretreatments necessary to protect ion-exchange and reverse osmosis operations from their interferences was presented by Crits (1989). The review also discussed analytical methods suitable for determining the presence of given contaminants and for assessing their removal.

The instruments need to assess extents of fouling are a feed pressure gauge, a product pressure gauge, and flowmeters for both the feed and product waters. Salt rejection can be measured by way of comparative conductivity.

The recovery should be held to 10 to 15% per membrane if a high velocity is desired to prevent (minimize) membrane fouling.

Scale Formation

Calcium salts, particularly calcium carbonate and calcium sulfate, are the most common scale formers, and the most frequent causes of RO problems. The tendency for calcium salts to produce scale can be managed in one of three ways: The water can be acidified to remove bicarbonate/carbonate; the calcium ions can be removed by water softening; or the water recovery can be limited to the point where exceeding the calcium salts solubility products is avoided.

The use of acidification entails the expense and hazards of handling acids. Furthermore, it requires the subsequent use of decarbonators (degasifiers) to remove the carbon dioxide formed by bicarbonate conversion. Water softening employing cation-exchange resins in the sodium form substitutes sodium ions for the divalent ions. The economic burden is generally tolerable. Moreover, any colloidal entities, such as may be present in surface waters, are stabilized in the RO concentrate stream against fouling the membrane because monovalent sodium ions replace the more destabilizing multivalent ions. Scale formation is thereby eliminated without the use of scale inhibitors.

Comb and Fulford (1991) presented the case for acidification. These investigators saw less risk in dependency on a chemical feed pump than on a water softener. The pump had less potential for failure and could be fitted with an alarm function involving a pH monitor-controller. Also, physically handling of the quantities of salt required in the softening seemed onerous. Finally, the demineralization by RO was more efficient for multivalent ions. In this regard, the substitution of sodium ions for calcium seemed to be a step in the wrong direction. The acid was directly fed from a concentrated (66 Baumé) 93% sulfuric acid source to a pH of about 5.6. This was seen to minimize operator attention.

While calcium and magnesium ions are the chief causes in scale formation because of their often generous presence, barium and strontium ions, usually in concentrations of as little as tenths of a ppm, are of a more baleful influence. The sulfates of barium and strontium, once deposited upon an RO membrane, are almost impossible to remove. Therefore, the analysis of the feedwater should be specified to quantify the presence of barium and strontium. Iron in its more oxidized ferric form also produces scale. The most effective scale prevention for RO is water softening. It gets rid of the metallic ions whose insoluble salts tend to produce scale. Softening will remove calcium and magnesium, but also barium and strontium, and even iron, manganese, and most trace metals and aluminum. Increasingly, RO units utilize softening pretreatment; the present usage is about 50%. It is possible, however, that for very large systems acid feeding would be less costly, softeners and large salt consumption being more expensive.

Solubility Product

Calcium sulfate can come to exceed its solubility product as a result of becoming concentrated by the RO action. The solubility product defines the maximum concentrations of calcium and sulfate ions that can coexist in solution. Any amounts of these ions in excess of those permitted by their solubility product can cause calcium sulfate to deposit as insoluble scale upon the RO membrane.

$$(Ca^{2+}) \times (SO_4^{2-}) = SP_{CaSO_4} \qquad \text{Eq. 9-2}$$

The same may come about for calcium carbonate and, more rarely, for calcium fluoride, barium sulfate, and strontium sulfate. Magnesium hydroxide and/or carbonate may also form scale if these salts become concentrated in excess of their solubilities as expressed by their solubility products.

Of greater concern are the salts (ions) in the reject stream leaving the RO unit. Since 75% of the feed stream usually emerges as permeate, the 25% making up the reject stream contains a fourfold increase in ion concentration. If water starts out with a salt concentration of 200 ppm, assuming a 99% rejection, after the first membrane the concentration is 4 × 200 or 800 ppm if the recovery is 75%; 5 × 200 or 1,000 ppm if the recovery is 80%.

Calcium carbonate and calcium sulfate may precipitate out. This can be prevented in one of two ways. The calcium (and other substances, including barium and strontium) can be removed, or their concentrations lowered by softening or by ion exchange. Otherwise, the carbonate may be removed and the sulfate be converted to the more soluble bisulfate by the acidification of the water. However, the use of sulfuric acid for this purpose would increase the risk of calcium sulfate scaling by its contribution of sulfate ions.

Acidification converts the carbonate and bicarbonate into carbon dioxide. This requires removal before RO is used because otherwise as much as 75% to 80% of the carbon dioxide will permeate the RO membranes, according to Everett (1976). Actually, no claims are made that RO removes any carbon dioxide; 100% is expected to permeate the membranes. The use of degasifiers for carbon dioxide removal has been discussed. (See page 325).

Calcium Sulfate Supersaturation and the Use of Antiscalants.
When the solubility product for a compound of limited solubility is exceeded, precipitation occurs. Some molecules exhibit the phenomenon of supersaturation, however. They remain in solution despite the fact that their ionic concentrations exceed the limits of their solubility products. Helpfully, calcium sulfate is one such compound. Moreover, materials have been found that, when added to calcium sulfate solutions, serve to promote the supersaturation effect. Several such adjuncts are available in the market as antiscalants.

High degrees of supersaturation can lead to spontaneous precipitate formation. Lower levels of supersaturation are amenable to the action of the commercial antiscalants. Low supersaturation may lead to nucleation of the supersaturated salt. Until they achieve a critical size, these nuclei may redissolve. Above the critical size, they grow into stable crystals that seed the solution to cause precipitate formation. The antiscalants inhibit the nucleation step, and so delay (or avoid) crystal and precipitate occurrence. Once the critical-size nucleation takes place, the rate of crystal growth is the same, whether antiscalant is present or not.

Amjad (1987) showed that the new antiscalant compounds distort barium sulfate crystals. The presumed built-in strains that result are hypothesized to lead to easier crystal fracture and removal. The polymeric antiscalant adsorbs into the growing crystal structure. This makes for irregular crystal shapes. The lack of regular surface planes inhibits orthodox crystal development. The consequences are cleavage lines that result in easier crystal disruptions.

The point being made is that the action of antiscalant additives need not necessarily function by influencing supersaturation. The antiscalant additives, it has been claimed, serve also to maintain some 85% of ferric iron (F^{e3+}) in soluble form, whereas it otherwise becomes precipitated as insoluble iron oxide, albeit in hydrated form.

Static systems are particularly susceptible to scaling. In extreme situations, permeate water is used to flush the concentrated reject water from the membrane surfaces. Temperature control, to avoid canceling out of supersaturation, is seldom used. Acid conditions, antiscalants, and softening are the most commonly relied-upon scalant controls. The Langelier Saturation Index (LSI) is very useful in this regard. (See page 528). Computer programs are supplied by the membrane manufacturers and the RO suppliers to guide the correct management of feedwaters in terms of such factors as hardness, SDI, and product-flow to minimum brine-flow ratios. These relate to the membrane warranties as they find expression in the RO design and its operation.

Antiscalant use obviates the need for acid addition. Typically, such compounds are used in waters with an LSI of about +2.0 or lower and pH of 8.0 or greater. Since the polyamide membranes have a wider pH tolerance than do the cellulose acetates, such additives are used largely with polyamide RO. A well water in Casper, Wyoming, contained 1,500 grains of calcium sulfate and a total dissolved solids value of 6,000. Its temperature was 110 °F. The water was cooled, and 5 ppm of a polyacrylic acid antiscalant was added prior to subjecting the water to RO treatment. The calcium sulfate did not deposit out upon the membrane, but stayed in solution in the reject stream. On the other hand, such polyacrylic acids are very bad foulants for ion-exchange resins, both for the cationic and anionic types.

The same polyacrylic acid product has been used to prevent silica from depositing upon RO membranes. In the area of Vancouver, Washington, water is obtained from 200-foot-deep wells that contain 200 to 400 ppm of silica. Hydroxyethyl phosphoric acid and disphonic acid have also been used.

Sodium hexametaphosphate in doses of 5 to 15 ppm serves the same purpose. It is reported to keep calcium carbonate as well as calcium sulfate in solution. Some report it as being less efficient than the polyacrylic acid preparation, presumably because its cyclic structure makes it less available for inclusion in crystal formation. The orthophosphates are linear and more effective, presumably because they become included in crystal structures. Polyacrylic acids, acrylic acid copolymers, and polymaleic acids are efficacious in 2.5-ppm concentrations to promote supersaturation, and hence to prevent scale formation; and in 2% to 5% strengths to remove scale formations once formed. In contrast, polymethacrylic acid of high molecular weight is not much adsorbed onto the crystal surfaces, and is therefore not comparably effective.

It bears being repeated that sodium hexametaphosphate can foul polyamide membranes. In one case a flux decline from 200 gpm to 150 gpm occurred.

Antiscalant Boiler Additives

Antiscalants are also used to prevent or minimize mineral depositions upon boiler tube surfaces in steam generating plants. Polymeric additives are also used for this purpose, as also are the chelants discussed on page 535.

These polymers have low molecular weights of from 1,000 to 10,000, and are negatively charged (anionic). They become associated with the suspended boiler sludges. This renders the deposits more fluid, and therefore more easily removed by bottom blowdown. It is hypothesized that the adsorption of the polymeric to the sludge particles makes these particles more hydrophilic in character. This promotes their wettability by water, and a greater fluidity results. By the same token, hydrophobic adsorptions to nonpolar boiler surfaces are minimized. As in the case of other antiscalants, incorporation of the polymeric molecules into the crystal lattice of the mineral alters the crystal's growth pattern by occupying growth sites, so that smaller crystals result. The resulting crystals may also be rendered weaker by the polymeric inclusions and be more easily disrupted. The polymeric charges may also restrict crystal growth by repelling ions that would otherwise become included in the crystal structure. Whatever their mechanism of action, polymeric additives of several types are effective: polyacrylic acid, sulfonated polymers, carboxylated structures, carboxymethylcellulose, and organophosphonates (Burris, 1987a, 1987b) (see Table 9-12).

Acrylic or methacrylic acid based antiscalants can combine with quaternarized coagulants, as may have been used to excess in the municipal water treatment plant, to produce difficult-to-remove precipitates from reverse osmosis membranes (Goodlett and Comstock, 1995). If the municipality employs such polymeric coagulants, non-acrylic or methacrylic acid antiscalants should be used.

Silica Fouling

Silica fouling is primarily a regional concern. Certain parts of the Southwest have waters containing 50 to 75 ppm of silica. Silica deposition is normally not a problem until the concentrations in the waste stream exceed 120 ppm. If the feedwaters contain less than 20 to 30 ppm of silica, the problem is not great. Concentrations of 50 to 60 ppm can be a problem. It is usually avoided by limiting the RO water recovery to under 50%. This escapes building up the silica content in the reject streams to problem proportions. While silica deposition on RO membranes is not a widespread problem, once deposited it is difficult to remove.

Table 9-12
Power Treatment of Chemicals

	Hardness	*Iron*
Synthetic sulfonated polymer	X	X
Synthetic carboxylated polymer	X	X
Poyacrylic acid	X	
Carboxymethylcellulose	X	
Organophosphonate		X

Burris (1987); Courtesy *Ultrapure Water* journal

Langelier Saturation Index

The Langelier Saturation Index predicts the tendency of a water to deposit scale, using calcium carbonate as the model compound. The LSI test is performed upon the waste stream, not upon the reject stream. (If precipitation of calcium carbonate were possible in the feed stream, the system's piping would soon be blocked.) While scaling materials may include various bivalent hydroxides, carbonates, and sulfates (e.g., magnesium hydroxide, strontium carbonate, barium sulfate, and calcium fluoride), the archetypical scalant may be taken as being calcium carbonate. For calcium carbonate to form deposits, the product of the calcium and carbonate ions must exceed the solubility product of calcium carbonate.

$$(Ca^{2+}) \times CO_3^{2-}) = SP_{CaCO_3} \qquad \text{Eq. 9-3}$$

The likelihood of the solubility product being exceeded therefore depends in part upon the carbonate ion concentration. It and the possibilities of calcium carbonate scaling can be diminished by removal of carbonate ions. This can be done by acidifying the solution to convert carbonate ion into bicarbonate ions or even, at yet lower pHs, into carbon dioxide in accordance with the following equilibria:

$$H^+ + CO_3^{2-} \text{<---->} HCO_3^- \qquad \text{Eq. 9-4}$$
$$H^+ + HCO_3^- \text{<---->} H_2O + CO_2 \qquad \text{Eq. 9-5}$$

Each of these chemical equilibria proceeds to a given extent, as defined by its ionization constant, or K value. The K value of the first equation defines the concentration of carbonate ion. Its relationship to the pH, the log of the hydrogen ion concentration, or the acidity level of a water, was established by Langelier to be the following:

$$pH_s = \log K_{sp}/K_2 - \log (Ca^{2+}) - \log (HCO_3^-) \qquad \text{Eq. 9-6}$$

From this relationship Langelier derived an index, called the Langelier Saturation Index (LSI), relating the pH of a water saturated with calcium carbonate and the pH of the water itself.

$$LSI = pH \text{ water} - pH \text{ water saturated with } CaCO_3 \qquad \text{Eq. 9-7}$$

This relationship can be used to forecast the potential of a water for scale formation. The LSI calculates the pH at which calcium carbonate scale formation is likely. To prevent this, a lower pH is arranged by the addition of acid.

Thus when the pH of the water (the brine or the water being treated) is lower than that of the water saturated with calcium carbonate, the LSI is negative in value, meaning that calcium carbonate scale will not form. If the LSI value is positive, it signals that calcium carbonate scale can form. In practice, enough acid is then added to bring the LSI value to zero, forestalling the possibility of scale formation.

When antiscalants such as sodium hexametaphosphate or polyacrylic acids are added, the mineral scalants form with greater difficulty. Thus waters of higher pHs can be tolerated, and thus, with sodium hexametaphosphate in concentrations of 20 mg/L, LSI levels of +1.0 are tolerable. Where a particular antiscalant product, AF-100 (BF Goodrich), is used in concentrations of 5.0 mg/L, LSI readings of +1.9 will still not produce scale (Kraft, 1985). The use of antiscalants, in effect, reduces the need for acid.

Of course, utilizing lower recoveries by the RO will also reduce the calcium and carbonate ion concentrations in the brine (the reject stream), to the discouragement of scale formation. However, this results in less permeate being produced and detracts from the economics of the operation. This approach is used only when calcium sulfate or barium sulfate formation is to be discouraged. The avoidance of calcium carbonate scale formation can be had by reliance upon acidification of the water to be treated as indicated by reference to the LSI.

Where the RO membrane is composed of cellulose acetate, acidification to pH 5.5 to 6 is practiced in any case to minimize that polymer's hydrolysis. This generates carbon dioxide, however, by conversion of the bicarbonate. The carbon dioxide can be removed by a degasifier or, as is more common in pharmaceutical applications, may be neutralized with caustic to be removed by subsequent demineralization. Degasification operations may be cheaper, but air degasifiers risk introducing organisms with the airstream. Where the RO is of polyamide, the pH can be brought to pH 8 to 8.5, and the bicarbonate ion can be rejected as such. At pH 5.5, 100% of bicarbonate permeates the polyamide membrane; while at pH 8.0, more than 97% is rejected. The pH adjustment in the case of polyamide RO is unrelated to considerations of polymer stability. Polyamide is stable over the pH range 4 to 11. To utilize the rejection of bicarbonate ion at pH 8 to 8.5 by polyamide RO, antiscalant may have to be added. The LSI reading can be used to determine the circumstances under which the desired pH level can be attained without causing scale formation. (Figure 7-9).

Actually, the antiscalants or sequestering agents are more expensive than acid. The desire to dispense with acid addition must derive from other than economic motives, possibly simply to reduce the hazards and liabilities connected with acid handling.

It is certainly possible that in the case of high TDS values, including much calcium and sulfate ions, even the use of sequesterants may not eliminate the need for acidification, as would be indicated by the Langelier Saturation Index. In such cases, the attainment of the pH 8 to 8.5 needed for bicarbonate rejection by thin-film composite RO would not be possible. If this were still desired, hardness reduction by water softening pretreatment could be used.

Suspended Matter: The SDI Test

Reverse osmosis membranes, being extremely retentive of collodial materials and other suspended solids are easily fouled in consequence. The silt density index test (SDI), also discussed on page 284, offers a measure of the fouling propensity of a feedwater. Performing SDI measurements, therefore, can provide a useful prognostication of the extent to which a water should be treated to reduce its filter-blocking suspended-material content before it is permitted to impinge upon the RO membrane. This can serve to prolong the service life of the RO, to reduce its downtimes to cleaning, and to promote the optimization of its function.

Two 500-mL samples are successively filtered through a microporous 0.45 µm-rated membrane, with the time required for the successive samples being noted. The SDI test is a must for reverse osmosis operations. It is the best means by which to predict what the RO cleaning frequency will be. It can be used to disclose whether the upstream carbon filter (if any) is removing or shedding particles, and to disclose whether the raw feedwater is varying in its quality. The SDI number has a special pertinence to RO operations because it is a measurement of the water's filterability.

There are those who have strong reservations about the silt density index, however, because there are numerous examples of very high SDI waters operating extremely well. It apparently depends upon exactly what the foulant is (Cartwright, 1991).

Paul and Rahman (1990) pointed out that suspended solids that foul the reference membrane in an SDI test wherein dead-end filtration is used, need not foul an RO membrane where tangential flow is employed. Likewise, these investigators stated that colloids passing through a 0.45–µm-rated microporous membrane may become destabilized to deposit upon an RO membrane by ion neutralization of their charges, occasioned by the concentration polarization of the RO process itself. Apparently, the fouling predicted by the SDI test eventuates when the offending particles most nearly fit the pore sizes of the reference membrane, and are not sufficiently removed by the tangential sweep. In this situation, pore plugging is presumed to occur.

Measurements of SDI are of definite value. They can be conducted on site; no outside laboratory services are required. They indicate whether particles are being generated or removed, and may therefore be utilized to assess the efficiency of a treatment or device intended to effect such removals.

The testing of a water's SDI before and after filtration can serve to assess the efficacy of the filter, and may even constitute a validation of its action. The SDI is inexpensive to perform. Zoccolante (1991) saw it as a highly underutilized analytical tool in water purifications. A very common use of SDI is to gauge the suitability of a water to undergo RO treatment. The higher the SDI, the greater the likelihood of early filter fouling. Manufacturers of RO units recommend maximum SDI levels for use with their devices. In general, there has evolved a reliable relationship industry-wide among SDI values, the flux (the gpd/ft^2) of a membrane, and the frequency of filter cleaning that will be required.

The SDI values are best not greater than 5 for spiral-wound RO units. Higher numbers presage more frequent cleanings, probably monthly; and SDI values of 1 would require less frequent cleanings, probably yearly. The more common values of between 1 to 5 will occasion about three RO cleanings per year. For hollow-fiber RO units, SDI values of even 3 or 4 are on the high side.

The SDI value of a water entering a multimedia deep-bed filter should be about 5. It should exit with a value of 5 at the most. Going into a carbon bed, a water's SDI value should be about 6. It should emerge with an SDI of 4.

Colloidal Fouling

Paul and Rahman (1990) dealt with the colloidal fouling of RO membranes. A chief factor would seem to be the colloidal stability. The colloidal particles of a stable colloidal suspension, as already discussed, do not settle out, because of their mutual repulsions caused by a like charge. Such colloidal particles could be retained by an RO membrane in a dead-end filtration mode, on the basis of size exclusion. In conventional RO devices employing tangential flow, this may happen only to limited extents, depending upon the percentage of recovery of the unit.

Essentially, particles will remain in suspension, stabilized by charge, size, and density (see Stoke's law). As reject fluid becomes more concentrated, however, the forced closer positioning of these particles, a consequence of concentration polarization, may overcome their mutual charge repulsions. Agglomeration will then occur. Colloids may also become destabilized by charge neutralization, depositing their constituent particles as an agglomerated fouling layer. Charge neutralization, as induced by coagulation aids (alum, ferric salts, polyelectrolytic polymer: see page 292) will also cause colloid destabilization. Most colloids are negatively charged. These charges may become neutralized by the bivalent ions (Ca^{2+}, Ba^{2+}) rejected by the RO membrane. The addition of hydrogen ions through acidification, to lower pH, can have the same effect. Positive charge concentration, then, can destabilize the colloidal particles to cause their agglomeration and deposition on the membrane.

Electrically Driven Fouling

In the case of electrically driven membrane processes such as electrodialysis and electrodeionization, additional aspects of membrane fouling, as induced by the electric current, are involved. The compartments in these devices, it will be recalled, are bounded on one side by a cation-exchange membrane (bearing the negative charges of anions, sulfonic acid groups), and on the other side by an anion-exchange membrane (carrying the positive charges of quaternary amine groups). The water flow through such a compartment makes for good mixing in the center regions, but inevitably this deteriorates as the surfaces of the membranes are approached. In the static boundary layers near the membranes ions become transported only by back-diffusion or by electrolytic transfer (Speaker, 1985).

Most foulants carry negative charges, particularly organics oxidatively altered to bear carboxylic acid groupings. Thus the positively charged anion-exchange membranes foul the most extensively. Another cause for precipitate formation and fouling develops at the anion-exchange membrane. As the ions in the dilution compartments become depleted, the current density decreases. This results in lysing of water molecules into hydrogen and hydroxyl ions. The latter, negatively charged, migrate through the anion-exchange membranes on their way towards the anodic electrodes. This leaves the depleting membrane surface at a lower pH, richer in hydrogen ions. These in turn repress the solubilizing dissociation of carboxylic acid moieties on the foulants, leaving them prone to precipitative fouling. The low pH also at least partially neutralizes the colloidal organics, usually negatively charged as well, and leads to their agglomeration and precipitation on the depleting side of the anion-exchange membrane.

At the concentrating face of the anion-exchange membrane, and at the depleting face of the cation-exchange membrane, there is an accumulation of hydroxyl ions; the pH rises. This causes the fouling precipitation of alkaline earth hydroxides. Speaker (1990) pointed out that a layer of oppositely charged material at the surface of any membrane bearing fixed charges produces a "sandwich membrane," characterized by alternating negative, positive, and neutral layers of varying thicknesses. This fouling impedes the passage of ions through the membranes. Thus in electrically driven membrane processes, the electrical resistance mounts exponentially with time, and necessitates the eventual replacement or refurbishing of the ion-exchange membranes. Ganzi (1991) disputed that hydroxyl ions accumulate at the cation membrane. He stated,

> There is no significant accumulation of hydroxyl ions on the diluting surface of the cation membrane. Dissociation of water is not catalyzed on the cation membrane surfaces commonly used in ED.
>
> Substantial pH shifts in ED only occur if normal operating voltages are exceeded or under fouling conditions. Fouling of anion membranes does not result in an exponential increase in electrical resistance of an operating ED module because water splitting begins to occur when the voltage loss at the membrane surface exceeds 0.83 volts. Instead there are large pH shifts in the concentrating and diluting streams.

In CDI, the salts do not need to travel from the water to the membrane; the salts travel from the resin to the membrane. Since there is a very large resin surface area, fouling is much reduced in CDI. Fouling is also reduced in the EDR process by polarity reversal. It is generally agreed that electrodialysis reversal fouls less than electrodialysis. There are a number of membrane fouling mechanisms. The most common, similar to ion exchange, is for high-molecular-weight weakly ionized compounds (too large to transfer) to bind to the anion membrane, preventing other anions from entering the membrane or resin.

The water that is supplied for electrodialysis or electrodeionization purifications may thus need pretreatment for the removal of alkaline earth elements (softening), and for the minimization of its organic contents. Otherwise these electrically driven membrane processes may be liable to compromise through fouling. Most ED and EDR systems do not use softener pretreatment. In electrodialysis, the equipment is operated below the limiting current density and at water recoveries that avoid supersaturation of the concentrate solutes. In EDR, any precipitate formed in one polarity cycle is dissolved when the polarity is reversed. Regenerable ion-exchange processes are in general equally as prone to organic fouling as most of the electro-membrane processes.

The modification of the surface properties of membranes to render them immune or resistant to surface fouling was reported by Speaker (1990). Ultrathin, molecularly oriented films or coatings that have low surface energies and that thus resist wetting and adhesion were the approach used. Optimization of the packing densities of the protective films further served to frustrate fouling. These coatings were said to alter radically the surface properties of the membranes without changing their bulk properties. The application to ion-exchange membranes intended for electrodialysis of one oriented molecular layer of fluorinated pyridinium bromide "effectively prevented increases in stack electrical resistance during 184 hours of operation" in the presence of humic fouling (Speaker, 1985). This investigation reported that one layer of fluorinated pyridinium bromide cut fouling-induced resistance-increase of a stack of electrodialysis membranes from 30 to 3.3 κW, and the ratio of final and initial resistances from 2.6 to 1.2. To date, however, the literature contains no accounts of such surface-modifying, fouling-defying treatments having received industrial trials.

Cleaning of RO Membranes

The pretreatment necessary to an RO operation depends upon the characteristics of the feedwater as disclosed by its analysis, and upon the membrane type that is selected. The purpose of the pretreatment is to avoid, or at least to minimize, the impairment of the RO membrane function that occurs as a result of fouling, scaling, or chemical degradation. Such interferences with the RO membrane operation are inevitable. Even the turbulent, tangential sweep of the flowing water cannot totally keep deposition layers from forming, or dislodge them. These layers, however thin, block or alter and thus detract from the membrane performance.

Cleaning and disassembling an RO filter can be undertaken when a 25% increase in differential pressure occurs because of blockage of the membrane area, whether from the accumulation of particulates or from scale formation. A 10% decrease in product flow is sometimes taken as the point where cleaning is initiated. A 1 to 2% loss in rejection is also used by some to signal the need for RO cleaning and disassembling. Cleaning may be performed on a maintenance schedule, particularly when an operational history has been developed for a feedwater of invariant quality. Actually, pressure increase, product-flow decrease, and rejection loss should all be monitored. The fouling mechanisms for different waters may variously assert themselves as one of these indicators. In any given situation, the relevant change will signal the need for membrane cleaning. If the feedwater is at 220 psig and the wastewater is at 180 psig, for a pressure differential of 40 psig, then a 25% increase in differential pressure caused by membrane blockage brings the reading to about 50 psig. At this point, RO cleaning is indicated to avoid irreversible damage to the RO unit. Normally, RO units should be cleaned once every 8 to 12 weeks at a maximum. Commercially available cleaners suffice. They may contain citric acid to help remove iron deposits by chelation, and detergents, enzymatic or otherwise, to help remove organic matter.

To detect when cleaning has become necessary, a pressure gauge is required ahead of the first vessel to register the feedwater pressure, and one is needed after the last one, ahead of the concentrative valve, to read the differential pressure through the system. (There should also be at least two flowmeters, for the product and concentrate.) From a comparison of the feedwater and concentrate pressure gauges, the differential pressure becomes evident.

The SDI of the RO feedwater should be measured. There is a correlation between the SDI levels and the frequency with which the RO requires being cleaned.

Paul (1994) advises that RO units should be cleaned when their flowrates decrease by 10% to 15%. He considers pressure drops to be too small to be useful indicators. Cleanings should be at high flowrates. Turbulence is required to flush out the foulants whose deposition upon the RO membrane was induced by the spacer-directed flow pattern. If the flows become too low because of blockage occasioned by excessive foulant depositions, cleansing becomes compromised. Accordingly, early and more frequent cleanings are advised. Cleaning temperatures can be important as the fluidities of the cleaning liquids are influenced thereby; increasing in direct relationships. The higher the temperature the better, to the level the RO membrane is capable of withstanding. The pump pressure per vessel is the consideration. As a generalization, the less foulant it is necessary to move through each 40-inch length the better. Therefore, each vessel should be cleaned individually, not the entire stage at once (Paul, 1994).

One reverse osmosis device manufacturer advises that the membrane should be cleaned as follows: Initially, an acid wash should be performed in order to remove mineral deposits. Citric acid at pH 3.5 is to be recirculated through the filter for 30 minutes. This is to be followed by a 30-minute soak, which is superseded by a 30-minute flush using deionized water to remove the last vestiges of the acid. Disinfection is then sought by means of a 1% Minncare® solution (a commercial, aqueous formulation of approximately 20% hydrogen peroxide,and 4% peracetic acid). This peracetic/hydrogen peroxide preparation is circulated through the RO unit at room temperature for about 30 minutes. A 30-minute soak succeeds this treatment, to be followed by an aqueous flush sufficient to remove all traces of the sanitizing agent. This last step also requires about 30 minutes. However performed, the cleaning technique relies upon scale removal followed by sanitization.

Chelates

Organic molecular structures have specific spatial arrangements as a result of their given atomic orders and constitutions. In certain cases, this molecular architecture positions two or more functional groups in such a manner as to create rather precise spatial dimensions between them. Within the field of force created by this functional group juxtapositioning, there exists an ability to bind other molecules or atoms. Metallic ions are particularly prone to becoming so fixed. This phenomenon is called *chelation*, after the Greek word for "crab's claw," implying by that very term the appositional holding arrangement of the two sections of the crab's pincers. The nitrogen atoms within each of the four pyrrole groups constituting hemoglobin thus chelate iron, whose presence serves, in turn, to bind oxygen; the same four nitrogen atoms within chlorophyll bind magnesium, to the same purpose.

Removal of Foulants by the Use of Chelates. The spatial positioning of the two carboxylic acid radicals of oxalic acid give it chelating properties for metals. It is thus used in surface-cleaning preparations to remove metals. The hydroxyl group and the three carboxylic groups of citric acid endow it with similar properties, hence its use as a metal cleaner in passivation practices. The four carboxylic acid groups of ethylenediaminetetraacetic acid (EDTA), situated within the close proximity of amine groups at each end of an ethylene chain, make it a strong chelating agent. The sequestering actions of the pyrophosphates relate to the same type of bonding that characterizes chelation. Their utility is thus in binding and removing metallic impurities, which in the usual applicational settings centers on iron. What is even more significant about chelation is that its binding of metallic ions so neutralizes the ionic character of the metal as to render it unresponsive to ion exchange. (See page 387 on the chelation of copper in ion exchange.) When, however, these chelates become disrupted, as by being deposited upon hot boiler tubes, the metallic entity is set free to work its corrosive (or other) mischief.

Chelation chemistry is applied to the purification of waters intended for the boilers of the power generation industry. Obligingly, chelates of calcium and magnesium are soluble. This permits the removal or sequestration of these elements free of the threat of deposit formations. As with all chelates, the chelating agent combines with more than one pair of the metallic element's electrons to remove it from the field of chemical reactions by forming a ring-structure complex.

Ethylenediaminetetraacetic acid, nitrilotriacetic acid (NTA), and mixtures of the two are widely used chelants. Of these, EDTA forms the most stable chelate. It remains integral at boiling water temperatures, although free EDTA decomposes under these conditions. The NTA is stable at boiling-water temperatures. Its use thus permits establishing a chelant residual in the boiler (Peters, 1987). According to Peters, EDTA should be fed to feedwaters downstream of any copper alloys after the deaerator but upstream of the boiler to allow time for reaction before the chelant is decomposed.

Unfortunately, residual chelant concentration in the boiler water cannot be determined because analytical testing is interfered with by the presence of iron. Therefore EDTA residuals are determined in the feedwater, while NTA residuals are measured in the boiler blowdown (Burris, 1987a, 1987b).

Several anions compete with the chelant for combination with metallic and hardness elements. Both hydroxide ions and silica successfully compete for magnesium ions, and phosphate ions win out in the competition for calcium ions. Chelants are ascendant over carbonate and sulfate ions for combination with calcium ions, however, thus avoiding calcium carbonate and/or calcium sulfate deposit formation. Despite the addition of chelant to the boiler, magnesium silicate deposits may form. Also, chelate addition may not sufficiently solubilize iron, as hydroxide ions may succeed in precipitating iron oxide. The latter may be preempted from forming deposits, however, by the addition of a dispersant (Peters, 1987).

Hardness contaminants are perhaps best controlled in boiler water applications by the use of chelants. However, excess chelant and chelant deposition products can contribute to corrosion. To thwart such an occurrence, an alkalinity residual of 200 to 500 ppm of sodium hydroxide is frequently retained in the boiler. Chelant treatment has been shown to be effective for industrial water boilers operating up to 1,000 psig. It has been employed, actually, at pressures up to 1,500 psig. At these higher pressures, chelant treatment has been in conjunction with feedwater demineralization, the use of phosphates, and the maintenance of low-alkalinity residuals (Peters, 1987).

Cleaning Agents for RO and UF Membranes

What is required in a cleaning operation is a tangential flow along the membrane surfaces to remove deposits. A low-pressure flow is indicated in order not to drive particulates into the membrane by a high transmembrane pressure. The data sheets on an RO unit will stipulate the correct cleaning pressures and flows, and these instructions should be implemented. The membrane service life of 6 to 8 years that, with proper handling and cleaning, is possible for RO units, may otherwise not exceed 1 to 2 years.

The sanitization of membranes was discussed in Chapter 2, page 116. The same sanitizing agents are usually used in greater concentrations, limited by concerns of membrane stability, in the cleaning operation. The rule, not too well enlightened by any great chemical rationale, is to use as strong a treatment as the membrane is likely to endure.

The removal of foulants from RO and UF membranes depends upon what the foulants are. For organics such as the tannins, lignins, and humic and fulvic acids typical of surface water seasonal turnover, removal can usually be accomplished effectively for cellulose acetate membranes by using up to 10% hydrogen peroxide, or from 100 to 500 mg/L of chlorine equivalence in the form of sodium hypochlorite solution. An enzymatic detergent is often effective in the removal of organic colloidal material. Turgidyne and ERA are said to contain proteolytic enzymes. Sodium hydroxide solutions with a pH of 12 are also used to remove TOC. For the cleaning of thin-film ROs, hydrogen peroxide and peracetic acid or combinations of both are effective. Peracetic acid in strengths of up to 4% has been increasingly reported to give beneficial results, though it is often applied in less than 1% concentrations.

Gagnon et al. (1995) documented a case wherein analysis of the spent cleaning solution indicated calcium, aluminum, and iron as being the principal ions removed during the cleaning operation. This strongly suggests that alum from the municipal water treatment plant may have reacted with polyacrylate-based scale inhibitor to form a gel upon the RO membrane, a not altogether unknown occurrence.

Alum-precipitated surface water foulants can be removed by a 30-minute contact with 3% to 5% sodium hydroxide to which sodium hypochlorite may be added. Alkaline detergents are difficult to remove, although an acid wash helps. Inorganic materials such as precipitated iron oxide can be removed using the chelating action of 0.5% ammonium citrate, or 5% citric acid at pH 9. Oxalic acid is often effective in removing iron-containing deposits. Recalcitrant deposits may be subjected to the more arduous attacks of 5% caustic soda at pH 11, 2.5% hydrochloric acid at pH 5, or 5% hydrochloric acid, or more usually, phosphoric acid. Acid treatment is more common in the Midwest for removing hard-water scale formations. Usually, alkaline cleaners are tried first.

Polyamide membrane cleaning is by 0.1% to 0.2% hydrochloric or phosphoric acid, by 2% citric acid, or by 0.1% to 0.2% sodium hydroxide. A 15- to 20-minute soak is followed by a 30- to 60-minute circulation prior to a water flush.

Silicone oils and silicone greases are particularly difficult to remove from membrane surfaces because of their extreme inertness to cleansing agents, the carbon-to-silicon bond being very stable. Silicones usually gain entrances to the system by way of being O-ring lubricants. At the risk of shortening O-ring life, the use of silicone gases and oils is advised against.

Aluminum ions, possibly forthcoming from an alum treatment, have been known to combine with monomeric silica to form aluminum silicate deposits on RO membranes. These can be removed, but with difficulty, using 2% hydrochloric acid.

The literature contains statements such as these: that "reagent A" will "lift off" biofilm, the all-pervasive microbiological foulant; or that "chemical B" will "destroy" biofilm. Except in the case of ozone, where experimental proof has been forthcoming from experiences in cooling-tower cleaning, these claims have been unsupported by experimental data and seem exaggerated (Merrill and Drago, 1980). Mittelman (1990) advised, however, that the ambient temperature administration of 50-ppm sodium hypochlorite solution for 2 hours sufficed to remove biofilm in potable water contexts where *E. coli* was the concern. However, the pH had to be below the pK_a value of 7.4 in order for hypochlorous acid to be present rather than the less effective hypochlorite ion. Failure of cleaning to restore the flux and the apparent reject rate indicate deterioration of the RO. A diminished reject rate accompanied by a high flux would mean the same.

Reverse osmosis performance should be monitored by way of the rejection rate and the downstream bacteria counts. Sanitization of cellulose acetate (not thin-film composite) RO membranes can be achieved with hydrogen peroxide. Certain Japanese semiconductor operations rely upon 1% to 2% hydrogen peroxide over a 24-hour period, used 8 times per year. Balazs (1987) recommended 10% hydrogen peroxide, 50,000 to 100,000 ppm. It degrades to a 5% strength going through the system. The peroxide was circulated for 25 hours, with the ion-exchange resin beds disconnected from the flow. Hydrogen peroxide has an electrode potential of 2.07 volts.

Mittelman (1986) listed a series of sanitizing agents, in decreasing order of effectivity on a mg/L basis for biofilm: ozone, sodium hypochlorite, iodine, quaternary ammonium compounds, hydrogen peroxide, formaldehyde or glutaraldehyde, ionic surfactants, and nonionic surfactants. He presented the dosage regime and duration required for different sanitizing treatments (Mittelman, 1985; see also Table 2-13, on page 109 in Chapter 2). He also presented evidence that planktonic organism populations are much more easily inactivated than are the attached (biofilm) or sessile organisms (Mittelman and Geesey, 1987; see also Figure 2-8, on page 99 in Chapter 2.)

Ridgway (1987) in his discussion of biofilms correctly observed that, "Virtually all of the commercially available cleaning formulations have been developed by empirical trial and error evaluations." Controlled laboratory comparisons are lacking. He advised the use of reagents that would disrupt the interactions between the organisms and the RO surfaces. Suggested specifically were the use of enzymatic cleaners, the mediation of surfactants to mask the hydrophobicity of the cell surfaces involved in biofilm adhesion, and the inhibition of biopolymer synthesis by metabolic inhibitors.

The use of surfactants in cleaning formulations seems logical given the prevalence of hydrophobic adsorptions in biofilm formation. Their inclusion is generally effective. However, Ridgway (1987) highlighted the complexities of surfactant/membrane interaction and urged caution. A study of such relationships does not easily lead to predictable results (Helenius and Simons, 1975). Thus strongly cationic or anionic surfactants may irreversibly combine with certain polyamide surfaces, whether caused by amine or carboxylic acid groups; and even nonionic surfactants may exhibit incompatibilities with RO membranes because of the presence of peroxides (Ashanti and Catraves, 1980; Chang and Bock, 1980). Whittaker et al. (1984) found a combination of urea and sodium dodecylsulfate to be an especially effective remover of biofilm. Unpublished data by Ridgway showed 6-molar urea, a strong protein denaturing compound, to partially solubilize the biofilm.

Unfortunately, cleaning of the RO membrane surface, even when effective, seems to lead eventually to even more speedy refouling. It seems best, therefore, to clean the membrane of its adhered bacteria, the biofilm, at regular and frequent intervals. (Ridgway (1987) suggested every 30 days.) The purpose is to forestall extensive biofilm formation; older biofilms seem more recalcitrant to removal (Argo and Ridgway, 1982; Whittaker et al., 1984).

It is generally assumed that in biofilm formation the membrane is a passive surface that does not contribute otherwise to the process. Jornitz (1991) indicated otherwise. He reported anecdotally that cellulose acetate membranes seem less fouled by organisms than are polyamide membranes. That proteinaceous adsorption to hydrophilic surfaces takes place less readily than to hydrophobic surfaces is known from biotechnology filtration experiences. Ridgway (1987) stated that pseudomonads adsorbed far more readily to polyamide RO membranes than to cellulose acetate RO membranes, and that different species of organisms adsorbed with different propensities to a given membrane type. The implications that polyamide RO membranes may foul more readily than cellulose acetate RO membranes seems therefore reasonable. Membrane surfaces may differ in the avidity with which they invite biofouling.

Some pattern, imperfectly formulated, emerges from the disparate means used to free surfaces from their adsorbed foulants. Oxidative destruction of the adsorbent may be attempted—with ozone where the inertness of the surface permits, with hydrogen peroxide and/or sodium hypochlorite where these are appropriate, and abetted by pH where possible. The hydrolytic destructive action

ommended are weekly treatments using 0.2% peracetic acid during a 1-hour exposure). An ion-exchange system can be hard-piped and, unlike RO, requires no storage tank. Tanks require proper maintenance, including periodic cleaning and sanitization. Their presence creates an atmospheric break in the system, which does usefully prevent pressure reversals. In this sense, RO units offer some risks, because the higher their operational pressures, the greater the magnitude of the pressure reversal, should it occur. Check valves are needed to prevent such reversals and to protect the RO units themselves from their effects. Otherwise the seals in the RO device can be damaged.

DI resin systems consume less water. Some 25% of the water fed to an RO device is discarded as the reject stream. Water costs are high; sewage costs can be even higher.

The DI/RO Choice: A Summary

The choice between DI and RO is not simply a balancing of TDS-removal costs. Water quality may be the determinant. Some applications are heavily based on membrane processes. In semiconductor usage, RO is usually relied upon to remove particles, colloids, and TOC. Chemical costs, safety, handling, and disposition are other factors. These favor RO. Water costs, particularly where the RO reject cannot gainfully be used, favor DI. Water availability and consumption may decide the issue where the economics of operations are the ultimate concern. The costs of electrical energy in different regions may lead to different conclusions. Where the cost of heating and pumping water is low, RO is favored. Where electricity, water, and sewage are expensive, RO is less attractive and the chemical costs of DI may compare favorably. The capital outlay requirements, previously discussed, are to be considered. Above all, the need to meet the required water quality must prevail.

If an ion-exchange system is rated for 50 gpm, it is possible to obtain 75 to 80 gpm out of it, provided the piping is not limiting. However, if an RO system is rated at 50 gpm, perhaps 52 gpm may be obtained. If the RO system is unduly stressed its chances for becoming fouled increase. Most RO systems still have ion-exchange following.

The water exiting a reverse osmosis treatment can be at 300,000 ohm-cm in its resistivity. A two-bed ion-exchange arrangement can yield somewhat better results, about 500,000 ohm-cm. An ionic equivalence of 4 ppm yields a resistivity of about 250,000 ohm-cm.

A System Designer's Approach to Selecting DI or RO

It may be of interest to consider how one systems design engineer* approaches the selection of DI or RO in the devising of relatively small-scale (up to 160-gpd capacity) demineralizing operations.

*Courtesy, George Laird, Systems Design Engineer, Water and Power Technology Inc., Salt Lake City, UT.

Four questions are first asked to learn the size system required, and the water quality needed:

- How many gallons per day constitute anticipated usage?
- What are the flowrate requirements?
- What quality water is needed: ordinary deionized water, WFI, low-organic water, or water filtered to a particular standard? Each degree of refinement necessitates an additional piece of equipment that contributes to the cost.
- Is the composition of the feedwater known; does it contain 30 ppm of TDS, or 600 ppm of TDS? (Feedwater in the Salt Lake City area has typically 200 to 500 ppm of TDS.) The higher the TDS level, the shorter the life of the deionizer. A TDS test meter is used to determine the actual water quality and temperature.

To give examples, some answers are assumed for the questions above. In the first instance, the requirement is for 5 to 10 gpd of deionized water. The source water is found to have a 300-ppm TDS content. Dividing the 300 ppm by the conversion factor of 17.1 ppm/grain yields 17.5 grains per gallon (gr/gal) of TDS. Service exchange deionizers come in different sizes. The smallest one has a 2,500-grain removal capacity. This so-called #1 deionizer is appropriate for laboratory use, and is small enough for on- or under-counter placement, being about 18 inches high and 8 inches in diameter.

Dividing 2,500 grains by 17.5 gr/gal means that approximately 140 gallons of deionized water will be secured before the unit's exhaustion. (In actual use, from 120 to 160 gallons may be produced, depending upon a more exact chemical analysis of the water.) At an average consumption of 7.5 gpd, this deionizer will last 19 days. This means that a tank exchange will have to be made about every 3 weeks at a cost of $45. The yearly cost, 52 weeks divided by 3-week intervals multiplied by $45, would be about $800.

The initial cost of the #1 deionizer is about $300, which includes inlet assembly, prefilter, interconnection assembly, quality control assembly, outlet assembly, and installation price. Some companies substitute a monthly charge for the initial purchase and replacement unit costs (for example,$10, $20, or $30 per month), and may or may not charge some fee at the time of a tank exchange. The leasing arrangements may also call for unit changes every 6 months, if not required sooner, whether the tank is exhausted or not.

The #2 deionizer has a 4,500-grain removal capacity. Dividing 4,500 by 17.5 grains per gallon means that this unit will produce 257 gallons before exhausting. Dividing 257 by 7.5-gpd consumption means that the deionizer will last 34 days, or 6.8 weeks on a 5-day basis. Fifty-two weeks divided by 6.8 says that 7.6 unit changes will be needed yearly. Each exchange costs $65, for a yearly total of

$497. The initial cost for the #2 deionizer is around $350.

The #3 deionizer contains 1.2 ft^3 of resin having a 12,000-grain removal capacity. Dividing 12,000 by 17.5 means that 685 gallons would be deionized to last 91 days between exchanges, or 18 weeks on a 5-day basis, for a total of 3 exchanges per year, each costing $95, for a yearly total of $285. The initial cost for the #3 deionizer is around $400 to $500. The large deionizer has a 5-gpm flowrate, compared to a 3/4-gpm flowrate for the smaller systems. It is larger and bulkier, however, being 8 inches in diameter and 48 inches high.

If the actual water consumption increases to 30 gpd or more, then reverse osmosis becomes a viable option. With DI resins, 685 gallons divided by 30 means that the 1.2-ft^3 unit will last only 23 days between exchanges, or 4.5 weeks for 11 or 12 changes per year, at $95 per change, for an annual total exchange cost of around $1,100 to $1,200. Depending upon the size of the RO unit, and upon the elaborations of its ancillary fittings, for the initial setup it can cost from about $2,500 for 100-gpd capacity, to $90,000 for 50-gpm capability. Thus it will pay for itself in less than 3 years.

At a water usage of 100 gpd, an RO unit is clearly mandated. Service ion exchange becomes cost-prohibitive. At such a water usage, the only alternative is an automated DI resin installation, a permanent bed unit automated to draw chemical regenerants every 2 to 3 days or so. However, this too comprises a capital expenditure of $3,000 and up.

Assume the water requirements to be 150 gpd. The need can be satisfied by several different sizes of RO units available in the marketplace. One supplier furnishes modularized units that incrementally process 60 or 80 gpd, and their multiples. An 80-gpd module can be expanded to 160 gpd by the addition of a second 80-gpd module; the rest of the system remains the same.

Installing an RO system also involves obtaining a water softener. A 10- or 20-inch prefilter is usually supplied with the RO. A carbon bed to remove chlorine from the water is needed if a thin-film composite membrane, usually composed of polyamide, is used. Alternatively, sodium bisulfite injection may be relied upon to remove the chlorine. The activated carbon may be utilized in disposable cartridge form or in permanent bed form (this latter ultimately to be discarded when spent, as it is too expensive to regenerate). Activated carbon is also supplied under service contracts. Also required for an RO operation is a storage tank, as the RO unit processes water slowly. A 160-gpd unit produces only 0.1 gallon per minute. Such volumes are not big enough to feed directly into a mixed-bed deionizer when one is used. A storage tank installation, in turn, requires a level-control system costing about $300 to turn the RO unit on and off, and to turn off the repressurizing pump if the tank goes dry as the water usage exceeds the rate of RO water production. The repressurization pump feeds the RO-treated water to whatever components require it, or directly to the point of use.

Because RO treatment significantly reduces TDS, the operation of an ion-exchange unit in subsequent conjunction with it notably prolongs the life of the DI resins, and so reduces the ion-exchange costs. It is for this reason that mixed-bed deionizers so often follow RO units, to polish the water to very high resistivities. If the deionizer has a 12,000-grain removal capacity and is fed with 1-gr/gal TDS water instead of 17.5-gr/gal TDS water, it will last approximately 17 times as long, correspondingly reducing the resin deionizer costs. Of course, the initial capital investment becomes greater. The RO system, depending upon its size, can range upward in cost from $3,000 for 100 gpd to $90,000 for 50 gpm units including the accoutrements. If, to the basic RO system, there is added a quality control monitor, a TDS or conductivity meter of different degrees of sophistication, a controller that shuts down on low feed pressure, a pretreatment interlock, and so on, then the price escalates. The main cost reflects, however, the cost of the RO unit's capacity. The RO membranes themselves become a continuing cost because their replacement becomes necessary after 3 years or so.

In any event, the foregoing sets forth the means whereby systems design engineers can arrive at decisions regarding the choice of DI resin installations, or RO units, or their combination. It is a decision reflective of the incoming water quality, and is addressed to the economics of the process as dictated by the volume and quality of the finished water product.

RO Laboratory Units

A number of companies supply small laboratory units that furnish high-purity water utilizing reverse osmosis and ion exchange. The water production is in the neighborhood of 150 liters per day. The water can be held to 18-megohm-cm resistivity,with a TOC level of less than 10 ppb. Indeed, arrangements exist for reducing the TOC to half this quantity. Coupling these units with ultrafilters, usually of 10,000 daltons, serves to reduce the pyrogenic content of the feedwater by 2 to 5 logs, depending upon whether RO pretreatment is involved or not. By means of such devices as replaceable cartridges of ion-exchange resins, RO units, ultrafilters, and activated carbon beds, small volumes of high-purity water are available at the laboratory for applications requiring some 30 to 50 liters per day.■

CHAPTER 10

DISTILLATION

Distillation as a purification procedure utilizes the volatilization of water as a means of separating it from its nonvolatile impurities; and the condensation of the volatilized water (steam) to isolate it from its more volatile impurities.

The distillation equipment in its simplest form, a one-stage still, consists of a boiler within which the water is vaporized, and a condenser by means of which the water vapor is condensed. The water is changed from liquid to gas by being heated, and reverts from gas to liquid through the agency of cooling or heat removal. By undergoing the changes in its states of matter that are occasioned by its evaporation and subsequent condensation, water becomes separated from its nonvolatile contents that cannot vaporize, and from its volatile components that cannot condense.

Where the impurities are organics other than nonvolatile solids, azeotrope formation with water is possible. In such cases, the separation of volatiles may not take place. Distillative fractionations would be necessary to effect such separations. Therefore, distillation is used primarily to separate water from its nonvolatile contents. As a practical matter, however, distillation is very effective in removing volatile impurities, among them low-molecular-weight organics, carbon dioxide, and oxygen. (See "Organic Matter," page 302).

In the design and operation of the boiler it is desired that the superheating of the water be minimized to lessen carryover of the non-volatiles by the entrainment of droplets. Additionally, the progressive concentration of non-volatiles in the boiler is limited by their periodic removal by way of blowdowns, now largely automated, of the stillpot contents.

The inevitable entrainment of mist (liquid particles) in the generated steam is countered by its separation from the water vapor using baffles, coalescing surfaces, cyclone separators, and certain stillpot design features. (See page 596). It is the purpose of these devices to prevent the carryover of the entrained non-volatiles into the condenser.

The water vapor is converted to the liquid state by its encountering the cooling surfaces of the condenser. However, to permit the separation of the water in its gaseous state from accompanying volatile contaminants, the cooling must be adequate but minimal. Higher degrees of cooling would encourage condensation of the volatiles as well. This means that the water exiting the condenser is still quite hot; it contains many calories. This heat can be used to preheat incoming feedwater to the still. Still-design importantly focuses on the economic reuse of this residual heat; the cost of heating the water being an important consideration in the distillation process.

States of Matter

It has been remarked that water is the only substance that is to be found in nature in each of the three states of matter: solid, liquid, and gas or vapor. What is significant about these states of matter is that their boundaries find definition in terms of distinct energy quanta.

Consider water in its gaseous state, consisting of individual water molecules isolated from one another. As the water temperature is lowered by the removal of heat, its disruptive thermal energy becomes reduced, permitting the attractive forces among the individual water molecules to assert themselves. The result is the liquid state, where the water molecules have attractive-bonding allegiances to one another. They are closer to one another than in the gaseous state. The resulting structure, albeit fluid, is thus denser than water vapor.

The degree of association among water molecules in the liquid state, augmented by hydrogen bonding, is apparent from a consideration of the boiling point of water. The boiling point of a liquid is usually rather directly related to its molecular weight. Consider, however, the combinations of hydrogen with each of three closely related elements: sulfur, oxygen, and nitrogen. Hydrogen sulfide (H_2S) has a molecular weight of 34. It boils at -59.6 °C. Hydrogen cyanide (HCN), with a molecular weight of 27, boils at 25 to 26 °C; and water, with a molecular weight of 18, boils at 100 °C. On the basis of molecular weight, water ought to boil at the lowest temperature, and hydrogen sulfide at the highest temperature of the three. The higher boiling point of water (and of HCN, although to a far lesser degree) is a result of hydrogen bonding among the individual water molecules. This creates a fluid, polymeric "gel" of water molecules. Extra heat must be supplied to liberate individual water molecules from their associative hydrogen bonds before they can be vaporized. The boiling point of water is thus inordinately high for a substance of its relatively low molecular weight.

If the liquid water is heated, thermal energy is absorbed by the water molecules until their resulting perturbations become large enough to disrupt their associative bonding. Additional thermal energy sets individual molecules free, converting the liquid water into steam or water vapor. Actually, water molecules exhibit some degree of association even in the gaseous state. That is why the ideal gas equation of state does not hold well for water except at extremely low pressures, below 10 kPa.

The heat required to effect this transformation between the states of matter is the latent heat of evaporation. It is the furnishing of this latent heat of vaporization that is central to the practice of distillation. This disruptive thermal energy is removed from the water vapor in the condensation step. Here it finds definition as the heat of condensation. Whether the heat is supplied or removed decides whether the water molecules can remain associated with one another or not, and determines whether water is a gas or liquid. When liquid water is cooled and the internal energy content of its molecules is diminished, they become even more responsive to their mutual attractive forces. The molecules approach one another even more closely. (Interestingly, water has a maximum density at 4 °C.) Given enough time for spatial alignment as the temperature is being lowered, as well as an overcoming of hypercooling, the water molecules will form regular spatial patterns, fixed molecular spatial arrangements of high stability. This is the crystal structure of ice. It will persist until disrupted by inflowing thermal energy. The heat that is surrendered by the water molecules as they form a crystal is the heat of crystallization. Its opposite effect is the heat of liquefaction, necessary to the thermal disruption of the ice crystal.

Hydrogen Bonding
Electromagnetic attractive forces can arise from dipole/dipole interactions, which is to say from the unequal sharing of the electron pairs constituting chemical bonds. That these electromagnetic forces can serve to adsorb or fix one molecule entity to another is shown in the special case involving the hydrogen bond. Given its low molecular weight of 18, water ought to be a gas at room temperature. However, because of strong dipole/dipole interactions, water molecules are joined by electrostatic interactions into a liquid polymer or gel. All water molecules in the liquid are each hydrogen-bonded to four neighboring water molecules, the intermolecular links being bent and stretched to produce irregular and varied networks. Within these arrangements, each water molecule offers two hydrogen atoms for bonding and accepts two in return, each oxygen atom having pairs of unshared electrons to provide (Tanford, 1980). (See Figure 10-1.)

The hydrogen bond, represented formally by three dashes, is weak enough to be broken easily by the molecular mobility of the liquid state, only to be reformed immediately with new neighboring water molecules. Facile though the bond may be, it represents a definite force. Because of its ability to form hydrogen bonds with other molecules, particularly oxygenated structures, water is a powerful solvent. Its high dielectric constant also gives it solvent properties, serving to lyse crystal lattices by the attenuation of their ionic attractive forces.

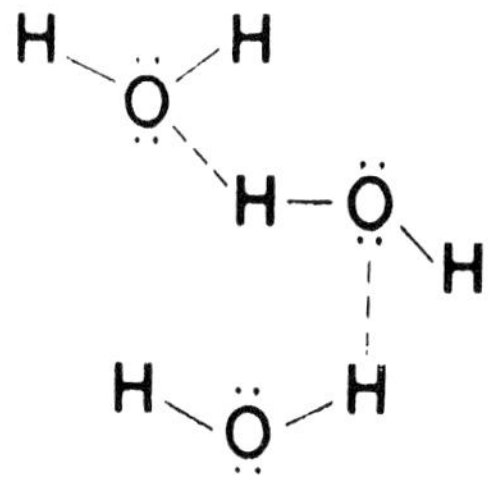

Figure 10-1. Hydrogen bonding.
Tanford, (1980); Courtesy Wiley Interscience.

Secondary Valence Forces

The valence bond responsible for the chemical union of two atoms consists of two electrons shared by these atoms. Were the two bonding electrons to be shared equally, the two united atoms would be electrically neutral. There would be no residual charges. This equitable arrangement is seldom realized. Usually, one atom or the other in the chemical couple possesses a disproportionate share of the two bonding electrons. This unequal sharing can be the result of any of several causes, usually induced by the influence of neighboring atoms. The electronic dislocation may be permanent or fleeting. In every case, however, one atom has in its vicinity a greater density of the bonding electrons than the other.

The condition is not one of ions, where one atom possesses both electrons and the other none, and where both ions, although bound electrically, are free to move independent of one another in their dissociated state. Rather, the chemical bond exists. Both atoms are inextricably joined to one another, albeit the electrons creating the chemical union are unequally shared. The electron being the seat of electronegativity, that atom possessing more than its share comes to bear a partial negative charge. Its deprived partner carries a partial positive charge. The partial electrical charges associated with the unequal sharing of the chemical bonding electrons are called secondary valence forces or Van der Waals forces. They serve to attract and bind entities of opposite charge. Being weak in nature, they operate only over small distances. Although weak, these secondary or residual chemical bonds are important in their influences.

Energy Considerations

Is is the formation and disruption of the bonding just discussed that is the effect of the thermal energy involved in distillation. Each kilogram of room-temperature water fed into a still requires 80 kilocalories (kcal) to become raised to 100 °C. However, to vaporize this quantity of water at the same temperature, 540 kcal must be added. In terms of mechanical energy, this is the equivalent of the lifting of 1 ton of water to a height of 750 ft. (230 meters). On this basis, the distillation of 1,000 kg of water per hour (250 gallons per hour [gph]) in a conventional still would require prohibitive expenditures of thermal energy.

The heat of vaporization required for water is 970 British thermal units per pound (Btu/lb_m), 8,080 Btu/gal, or 2,255 kilojoules per liter (kJ/L), at 1 atmosphere (absolute) of pressure. The furnishing of this much heat constitutes the chief economic drawback to the use of distillation. The heat involved in vaporizing water is released when the water is condensed. (This is the heat of condensation, which must be removed in order for the water molecules to be able to associate with one another in the liquid state without disruption). Efforts are made to recover and utilize as much of this released heat as possible to minimize the economic costs of distillation. Energy recovery is approached in a number of different ways, largely in different still designs.

The Performance ratio (R) of a still (Disi, 1995) is defined as the amount of distillate produced in relation to the amount of steam consumed and is given by:

$$R = Md \div Ms \qquad \text{Eq. 10-1}$$

Where R is the performance ratio, Md is the mass of distillate produced (lb), and Ms is the mass of steam consumed (lb).

Another way to measure the performance of a still is often stated in terms of thermal economy (E). This is defined as the amount of distillate produced in relation to the amount of energy input and can be given by:

$$E = Md \div 1{,}000 \text{ Btu heat input} \qquad \text{Eq. 10-2}$$

One-Stage Stills

In theory, a simple one-stage still (Figure 10-2), consisting of a boiler to vaporize water, a disentrainment device to free it of contaminant-containing droplets, and a condenser to liquefy the purified water vapor, ought to serve adequately to purify water by distillation. The conventional or one-stage still is energy-intensive, however, requiring 9 pounds of steam and some 9 to 12 gallons of cooling water to produce each gallon of distillate. Despite the excessive costs and water consumption, such stills are used where the quantities of water being distilled are small. Lower capital costs offset the higher energy costs to make the overall costs acceptable in such cases.

Nevertheless, the quantities of cooling water required for conventional stills are wastefully excessive. The cooling water may enter the still's container at 5 °C. It cannot, however, leave at temperatures above 70 °C (Kuhlman, 1994). Although the water effluent from the condenser is large in quantity, its tempera-

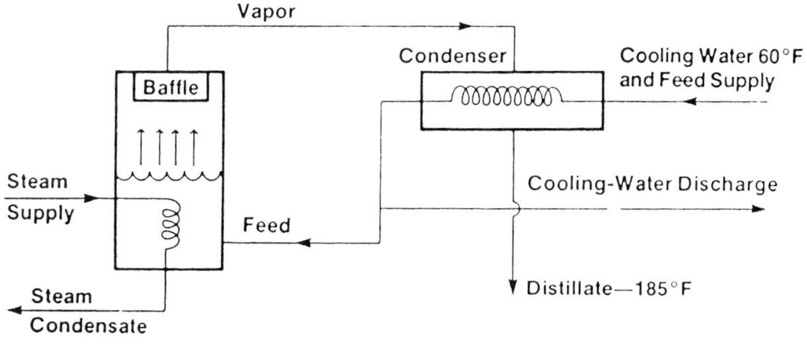

Figure 10-2. Single-effect distillation process.
DiSessa (1980); Courtesy, *Pharmaceutical Technology*

ture is too low to effectively heat larger stills. One kilograin of water at 5 °C will remove 65 kcal of heat from water at 100 °C. Another 8 kg of water at 5 °C will be needed to remove the heat of condensation. Given heat-exchange inefficiencies, from 9 to 12 kg of 5 °C cooling water are necessitated for each kilogram of distilled water produced.

If the heated condenser water is not utilized to feed a still, it may be employed as rinse water wherever its ionic content permits. Otherwise, it may first be demineralized, as by twin-bed ion exchange, and/or by mixed-bed ion exchange.

In the single-stage still, the heat of condensation, the heat that must be withdrawn from the water vapor to cause it to condense, is removed by cooling water within coils on whose outer surface the vapor condensation occurs. The cooling water thus becomes heated prior to itself being distilled. This preheating of the water intended for distillation conserves energy (Otten, 1976). The preheated water is subsequently used as still-feed water. If not, a separate preheater is recommended.

Single-stage stills rarely exceed 200 gallons per hour (gph) (760 liters per hour [L/h]) in capacity because of their relatively high energy requirements and costs of operation. Different still designs are involved to provide practical distillation operations.

Multiple-Effect Stills

In the single-stage still, a small amount of energy can be conserved by using the distilled water vapor in the condenser to preheat the water to the evaporator. In the process, the water vapor itself is cooled and condenses. An alternative is to use the hot uncondensed water vapor to heat the water in the evaporator of a second still that is under a lower pressure. The result is an energy savings, accompanied by the distillation of water in the second stage, or effect, roughly equivalent in volume to the water boiled in the first effect. The second effect will operate at a lower temperature, dependent on the equilibrium at the reduced pressure.

The condensate from the second effect is collected as purified distillate. The vapor produced in the second effect is transferred to the condensing side of the third effect, and the procedure is repeated. Condensate from the third effect is collected as purified distillate. This cascading procedure is repeated for as many effects as are in the still. Consequently, the net energy requirement for a typical six-effect still with a top operating pressure of 116 psig is 238 Btu/lb_m, as opposed to 970 Btu/lb_m for single-effect evaporation. The addition of effects requires higher operating temperatures and pressures to provide the necessary temperature/pressure difference between effects. A six-effect still, for example, typically operates at 140 °C (285 °F) in the first effect. The pressure in the first effect of a multiple-effects (ME) still may begin at 10 bar. The last effect is at atmospheric pressure (Figures 10-3 to 10-5).

Provided that one has sufficient inlet steam pressure available to provide a temperature difference across each effect of about 11 °C (about 20 °F), the still can be expanded to incorporate the number of effects dictated by the thermodynamic properties. Since the additional effects cost money, the number is usually limited to the minimum as dictated by the economics of the operation.

With each added stage, there is a lowering of the variable cost occasioned by an increase in the energy recovery and savings. This, in turn, is offset by the added fixed cost of each additional stage. Each added column will cost more but will save less energy than the previous one. There will thus be an optimum configuration, depending on the variable versus the fixed cost. Advantageously, the first stage of such a still serves as a pure-steam generator (DiSessa, 1981; Kuhlman, 1982). By definition, pure steam is steam free of endotoxin content.

Multiple-effect stills became popular as a result of the good manufacturing practices proposed for large-volume parenterals by the FDA in 1976. Although never formally finalized, (and were withdrawn in 1994) these proposals stipulated that WFI stored at room temperature would require being discarded after 24 hours. Indefinite storage could be maintained at 80 °C under conditions of circulation. With the exception of the pharmaceutical companies making very large quantities of parenteral solutions (3,000 to 10,000 gph or 11,300 to 37,800 L/h), most companies usually keep the stored water above 80 °C. The ME stills

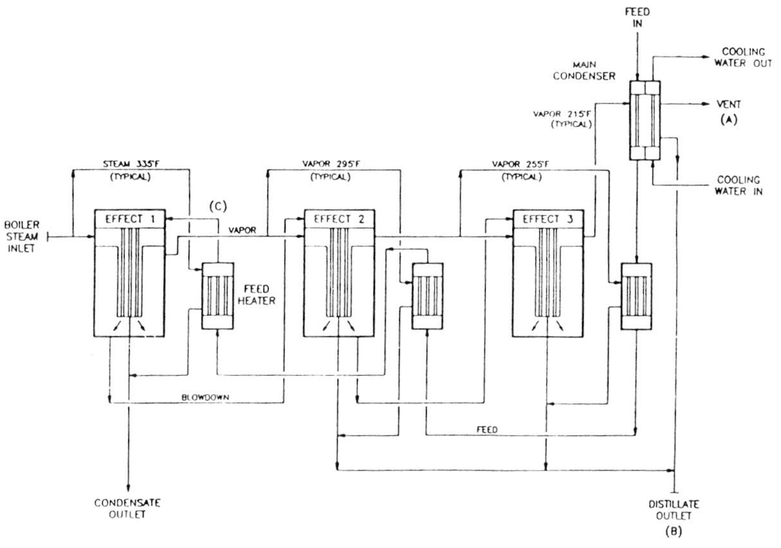

Figure 10-3. Simplified flow diagram, traditional multiple-effect distiller.
Courtesy, Aqua-Chem Inc.

can be equipped with from two to nine stages. The optimum number is selected and defined on the basis of present or future energy costs. The operation of an ME still requires the availability of high-pressure steam. Operation at maximum capacity necessitates about 110 psig. Maximum capacity is usually double the minimum capacity. The latter requires about 45 psig of steam pressure. Multiple-effect stills cannot be operated on low-pressure steam. (As Smith [1991] pointed out, the efficiency of a multiple-effect still actually depends upon the number of effects. The Office of Saline Water studied ME stills having as many as 100 effects. They were outstandingly efficient). The ME still has no moving parts and can, therefore, be expected to be relatively maintenance-free. It is made of 316L stainless steel, so it can be cleaned in place by way of recirculated descaling solution. Its cooling water consumption is very small. and decreases with the number of stages. The temperature of water emerging from ME stills, in the vapor phase, is at about 85 °C.

Vapor-Compression Stills

Compression of the water vapor that is formed in a still offers a means of minimizing energy expenditures. The compression of a gas results in a temperature elevation of the gas, and an increase in its thermodynamic enthalpy. The component water molecules, in undergoing compression, approach one another

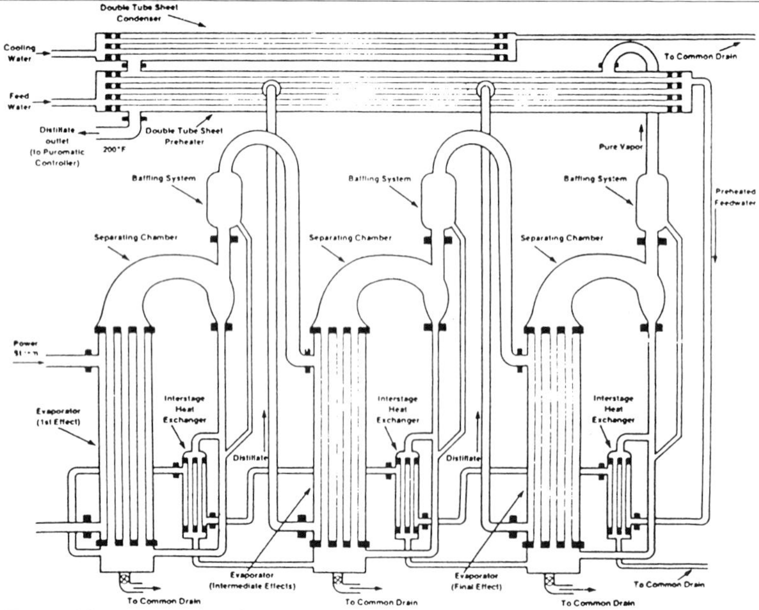

Figure 10-4. Typical multiple-effect still.
DiSessa (1980); Courtesy, *Pharmaceutical Technology*

more closely, and their mutual attractive forces begin to assert themselves more strongly. As a result of this thermodynamically more stable condition, the energy that had served to disrupt this closer intermolecular arrangement prior to the imposition of the pressure is emitted by the vapor molecules in the form of heat. The compression of the water vapor formed in a still thus serves to elevate its temperature, and convert it to usable heating steam. The mechanical energy required in the compression is quite small. The steam thus formed is used for heating water in the evaporator. Upon its becoming simultaneously cooled, it becomes converted to the condensed water that is the object of the distillation. The end effect of the vapor-compression (VC) still design is that no cooling water is required; more than 90% of the energy requirement is neutralized (Kuhlman,

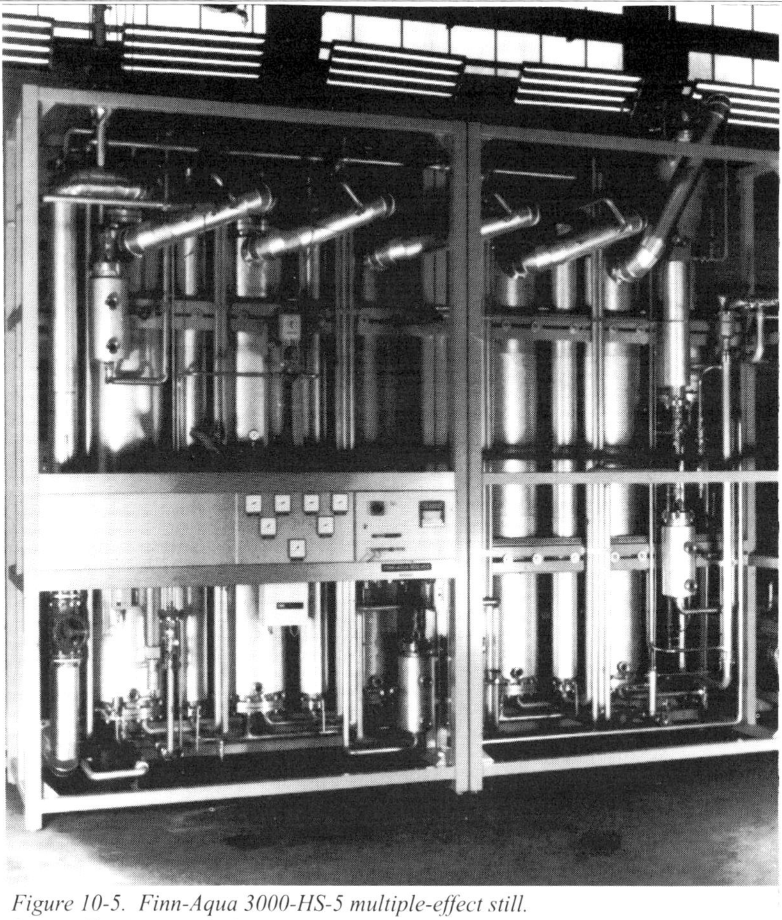

Figure 10-5. Finn-Aqua 3000-HS-5 multiple-effect still.
Courtesy, Finn-Aqua America Inc.

1981; DiSessa, 1981) (Figure 10-6).

Vapor-compression stills are designed to recycle the latent heat of vaporization of the produced steam. When the steam is condensed, the heat evolved is used to vaporize additional water.

In the conventional type of VC still, the feedwater enters the heat-transfer unit, where it is heated by the distillate. Then it enters the evaporator/condenser to be further heated to vaporization. The steam enters the condenser/evaporator, also a heat exchanger, where it condenses while preheating the feedwater. Additional energy efficiency can be achieved if the feed is also preheated using the blowdown steam within a counter heat exchanger.

Downstream of the evaporator in a VC still is a mechanical compressor that raises the saturation temperature and pressure of the vapor so that it can serve as a heat source for further evaporation. As the compression of the vaporized water molecules brings them closer together, their mutually repulsive forces are overcome. This results in the release of heat; just as the separation of the water molecules in close proximity requires the inflow of heat, to disrupt the Van der Waals attractive forces. Vapor compression stills operate on a pressure differential of 2 or 3 psig (about 1/5 bar). This produces a temperature rise of from 8 to 10 °F (about 2.8 °C).

The net energy requirement is the difference between the enthalpies of the vapor on the suction side of the compressor and the vapor on the discharge of the compressor. This enthalpy difference is much less than 970 Btu/lb_m, the heat of condensation. For the Aqua-Chem falling thin-film type of VC still, wherein the water is sprayed onto the tubes, it can be as low as approximately 142 Btu/lb_m of produced distillate if the distillate is discharged hot at 82 °C (180 °F) from the still, or about 52.6 Btu/lb_m if the sensible heat of the distillate is recovered and the distillate is discharged at 33 °C (92 °F) (Jackman, 1989). The Meco VC stills, wherein boiling water is on the inside of the tubes, give lower numbers. Smith (1991) suggests vapor-compression operating Btus in the range of 25 per lb_m. He gives 170 Btu/lb_m for a six-effect still; Jackman uses the figure of 238 Btu/lb_m for a top operating pressure of 116 psig.

Vapor compression stills can be arranged to discharge the distilled water at any temperature ranging from just below the boiling point (90 to 95 °C), down to nearly ambient temperatures of about 30 °C. The desired discharge temperature can be maintained by controlling the relative mass flowrates of distillate and feedwater within the feedwater preheater. In essence, a VC one-stage evaporator will deliver the water at about 95 °C., around 5 to 10 °F (3 to 6 °C) above the incoming feedwater temperature. Disi (1995) uses slightly different figures, namely, a low-temperature product water at 95 °F (35 °C), about 25 °F. (14 °C) above the feedwater temperature of 70 °F (21 °C). High-temperature product water is usually at 180 °F (82 °C). This accords nicely with the FDA preference for hot WFI water. If, however, additional energy is saved by the use of auxiliary heat exchangers, the outflowing water can be produced down to room temperature.

There is a perception, perhaps not entirely free of rival marketing inputs, that while the energy consumption of VC stills is low, the maintenance costs can be high because of the large number of moving parts such as compressors, gears, and belts. Furthermore, certain nonsanitary components of the compressor are in contact with the distillate. There is said to be a heightened possibility for contamination caused by wear and even by oil. The latter impurity may be insidious, its presence not being signaled by resistivity, the conventional testing. The newer VC stills meet Good Manufacturing Practice requirements, however, and do not have significant problems with their compressors, gears, belts, or pump seals (Smith, 1991).

There are two general types of vapor-compression stills. The Aqua-Chem type uses a thin falling-film evaporator; a pump is used to spray the feedwater over the pipe bundles. In the Aqua-Chem operations, the water enters at 40- to 50-psig pressure. It is designed for a 10:1 feedwater-to-blowdown ratio. Figure 10-7 illustrates this type of horizontal spray film VC still. In the Meco design, the pipe bundle carrying the product water heats the feedwater by being immersed in it. Figure 10-8 shows a calandrial-type vertical tube VC still. Partisan claims are made for each design.

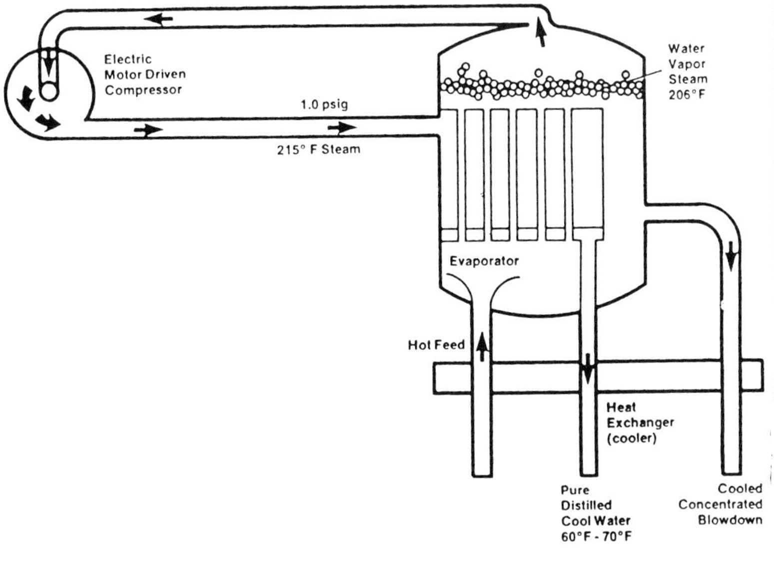

Figure 10-6. The principle of vapor-compression distillation.
DiSessa (1980); Courtesy, *Pharmaceutical Technology*

The Zyclodest Still

In a second type of VC design, called the Zyclodest, water is used continuously as a heat-exchange medium in a separate loop, helping to condense the steam produced by adsorbing its heat. It becomes vaporized thereby. It is then compressed to become even hotter before being allowed, in a heat exchanger, to heat and evaporate the incoming feedwater. The water used as the heat-exchange medium, now condensed to liquid, flows back through a pressure-reducing valve to where it again becomes vaporized by the heat it picks up, in a heat exchanger, from the vapor that it thus serves to condense. Then the cycle is repeated.

The Zyclodest process has been said to have a several advantages (Mahoney, 1982): 1) Operating at higher temperatures, above 100 °C, it is more efficient than other still types at removing volatile gases from the water being distilled. 2) It can be used to produce pyrogen-free steam for self-sterilization. 3) A cyclone design serves to free the rising steam vapors from entrained water droplets, thus eliminating liquid carryover. 4) The distillate is delivered under pressure, up to 20 psig (1.3 bar). Therefore, no pump is needed to transfer the distillate to the storage tanks. 5) Advantages are seen to derive from the design and construction itself; no moving mechanical parts are in contact with the distillate. It is, in effect,

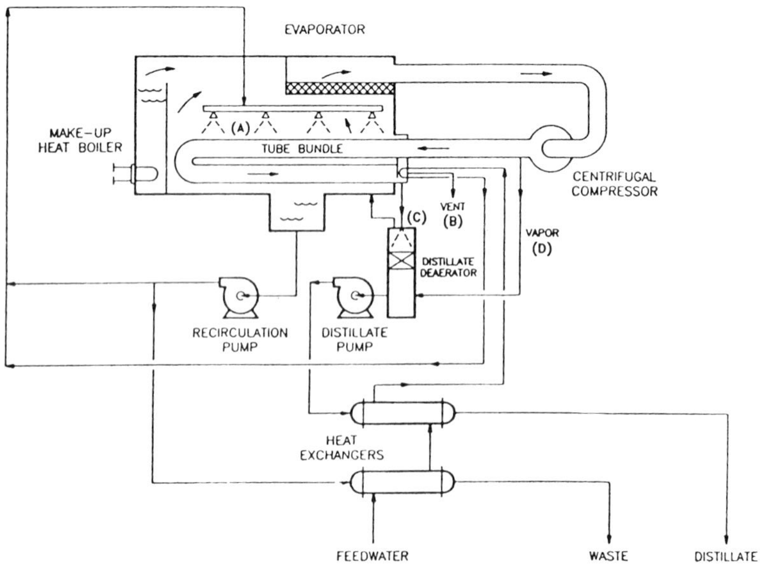

Figure 10-7. Simplified flow diagram, horizontal spray film vapor-compression distiller.
Courtesy, Aqua-Chem Inc.

a double-stage VC still (Smith, 1991).

The Zyclodest still is still being sold in Europe, albeit in small numbers. Only one such still is said to be operating in the United States (Figure 10-9).

Indirect VC Heating Cycle Design

In not-necessarily disinterested critiques, the single-stage still has been characterized as being simple in design, reliable in performance, relatively inexpensive to acquire, but intensive in its use of energy. The multiple-effects design has been viewed as offering a significant improvement in energy efficiency. The high-pressure steam requirements are considered, however, as being conducive to corrosion, as requiring expensive pressure vessels and interstage controls, and as heightening the risks of scaling and increasing the needs for maintenance.

Topper (1991) saw the VC still as being even more energy-efficient than the ME design, and some six times as efficient as the single-stage still. Considered as the VC still's greatest shortcoming, however, was the nonsanitary contact of the compressor with the pure water vapor during the transfer of compression-released thermal energy through a heat-exchange surface to the water. In an

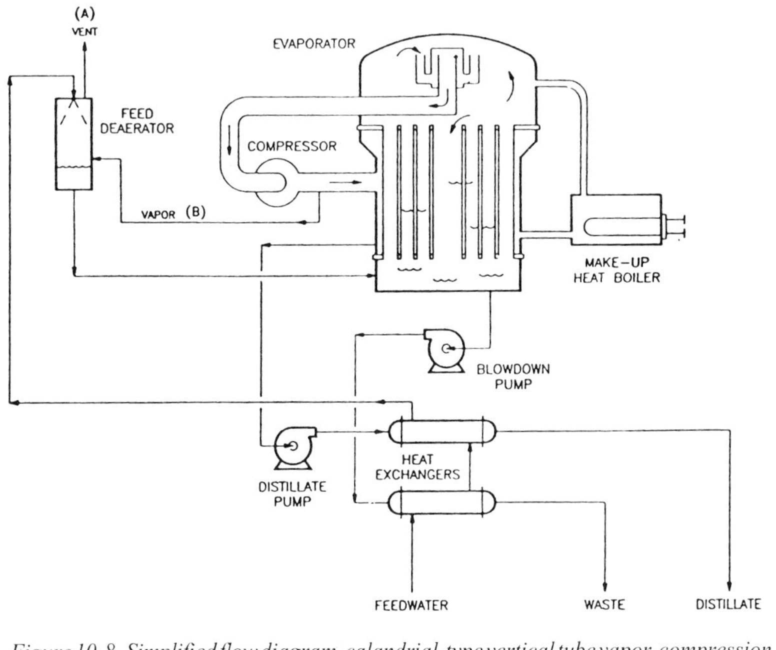

Figure 10-8. Simplified flow diagram, calandrial-type vertical tube vapor-compression evaporator.
Courtesy, Aqua-Chem Inc.

indirect vapor-compression heating-cycle design by Topper (1991), boiler feedwater was passed to a condenser where its latent heat was transferred to a secondary evaporating fluid. The compression of the vapors of this secondary fluid surrendered their latent heat to the boiling of the feedwater in a water vaporizer.

The principle involved is that common to heat pumps. It offers the advantage of using the secondary fluid to mediate the latent heat transfer. It is the vapors of this fluid, not those of the distilled water, that encounter the nonsanitary compressor. The use of positive displacement compressors with their high compression ratios becomes possible because lubrication cannot contaminate the distillate. Higher compressions yield higher temperature differences; this permits the use of smaller heat-transfer surface areas. Topper (1991) stated that the heat of compression was entirely used by this process.

The indirect VC heating-cycle design has an interesting lineage. In the 1950s work was performed at the University of Florida on this concept using a secondary Freon cycle. More recently, Australian stills have been designed using such a Freon refrigerating cycle (Smith, 1991). Topper (1991) projected the commercial application of his still design to the successful preparation of WFI-grade water.

Thermocompression Still

A variant on the vapor compression scheme was the Thermocompression Water Still.* Its advantage was that it required fewer moving parts, and no pump or compressor to remove the water vapor from the still. Rather, it used a steam-driven eductor operating on the venturi principle to create the compression, and the consequent temperature rise of the distilled water vapor. Because of the venturi effect, a partial vacuum was created on the boiling water surface in the evaporator, thus lowering its boiling point to 98.3 °C (209 °F) and facilitating its vaporization (Otten, 1976; DiSessa, 1980).**

The Thermocompression Water Still design (Figure 10-10) was roughly equivalent to a three-and-a-half effect still from the thermodynamic standpoint. Critics of its design stated it to be somewhat impractical, however, since an increase in the fouling factor or the tendency to form scale on the heat-exchanger surfaces cut the capacity exponentially. This negative scale effect was said to be caused by the reduction in the heat transfer which caused a slight back pressure on the steam coming from the eductor outlet. Thus the vacuum created by the

*Vapor compression stills are called thermocompression stills in Europe. In the United States, the identity is blurred because the term "Thermocompression" is copyrighted.

**Water vapor is in equilibrium with liquid water at any temperature. The quantity of water vapor, or its partial pressure above the liquid, increases, however, with rise in temperature. By definition, the boiling point is that temperature at which the pressure of the vapor equals 760 mm of mercury, the standard for atmospheric pressure at sea level. If the atmospheric or ambient pressure is lowered, however, the transition in the states of matter (the lower vapor pressure needed to define the lower boiling point) occurs at a lower temperature.

eductor was reduced and, of course, the temperature required to boil the water was increased.

The Thermocompression Still had a lower energy consumption than conventional stills, but higher than the vapor compression still. The capital cost was high. In any event, only a few of these stills were placed into operation, and some small number of these may remain in service. They seem no longer to be manufactured.

Useful details concerning still designs, operational considerations, and performances were given by Saunders (1981).

Stills should be equipped with visual or automatic temperature and high water level indicators. A level indicator should be present in the condenser. The stills should be provided with proper drainage and blowdown controls. On-line conductivity sensing devices should be employed in conjunction with automatic

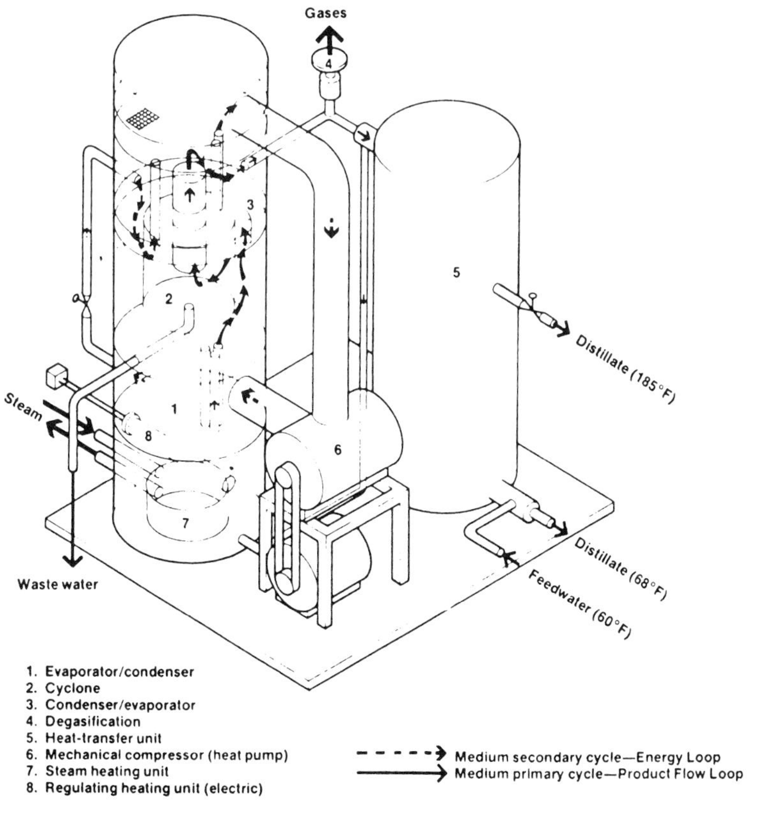

Figure 10-9. Zyclodest vapor-compression distillation system.
DiSessa, (1980); Courtesy, *Pharmaceutical Technology*

diversions to drains for those instances where the distillate is of unsuitable quality.

Some Specific Design Features

In the Finn-Aqua Still, the evaporator consists of a heat exchanger wherein steam encounters the shell side, and water to be distilled becomes heated thereby on the tube side. The heating vapor generated within the tubes exits from the evaporators along with heated but unvaporized water. The unconverted hot water flows into a chamber and out of the bottom of the evaporator and then out a drain, to be subjected to further vaporization in the succeeding still stages. The water vapor flows out the top. The water vapor formed in the evaporator flows into the plenum or chamber along with the heated but unconverted water. Being vapor, however, and hence of a lower density than liquid water, in the last stage it rises to the top of the chamber and out into the condenser.

Stills produced by Vaponics, Finn-Aqua, and others incorporate the same fundamental thermodynamic design. However, the design details differ. Some, like Finn-Aqua, incorporate tube sheets. In the Finn-Aqua, the tubes are fed from the top using a "falling film" heat-transfer principle; whereas others boil the water inside of the tubes of the tube sheet. This "falling film" evaporator design reduces the requirement for area, but also increases the relative effect of the fouling factor observed when a small amount of scale develops on the tube surface. Because the scale formation on both the Finn-Aqua and similar stills develops on the insides of the tubes, cleaning these tube surfaces would seem to be difficult. However, with surfaces made of 316L stainless steel, it is possible to circulate descaling solution without disassembling the still.

Vaponics uses the principle of boiling the water in individual evaporators. A return-bend tube sheet configuration is used. This allows the scale to develop on the outside of the tubes instead of the inside. Because of this, the scale tends to flake off the tubes when the tube cools down. A high-purity chamber, located in the bottom of the condenser, is included as part of the standard equipment. This feature reboils the condensed distilled water, removing volatile impurities continuously, and ensures that the water coming from the condenser is at the boiling point. Because of this feature, the purity from the Vaponics stills generally ranges between 8 and 18 megohm-cm of resistivity, temperature-corrected to 25 °C. In the Finn-Aqua still, the same effect is sought by maintaining the condenser under slight pressure, and at a temperature of somewhat above 100 °C. The problem is that there is difficulty in removing volatiles like carbon dioxide unless they are vented to the atmosphere.

Vaponics employs titanium as the preferred material of construction of the tube bundles. Prevention of corrosion of the evaporators of stainless steel fabricated stills, said to be possible, is sought. Titanium is also incorporated in the fabrication of the condenser coils as a standard material of construction.

Carryover of Impurities

Proper still operations are called for, otherwise solids may be carried over with the vapor, and volatile entities may remain in the condensate. Still design is addressed to the problem of entrainment.

The manner and rate at which heat is supplied to a volume of water in an evaporator will, among other things, govern the vigor of the vaporization process. Too ebullient a vaporization may serve mechanically to entrain nonvolatile particles along with the steam, thereby contaminating it. It would seem best, from this point of view, that broad but moderately fired heating expanses be used. Intense point heating could lead to the superheating of the water, with attendant carryover potential. Such intense point heating with its associated large temperature differential across the evaporator also increases the likelihood of scale formation.

Foaming is a potential problem in distillations. Jackman (1989) stated:

> Organics can promote foaming, allowing liquid to climb the walls of the still and carry over into the distillate. Foam affects both cyclone separators and mesh pad separators. However, the result is worse for the cyclone separator. Foaming is seldom evidenced by bubbles visible in the sight glass of a still. Any significant decrease from the surface tension of pure water, as caused by organics, can be defined as foaming, whether actual foam is visible or not. Such a surface tension decrease results in smaller entrained droplet sizes and hence lower distillate purity. Because foaming

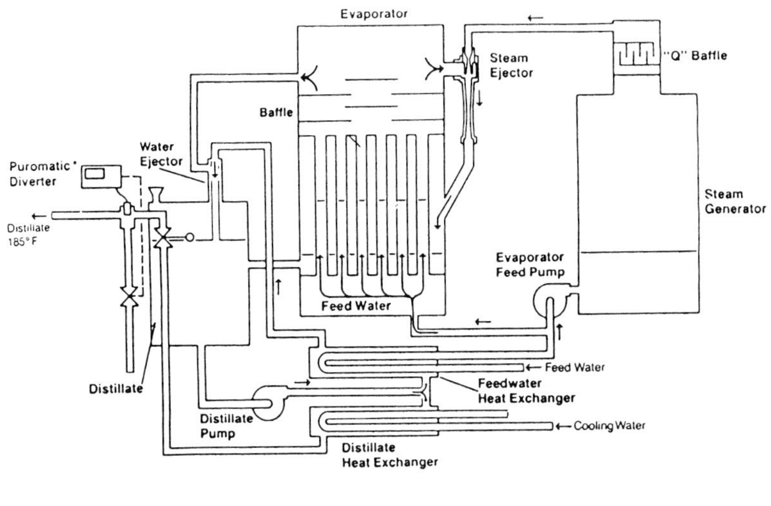

Figure 10-10. Schematic diagram of thermocompression distillation system .
DiSessa (1980); Courtesy, *Pharmaceutical Technology*

is seldom visible and may not be obvious, excess organics in the still feedwater can be a difficult-to-identify cause of water quality problems in a still. This is compounded by the fact that the presence of high organic levels is often intermittent due to the intermittent nature of bacterial excursions.

Smith (1991) believes that sodium ions in conjunction with organics could cause foaming. Some believe that the thermal decomposition of bicarbonates to carbonates, thereby producing carbon dioxide, is a cause of foaming. Indeed, it is often easier to distill seawater than freshwater containing organics or bicarbonate. Many waters contain as much as 10 grains of hardness and much bicarbonate; North Dakota waters are especially hard.

The concern in still design is with the rising water vapor, with its abilities to become separated from entrained water droplets, undistilled and therefore unpurified, that may accompany it on its upward flow toward the condenser. Condensation of such droplet-bearing vapors would inevitably contaminate the distilled water with the impurities resident in the entrained, unvaporized liquid water droplets. The three most common mist elimination devices are wire mesh pads, cyclone separators, and the "Q baffle." The wire mesh pads furnish surfaces upon which the entrained droplets can impinge to form liquid films that drain downward. The cyclone separators with their expansive chambers slow the velocities of the vapors, permitting their separation from droplets and particles.

The baffle system may involve the vapor steam impingement upon either dry or wetted surfaces (the latter are preferred); or the coalescence of small droplets into large, with their eventual removal by gravity. The volume variations caused by pressure or velocity changes serve to separate the water vapor from droplet and particle carryover.

In the Finn-Aqua still, the vapor rising through the annular space around the heat exchanger is forced to rotate by built-in guide members. Indeed, the rising, droplet-bearing vapors attain a strong centrifugal force in the process. This serves to fling the microscopic droplets with their contained impurities across a short space and through apertures in the surrounding wall, whereby they become separated from the ever-rising vapors. The centrifugally-separated droplets coalesce to a liquid film that runs down the wall to return to the still pot. The vapors continue upwards, eventually to become condensed (Figure 10-11).

Some stills that operate as typical evaporators are designed with a maximum possible disentrainment distance. This provides a vertical separation between the liquid level in the still and the point where the vapor stream is removed for condensation. The farther above the liquid level this removal point is, the greater the opportunity for liquid water droplets to drop out of the vapor stream under the force of gravity.

Low-vapor-velocity still designs utilize an evaporator of such sufficiently generous dimensions as to ensure that the vapor velocity generated is kept between 1 and 2 feet per second (ft/sec) (Figure 10-12) (DiSessa, 1980). Smith (1968) recommended a velocity of 0.5 ft/sec with water of tap water purity. For large-capacity stills, however, it could be impractical to incorporate the proportionately large evaporators that would be required for such low vapor velocities. Instead, stills in excess of 15 gph (57 L/h) and up to 2,900 gph (10,977 L/h) capacity depend on high-vapor-velocity design (50 to 200 ft/sec) [127 to 508 cm/sec] at the water surface, where the centrifugal forces inherent in cyclone

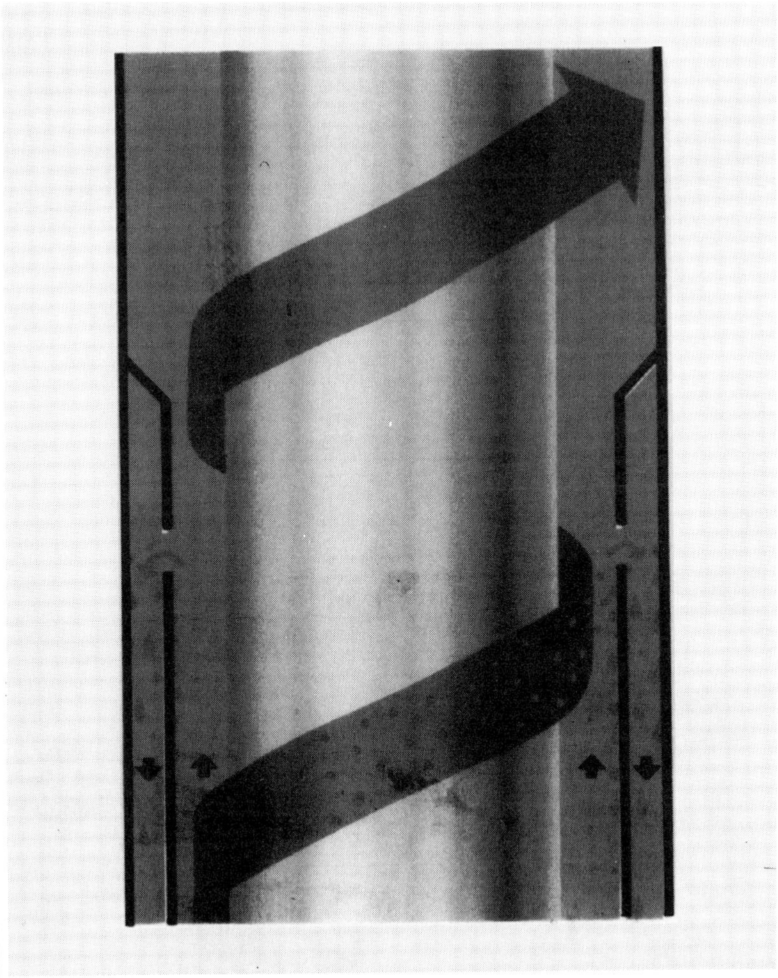

Figure 10-11. Finn-Aqua baffle arrangement.
Courtesy, Finn-Aqua America Inc.

separators serve to remove entrained droplets and particles from the water vapor stream (DiSessa, 1981; Saunders, 1981). Stills operating on the high-velocity "thermal siphon" principle do not have a maximum disentrainment distance (Figure 10-13).

As is presented by Jackman and Sneed (1990), the "theoretical efficiency of mist elimination devices is measured as the decontamination factor, DF, which is defined by

$$DF = \frac{\text{concentration of solids in feedwater}}{\text{concentration of solids in the distillate}} \qquad \text{Eq. 10-3}$$

"(Theoretical Decontamination Factors are usually measured in test systems operating on inorganic salts and therefore do not take into account the deleterious

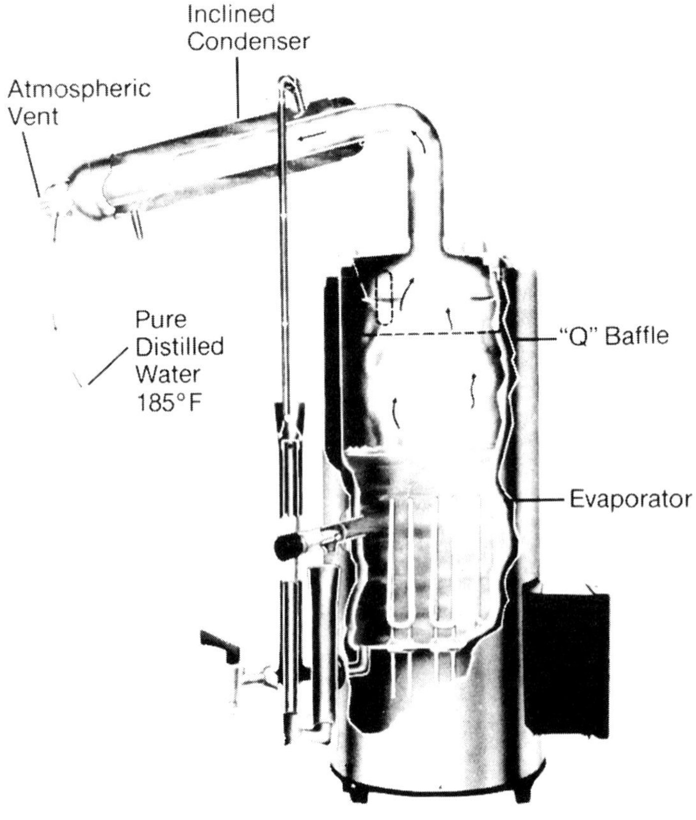

Figure 10-12. Low-vapor-velocity distillation principle.
DiSessa (1980); Courtesy, *Pharmaceutical Technology*

effect that foaming [caused by organics in the feedwater] can have on distillate purity.)"

Wire mesh pads can have decontamination factors of between 1.5 x 10^4 and 3×10^4. Finn-Aqua, which uses cyclonic separators on its stills, guarantees a reduction from 25 EU/mL to 0.125 EU/mL. This yields an effective *minimum* DF of 2×10^2 for cyclonic separators. Both types of mist eliminators normally produce water with better than 0.5 micromho/cm of conductance. (It should be noted that not all experts agree with these numbers.)

The still should be maintained properly to promote the correct performance

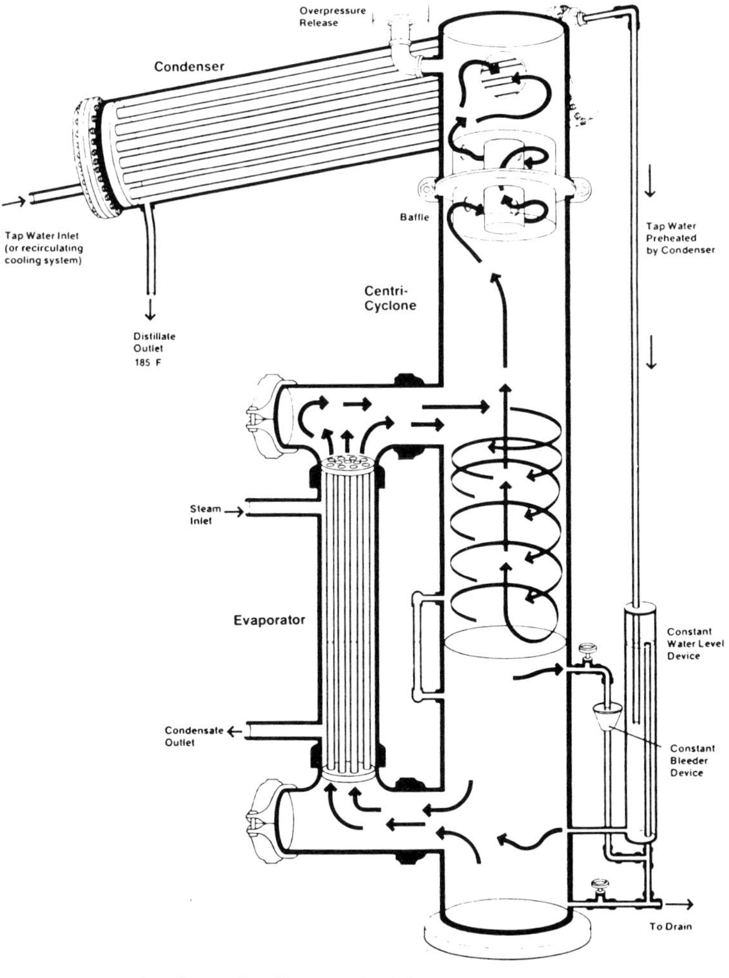

Figure 10-13. High-velocity distillation principle.

of mist elimination devices and the pretreatment system. Mist eliminators should be checked periodically for proper positioning and for corrosion.

The consequences of carryover would be aggravated by the fact that the impurities in the water concentrate at the liquid/air interface, which is the foam. The use of properly treated water ought to obviate completely such an occurrence. Nevertheless, some still design includes evaporation at a low vapor velocity, as well as the continuous removal of a foam by an internal foam dam and skimmer. The use of softened and deionized feedwater is the best solution (Smith, 1969), and serves to keep foaming from becoming a problem.

Despite the best still design, proper manipulation is required to secure desirable results. Instances have been reported where distilled water was found to be pyrogenic, presumably a result of droplet entrainment. For desirable results, a conjunction is required of the still, its operational manipulations and upkeep, and of the water fed it.

Condensate Feedback Purifiers

Smith (1988) pointed out that using a condensate feedback purifying system based on ion exchange is an especially effective way of pretreating feedwaters for single-stage stills. The purification train consists of twin-bed ion exchangers plus an organic-removal column through which the cooled raw steam condensate is passed. This serves also to remove amine impurities. The impurities are generally so low in concentration that the purification train is long-lasting. This makes it feasible to use disposable purification capsules even for single stills having capacities up to 50 gallons per hour. The feedback purifier system cannot be used on multiple-effect stills unless there is an additional source of condensate, because the raw steam condensate in such stills constitutes from 15% to 50% of the feedwater requirements. Smith (1988) also advocated the use of a condensate feedback purifier system as a pretreatment technique ahead of pure steam generators. These, to all intents and purposes, operate similarly to single-effect stills.

Reverse osmosis can effectively be used in a pretreatment mode for a distillation operation. To minimize the need for a pretreatment train for the RO itself, a very low recovery is used, about 10% instead of the customary 50% to 75%. This sharply reduces the prospects of scaling of the RO by reducing concentration polarization and maximizing the crossflow velocity. If a thin-film composite RO is used, chlorine must be eliminated. If a cellulose acetate RO is employed, the pH requires control. The reject water, in a ratio of 9:1 to the product water, is sufficient to operate the condenser without an additional requirement of cooling water to the still. The use of RO for this purpose is the subject of patents (Smith, 1988). Indeed, while RO treatments of water in combination with other cleansing practices can be used directly to produce Water for Injection, it has become increasingly the practice to utilize RO to treat water prior to its distillation (Smith, 1982).

Blowdowns

In any still, regardless of the feedwater purity, there is an inevitable buildup of residue in the evaporator, whether as a colored sludge or as scale. The scale interferes with heat transference and can result in damage from local overheating. To avoid a buildup in the concentration of the still-pot residues, most still manufacturers recommend that the evaporator contents be drained or blown down at regular intervals, and also whenever the still is shut down.

In single-stage stills, because of the latent heat characteristics of steam, the condensate volume always exceeds the production value by about 5%. This makes it possible to use 5% of the feedwater to continuously blow down the still evaporator. The blowdown purges the evaporator or still pot of its accumulated solids. A continuous blowdown makes it unnecessary to use periodic shutdowns between operations to achieve this purpose. When calculating the amounts of feedwater needed for a still, the volume required for blowdown should not be omitted. High-quality feedwaters prepared by RO or ion exchange may require 7% to 15% of the distilled product water for blowdowns. Most still designs include automatic continuous blowdowns. Softened feedwaters may require as much as 30% to 50% (Kuhlman, 1991). Effective blowdown operations are important. As scaling progresses, pieces of scale may break off and lodge in orifices to cause their becoming blocked. Flooding and spillover of the still by the feedwater may then result. Such hazards can be avoided by proper blowdown manipulations. The reduction of the need for extensive or frequent blowdowns depends, in turn, upon the purity of the feedwater.

Comparison of ME and VC Stills

It is not possible to compare directly the costs of operating a multiple-effects still with those of a vapor-compression still. Each has its advantages and limitations, and each has its partisan advocates. Aqua-Chem, a manufacturer of VC stills, offers its views of the comparative situation in Table 10-1. Jackman (1990) in Tables 10-2 and 10-3 presents typical operational and performance parameters for VC and ME stills, respectively. At present energy costs, if hot distillate i required, a VC still equates with a six-effect ME still. The vapor compression costs will be lower for cold distillate, the expenses for the heat-exchanger operation being absent.

According to Kuhlman (1991), the most important differences among ME still designs are as follows:

- Mueller "Pyropure" and Vaponics use the traditional method of boiling a fairly large amount of water into steam, while Finn-Aqua uses a "dry" distilling method with almost no water at the bottom of the evaporators.

- Mueller "Pyropure" uses the same Q-Baffle that they use on the single-effect Thermodrive stills. Finn-Aqua and Vaponics use centrifugal separation systems. The Finn-Aqua centrifugal separation takes place in the evaporator, and "planers" are used to shave off the impurities forced to the outer layer of the rotating steam pillar. Vaponics uses separate cyclone separators that function without planers. The Mueller "Pyropure" uses both a centrifugal separation system and a Q-Baffle that forces the steam to make a number of 180° turns.

- Mueller "Pyropure" and Finn-Aqua use double tube-sheet condensers while Vaponics uses double concentric tube-type condensers. Stilmas uses two condensers—one cooled with feedwater and one with cooling water. Finn-Aqua, Mueller "Pyropure," and Vaponics each use one condenser with separate tubes for feedwater and cooling water.

The primary difference between VC and ME stills vis-a-vis pretreatment is in the levels of various contaminants that can be tolerated by each still type without adverse effects. Generally speaking, ME stills are more sensitive to scaling and chlorine-induced corrosion than VC stills because ME stills operate at a higher top temperature, approximately 141 °C (285 °F), as opposed to 104.5 °C (220 °F).

Table 10-1
Relative Advantages and Disadvantages of VC and ME Stills

	Advantages	*Disadvantages*
Multiple-effect (six-effect); top pressure = 16 psig	1) No compressor requiring maintenance	1) Less energy-efficient than VC (238 Btu/lb_m vs. 142 Btu/lb_m thus higher costs 2) Requires greater pretreatment to prevent scaling because of high top temperatures and pressures. Fifth effect is especially subject to scale formation if blowdown in sixth effect is insufficient, thus higher pretreatment capital costs. 3) First effect sensitive to stress cracking and corrosion because of high temperature.
Vapor compression	1) More energy-efficient (142 Btu/lb_m vs. 238 Btu/lb_m) 2) Less stringent pretreatment requirements, runs "colder" than ME.	1) Has compressor that requires regular maintenance.

Courtesy, Aqua-Chem., Inc.

The VC stills may tolerate up to 0.5 ppm of chlorine (Jackman, 1991). The solubility of scaling salts decreases at higher temperatures. Depending on the raw water quality, pretreatment to a ME still may need to consist of a DI system; whereas pretreatment to a VC still may need to consist of only a softener. Even so, the still may have to be descaled periodically. Additionally, if the softened water contains bicarbonates, the still must be designed with cyclone separators, at added cost, to accommodate the droplet entrainment caused by the carbon dioxide formed by the thermal decomposition of these salts. The evolution of carbon dioxide causes foaming in the still. Its presence in the distilled water may lower the pH below the levels stipulated for the product water. A complete demineralization of the feedwater is obviously best from a technical point of view. Its costs require justification, however.

The VC stills are noisy, which may cause them to be located in relatively out-of-the-way areas, necessitating long reaches of water-distribution piping. Distribution has its own problems, as will be discussed, and shorter distribution systems can be more desirable.

Figure 10-14 is a photograph of an Aqua-Chem VC still; Figure 10-15 is a flow diagram of its operation. Vapor-compression stills that utilize thin-film evaporation mechanisms (e.g., Aqua-Chem) have greater deaeration ability than do certain makes of ME stills (Tom, 1990). The thin-film evaporation process acts as an air stripper and can remove low levels of VOCs without the need for special pretreatment. Volatile organic compound levels as high as 10 ppb can be stripped by this type of still. Levels remaining in the distillate are nondetectable by gas chromatographic analysis. Hence, use of a still with inherent deaeration capability may allow elimination of a carbon filter from the pretreatment system (Tom, 1989). Carbon beds may, however, be indispensable where trihalomethanes are to be removed. Distillation normally does not suffice for their elimination (Smith, 1991).

Despite those useful features of the Aqua-Chem type of VC still, the competitive MECO-design VC still has dominated the pharmaceutical market. Whether this is because of technical or for marketing reasons, it is difficult to say.

Feedwater Flows

Many stills require an even pressure and its resulting even flow of feedwater. Indeed, this situation is, in any case, preferred. Flows emanating from reverse osmosis units are generally not even. The use of a surge tank to provide even pressure to a booster pump inlet can be helpful. A more efficient still operation will result (Kuhlman 1994).

Feedwater Quality Requirements

Distillation is not an absolute process. The quality of the distilled product water bears a relatively proportionate relationship to the purity of the feedwater. The prevailing rule is, "The cleaner in, the cleaner out." Topper (1991) stated that distillation effects a hundredfold increase in the treated water purity. The 100-to-1 ratio was long ago developed as a guide for still operations. Smith (1991) pointed out that a feedwater containing 1,000 milligrams per liter (mg/L) of impurity will, indeed, produce water containing less than 10 mg/L, a 100-to-1 reduction. However, the average stills are fed waters containing 10 mg/L rather than 1,000 mg/L of impurity, and produce waters containing impurities in the range of 10 parts per *billion*. This is equivalent to a thousandfold increase in purity (Smith, 1991). It is evident that distillation can be an effective purification process. However, feedwater resistivity for stills should at least be one megohm-cm quality.

The purity of the feedwater, in addition to influencing the quality of the distilled water, may affect the integrity of the still itself. Proper still operation and maintenance requires the elimination or control of certain feedwater ingredients. The water must be free of components such as chloride and sulfate ions, which will cause corrosion; chlorine and ammonia, which will volatilize; hard or temporary hard-water components, or silica, (either colloidal or dissolved), which will result in interfering deposits on the evaporator surfaces; and organic substances, which will volatilize along with the water or which may cause foaming. According to Jackman and Sneed (1990), the TDS of the feedwater should be below 4 ppm.

Most of the stills used in industry today have significantly sophisticated pretreatment. Practically speaking, problems caused by feedwater impurities are

Table 10-2
Typical Operational and Performance Parameters for a VC Still (Aqua-Chem P600 VC Still)

Rated capacity	600 gph
Operating temperature	212 °F
Decontamination factor	1 x10^4 - 3 x10^4
Energy consumption	142 Btu/lb_m distillate produced (distillate discharge T = 180 °F) 52.6 Btu/lb_m distillate produced for distillate @ 92 °F.
Pretreatment Requirements:	
Langelier Saturation Index	negative (usually achievable with softening)
Silica (total)	6-10 ppm
Chlorine	0.5 ppm
VOCs	10-50 ppb

Recommended Preventative Maintenance:
1) Periodic compressor inspection required
2) Periodic cleaning for scale removal

Jackman (1990); Courtesy, Aqua-Chem., Inc.

relatively rare.

As stated, Jackman holds that soluble organics lower the surface tension of water, resulting in smaller than normal droplets existing in the two-phase mixture present in the hotwell of the still. These are too small to be retained by the effective pore size of the demister. Feedwater entrainment is the result.

Distillation, not being an absolute process, depends importantly upon the feedwater quality for the acceptability of its results. Most entrainment is inevitable. Its amelioration is a purpose of still design. The less pure the feedwaters, the more likely the carryover of the dissolved solids, and the lower quality of the distillate. Indeed, if the feedwaters are sufficiently high in TDS the demisters may be overwhelmed by scale formation. Such a buildup would alter the vapor flow pattern and velocity through the demister. Since the correct functioning of a demister or cyclonic separator depends on the proper velocities through the device, a narrowing of the flow channels could cause a short circuiting through the demister device. Higher than normal blowdowns, perhaps an increase to 20% from 10%, may help by reducing the impurities within the stillpot. Actually, an adequate pretreatment of the feedwaters must be relied upon. It should include ion-exchange or RO treatment. A good first approximation would aim for feedwaters having one megohm-cm resistivity. Less pure feedwaters can compromise the distillate quality.

A possible problem in distillation operations is the formation of scale on

Table 10-3
Typical Operational and Performance Parameters for an ME Still (Finn-Aqua 6-Effect Model 1000H)

Rated capacity	580 gph
Operating temperature	265 °F
Decontamination factor	25 EU/mL (feed) => 0.125 EU/mL distillate) => DF effective = 2 x10^2
Energy consumption	238 Btu/lb_m distillate (distillate discharge T = 210 °F)
Pretreatment requirements:	
Langelier Saturation Index	Negative
Conductivity	≥ 5 micromhos/cm (requires DI or RO treatment to achieve)
Silica (total)	≥ 1 ppm
Chlorine	0 ppm
VOCs	0 ppm

Recommended Preventative Maintenance Schedule:
(1) Cleaning for scale removal: 2-6 /yr, depending on quality of feedwater
(2) Metal stress inspections: Equipment teardown required if metal stress cracking or corrosion detected.

Courtesy, Aqua-Chem Inc.

heating surfaces. This can cause the local overheating and failure of electricity- or gas-heated tubes. For this reason, the dissolved-solids content of the feedwater is important. Deionization and demineralization of the feedwater to where its TDS is between 6 and 10 ppm (depending upon the still type) will avoid scale formation. The spontaneous cracking and falling off of scales will occur when convex scale-bearing heating surfaces cool and contract. This is sometimes promoted by the use of chilled-water sprays. For this reason, relatively large horizontal steam coils are used wherever possible (Smith, 1975). In the case of ME and VC stills, however, the heated water is usually contained inside the heat-exchange tubes in order to offer a large expanse of heat-exchange surface. Scale formation, whether adhering or not, could block the tube interiors. For such stills, the use of pretreated waters is essential.

There is a belief, perhaps reflective of marketing influences, that scale is more easily removed from vapor-compression stills than from their multieffect counterparts. Operating at higher temperatures, the ME stills, when they acquire silica deposits, convert them to difficult to remove vitreous coatings. The deposits formed on vapor-compression still surfaces are of a more mixed composition, being formed from less pure feedwaters. In consequence they are less glass-like and easier to remove.

The possible formation of scale in the boiler is well understood. Less widely

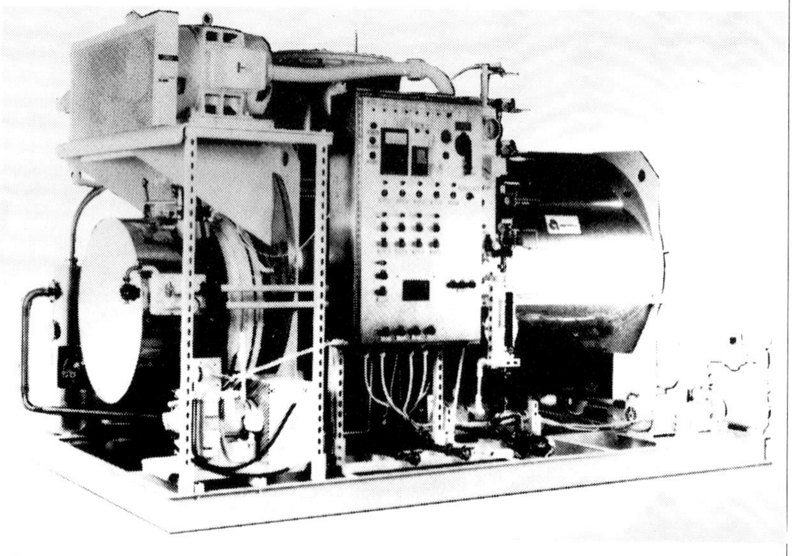

Figure 10-14. Aqua-Chem VC still.
Courtesy, Aqua-Chem, Inc.

comprehended is that the cooling water may form scale upon the surfaces of the cooling water coils. To avoid this possibility, the cooling water should be softened. Chlorides should also be removed from the cooling waters, as they may otherwise cause pinhole corrosion. This would permit cooling waters to mix with the distilled product water. The contaminated water would be manifest by an elevated endotoxin level and a lower resistivity in the product water. The avoidance of such corrosion requires the removal of chloride ions from the cooling water, as by ion exchange.

Kuhlman (1994) suggested that most failures of WFI preparation by distillation stem from improper feedwater pretreatment. In many cases such failures are obviated by the use of Purified Water as the feedstock. Ion-exchange produces better quality water than does RO. Kuhlman prefers the use of two-bed units over mixed beds. A two-bed strongly-basic unit produces better than 1-megohm-cm resistivity water. A valve leaking regenerating hydrochlorine acid may cause this corrosive agent to enter the product water. In two-bed systems such contamination is distanced from the still by the anion-exchange tower. Where mixed-beds are used, the still-corroding acid may directly access the still itself, to cause extensive damage. Kuhlman (1994) holds that reverse osmosis, even two-pass RO, is not always capable of producing feedwater of a quality adequate

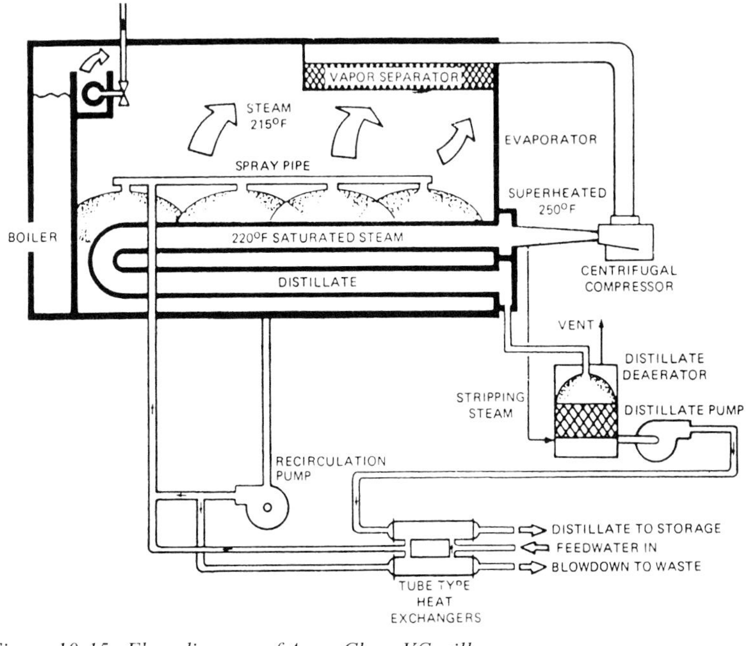

Figure 10-15. Flow diagram of Aqua-Chem VC still.
Courtesy, Aqua-Chem, Inc.

for stills. He advocates the use of electrodialysis followed by ion exchange, or reverse osmosis followed by ion exchange. The second of these arrangements is preferable because of its ability to remove silica and its scale-forming problems.

Ion-exchange resins can exhaust their silica-removal capabilities before they signal their lack of ion-exchange capacity. Kuhlman (1994) recommends therefore, that empirical determinations be made of the "gallonage" exhaustion of silica-removal capability, and that such experiences form the basis for ion-exchange regeneration.

Cleaning of Still Surfaces

Soluble silica can be distilled at very high temperatures along with the water vapor. Upon condensation, it can form a vitreous coating on the still surfaces. Interference with heat transference and still efficiency will result. The soluble silica should be removed by strong anion-exchange action. The boiler scale can be removed by an acid cleaning in place. Removal of silica will require treatments with an even stronger acid reagent. Concentrations of 0.1% to 0.15% ammonium bifluoride at 60 to 80 °C for 6 hours or so are required, depending upon the severity of the problem. Some use 10% phosphoric acid at 160 to 180 °F (70 to 80 °C). Others use citric acid, sulfamic acid, or mixtures of the two to remove rouge. Gsell and Disi (1994) believe, however, that 10% oxalic acid may etch the stainless steel surfaces if used in excess of 30 minutes. On occasion, reducing agents, such as sodium hydrosulfide, are also tried. Smith (1991)

Table 10-4
The Effects of Incomplete Degasification of Still Feedwater.

Dissolved Gas	*Carbon Dioxide (CO_2)*	*Ammonia (NH_3)*
Effect	Low pH distillate	Low pH distillate if present along with dissolved CO_2
Mechanism	(1) $Ca(HCO_3)_2$ <----> $CaCO_3$ + H_2O + CO_2 (2) $H^+ + CO_3^{-2}$ <----> HCO_3^{-1}	$P_{vent} = P_{steam} + P_{CO_2} + P_{NH_3}$; $P_{steam} >> P_{CO_2}, P_{NH_3}$; P_{steam}, P_{vent} are ~ constant ; P_{CO_2} = Constant - P_{NH_3} $\therefore P_{CO_2} \downarrow$ as $P_{NH_3} \downarrow$
Solution	CO_2 stripping using deaeration tank	Remove ammonia upstream using activated carbon or breakpoint chlorination oxidation to N_2

recommends the use of caustic in combination with EDTA. Dilute acids may be used, but they require circulation over longer periods of time. From the wide scope of cleaning agents that are variously used and recommended, it is fair to conclude that the problem of still-surface cleaning is complex and has no single solution.

The handling of such cleaning reagents has its risks. These were best avoided. It is preferable to remove the feedwater hardness and the soluble and colloidal silica before the water enters the still.

As will be described, in one situation silica was allowed to deposit upon the still surfaces. It did not accumulate beyond a certain thickness; added deposits broke off. The coating did decrease the still efficiency as regards heat utilization. However, the decrease in the still's output from about 3,000 gph to 2,800 gph was considered less expensive than the strongly basic ion exchange needed for removal of silica. Such deposits, often vitreous, are generally avoided as they can decrease the capacity of a still (by as much as 90%). At other times, the silica accumulates in the evaporator as a colloidal powder.

Amines

Among the organic compounds particularly to be considered in still operations are amines. These may have their origins in the thermal decomposition of strongly basic anion-exchange resins, or arise as residues from the manufacture of anion-exchange resins, whether strong or weak. Amines such as trimethylamine impart a fishlike odor to their aqueous solutions. Most of the amines commonly encountered are volatile, and are removed by distillation. Others may, however, condense with the water and not become separated. Even the amines that are too high in molecular weight to be volatile may codistill with the water vapor and recondense with the distillate. Such objectionable compounds must be removed, as by adsorption onto activated carbon, before the feedwater enters the still (Kuhlman, 1991; Smith, 1988).

Volatile Impurities

Such volatiles as carbon dioxide, chlorine, ammonia, and amines should be removed from the feedwater. Otherwise the high volatility of these substances will cause them to emerge from the still along with the condensed water, and to contaminate it.

It is sometimes the practice to have a wisp of steam emerging from the condenser to help carry off entrained volatiles.

For feedwaters with relatively high levels of dissolved gases, ammonia, or carbon dioxide, the deaeration or chemical removal upstream is important for optimum operation of either type of still. The presence of significant levels of dissolved carbon dioxide can produce distillate with low pH. The presence of ammonia will result in high pH. If ammonia is present along with carbon dioxide, however, the distillate may have a low pH (Table 10-4).

The probable presence of ammonia in waters containing chloramines has been remarked upon (see page 332). Its influence upon conductivity is profound; 1 ppm causes a reduction of 8μS/cm.

Organic Impurities

The literature references the possibilities for foaming to occur in still operations. However, it seems to have been a greater problem in the past than it is now. Nevertheless, its possible occurrence requires address.

Organic impurities can be of such a variety as to threaten corrosion of the still itself, as well as the quality of the distilled water. Distillation of soluble organic substances can occur in accordance with the rules of binary solution distillations. The constitution of the condensate may reflect ideal vapor/solution composition relationships, or yield the azeotropes of minimal or maximal vapor/solution situations. In any case, organic material may codistill with the water vapor.

Organic compounds that are not soluble in water but have a fair vapor pressure at elevated temperatures can steam-distill. For example, at some given temperature below its boiling point, the water may have a partial vapor pressure of, say, 690 mm of mercury (Hg) (below the 760 mm of Hg partial pressure necessary for its distillation). But if at this temperature the insoluble organic impurity has its own partial vapor pressure of as much as 70 mm of Hg, then the sum of the two partial pressures, exceeding 760 mm of Hg, will be enough to cause distillation of the mixture. The condensed water will contain the steam-distilled organic compound as a contaminant. In preparative organic chemistry, steam distillation is a useful device for isolating certain water-insoluble organic compounds from their reaction mixtures. The need to avoid its complications in WFI manufacture is, however, self-evident.

To eliminate problems with such organics, their chemical digestion with alkaline permanganate or phosphoric acid is recommended. Depending on the circumstances, the oxidative or hydrolytic destruction of such organics may be speedy, or may require as much as 48 hours. Interestingly, in multiple stills, the water being treated can be fed along with a digestive chemical into the first stage of the still for simultaneous organic destruction and distillation. Smith (1968) recommended that where two chemicals are involved in the degradative destruction of the organic impurities, the water be distilled three times at each of three different stages to avoid carryover. Particularly low vapor velocities are indicated for such procedures: less than 0.1 ft/sec (3 cm/sec) to accommodate the foaming tendencies of alkaline permanganate in the first stage, and not more than 1 ft/sec (30 cm/sec) in the final stage.

Recommendations can be found in the literature for removing small quantities of organics from waters that are pending distillation, or from the distilled water itself, by the use of "organic" traps, macroreticulated ion-exchange resins. (The use of these resins has also been suggested for the "self-sanitizing" of stored water [Kladko, 1982].) Interestingly, those relatively versed in these resins suggest their use before distillation, comprehending, no doubt, that these chemically modified, cross-linked polystyrene-based resins do inevitably leach organics. Their faith is in distillation as the final water-purifying treatment. Some whose expertise is in distillation, apparently aware of its limitations, pin their hopes on the "organic trap," of whose limitations they are less informed. Polymer chemists, it is suggested, would see the macroreticular ion-exchange resins as sites for organic adsorption and ion exchange, but also as loci for an inevitable, if small, leaching of organics.

The use of such deionizing resins in the preparation of WFI following distillation would, in any case, seem to be a violation of the USP regulations regarding WFI manufacture.

The removal of trihalomethanes by distillation is also difficult. These molecular species are so low in their molecular weights as to have vapor pressures similar to that of water. They are among the organics that constitute VOC (volatile oxidizable carbons), actually, volatile organics. Therefore, they substantially vaporize with the water and condense with it during the distillation process; separation is thus compromised.

Tom (1990) stated that the removal of THMs from ME stills requires the use of one or more highly efficient deaerators. These would serve to remove the THMs, other VOCs, and carbon dioxide as well. According to Tom (1990), the VC stills that boil the feedwater in vertically positioned tube (calandrial type) bundles are vented only at the feed deaerator. Depending upon the VOC and carbon dioxide content of the feedwater, more volatiles, including THMs, may become liberated subsequently but, not being able to escape, may be carried over into distillate. Tom (1989) stated, however, that a more efficient removal of volatiles (such as VOC and carbon dioxide) is managed in vapor compression stills incorporating horizontally positioned bundles. He ascribed this to the particular still design that encourages the liberation of volatiles.

Using a feedwater deaerator in conjunction with an ME still, Kroneld et al. (1989) achieved a removal of 98.4% of chloroform, 41.7% of benzene derivatives, and over 90% of the VOCs. The use of two feedwater deaerators gives better results. Employing a distillate deaerator may be better yet. Tom (1990) claimed, however, a complete THM removal from a level of over 100 ppb without special feedwater treatment using a horizontal-bundle VC still. Feedwaters varying in their THM content from 9.7 to 102 ppb yielded distillate free of THM. The detection limit of the gas chromatographic analysis is 0.5 ppb of THM.

Bacterial Endotoxin Removal

Distillation of a properly treated water should serve to prevent its endotoxin content from entering the product water. Distillation has been shown capable of removing bacterial endotoxins.

Varying quantities of pyrogenic material were separately fed to a standard three-effect Finn-Aqua still (Saari et al., 1977). The pyrogen sources used were 2.4 mg of *E. coli* endotoxin per 100 liters of softened water; 700 mL of *E. coli* culture medium per 100 liters of softened tap water (the limulus titer was 1:500); and increasing aliquot quantities of sewage sluice with 2,000 liters of softened water. The total distillation time was 5 hours. Samples were collected at hourly intervals, and their pyrogenic content was assayed by both rabbit and limulus amebocyte lysate (LAL) tests. Only in those trials involving some 8% of sewage sluice, when the limulus titer of the feedwater was about 1:5,000, was pyrogen carryover evident. At concentrations of as high as 6% of sewage sluice, pyrogen-free distilled water was produced repeatedly. Jackman (1991) advised that similar results were obtained with endotoxin challenges using VC stills.

Nevertheless, experiences exist where pyrogens have presumably been carried over in the distillation process. Still operations should not be taken for granted, nor the cleanliness of the feedwater neglected. Conceivably, bacterial endotoxin carryover results from foaming. This occurs when organics and organisms are allowed to accumulate in the feedwater. Proper organic removal should be instituted, and the correct sanitization of the pretreatment components should be practiced.

The work by Saari et al. (1977) notwithstanding, distillation, as other water purification processes, is not an absolute. It can be depended upon, however, to reduce the concentration of pyrogenics by 3 to 5 logs when properly performed.

Avallone (1992) called attention to the occasional spiking of bacterial endotoxin concentrations to levels of 250 EU/mL in the feedwaters intended for stills. This is presumably caused by the unloading of endotoxins by ion-exchange beds used to prepare the feedwaters. This, incidentally, is one reason why the preparation of WFI by the use of ion exchange is not permitted. Avallone related that each of three new stills, including multi-effects, were found periodically to produce WFI with bacterial endotoxin concentrations in excess of the stipulated 0.25 EU/mL maximum. Avallone, then an FDA investigator, concluded that the proper pretreatment for still feedwaters should include devices or operations capable of reducing endotoxin concentrations to below the quantities that still manufactures are willing to guarantee as results from the performance of their instruments. Such endotoxin reducing or eliminating agencies can be ultrafilters, usually of 10,000-dalton specifications, or charge-modified microporous membranes. It bears being stressed that the charge-modified filters remove oppositely-charged entities such as bacterial endotoxins on a stoichiometric basis; that such filtration conditions as flowrate, differential pressure, endotoxin concentration, and the pressure of competing molecules govern their endotoxin removal efficiencies; and that their exhaustion, unlike that of other filters, is not signaled by pressure buildups. Charge-modified filters can perform well. Their proper usage, however, requires their being appropriately managed. They should be arranged as described on page 210.

More importantly, Avallone (1992) concluded, "Unless a firm has a satisfactory pretreatment system, it would be extremely difficult for them to demonstrate that the system is validated."

Still manufacturers are reluctant, for competitive reasons, to stipulate bacterial endotoxin log reductions. One still manufacturer does guarantee a 5-log reduction. Generally, guarantees of 4 to 5 log reductions can be obtained for still performances either at the still manufacturer's plant or at the use-site, provided the feedwaters contain no detergents (foaming), or volatiles including chlorine and ammonia; and have a conductivity of greater than 5 micromhos, the reciprocal of 5-megohm-cm resistivity. Certainly, the feedwater stipulations require no less than 1-megohm-cm of resistivity. Stills are tested with feedwater spiked to between 100 and 1,000 EU/mL bacterial endotoxin units per milliliter. Vapor compression stills specify feedwaters free of volatiles and of hardness.

Finally, the feedwater whose quality is imperiled by a blow-through of bacterial endotoxin laden product water from the ion-exchange resins would almost certainly signal such an occurrence by a high conductivity, and the product water from the still would probably show the high conductivity of high CO_2 contents.

Whatever the situation, the feedwater to the stills requires being guarded against excessive bacterial endotoxin concentrations.

The conjunction of stills and RO optimizes the precleaning of feedwaters, and contributes to better still operations. USP Purified Water offers advantages as a feed for still operations. Its limited organism population serves to minimize its endotoxin level, rendering endotoxin carryover less likely. Also, it minimizes problems associated with scale formation within the still.

Distillation of the pretreated water should serve to eliminate the pyrogens from the product water.

Pharmaceutical Applications

The *USP 23* monograph on Water for Injection says that WFI may be produced either by RO or by distillation. Japan, in its domestic market, permits WFI prepared by reverse osmosis, ultrafiltration, or distillation. For its exports to the United States, it uses WFI manufactured by distillation (Jackman, 1991). This is in recognition of the FDA's strong preference for WFI prepared by distillation. Distillation is generally seen as being more troublefree than RO. Indeed, were WFI to be prepared by RO in the United States, the FDA would insist that it be accomplished by double-pass RO, product-staged.

Neither RO nor distillation, the two accepted methods for producing Water for Injection, can be relied upon automatically to guarantee the desired product quality independent of a maintenance-free operation. Distillation is favored, not necessarily because of any inherently greater reliability on its part, but because it involves heating the water, and producing it at elevated temperatures. As a result, the threat of organisms is eliminated, or at least sharply reduced.

Distillation is seen as a self-sanitizing process. At 80 °C, only spores and extreme thermophiles can survive; most thermophiles will not grow above 73 °C. Most waterborne organisms are killed at 60 to 80 °C. Most pathogens will not grow above 50 to 60 °C. Moreover, purified waters do not supply them the nutrients they require. Vegetative organisms will not grow above 60 °C, and mesophiles and psychrophiles will not grow above 50 °C. *Legionella pneumophila* is reported as sometimes surviving at 50 to 55 °C.

The FDA recognizes that water emanating from stills can be bacterial endotoxin-free. However, more than the mere use of a still is involved. Still operations can be mismanaged so that bacterial endotoxin becomes entrained into the distillate; this despite the fact that at least some stills can be operated to give endotoxin-free effluent from sewage water (Saari et al., 1977). What is required are such proper practices as are known to deliver WFI (in other words, an accordance with GMP).

It is very important to test the water produced as it exits from the still and before it enters its storage tank. In some cases where bacterial endotoxin has been found downstream of stills, it was found to have been caused by carryover in the water vapor. In at least one case, it leaked through pinholes that resulted from corrosion of the walls of the heat exchanger, purposely made thin to promote heat transfer, and thus liable to easier breaching through corrosion.

Although WFI need not be sterile, it is known that the use of stills according to manufacturer's instructions will dependably yield sterile water. The finding of organisms or endotoxins in the water exiting from the still will be taken as evidence of a serious dysfunction, whether of the still, and/or of adherence to pertinent GMP, or both. Such a judgment is independent of the utilitarian suitability of the water, as for nonsterile dosage forms, for instance.

A still operated under GMP is intended to yield sterile water. A still that yields nonsterile water, endotoxic or not, is outside the use sanctioned by GMP, and the FDA would deem the operation out of control.

Most of the stills used in the United States as well as elsewhere in the world are used in laboratories for the ordinary production of pure water for laboratory purposes. With the advent of ion exchange and RO systems, the emphasis on small stills has become reduced. Nevertheless, sales of stills producing 1 gallon per hour continue to be robust.

Water for Injection is prepared almost exclusively by distillation, and the use of distillation is heavy in applications allied to the health industries.

In a parenteral operation, only about 10% of the product water is used in formulations. Most of the remainder is used for the final rinsing of components and vessels, as required by the FDA. Often WFI-quality water is used for the entire wash cycle, to avoid the handling of different grades of waters. In applications where it is feared that expensive products may be jeopardized by unknown water impurities, distilled water may be used even though it is not mandated by any regulation. This is frequently the case in biotechnology settings and in diagnostics work. On occasion, WFI is used even where USP Purified Water would suit simply because in its representation of pharmaceutical purity the WFI, invariably prepared by distillation, assures against any uncertainties regarding its quality.

An example can be given of a parenteral manufacturer who distills WFI by way of VC stills of some 3,000-gph capacity. The stills are equipped with heat exchangers to yield hot WFI as required. The water produced is stored in 35,000-gallon tanks.

The plant's feedwaters originate from wells going as deep as 300 feet, and having flows as high as 500 gpm. The water contains 48 to 70 ppm of silica, 88.5 ppm of TDS, some bicarbonate hardness, and has a pH of 7 to 7.2; the wells differ somewhat in their water characteristics. A chlorine analyzer controls the addition of chlorine at 2 ppm to the raw water storage facility of about 50,000-gallon capacity, from which water of potable quality is flowed into the plant by a booster pump at 80 psig. The daily water consumption can be in excess of 350,000 gallons.

The water is flowed through carbon beds whose management is described on pages 374, Chapter 7. It is then deionized in a series of twin-bed ion exchangers. The rate of water flow through an ion-exchange column is about 45 gpm. The ion-exchange beds undergo triple regenerations to insure their maximum capacity. The cation-exchange bed is regenerated every 250,000 gallons, which equates to about every other day. A two-stage process uses 2% sulfuric acid followed by 4% sulfuric acid. The anion-exchange bed is weakly basic resin, for its ease of regeneration. It is regenerated when its effluent waters show a conductivity of 13 micromhos/cm. This equals a resistivity of 750,000 ohms-cm.

Before bed regeneration, the cation-exchange resin is backwashed with 145-gpm flows for 15 minutes to loosen the bed. The anion-exchange backwash of 15 minutes for the same purpose is at a flowrate of 85 gpm.

The pH of the water coming off the anion-exchange beds is around 4, because of the release of carbon dioxide from the bicarbonate present in the water. The carbon dioxide is removed by a steam degasifier before the still. The TDS of the effluent from the ion-exchange beds is 36 ppm (compared with the 88.5 ppm of the raw water). The endotoxin content of the feedwater can be as high as 20 EU/mL, but is usually lower. The water is analyzed daily for organisms, and weekly for endotoxins. The alert limit is 300 cfu/mL; the actual count is usually zero.

The silica content of the raw water, not removed by the weakly basic anion-exchange resin, enters the still, as does its small hardness component. Scale forms, but does not continue to accumulate. After a thin, vitreous layer forms, the remaining scale drops off. The stills are cleaned annually, using sulfamic acid. The scale that does adhere is not a problem. It manifests itself by diminishing the heat transference, so that perhaps 2,700 gph rather than 3,000 gph are produced. This is considered a tolerable price to pay for the ease of regenerating weakly basic resins. The water entering the still contains 36 ppm of TDS, and the distilled water contains 3 ppm of TDS.

The distilled water analyzes daily at zero cfu/mL, and at well less than 0.25 EU/mL in endotoxin. It is stored hot at 85 °C in a recirculated mode within the WFI storage tank.

The FDA's "Guide To Inspection of High-Purity Water Systems" (1993), the following remarks appear about stills:

> Most of the new systems now use multi-effect stills. In some of the facilities, there has been evidence of endotoxin contamination. In one system this occurred, due to malfunction of the feedwater valve and level control in the still which resulted in droplets of feedwater being carried over in the distillate.
>
> In another system with endotoxin problems, it was noted that there was approximately 50 liters of WFI in the condenser at the start-up. Since this water could lie in the condenser for up to several days (i.e., over the weekend), it was believed that this was the reason for unacceptable levels of endotoxins.
>
> More common, however, is the failure to adequately treat feedwater to reduce levels of endotoxins. Many of the still fabricators will only guarantee a 2.5 log to 3 log reduction in the endotoxin content. Therefore, it is not surprising that in systems where the feedwater occasionally appear in the distillate (WFI). For example, recently three new stills, including two multi-effect, were found to be periodically yielding WFI with levels greater than .25 EU/ml. Pretreatment systems for the stills included only deionization systems with no UF, RO or distillation. Unless a firm has a satisfactory pretreatment system, it would be extremely difficult for them to demonstrate that the system is validated.
>
> The above examples of problems with distillation units used to produce WFI, point to problems with maintenance of the equipment or improper operation of the system indicating that the system has not been properly validated or that the initial validation is no longer valid. If you see these types of problems you should look very closely at the system design, any changes that have been made to the system, the validation report and the routine test data to determine if the system is operating in a state of control.

Steam

The distillation of water creates steam that, being a gas, enables its separation from nonvolatile matter. The condensation of water vapor, steam, transforms it into the water that is the subject of this writing. However, steam as such finds important applications in pharmaceutical processing as well. It is much used for its heat transference properties.

Service steam. Steam is used in the pharmaceutical industry in at least two ways: first, as plant or service steam for general heating purposes, as generated in steam boilers; and second, specifically to achieve the sterilization of the surfaces it is led to encounter. The generation of steam in steam boilers must contend with corrosion of the boilers and of the piping used to convey it, generally of iron or carbon steel, particularly in older installations. The valves and instrumentation in such systems are often of bronze or brass, also subject to corrosion. Such service steam may be contaminated with imperfectly removed dissolved constituents of the feedwaters, or of the water treatment chemicals, the feedwater additives, utilized to purify the boiler water. Rust and scale attendant upon corrosion and the deposition of insoluble materials are usually also present in plant steam. In addition, such steam entrains volatile organic additives, usually amines, ammonia derivatives utilized for their basicity to prevent corrosion.

Filtration of service steam to remove solid particulates is often employed using woven wire, sintered, or matted metal filters. However, borosilicate glass fiber filters are also used for this purpose. Usually, 0.5-μm- or 1.0-μm-rated filters composed of 316L stainless steel are used. When such filters are used, they should be replaced for cleaning when the pressure drop increases by 50% (Lukaszewicz et al., 1984). Such filters are incapable, however, of removing the volatilized organics. The impurities present in service steams are usually pyrogenic in character (Forster, 1982). The use of service steam for the sterilization of surfaces meant to encounter pyrogen-free pharmaceutical preparations is, therefore, eschewed.

Clean steam and pure steam. The distinction between clean steam and pure steam is not too widely agreed upon. Some see "pure" steam as signifying its preparation in conformity with GMP requirements, while "clean" steam, albeit also free of additives, may have been prepared in equipment containing features including threaded connections. In this view, clean stem is not in accord with GMP; it is equipment dependent. Others define clean steam in different terms, namely, as steam generated by boilers.

In the vaporization of water, the purity of the water vapor, and hence of its condensate, may be compromised by the mist or water droplets that may become entrained. When a boiler is used, that is what inevitably happens. Clean-steam generators are boilers. Therefore, the water vapor they create (clean steam) is essentially of the same quality as the feedwater whose droplets are entrained.

The vapors emanating from the first stage of a multistage still are free of mist and droplets because of the demisting action inherent in the still design. This steam is pure steam. Its condensate is Water for Injection. It is free of the impurities present in the feedwaters. Pure steam is pyrogen-free.

Clean steam is defined by Latham (1995) as that which is generated from treated waters free of volatile additives such as amines and hydrazines. It is presumably free of droplet entrainment. It may, therefore, be used for introduction into autoclaves, piping, and other production equipment in efforts to sterilize and disinfect same, or to humidify clean rooms. It is its chemical purity that differentiates it from plant steam. Clean steam meets GMP requirements to avoid product contamination.

Where the clean steam condensate is equivalent to the quality of WFI, it may be called pure steam. Essentially, pure steam, in addition to having the chemical identity of clean steam, is free of pyrogenic agents. Pure steam is required where the use of WFI is indicated, as in the aseptic processing of ophthalmics and parenterals, and in the sterilization of WFI systems and their distribution loops.

Smith (1995) is in agreement with the above definitions and descriptions, but indicates, as well, that the appellation "clean steam" is sometimes extended to plant steam treated by way of a high-efficiency filter to remove particles to a given specification. Volatiles, if constituents of the feedwater, will not be removed.

Increasingly, pure steam is derived from stainless steel stills fitted with stainless steel condensers and tubing, and operating on feedwaters suitably demineralized and prepurified. When multistage stills are used to prepare Water for Injection, the first stage of each such device lends itself for use as a pure-steam generator. There is no need, therefore, to rely on the plant steam to achieve pyrogen-free steam sterilizations.

Steam can be withdrawn from the first stage of the multistage while it is in operation making water. In other cases, clean steam may be produced only when WFI production is stopped. However, if too much steam is withdrawn, the mass effects in the second stage may become disturbed. The design of the orifices in the several stages requires that a certain minimum flow be maintained through them.

Steam sterilizations are usually accomplished by maintaining the item to be sterilized at 121 °C for 15 minutes. In such practices it is necessary to validate that the equipment or article being steam sterilized was actually at 121 °C for the requisite period of time. The time interval involved in bringing the object up to that temperature is not considered part of the sterilization cycle.

Pertinent properties of steam. Heat flows from conditions of high temperatures to those of low. In this regard heat is like a fluid that flows or diffuses in response ot gradients, whether of concentration or pressure. Thus, a hot object in contact with a colder object will lose heat to it, the temperatures of both articles tending to equilibrate. The transfer of heat through various media is, however, subject to the heat transfer properties of the media (as measured by their heat transfer coefficients) or inversely, to their insulating properties.

To sterilize an article at 121 °C, it would, in principle, suffice to encounter it with heated air. However, air has a low heat transfer coefficient, approximately 5 to 50 Btu per hour per square foot, per °F, as compared to 1,000-8,000 for steam. It would, therefore, require air heated to about 4,000 °F. to deliver an amount of heat furnished by steam at 250 °F. (121 °C) (Forster, 1982).

Because steam, unlike heated air, undergoes a phase change from gas to liquid at 100 °C, it has a latent heat content. (At 250 °F (121 °C), it is 945 Btu/lb compared to zero for air.) When the steam condenses, the water molecules comprising its gaseous state are brought into the much more stable thermodynamic condition. Therefore, the internal energy common to the more disruptive situation of the gaseous state, the latent heat of condensation, becomes available for heat transfer purposes, as in the case of steam. The water formed by the steam condensation must, of course, find accommodative removal. It is for this reason that steam is so suitable as a heat transfer agent, a means of effecting sterilizations.

Coalescing filters and cyclone demisters. The carryover of liquid droplets by the steam vapor may serve to contaminate the clean steam with whatever impurities characterize the feedwaters of the still. Therefore, removal of the

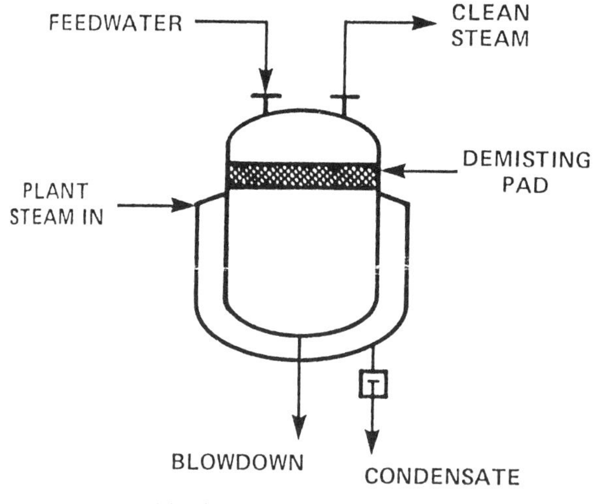

Figure 10-16. Jacketed-kettle steam generator.
Forster (1982); Courtesy: Stearns Catalytic Corp., Philadelphia, PA; and *Pharmaceutical Technology*.

entrained mist is important. Coalescing filters, usually but not necessarily mats of 316L stainless steel fiber, are used to provide extensive surfaces on which the water droplets can deposit by inertial impact, and coalesce into drops large enough to separate out as a flowing liquid film in response to gravity. The principle of action is that the porous medium in the coalescing filter is wettable by the entrained discrete water droplets. This serves to overcome their surface tension, with the result that the droplets form a liquid film that drains away. In clean-steam generators, opportunities for water droplet coalescence are provided by internal baffle designs, and by the use of woven mesh demister pads that perform on a velocity liquid scrubbing principle (Forster, 1982).

The internal baffle designs of clean steam generators (stills) may also create centrifugal forces that serve to separate entrained water droplets from the steam. Such cyclone designs can produce an acceleration of about 500 g to the generated steam vapor. This high centrifugal force arises from the geometry of the flowpath. In principle, the steam feed is introduced tangentially into a cylindrical portion of the apparatus. A rotational motion is imparted thereby to the vapor, which throws the entrained droplets outward to the walls where they form a thin liquid film that drains away at the bottom while the demisted steam escapes from on top (Purchas, 1981; Forster, 1982).

By means of such devices, clean steam may be prepared free of entrained water droplets, and hence be in a pyrogen-free condition for use in pharmaceutical steam sterilization settings.

Clean steam generators. Clean-steam generators are available as packaged units. These usually include all the necessary accoutrements including the feed-water pump and the relevant instrumentation. Mention has already been made of the use of the first stage of a multistage still to serve as a clean-steam generator. Pure steam generators are of the same design as the clean-steam devices. They use WFI as their feedwater.

Largely, clean-steam generators fall into two design types. In one, steam is generated from water contained in a jacketed kettle. The steam arises through a demisting pad to be conducted to its point of application (Figure 10-16). In the second design, called a shell-and-tube heat exchanger, the water to be converted to steam is fed into a container. It is vaporized by means of plant steam contained and circulated through tubes led into the water-containing shell. The generated steam exits through a demisting pad to its applicational site (Figure 10-17).

In both design types, provisions are made periodically to blow down, and hence clean, the water-containing vessel of liquid that has become rich in concentrated impurities left behind by the steam evaporation (Forster, 1982). Clean (pure) steam generator designs and systems are treated by Latham (1995), and particularly by Smith (1995).

Operational requirements. Lukaszewicz et.al., (1984) summarizes the requirements for clean steam generation and distribution:

1. Only nonvolatile boiler additives, if any, should be employed to reduce corrosion by lowering the oxygen content of the distribution system, and to reduce scaling and corrosion of the boiler.
2. The boilers, as also the distribution piping should, as in the case of Water for Injection manufacture, be of 316L stainless steel and of welded construction.
3. Ball-type valves should be used in the steam lines.
4. Steam condensate should not be returned to the boilers. Hence, the boilers should not be fitted with integral condensers. The condensation of the steam is to be managed subsequently in a separate stage of the process.
5. Final point-of-use filters of stainless steel rated at 0.5 to 1.0 μm should be employed to remove particles that may have become generated in the system upstream of the boiler.
6. The point-of-use filters should be cleaned when they have undergone a pressure increase of some 50%.
7. Sampling ports protected by 0.2-μm-rated Teflon membrane should be used daily to monitor the steam both microscopically and chemically for possible impurities. Contamination sources should be addressed.

Pharmaceutical uses of clean steam. Pure steam is used extensively in the pharmaceutical industry. It is used to sterilize the surfaces of equipment and

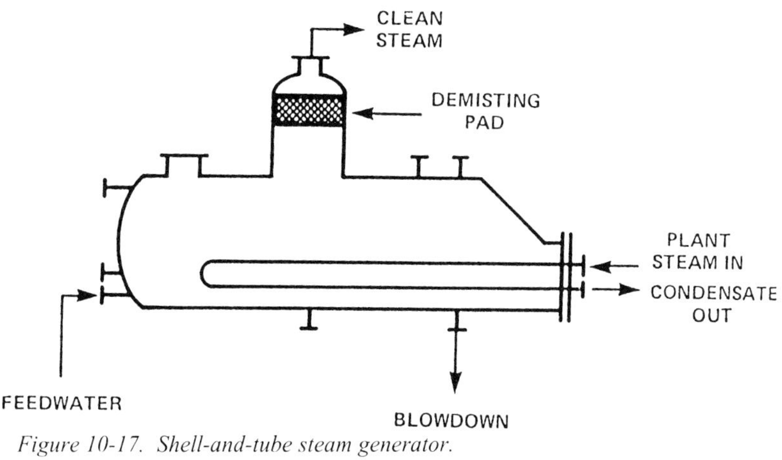

Figure 10-17. Shell-and-tube steam generator.
Forster (1982); Courtesy: Stearns Catalytic Corp., Philadelphia, PA; and *Pharmaceutical Technology.*

containers intended for contact with sterile, pyrogen-free preparations. Clean steam is used in the sterilization of such small equipment parts as small containers and filling-machine heads. The steam-in-place sterilization of formulation tanks, the attached pertinent pipes for conducting the compounded preparation, the filters intended for the purification of the solution, the vent filters, and even of the filling machine may all be accomplished using clean, live steam at 121 °C. The term *live steam* identifies steam heated to temperatures above 100 °C, steam under pressures above atmospheric.

Large sterilizers utilizing large volumes of steam are employed in terminal sterilizations of product, as of large-volume parenterals. In such situations, the product water inside the glass container equilibrates to the same vapor pressure as the surrounding, sterilizing steam. Therefore, there is no glass container breakage caused by pressure differences.

Clean steam is also used to introduce necessary degrees of humidification in particular pharmaceutical manufacturing contexts. One such circumstance relates to the control of the proper relative humidity in filling rooms by way of heating, ventilating, and air-conditioning (HVAC) systems. Another is the humidity level required for ethylene oxide sterilizations.

Clean steam is used in these various settings to help achieve the requisite degree of sterility necessary to pharmaceutical processing.■

CHAPTER 11

DISTRIBUTION AND STORAGE, MATERIALS OF CONSTRUCTION, AND CORROSION

In order to achieve high quality at the point of use, the materials used in the construction of water storage and distribution systems should be selected in accordance with certain design criteria, and they require being assembled by appropriate techniques. Succinctly stated by Sanders and Furne (1986), such considerations include the following:

- Wetted parts and materials require smooth, nonporous surfaces.
- Jointing methods (either piping or linings) should minimize crevices and discontinuities.
- Materials should not contain biologically degradable substances that can be nutrient sources.
- Materials should not contain leachable additives such as pigments.
- Jointing methods should minimize or eliminate the use of glues or solvents capable of migration into the water.

In the pharmaceutical industry, the stainless steels have been the materials of choice although polymerics are widely used, and are sometimes preferred or even necessitated. In the semiconductor industry, the polymerics largely constitute the materials of construction. Early on, PVC was widely used; PVDF, among other fluoropolymers, is a more recent selection.

Hungry Water

High-purity water, particularly because it has been freed of ions, is very corrosive. It is described as "hungry water," a characterization of its corrosivity. Deionized water displays a neutral pH (7.0) only at 25 °C. At elevated temperatures, the pH is increasingly below 7.0. The water is thus more avid in its acidic attack on metals at higher temperatures because of the presence of greater concentrations of hydrogen ions.

The presence of minerals in normal water often results in the deposition of protective coatings on metal surfaces. These coatings serve to shield such areas from further corrosive contact with the water. Deionization, or even the softening of water, removes the minerals that offer such mediating interfaces; and exposes the metal to normal but relentless corrosive attack by the water, seemingly more aggressive because it is unremitting.

Both high-purity water and the trace amounts of the components it contains exhibit chemical behavior different from that manifested by higher constituent concentrations (Lerman, 1988). Because highly purified water is chemically aggressive, the materials of construction of the tanks used to contain it and of the pipes employed to convey it are important.

Stainless Steel Composition

Austenitic stainless steel containing both chromium and nickel is usually used in one or another of the several alloy forms constituting the series. In the United States, four types of stainless steel predominate: 304, 304L, 316, or 316L (American Iron and Steel Institute, SS601-477-25M-GP, 1977).

The composition of the steel is significant in at least two respects. First, it must be capable of withstanding corrosion; and second, it must not cause changes in resistivity properties consequent to being welded. For high-purity water and pharmaceutical-product installations, concerns with materials of construction center largely on corrosivity. Because of their relatively high resistance to corrosion, the stainless steels are used in the fabrication of stills, tanks, and their interconnecting tubing.

For a stainless steel grade, the designation L signifies a low carbon content, particularly desired where welding operations are to be employed. The heat required for welding of stainless steel causes a segregation of its carbon content within the heat-affected zone. There the carbon forms carbides with the metallic components (for example, chromium carbide). These carbides are particularly susceptible to intergranular corrosion in a way that a metallic component itself (for example, chromium) is not. Thus the steel's resistance to corrosion is lowered.

To minimize the opportunities for carbide precipitation, the amount of carbon is restricted in the L-grade stainless steel formulas. Both 304 and 316 can contain as much as 0.08% carbon. Their L grades can be composed of less than 0.03%. Other properties of the stainless steels are also affected, some adversely so, by the formula changes involved in the lowering of the carbon content. Price differentials result also. There is room for individual evaluations to be made. If, say, standard 20-foot (600 cm) lengths of stainless steel tubing are to be clamped together rather than welded, then a lower carbon content may be unnecessary.

The clamped sections of pipe cannot simply be interchanged with the welded. Fittings that are clamp-ended may not be L grade. They may well have a different metallurgy. The clamp ends are welded onto pipe. This may require being followed by an annealing or other treatment.

The chief difference between 316 and 304 is the molybdenum content (about 2.5% in the 316 grade). Molybdenum is regarded as conferring greater corrosion resistance, as it minimizes chromium carbide formation. This facilitates the formation of chromium oxide, whose inertness is the object of using stainless steel. It may well be, however, that in particular contexts the resistivity of 304 stainless, in widespread use because of earlier reliance placed on it, is more than adequate.

In practical situations, cost/benefit analyses should be made before the grade of stainless steel is designated. Indeed, in a recent major pharmaceutical installation, 316 tubing was chosen for contact with deionized water, while 304 tubing was selected for the conveyance of distilled water. The reasoning was that 304 stainless steel is considered more corrosion-resistant at low temperatures, while 316 stainless steel is judged to be better under hot temperatures. Tanks and tubing may be exposed to different temperatures. Usually, the tanks face a more demanding environment and are often fabricated from a higher, more resistant alloy. The tendency in this country is toward welded systems of continuous running lengths of tubing and fittings, although some clamp joints may exist to enable the servicing of particular items of equipment. In such installations, 316L stainless is the material of choice. Valley and Rathbun (1977) recommended that 316L be used for all equipment surfaces that come in contact with deionized or distilled water. However, neither opinion nor practice is unanimous in the industry.

It is said that 316L stainless steel has better resistance to pit corrosion than does 304L, and that the latter is more difficult to weld. More importantly 304L is not standard in all sections. The use of two differing metals can more likely be avoided therefore if 316L is used because valves and other parts are more readily available in this composition. The mixing of metals is believed to predispose to corrosion.

A superior resistance to corrosion is shown by 309 stainless. It is used for high-temperature strength and scale resistance. Grade 310 is similar to 309 but has a higher alloy content to give even higher improved high-temperature strengths and scale resistance than 309. Stainless 316 has the best corrosion resistance of all the grades. It resists pitting and is inert to most chemicals. The 316L grade is an extremely low-carbon stainless steel, as corrosion-resistant as 316. Grade 321 contains titanium, which stabilizes welds even under conditions of severe corrosion. It gives no carbide precipitation during welding, and shows excellent resistance to corrosive chemicals (Combs and Veloz, 1990).

In short summary, 304 stainless is corrosion resistant enough at low temperatures. Higher temperature levels require the 316 grade. The 316L type, having a lower carbon content, is more suitable for welding. Its resistance to corrosion is not greater than that of the 316 stainless steel.

In Europe the trend has been to 316 Ti, a titanium-containing stainless steel—

more costly and harder to work, but said to be more resistant to intergranular corrosion after welding. Because of its toughness, 316 Ti stainless steel does not lend itself to finer mechanical finishes. Table 11-1 compares the composition of 316L and 316 Ti stainless steels.

Welding of the Stainless Steel

Welding is the preferred method of joining the stainless steel sections, whether of tanks or tubing, because it eliminates the intrusion of cements or fillers and avoids the introduction of interstices that are the result of clamping sections together, albeit in conjunction with gaskets. Welding, properly performed, presents a smooth, unbroken, corrosion-resistant surface. The smoothness is important, for pinholes and crevices are seen as locations wherein microorganisms may lodge and flourish. The purity of the metal used in the welding is obviously important, and first-rate welding skills on the part of the welder are essential.

Tubing versus Piping

The choice between tubing and piping is generally made on the basis of which is more suitable for the welding process. Tubing has both its inner and outer diameters specified; while piping has only its outer diameter given, and that only nominally. The tighter specifications for tubing, making for a more reliable welding practice, explain its widespread usage. Piping will more markedly vary in its dimensions than tubing (ASTM A-269, ASTM A-270). Thus, pipe has only a nominal outer-diameter (o.d.) specification. A 2-inch o.d. (5.08-cm) pipe can actually be 2.28 inches (5.79 cm). Stainless steel sanitary tubing of a 2-in o.d. (5.08-cm) will be within 0.002 inches (0.0051 cm) of specification.

Variations in outside/inside diameter, in wall thickness, in ovality (out-of-roundness), and in concentricity all influence the welding operation and its outcome. Dimensional irregularities at pipe joints may serve to harbor organisms. Smooth-welded joints, highly regular transitions from one pipe length to another, are therefore what is desired. Once a welded joint is made of two 20-foot (610-cm) tubing lengths, there is no easy means by which the inside surface of the joint can be polished. The disposition to joint smoothness is ensured by the use of stainless steel sanitary thin-wall tubing.

Ease of welding is not the only factor in choosing between pipe and tubing. Pipe is difficult, if not impossible, to polish adequately. Moreover, sanitary fittings are tube-o.d.-sized, leaving virtually no option other than the use of tubing. Tubing need not necessarily be thinner than pipe. Schedule 5 pipe has the same wall thickness as 16GA sanitary tubing (Manfredi, 1991).

Tubing Welds

For butt-end welding of tubing in sanitary installations, the use of filler metal is avoided. The ends of fittings are usually true and square as manufactured. The tubing may be further cut at the construction site, by an abrasive cutoff wheel, and its end made true by facing with a belt grinder. However, abrasive cutoff and belt grinding are normally not acceptable for sanitary installations since inclusions may be imparted by this technique, and the heat engendered can alter the metallic structure. Another method is to use a low-rotations-per-minute (30 to 40 rpm) radial-type saw, lubricated, to effect the squaring cut. Facing is then often not required, but can be made if necessary, such as by abrasive grinding. In any case, any abrasive cutoff or end preparation should be finished by facing and/or machining.

The trued tubing ends (or tubing and fitting ends) can be welded together without the use of filler metal.

Welding is a skill, and as such its outcome is a product of the particular welder's abilities. Prudent establishments qualify their welders. Samples of welds are required beforehand. Standards are set. Welds performed on the job are inspected, whether by borescope or even by actual, if occasional, excision. Efforts should be made to secure qualified mechanical contractors.

Welded tubing can be inspected for smoothness of the weld by use of a borescope with fiber optics that permits examinations of the tubing throughout its 20-foot length. Welds are often numbered, and each completely characterized by a series of three photographs. At least one camera company, Olympus, offers a flexible borescope and camera for this purpose. A permanent record of each weld results. The use of a video scope and videotaping is currently replacing the borescope. Welch-Allyn is an industry leader in this practice.

The quality of a weld can be probed in several ways. A visual examination of its external surfaces, such as by borescope, may be revealing, particularly to an experienced observer. The use of a dye bath to disclose subtle penetrations such as pinholes and microscopic cracks may be helpful. However, the use of dye is best avoided, for the dye must then be removed by cleaning. X-ray examinations made from various angles may, by a lack of uniformity in the X-ray image intensity level, disclose porosity or other insufficiencies in the metal fusion process.

Table 11-1
Compositions of Stainless Steel

	316L	*316 Ti*
Carbon	<0.3	<0.06
Chromium	17.0-17.5	17.0
Molybdenum	2.2-2.8	2.2
Nickel	11.5-14.5	11
Titanium	0.0	>5% carbon

Courtesy, *Survey of Stainless Steel Grades*, Vereinigte Edelstahlwerke, AG, Vienna, Austria

Increasingly, particularly in the pharmaceutical industry, the tendency is to utilize automated welding devices to reduce operator subjectivity and its variability. (Presumably, however, the essence of skill is to know when to make those departures from a standard procedure that are required by particular circumstances. Indeed, this is seen as the great advantage of customizing.) In any case, there are automated welders that rotate the torch around the joint to be welded. Some of the devices are computer-programmed to take into consideration the wall thickness of the tubing, to make certain the sameness of duration of the welding-torch action per given arc of the joint, and to ensure the proper flow of argon or other inert gas. Overall, the intent is to derive a proper, smooth weld without the overheating that would be conducive to unnecessary carbide precipitation. An advantage of this automated welding machine is that it can have a callback and printout feature to see whether the actual welding action did indeed conform to the programmed intent. The printout has utility, possibly along with photographs of the internal weld surfaces, as a hard-copy audit, often kept as part of a permanent record. Such printouts and callbacks are optional. Their inclusion is based upon the equipment used and the job specification.

The welding is performed in the absence of oxygen to avoid the oxidation of the stainless steel components. The general term for this type of welding is TIG welding, for tungsten inert gas, although other weld methods are also performed in the absence of oxygen. Argon is the inert gas most frequently used. Helium is not recommended for stainless steels. A mixture of 95% argon and 5% hydrogen for the torch gas can reduce the heat required by as much as 15% (Manfredi, 1991). Arc welding is a means of focusing and concentrating the heat on a given spot, thereby avoiding the unnecessary overheating of a more general area. The use of inert purge gases on the insides of the tubes greatly reduces oxide buildup, and results in a smooth inside weld joint (American Iron and Steel Institute, SS803-479-25MGP, 1977; Artiss, 1982b).

Fabrication of Stainless Steel Tanks

The thickness of stainless steel tank walls reflects the intended duty cycle, the mechanical stresses for which the tank is designed. It will make a difference in tank wall thickness whether the tank is to be of a vertical or a horizontal geometry; whether it is to support agitators and where they are to be positioned (top, bottom, or side); and whether the tank is to withstand vacuum or pressure, and to what level. The heat transference properties of jacketed walls need to be considered as well. It is possible that the tank walls may be so thick as to resist the degree of heat penetration necessary to the melting of the stainless steel during welding.

The large steel sections required for tank fabrication may make it impossible to correctly true and square all edges. In such circumstances, the welder may use fill material from stainless steel welding rods. One concern with filler metal is its composition. It is possible to secure welding rods that contain such impurities as will predispose the weld to corrosion. The source of the filler metal should be known with reliability. While it is an object of skillful welding to secure smooth welds, the use of an even overlay of "smear metal" is considered undesirable, as it may create hard-to-reach crevices where impurities, bacterial and otherwise, might become lodged and difficult to remove. Very thick material is beveled and welded in stages, and filler metal is required for this procedure. Virtually all joint configurations over 0.109 inches thick are thus performed (Manfredi, 1991).

The securing of good welds, in addition to considerations of contamination sites and cleanliness, can have economic value as well. Tanks can be made of less costly, thinner metal if their sufficiency of structural strength can be ensured.

Thinner metal necessitates that fewer tank apertures be used. It is advisable to use multipurpose tank inlets. Considerations of ease of cleaning also impinge on tank design and affect the metal thickness and welding practices necessary to tank fabrication. Standard tanks are the least expensive because the fabricator already possesses the tools and designs. Additionally, the required amount of welding is minimized. In such standard arrangements, low-profile manways are used for ease of cleaning and serve also as common inlets for multiple fittings.

Stainless steel is susceptible to the catastrophic failures of stress cracking as induced by contact with chlorides. Therefore, the insulative lagging used to minimize heat loss on pipes and vessels should be made with chloride-free materials. Cera wool, one such substance, is available from Manville Filtration and Minerals, Denver, CO, for this purpose.

Coupling a storage tank with a jacket that permits heating in effect converts it into a heat exchanger. A jacketed tank both heats the tank contents and provides for storage, saving part of the cost of a heat exchanger, which itself often is a vessel with a heating jacket. However, the stresses imposed upon a tank by heating and cooling considerably shorten the life of the tank. When failures occur, they usually take place in the jacket rather than in the tank itself.

Jackets are affixed to tanks in any of several ways. The jacket or outer shell may be welded to the inner tank all along its outer borders. The inner, circumferential space makes room for circulation of the heating fluid. In a second type of joining, the shell is dimple-welded to the inner tank walls, with spot welds replacing the peripheral welds. A third type of welding the jacket to the tank is a blend of both methods. However performed, the welding tremendously works the walls of the inner vessel, and distorts them with the stresses and strains caused by the welding. There is the possibility of tank failure at such stress points. Usually, however, system redesign dictates the replacement of tanks long before they fail (Manfredi, 1991).

Passivation and electropolishing treatments are made to protect tank and pipe surfaces against corrosion. Tank surfaces, because of their large expanses and the thinness of the metal, are often in a dynamic mode. They are given movement by cyclical temperature experiences and by the flexing caused by evacuation pumps. Passivation coatings can thus become shed or abraded, as by water scouring at pipe elbows.

Surface Finishes

Surface finishes of the stainless steels are seen to be very important. Crevices and crannies may shield impurities against removal, and rough surfaces are considered more encouraging to biofilm formation than are smooth surfaces, despite evidence that organism attachments speedily and inevitably form in either case. There are various ways to impart mechanical finishes: mill roller finishes (productive of a matte appearance); bead blasting; and various abrasive finishes, progressively applied. Mechanical finishing is extremely variable in quality and very dependent upon the application technique. Furthermore, mechanical finishing can trap impurities, may mask blemishes, and increases the exposed surface area. Chemical or electrochemical finishing, commonly called electropolishing, is considered better (Manfredi, 1991).

Abrasive Polishing

Polishing treatments bear numerical designations that imply the number of grit lines per inch; the higher the value, the smoother the surface. The final grit finish—for example, 260—should be approached progressively; first treatment uses 60 grit, then 80, 120, 180, and so on until 260 is reached. The surface should be brought down consistently from that of the raw stock. Curiously, a more reflective finish, although not so smooth a surface, may result from omitting intermediate steps. This is sometimes done to cut costs in the mistaken belief that the better-appearing surface is the smoother. The modes of mechanical polishing can differ, as also their effects. The polishing can, for instance, be applied radially, longitudinally, or circumferentially.

Table 11-2
Surface Measurements Comparison

RMS (Microinch)	*RMS (μm)*	*RA (Microinch)*	*RA (μm)*	*Grit Size*
80	2.03	71	1.80	80
58	1.47	52	1.32	120
47	1.20	42	1.06	150
34	0.86	30	0.76	180
17	0.43	15	0.38	240
14	0.36	12	0.30	320

These values are the average data of many tests. Therefore, slight deviations from the norm do exist. However, because of the number of tests performed, reasonable accuracy is assumed. Because of the many variables that create this data, deviations of ± 5% would be considered well within good measurement parameters.

DCI, Inc. *Bulletin on Material Welds and Finishers,* (WF, 890-1);Courtesy, DCI Inc., St. Cloud, MN

The ability to characterize large surfaces by measurement of very small areas requires statistical considerations that are very seldom met, though the standards for surface finishes and their measurement have improved. Meeting those standards is still an art. Microinch, roughness average (RA), and RMS finish specifications are checked by use of a profilometer, a stylus device used to trace across the surface profile. Such measurements more accurately reveal the surface RA, and are used to evaluate surface finishes (Tables 11-2 and 11-3). Figure 11-1 reflects surface smoothness measurements relative to biofilm adhesions (Vanhaecke and Van den Haesevelde, 1991).

Electropolishing

The use of abrasive particles to remove gross imperfections from stainless steel surfaces inevitably induces scratches, potential refuges for organisms, in those surfaces. It is said also that in mechanical polishing, such as with the aid of an abrasive wheel and polishing compound, there exists a possibility of mechanically folding over or bending down of protruding metal roughnesses in such a way as to hide cracks and scratches and to imprison within them, for slow release, the corrosion products of the debris of construction they contain. This is objectionable (Artiss, 1982a).

Electropolishing, essentially the electrolytic reaction opposite to the electrodeposition of metal, is preferred. The practice employs phosphoric acid in an acidic electrolyte solution. Electropolishing is performed after mechanical polishing. It preferentially removes protruding metal, thereby smoothing roughnesses. It also tends to even out scratches and crevices by making them

Table 11-3
Microinch Surface Roughness Versus Abrasive Grit Finish for Tri-Clover Finishing Processes

Surface Roughness (Microinch Finish, AA [RA]) Maximum	*Nominal (Approx.)*	*Approximate Equivalent Abrasive Grit Finish*
10	7	500
12	8	400
15	10	320
20	13	240
26	16	180
32	20	150
45	26	120
83	45	80
140	75	60

Proper electropolishing will reduce roughness of grit finishes (exclusive of surface imperfections) by approximately:

40% at microinch finishes greater than 20

30% at microinch finishes greater than 20

Courtesy, Kalamazoo Electropolishing, Kalamazoo, MI

more shallow and less abrupt. It thus conveys a higher degree of polish to the metal surfaces. To some small but significant dimension, possibly 1 mil, iron is preferentially removed from the stainless steel surface by electropolishing. This endows the finished coating with the character of a nickel/chromium oxide cladding that exhibits enhanced resistivity to corrosion.

Electropolishing is particularly effective in removing smear metal from welds to reveal the true character of the underlying surfaces. The use of electropolishing to avoid the folding of metal over fissures or scratches, such as may occur in mechanical polishing, is considered one of its advantageous features.

Yet electropolishing, although it has its strong advocates, is hardly universal in practice. It is an expensive process and may find restrictions in its application on the basis of cost-benefit study analyses. Thus, as one study has it, the imposition of a 2B finish by the use of glass bead abrasions adds some 10% to the cost of the stainless steel. The conferring of a number 4 finish would add 25% to the cost; and electropolishing would add 50%. Some estimates place electropolishing as constituting 80% of the total cost of all finishes.

In the electropolishing technique, the metal being electropolished is attached to the positive pole of a direct current source. Using as electrolyte a solution mainly of sulfuric and phosphoric acids, the electric current is passed from the workpiece to the cathodic electrode. Metal dissolution occurs at the workpiece anode; more takes place at surface peaks and irregularities. A smoother workpiece results, less likely to provide crannies hospitable to shielded organisms. Microscopic burrs and fissures as well as embedded particles become removed by the electropolishing that confers a high gloss to the treated metallic section (Mangan, 1991). A reduction in surface area results.

Electropolishing can be considered a form of passivation in that the resulting surface is chromium-enriched, a result of the removal of inclusions, cracks, and tears, all sites promotive of corrosion. Moreover, electropolishing, being an anodic process, generates oxygen, the action of which may in itself contribute to the formation of the passive chromium oxide layer on the stainless steel. According to Mangan (1991), electropolished surfaces examined by electron spectroscopy for chemical analyses (ESCA) and auger analysis show higher chromium oxide contents than do nonelectropolished areas. Mangan cited work done with radioactive bacteria and with sucrose solutions to attest to the more ready cleanable surfaces derived from electropolishing.

Although the surface finishes may well influence the ease of attaining the requisite degree of cleanliness and the avoidance of contamination, the overriding governances are the upkeep and maintenance protocols that are practiced daily.

Field Usage

There is no universally accepted standard for surface finishing for stainless steel.

Tubing in the United States is usually of an interior 180-grit finish (Giorgio, 1978). More recently, Manfredi (1991) held that 150-grit interior finishes predominate. But in the Chicago, IL, area alone, two large pharmaceutical manufacturers rely on 150-grit finishes, one on a 180-grit finish, and one on a 180-grit finish following by electropolishing. Stainless steel pipe having lengths of 20 feet and diameters of 1/2 to 4 inches can be had in electropolished condition. Water for Injection is usually flowed through pipe finished to a 240- to 320-grit

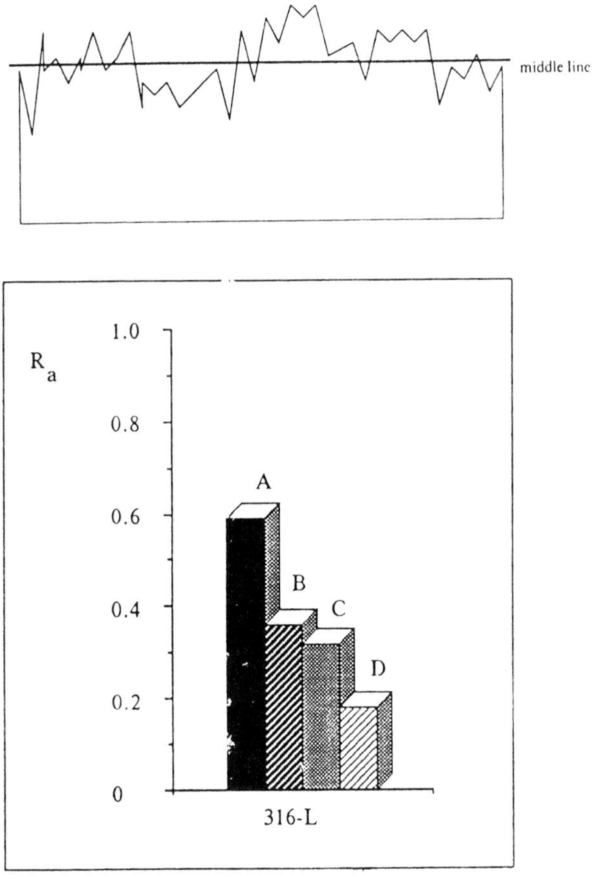

Figure 11-1. TOP: Surface roughness profile of an unelectropolished stainless steel material as measured by a perthometer. BOTTOM: R_a values of a 316-L stainless steel. A, B, C, and D, respectively: 120, 320, 400 grit, and 320 electropolished.
Vanhaeke and Van den Haesevelde (1991); Courtesy, Interpharm Press

surface. (Manfredi [1991] has disagreed, however, that this is the usual situation.)

Mirror-finished electropolishing usually results after a surface has been prepared by 240-grit-or-above mechanical finishing, though some facilities apply it after a 150 or 180 finish. If a grit finish of 150, 180, or even 220 is used, however, subsequent electropolishing may still evince underlying marks of the mechanical finishing process. The 3A standard operative in the dairy and food industries depends on a 150-grit finish. At least one midwestern pharmaceutical manufacturer insists on mirror-finish electropolished surfaces for parts such as pipes and tanks, and checks the attainment of such quality by use of a profilometer.

The present status seems to be that 316L stainless steels with mechanical finishes are widely accepted. There is, however, at least an intellectual acknowledgment of the utility of electropolishing, however deferred in practice.

The FDA does not stipulate any particular type or grade of surface finish as being required for stainless steel in contact with pharmaceutical waters, or drug or food products. No case of FDA rejection because of the finish is of common record.

Bringing the steel to a high luster by buffing alone has its dangers. The steel surface normally consists of ridges or plates, often referred to as "fish scales." Buffing, in its smoothing action, may fold these surface features over, and imprison beneath them the waxes of the buffing compounds and the iron oxides generated by the buffing friction. This would make for a slow, prolonged release of impurities from the buffed steel despite its attractive appearance. Such a situation is highly undesirable.

An acceptable treatment is buffing, after grit-polishing to remove the "fish scales." to be followed by electropolishing. Electropolishing has its expenses, although the attractive appearance of the electropolished metal has its psychologically appealing side. The several aspects of Figure 11-2, courtesy of Gulliford (1997), show in SEM #18425 a stainless steel with a typical #4 finish obtained by using 150- to 180-grit polishing. SEM #18433 illustrates the same stainless steel specimen after buffing. SEM #18427 displays that buffed stainless steel after an electropolishing treatment. In SEM #18434 is shown a composite of the three different finishes. A semiconductor manufacturer found acceptable a stainless steel brought to an electopolished finish by way of a 150- to 180-grit treatment followed by buffing.

Any finish finer than 150 is commonly considered sanitary. Most finishes today are 180 or 240 grit.

Passivation of Surfaces

Whatever their degree of smoothness and relative inertness, stainless steel surfaces are amenable to chemical attack—particularly where iron or its metallurgical combinations are exposed.

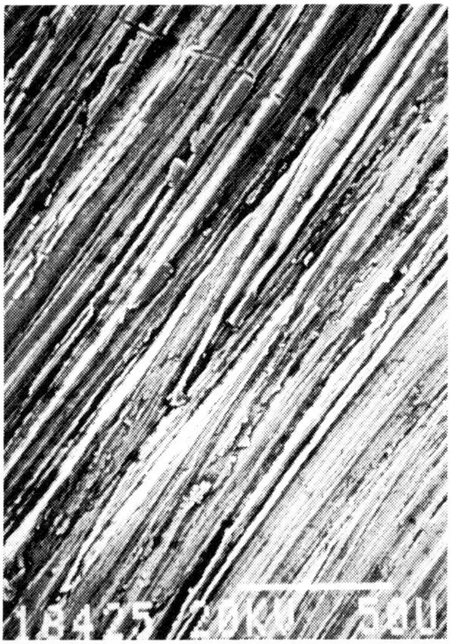

#18425. Typical #4 finish using 140-180 grit to RA<10

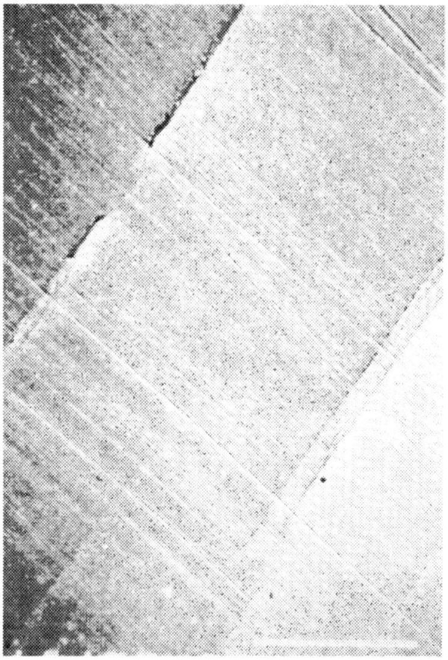

#18433. After buffing to RA<5

#18427.

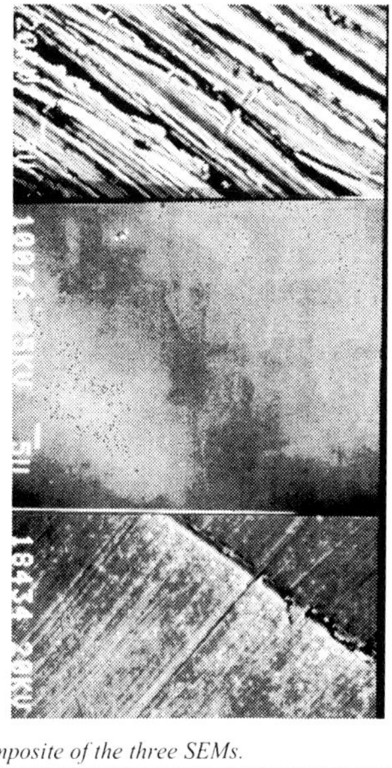

Composite of the three SEMs.

Figure 11-2. Scanning electron micrographs of stainless steel finishes used in WFI contacts.

Gulliford (1994); Courtesy, Gelman Sciences Inc., Pleasanton, CA.

Passivation of these surfaces removes iron, usually by the action of warm nitric acid over a period of 20 minutes to 4 hours (as variously practiced), to leave a surface of chromium and nickel that is converted by the oxygen of the air or by the oxidizing action of the passivating agent into impervious chromium oxide. The use of warm 20% to 40% nitric acid is generally relied on (20% is the more commonly used strength). In any event, passivation permits deposition on the metal surfaces of a coating of the interaction product of metal and oxygen, molecules thick, so tightly adhering as to protect the underlying metal against contact with and corrosion by water. The protection conferred by passivation requires renewal from time to time, as when the surface becomes scratched and newly exposed.

Generally, any of several different regents is used to effect passivation. Citric acid, often in the form of mixed chelants wherein ammonium citrate may be present, is often employed. Phosphoric acid is also made use of. Nitric acid operates through the solubilization and removal of iron. The citrates are chelants for iron, and serve to solubilize it by chelation (see page 535). Some utilize phosphoric acid to effect passivation, although according to Banes (1995) its performance is not documented. There are also proprietary reagents that are used to induce passivation.

Reagent concentration, the duration of the application, and temperature govern the passivation reaction. Temperature is the chief determinant, in keeping with Le Chatelier's principle that the rate of a chemical reaction doubles with every 10-degree rise in temperature. Nitric acid is more aggressive than is citric acid and therefore requires lower temperatures for its passivating action. Nitric acid, most commonly in a 20% concentration, is usually flowed or recirculated through the stainless steel equipment at temperatures from ambient to 140 °F (60 °C). At 140 °F the contact time is about 3 hours. When utilized at the temperature range of 140 to 160 °F (60 to 71 °C), the required contact time is shorter; possibly 20 minutes at the higher temperatures. At lower temperatures, the contact times may extend to 12 to 18 hours. It is possible for the passivating action to be too aggressive, to be used at too high a temperature. Stainless steel surfaces are not necessarily produced free of blemishes, from whatever causes. The removal of a localized flaw by passivating reagent carried too far may result in the development of a pit. Such pits, resulting in differential oxygen concentrations across the steel surface, may promote corrosion and rouge formation. The use of nitric acid in higher strengths at temperatures above 100 °F (38 °C) may sometimes be too aggressive over longer periods of time. Where passivation is concerned, stronger is not necessarily better (Banes, 1995).

Citric acid or its mixed chelants is often used at 140-160 °F (60 to 71 °C) in strengths of 10% to 15% by volume over a 3-hour period. Being weaker in its action than nitric acid, it requires higher temperatures. When ammonium citrate is used it is logically better to prepare it prior to bringing it on site. This minimizes the need for on-site manipulations.

The term "passivation" suffers from ambiguity. Passivation is the last treatment given the assembled units of a liquid-conveying system prior to its use. Constructed on-site and exposed to contamination by all sorts of particles and even protective oils, a system requires a thorough cleansing away of debris before its initial use. Ferrous particles from general construction deposited loose upon stainless steel surfaces will rust and will cause pitting to occur under them. To avoid this pitting, the system should be cleansed immediately after water has been introduced.

There is a growing use of citric acid treatments for stainless steel. Others employ phosphoric acid. Such acid treatments are also referred to as passivation, although most regard the citric acid treatment as part of the cleaning-in-place of the installation, rather than as a form of passivation. The ASTM Standard A380 (1980) referencing passivation refers to citric acid and the mixed chelants based on it as "cleaning acids," possible because these reagents are not oxidants, as is nitric acid. Sodium hydroxide washes are also used to help remove polishing compounds, construction dirt, and the oil that is initially protective of the metal surfaces against moisture and condensate. True passivation requires that some 12% to 14% of chromium be present in the steel. Passivation with 20% nitric acid has the advantage over air passivation in that it removes iron from the stainless surface, such as may have been deposited by scratching it with a carbon-steel implement during its fabrication.

Such "self-healing" passivation by oxygen is reassuring, given the ubiquity of air in most processing contexts. Nevertheless, repassivation on a maintenance schedule is advised because even passivated surfaces are not completely impervious to chemical attack and must from time to time be renewed.

Passivation, then, is a means of conferring upon stainless steel surfaces a degree of inertness against corrosive attack. By one means or another a relatively inert anodic film, an oxide layer, is substituted for the more corrosion-prone metal alloy layer. The passivation treatment is seen to consist of two actions where the stainless steels are concerned. Whether by the technique of electropolishing (the reverse of electrodeposition), or by treatment with suitable dilutions of nitric acid, iron molecules are removed from the metal alloy surface, to a depth of tens of angstroms. The treatment's anodic action simultaneously oxidizes the remaining chromium and nickel surface into impervious chromium oxide. Thus, Nishimura and Judo (1988) found that the oxide-film composition was richer in chromium and poorer in iron than the metal alloy itself. In the case of 316 stainless that contains molybdenum, the chromium enrichment was greater and more uniform than for the 304 stainless, from which it was concluded that the molybdenum enhanced the chromium enrichment. Curiously, molybdenum alone does not promote the passivation of iron. It does so only in combination with chromium (Olefjord, 1980).

Increasingly, biodegradable organic chelating agents, of various competitive origins, are being advocated for passivation purposes. Balmer and Larter (1993) describe an evaluation of the efficiency of one such related chelant composition using Auger spectroscopy. Commonly used chelates are polyfunctional carboxylic acids and their salts containing hydroxyl and amine substituents. (See page 535 on chelants). Because of their molecular architecture, chelants strongly bond to particular metals, such as iron, and are in consequence effective in removing them from their less strongly bonded situations.

Testing for a passive surface usually entails looking for traces of free iron on the metal surfaces. The ASTM Ferroxyl Test is usefully employed for this purpose (ASTM A-380, 1988). The testing solution having been applied to the surface, a blue color appears within 15 seconds when free iron is present (Banes, 1990). The need for passivation or for repassivation thus becomes signaled. Passivation may also be assessed by an electrochemical spot test utilizing a 9-volt battery. The degree of passivation is defined digitally on a scale of 1 to 10. The use of copper sulfate solutions may be made to produce color, as caused by the plating out of copper metal. The presence of iron can also be tested for directly by X-ray photoelectron spectroscopy (XPS).

Balmer and Larter (1993) state that the chromium-rich passivation layer is from 0.5 nm, about 5 angstroms, to 10 times that thick from one to ten molecules in depth. These authors suggest that the ratio of chromium to iron in the passivation layer will become targeted at 1.5 for the electronics industry. No such standard is in the offing for the stainless steels being used in the pharmaceutical industry.

Specific protocols for passivation, including assessment of the adequacy of the surface's cleanliness, the testing of the completeness of the passivation treatment, and the means of disposing of the waste solutions that are generated, were given by Banes (1990). Tests for pertinent corrosion, spectra and scanning electron microscopic analyses, and a discussion of field case observations related to passivation were presented by Coleman and Evans (1990).

Disposal of spent passivation solutions may pose a problem. The acids can be neutralized. The heavy metals require proper disposition.

In the power industry in the United States, carbon-steel passivation is achieved by the use of amines such as hydrazine. With hydrazine, temperatures of at least above 121 to 149 °C (240 to 300 °F) are required for rapid passivations to occur. A carbohydrazide-based amine, said to passivate at lower temperatures, is sold under the trade name of Liminox. Passivation of carbon steel surfaces results in the formation of a uniform, tightly adhering oxide layer that shields the underlying metal surface against chemical attack. Above about 177 °C (350 °F), passivation of carbon steel surfaces occurs spontaneously, possibly due to the dissociation of water and its consequent chemistry above that temperature (Cutler, 1991).

Gold EP Electropolishing

In the semiconductor industry, freedom from metal ions such as would result from the corrosion of stainless steel is essential. Ushikoshi et al. (1991) described a new method of passivating stainless steel intended to impart to it an improved, smooth, and leach-proof surface. Ordinary passivation films have depths of tens of angstroms thick when formed by electropolishing. Ushikoshi et al. (1991) process their austenitic steel surfaces by electropolishing, followed by heating at 400 to 500 °C in an oxidative environment, to yield a passivated oxide coating that is 100 to 200 angstroms thick. The resulting surface glitters in the interference colors of gold, and hence has been named "Gold EP" by its inventors. Its surface, as measured by SEM-derived technology, has a roughness of 0.01 μm. According to Ushikoshi et al., Gold EP has a far stronger corrosion-resistance than have stainless steels passivated by electropolishing or by mechanical polishing.

Figure 11-3 illustrates the comparative corrosion losses incurred, respectively, by stainless steels buffed by #320 grit, electropolished, and Gold EP

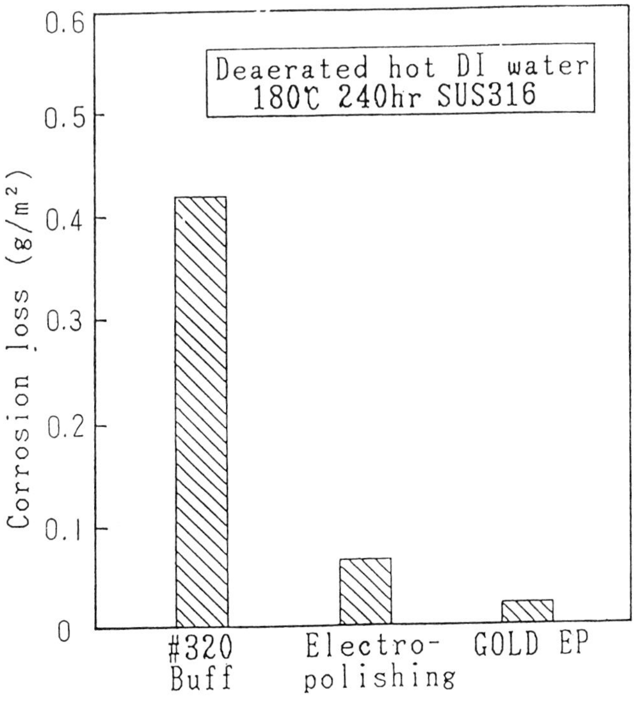

Figure 11-3. Comparison of corrosion loss by surface treatment method.
Ushikoshi et al., (1991); Courtesy, Semiconductor Pure Water Conference

treated. The Gold EP shows the least corrosion when immersed in deaerated high-purity water at 180 °C for 24 hours. Figure 11-4 shows a like superiority for Gold EP austenitic steel when the degree of leaching of TOC, iron, nickel, manganese, chromium, and sodium were compared to stainless steels passivated by mechanical polishing or ordinary electropolishing. The leaching medium used was high-purity water at 80 °C over a 5-day period. Ushikoshi et al. (1990) referenced reports that Gold-EP-treated pipes have lower leachabilities than do plastic pipings composed of perfluoroalkoxy resin (PFA), PVDF, or polyetheretherketone (PEEK).

Whatever the merits of Gold EP, its present practicality may be questioned. The pipe section welds could not be of this composition. Arc welding would completely rearrange the metallurgical structure to yield a non-Gold EP joint every 20 feet, and at every fitting and elbow. The promise of Gold EP would thus seem to be deferred.

Auger electron spectroscopy reveals the Gold EP passivation film to consist of two layers, namely, a first layer of iron-dominated material overlying a second layer of chrome-dominated structure. While sufficiently corrosion-resistant in this two-layer manifestation, the inertness of Gold EP can be enhanced by the acid-pickling removal of the iron-rich layer. This improvement is the subject of Japanese and American patents (Takahashi et al., 1988). Figure 11-5 outlines the process for producing Gold EP passivation.

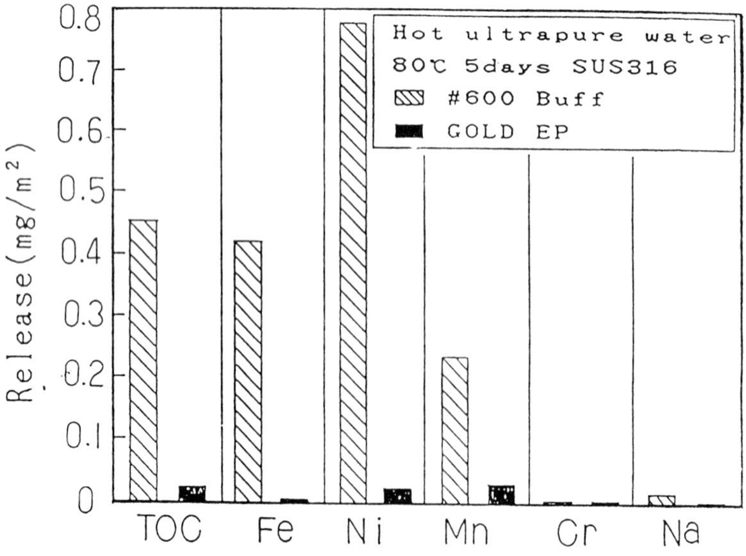

Figure 11-4. Leach-out test in hot high-purity water.
Ushikoshi et al. (1991); Courtesy, Semiconductor Pure Water Conference

Rouging

From time to time, a deposit of rouge, red iron oxide, is detectable on an expanse of tank surface or on valve faces. It is the product of, and evidence for, the rusting of iron. Its origins are not really understood and may be various. Its discovery on tank walls does not necessarily signify that it was formed there; it may have been pumped into the tank from other locations. Rouging is often detected upon Teflon diaphragms, onto which it has flowed, made evident by their whiteness.

There is an understandable reluctance on the part of some to accept that the stainless steels can and do rust, albeit at a slow rate. Rouge is the product of that corrosion. Some rationalize its presence as evidence of "bad metal" somewhere in the system, as proof of poor welding, or as the inevitable accompaniment of carbon-steel impurities or debris not completely cleansed from the system. If possible, the cause of the rouging should be found and eliminated. It is not necessarily an innocuous occurrence. The rust may be in colloidal form. Being

Material checking
↓
Electropolishing
↓
Pure water rinsing
↓
Acid pickling
↓
High-purity water rinsing
↓
Drying
↓
Heat treatment
↓
Acid pickling
↓
High-purity water rinsing
↓
Drying
↓
Packing

Figure 11-5. Working process of Gold EP.
Ushikoshi et al. (1991); Courtesy, Semiconductor Pure Water Conference

insoluble, its presence will not be revealed by the conductivity meter. If not eliminated, it may eventually contaminate the drug product. Deposited on stainless steel surfaces, it may cause pitting. If the creation of space is essential, substitute for the bracketed paragraph on Page 610. The cause of rouging being complex, its occurrence is unpredictable. Its prevention is often attempted prophylactically by annual repassivations. The system should be monitored in establishing the repassivation schedule, although rouging may not necessarily become reveallled. It is necessary first to derouge, as with phosphoric acid. Indeed, this should perhaps be done every six months in any case. Then repassivation should be performed. Depending upon the size of the system, the operation can require one to two days.

Evans (1994) states that new austenitic steels of the 300 series (304,304 L, 316, 316 L) are made largely from recycled sources of "lower alloys" such as 400 ferritic or martensitic materials to which nickel and chromium, and in the case of 316, molybdenum are added. Interestingly, he points out that aluminum is often added to American Austenite to "deoxidize the melt." This is intended to remove oxygen and prevent porosity. However, this practice also predisposes to corrosion-inducing inclusions. Moreover, the composition of the steel aside, its surface finishing by way of mechanical buffing or abrasion or even by use of electropolishing solution, often impure, may impregnate the stainless micro-structure with contaminants. Opportunities therefore exist for the stainless steels to undergo some degree of corrosion. Rouge, the complex oxide that forms, is the result.

Coleman and Evans (1991) stated that rouging can be caused by a number of situations: by the presence of carbon or marstenitic steel in an otherwise stainless steel system; by the mechanical polishing involved in surface preparations; by the production of excessive heat tinting during welding; and by improper passivation techniques.

Manfredi (1991) has observed the more ready appearance of rouging in dispositions involving temperature differentials. Rouge seems more evident upon the cooler pump surfaces of heat-lagged hot-water systems. High temperatures and the presence of oxygen are seen to promote the rusting of the steel. The rouge may assume different colors. Traditionally the red rouges are most common in high-purity high-temperature water systems, while the blue/black rouges are typically found in clean-steam systems. In general, it has been observed that the better the grade and finish of stainless steel, the slower the development of rouging. That is to say that under the same conditions 304 will probably develop rouge before a similar finish that has been electropolished. When new systems are constructed, the highest-quality materials available should be used, avoiding dissimilar metallurgy. This will minimize the disposition for rouging and other corrosion phenomena (Banes, 1995).

Passivation, the removal of iron from the metallic surface, is the recognized way of avoiding or minimizing rouging. Various degrees of rouging are manifest by progressive deepening of color. Different rougings adhere to the metal with different degrees of tightness. The blue-black tints adhere so closely as to serve, perhaps, as rouge claddings protective of the underlying metal. The greater concern is with the nonadhering, suspended varieties.

Rouging may manifest itself as a very faint dustlike reddish color. In more severe situations or over longer periods of time, it becomes deeper red, brown, and even purplish in color. Auger electron spectroscopy reveals the outer surface of rouge to be rich in carbon, conceivably organic in nature. This overlays an iron- and oxygen-rich material, presumably an iron oxide (Jabblar, 1989). Banes (1990) suggested that the organic layer may account, at least in part, for the failure of common cleaning agents and even passivating acids to remove the rouge film. Strong reducing agents such as sodium hydrosulfite do remove it, as does also phosphoric acid to some extent.

Coleman and Evans (1991) stated that rouge appears in many colors and forms. They have observed it as a layering of a yellowish-green powder over a dense brown deposit, itself superimposed upon a tenaciously adhering ingrained black layer. Most often, according to Coleman and Evans (1991), it appears as a dense reddish brown coating above a black substrate. These investigators have also observed rouge as a gelatinous and hence apparently hydrated layer underlying an upper dry crust, the surface of which was pocked with craters and littered with a white dust.

When analyzed by Auger electron spectroscopy, the white specks were seen to be composed of iron, chromium, nickel, nitrogen, carbon, and oxygen. Also present were oxides of silicon and aluminum. Contained within the craters were oxygen, chromium, carbon, and iron. White crystals at the edge of the craters were composed of oxygen, carbon, iron, chromium, and small quantities of nickel. By contrast, Auger electron spectroscopy showed electropolished 316L stainless steel to contain a much lower iron-to-chromium ratio than did the corroded sample (Coleman and Evans, 1991). These investigators believed that the surface pitting indicated sites where the passivated layer had been breached. The surface corrosion products were then enabled to attack the underlying dynamic metal phase and the base metal to produce the observed particles and crystals. Coleman and Evans (1991) believed that rouging is a self-catalyzing corrosion, an ongoing dynamic process that leaches the constituents of the corroded stainless steel. In their view it requires serious and prompt address. Its removal and amelioration can be managed by the application, they stated, of a proprietary mixture of "mixed chelates," a preparation of ammonium citrate and ethylenediaminetetraacetic acid (EDTA) in undisclosed proportions (Coleman, 1991).

Because of the organic films associated with rouge, the first-step cleaner used in repassivations is aqueous detergent solution, followed by a water rinse. The passivating acid solution is next applied to remove free iron, residues, and oxide films. The passive oxide film forms by anodic oxidation following flushing of acid from the surface and its free drainage.

The welding of stainless steel usually results in the formation of some iron oxides, as revealed by a darkening of color of the steel within the heated zone. The belief is that this region of color formation is forever after especially prone to rouge formation; the darker the color, the more severe the potential rouging. In the welding operation, the development of straw-colored tints is considered inevitable. The development of darker tints is to be avoided. The artfulness and experience of the welder is heavily depended upon. It is tested by close inspections of samples of welding performed by the very welder prior to assigning him the actual work. The correct use of purge gases and the proper art of welding stainless steel are requisites to minimizing rouge formation. However, the subsequent exposure of the steel to clean steam or to 80 °C water is seen as inevitably leading to rouge formation.

That rouging is an ineluctable consequence of exposure to higher temperatures is a disadvantage of hot-water systems, regardless of their beneficial microbiological influences. Waters protected by ozone have the advantage of being operated at ambient temperatures. Moreover, ozone decomposes to oxygen. Oxygen is required for the maintenance of a passivation film. Thus, areas that are shielded from oxygen, as under gaskets, are found to lose passivation and to corrode. Rouging is not found in ambient water systems (Banes 1995), nor where water is stored under ozone even after one year. (See page 71).

Piping Materials in Distribution Systems

The high-purity water, after production, must be piped and distributed to its areas of use, often several hundreds of meters distant. There may well be numerous points of use. Distribution loops involve a like extent of return piping. What is desired of the piping is that it be inert to the action of the water it conveys at each and every stage of water purity, that it not leach any of its components into the water, and that it withstand the sanitizing reagents periodically used to combat the biofilm inevitably formed upon its inner surfaces. (We now comprehend that biofilm will inexorably form upon wetted pipe surfaces regardless of their compositions. See previous section on Biofilm, page 90).

The piping must be of a composition that will permit its erection in sag-proof dispositions, so as to prevent the formation of stagnant pools. The piping must also be impervious to its outside environment, so as to have a long service life. It should not permit the permeation of air or other gases, nor of ultraviolet or other radiation. All of the above requirements should be met, furthermore, with due regard to economic considerations, including costs of installation and maintenance. Above all, the piping must preserve the purity of the product water being conveyed by it.

The FDA permits plastic piping, despite its having been proscribed in GMP/LVP 212.49. However, it must be validated with respect to extractables, and its method of being joined must not yield crevices and must withstand the necessary elevated temperatures.

Stainless steel. In pharmaceuticals, the material of choice for piping is stainless steel. Older systems may be composed of polyvinyl chloride (PVC), and newer distribution arrangements utilize polyvinylidene fluoride (PVDF). In the semiconductor industry PVC is being replaced, almost always by PVDF. Overall, PVDF is used almost exclusively in semiconductor installations.

Certification of finishes, of mill test reports (MTRs), and of mechanical background are all available for stainless steel. Because stainless steel, by its very nature, is a potential source of metallic ions, its use has largely been eschewed in electronics waters. However, the use of passivated stainless steel piping is on occasion seen as worthy of consideration, particularly where mechanical strength is required (e.g., at pump discharge locations). In some such cases, slow-closing valves lead to stainless steel headers that are followed by PVDF piping. As discussed earlier in this chapter, many stainless steels are available in the market.

The advantage of the competitive polymeric piping is that it minimizes opportunities for heavy-metal pickup by the water. The disadvantage is that it is not so strong. Polymeric piping requires the installation of much more support to prevent the pipe sagging that would lead to poor drainage and difficulty in cleaning. Stainless steel piping is supported every 8 to 10 feet, while plastic piping may require being supported every 4 or 5 feet. This can double the installation costs (Manfredi, 1991), but not necessarily. Continuous rigid supports such as angle irons may be used, and these are less costly.

One pharmaceutical operation eschews the use of stainless steel in order to avoid the possibility of contamination with nickel, chromium, and zinc ions inimicable to its antibiotic preparation. Its WFI is prepared by two-pass RO (actually triple-pass). The piping used is PVDF and the sanitization is by intermittent ozone administration. Reverse osmosis water storage is in a fluorocarbon-lined tank.

Polyvinyl chloride. Early on, PVC was used as piping material for water systems. The term "polyvinyl chloride" refers to a polymer; essentially it is a polyethylene, every alternating carbon atom of whose chain bears a single chlorine atom substituent. The chlorine groups confer some oxidative stability over the corresponding hydrogen substituents. However, the chlorine atoms, particularly in tertiary positions at points of polymer branching, are extremely heat- and ultraviolet-light-labile. They are split from the PVC, in conjunction with hydrogen atoms, to form hydrogen chloride. The dehydrochlorination reaction introduces color-producing unsaturation in the remaining polymer. The polymer is compounded with stabilizers, often organometallic in nature, to protect these molecules against dehydrochlorination; with activated carbon, to confer better mechanical properties of rigidity and impact strength and to protect against UV light; with fillers to add opacity and color; and with plasticizers for formability. Indeed, PVC cannot survive most molding, extruding, or other forming processes without the addition of stabilizers against dehydrochlorinations. What is actually used in pipe fabrication is not PVC polymer but PVC compound. The composition of the particular compound in the United States is defined in accordance with ASTM standards. In other countries, different standards may be used. Thus, in Japan there is available a “Clean PVC.”

Because PVC piping may contain, and hence leach, the added compounding materials, it is progressively being replaced by other piping materials. The chief concern is the metallic (usually heavy metal) stabilizers and their leaching into the water. Stainless steel has largely replaced PVC in pharmaceuticals; PVDF has been and is replacing it in the semiconductor industry. Where PVC is still used in the electronics industry, it is largely in the makeup portion of the water system. Once the water achieves high purity, it is usually conveyed in PVDF piping.

When PVC piping is used, it should be constructed of high-grade polyvinyl chloride compound intended for quality pipe. It should contain no metal stabilizers and as little plasticizer as possible. The pipe should be precleaned prior to its installation. Only pipe cutters should be used in cutting it to length; hacksaws are unsatisfactory because they create particles. The edges of the pipe should be beveled. The art lies in the pipe assembly. No lubricants should be used, and pipe ends should be butt-ended with a minimum of glue line. Threaded pipes are unacceptable in any situation requiring sterility, as organisms may become ensconced within the threads. Sealants such as polytetrafluoroethylene (PTFE) tape or suitable liquid glues are relied on.

Polyvinyl chloride offers limitations in terms of extractable plasticizers, residual monomer, and leachable stabilizers intended against thermal and UV light dehydrochlorinations. Nonpigmented and nonstabilized PVC has a shorter service life than the protected variety. However, the more sophisticated the water purities, the more the ordinary utility of PVC may become overlooked. Polyvinyl chloride and polypropylene (PP) cost only about one-third the price of stainless steel. Polyvinyl chloride piping does not require a high level of skill to install, and accepts a wide variety of fittings such as gauges, valves, and flanges. Piping of PVC is suitable for plating-shop operations, and suffices for the more ordinary high-purity waters.

It is only fair to state that some PVC pipe manufacturers do believe they have demonstrated their product to be suitable for the conveyance of high-purity waters. Sinha and Van Winkle (1993) found extractables from such PVC pipe rinse out to equilibrium impurity levels in less than 30 days, even in the presence of additives and solvent from the pipe-joining process. The subject study involved resistivity and TOC determinations, and investigated surface elemental analysis and surface roughness studies, along with extractables analyses.

The FDA in its "Guide to Inspections of High Purity Water Systems" (1993) emphasizes the concern about extractables: "Most of these systems employ PVC or some type of plastic tubing. Because the systems are typically cold, the many joints in the system are subject to contamination. Another potential problem with PVC tubing is extractables. Looking at the WFI from a system to assure that it meets USP requirements without some assurance that there are not extractables would not be acceptable."

Extractables and Biofilm Formation

PVC is often denigrated because it yields extractables. All polymerics yield some extractables. Not knowing their effect, one seeks, instinctively, to minimize the quantity of extractables. The real question, however, is not the quantity of extractables, but whether these are harmful. It had also been feared that organic extractables could serve as nourishment for organisms, encouraging their growth and biofilm formation. It has not been found, however, that such is the case. The Gram-negative organisms native to water systems need so little nutrient to grow that they flourish even in the purest waters. There is no evidence that the extractables from PVC, or other polymeric materials, encourage biofilm formation. In any case, in pharmaceutical water contexts the accepted permissable level of organic material (TOC), whether from extractables or otherwise, is 500 ppb. Water systems based on PVC accord with this requirement.

Of significance is the fact that none of the studies on bioflIm formation has quantitated the amount of biofllrn as being related to the nature of the surface, whether stainless steel, PVC, or whatever. As Vanhaecke and Van den Haesevede found, stainless steel is not impervious to biofilm formation by *P. aeruginosa*, and that organism in its hydrophobic manifestation readily colonizes electropolished stainless. There are no published studies that show PVC to be more susceptible to biofilm formation. Anecdotal accounts indicate that no difference exists.

Polyvinylidene fluoride. In the quest for chemically inert polymeric piping, the fluorocarbons have been targeted because the carbon-fluorine bond has great stability to heat and oxidation. Its inertness to oxidation and aggressive chemicals far exceeds that of the various carbon-hydrogen bonds that are common constituents of most polymers. The most resistant fluoropolymer would be PTFE. All of the atomic appendages of its carbon-to-carbon chain are fluorines. Unfortunately, PTFE has thus far proved intractable to formation into pipes. Polyvinylidene fluoride consists polymerically of repetitive units of two carbons, one of which is bonded to two fluorine atoms, and the other to two hydrogen atoms. While highly resistant to chemical attack, PVDF is not so inert as PTFE. It is, however, amenable to being fashioned into piping with smooth inner walls. Recently, techniques have been perfected to join lengths of PVDF piping with crevice-free smooth welds. It is not surprising, therefore, that PVDF piping has received a good reception in the electronics industry. It should prove equally serviceable in pharmaceutical applications.

Polytetrafluoroethylene, PTFE, can be considered a fully fluorinated derivative of polyethylene (or polymethylene) wherein fluorine atoms are substituted for all the hydrogen atoms of the polyethylene. Partially fluorine-substituted polymers are possible; PVDF is one such. Chemical inertness and mechanical intractability (stiffness, or high modulus) both derive proportionate to the degree of fluorine substitution. These two consequences cannot be separated. Some suppliers offer a "flexible PVDF." There is no such material. There are PVDFs so modified with admixtures of other polymers as to give flexible compositions. Nevertheless, however useful their flexibility, these polymerics inevitably compromise the chemical inertness of the PVDF (Seiler and Barber, 1989, see page 633).

As with many polymers, PVDF can be formed by suspension polymerization or by emulsion polymerization. Each type is championed by its manufacturers as being the better product. Evaluations are sometimes performed using the

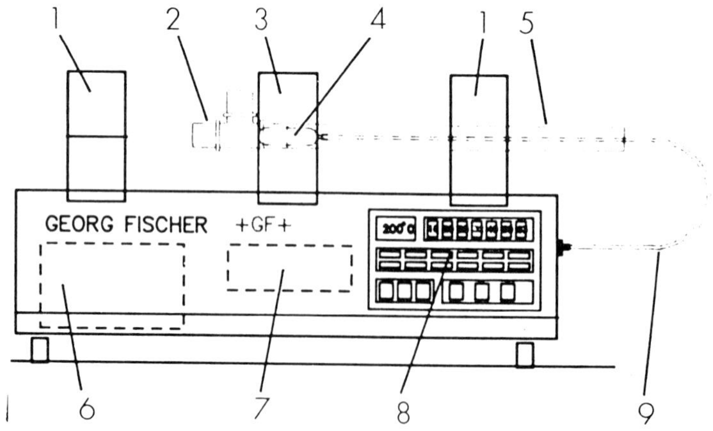

Figure 11-6. Sketch of the welding equipment necessary for bead- and crevice-free welding. The device is a tabletop unit consisting of pipe support clamps [1], fitting [2], heating element [3], internal inflatable bladder [4], pipe [5], air compressor [6], cooling fan [7], self-contained controls [8] and bladder hose [9].
Sixsmith and Hanselka (1989); Courtesy, *Ultrapure Water* journal

polymer pellets from which the PVDF pipe is formed by extrusion. Some have considered judgments and comparisons to be meaningful when performed on the pipe itself (Maquet, 1988). That investigator concluded that both PVDF grades comply with the most stringent specifications required for high-purity water.

Sixsmith and Hanselka (1989) described their method for the production of bead- and crevice-free PVDF pipe-bonding joints. These investigators employed welding of PVDF pipe ends in close contact and firmly held in place. An inflatable bladder positioned at the weld area inside the pipes served to make smooth the inner weld surface, eliminating beads. Given the restriction of the pipe movement by clamping, the heat of expansion caused the heat-softened PVDF to flow together compressively at the joint to form a crevice-free weld. An externally applied heat source was used in conjunction with the reusable inflatable bladder. Figure 11-6 illustrates the fusion device. Figure 11-7 is a cross section of such a weld area as shown by polarized light photography. In contrast, thermoplastic butt welding and socket fusion of PVDF pipe ends are inherently prone to bead production and possibly to crevice formation as well.

As with all materials, PVDF has its limitations, chiefly some susceptibility to free-radical attack, albeit far less than do most polymers.

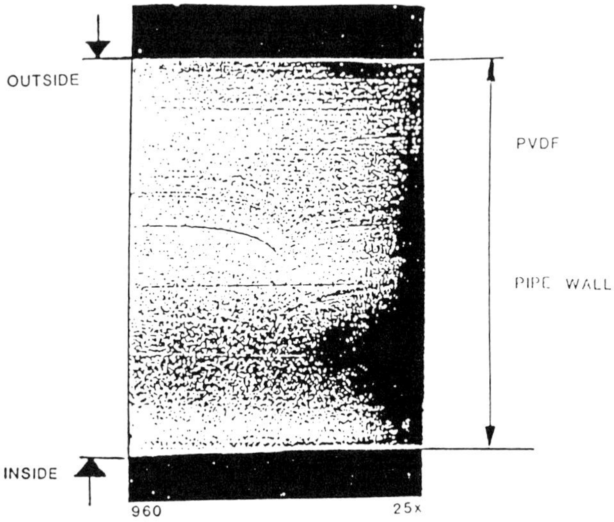

Figure 11-7. A cross section of a bead- and crevice-free weld through the joint area using polarized light photography. As can be seen in this photograph, there are no internal beads or minute crevices on the inside pipe wall for microbial growth. Smooth flow lines are evident, indicating a relatively stress-free weld.
Sixsmith and Hanselka (1989); Courtesy, *Ultrapure Water* journal

Stainless steel is not damaged by ozone. Indeed, one may speculate that ozone would induce passivation. Polymeric materials are not so impervious. Polypropylene and polyvinyl chloride will undergo oxidative degradation because of the susceptibility of their carbon-hydrogen bonding. Polyvinylidene fluoride should also be responsive to ozone, albeit at a lower rate of attack. Burkhart et al (1996) state: "PVDF piping to be resistant to ozone exposures of 30-50 ppm even after 2 years. Unlike stainless steel, its metallic extractables are minimal. There is no significant difference in the encouragement of bacterial growth. PVDF is a suitable material for high-purity water systems. Zahka and Smith (1989) stated that PVDF filters do withstand at least 30 hours of 1 ppm of ozone without ill effect; and Zahka and Vahkshoori (1990) demonstrated that a particular PVDF ultrafilter withstood at least 600 ppm-hours of ozone with no loss of functionality. A paper by Pate et al. (1990) presented information on PVDF piping in close proximity to a high-intensity UV sterilizer. After 1 year of use, a significant degree of degradation developed at the PVDF joint directly above the UV sterilizer light units. A multitude of stress cracks were observed on the interior bead of the butt-weld joint. Discoloration of the pipe wall occurred.

Imbalzano and Kratzer (1986) reported on the development of discoloration of PVDF, accompanied by fluoride ion release. Balazs (1991) stated that fluoride ion is found in all systems using PVDF piping. The explanation attributed the darkening of the polymer and its loss of fluoride to a dehydrohalogenation reaction. Similarly, chlorine is abstracted from polyvinyl chloride under free-radical attack. A hydrogen atom is then abstracted to form hydrogen chloride and to introduce a double bond into the polymer structure. The subsequent development in like fashion of other unsaturated linkages creates a conjugated double bond system. The depth of color developed by the polymer reflects directly the extent of the double bond conjugation. An 8% degree of conjugation is productive of color generation (Pate et al., 1990).

The carbon-fluoride bond is not so labile as the carbon-chlorine bond. However, the double substitution of the vinylidene structure does increase the carbon-fluorine instability. In any case, PVDF seems definitely to lose fluorine, manifested as the fluoride ion; and develops color under conditions where free radicals are generated, (i.e., by high-intensity UV lamps). The analogy to the known dehydrohalogenation of polyvinyl chloride under free-radical conditions seem reasonable. Pate et al. (1990) ascribed the stress cracking of the PVDF to the increased brittleness of the degraded polymer. These investigators also attributed some of the color formation to the presence of altered methyl cellulose. Added in 10-ppb quantities to the PVDF formulation as a "seed" during the polymerization process, methyl cellulose also undergoes degradation under free-radical attack. The long-term implications of PVDF susceptibility to free-radical attack are uncertain. Its reported generation of fluoride ion bears being noted.

According to Balazs (1991), low quantities of fluoride ions can etch the wafer surfaces in semiconductor settings.

Hanselka (1991), in commenting upon the mechanical failures of PVDF piping in circumstances where welds with their inherent stresses had close propinquity to ultraviolet light, correctly indicated that PVDF does satisfactorily endure outdoor UV and ambient sunlight. The sources of the stress/UV deteriorations are not fully comprehended. Polymer stability reflects more than a counting of the carbon-fluorine bonds of fluorinated polymer structures. The free-radical ambiences involved are unknown. Thus, the much-vaunted ultrastability of the carbon-fluorine bonds of PTFE is notoriously unstable to ionizing gamma-ray irradiation. Fluorine is released. It has a cannibalistic effect upon the carbon-carbon bonds of the remaining polymer. Also, PTFE, ordinarily impervious to sunlight and/or UV light, will undergo loss of fluorine when flashed by very-high-intensity light. Additionally, the presence of two fluorine atom substituents on the same carbon, the vinylidene structure, renders their attachments less secure than if they each separately occupied sites on two adjacent carbons.

An evaluation of the real-life failure modes of polymers was made by Hanselka et al. (1987). Degradations of PVDF by high-intensity UV light were described by Pate et al. (1990). These latter investigators stated that PVDF will undergo loss of hydrogen fluoride (analogous to the dehydrochlorination of PVC); that thermally stressed joints have a higher susceptibility; and that mechanical stressing increases that susceptibility. For this very reason the chief supplier of PVDF tubing advised that their tubing be so positioned as to insure its shielding from UV light, with a PFA-lined weir-type diaphragm valve to be used downstream from the UV lamps. This will reflect the UV light around the weir. The diaphragm valve leads to the PVDF tubing, now shielded from the UV light emanations.

Some safety concerns may attend the use of PVDF piping where steaming is used. The maximum applicational temperature is at about 140 °C. This does provide a margin against steam at 125 °C. The safety issue could arise where overheating conditions and/or pressure regulator failures might be involved.

Other polymeric piping. Clean piping of acrylonitrile butadiene styrene (ABS) polymer is used at room temperature. Polyethylene (PE), polypropylene (PP), PEEK, PFA and Clean-PVC are also used. The polyethylenes are oxidation-prone. Polypropylene may be regarded as methylated polyethylene; nevertheless, PP piping is used. The methyl substituents create tertiary hydrogens, which are very susceptible to oxidative attack. Polypropylene must be stabilized by additives against this occurrence. As the polypropylene chain undergoes its oxidative free-radical attack, it suffers both chain scission and cross-linking. As a result, the long, flexible, linear polymer is transformed into short, stubby, multibranched molecules. This results in the creation of particles.

Japanese investigators compared a relatively new polymer in pipe form with PVDF, PVC, PP, and PFA. The new material, PEEK, is described as a polyetheretherketone.

The PFA bears a single alkoxy substituent, an alkylated ether linkage, about once for every ten possible fluorine atoms. Strictly speaking, it does not merit the "per" appellation, which implies the ultimate degree of thoroughness, here of fluorination. Yet this polymer is more fluorinated than any currently available except PTFE. The alkoxy group renders it more tractable to heat than PTFE. Consequently, it can be fashioned into pipe. It is, however, an expensive polymeric material.

Motomura and Yabe (1991) illustrated in Table 11-4 the comparative me-

Table 11-4
General Characteristics of Piping Materials

	Polyvinyl Chloride (PVC)	*Poly-propylene (PP)*	*Polyvinyl-idene Fluoride (PVDF)*	*Perfluoro-alkoxy Vinylether (PFA)*	*Poly-etherether-ketone (PEEK)*
Molecular structure	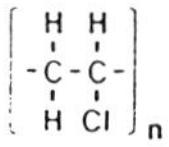	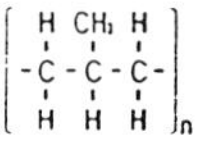	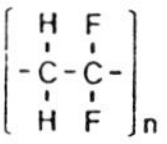	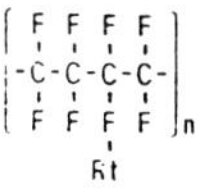	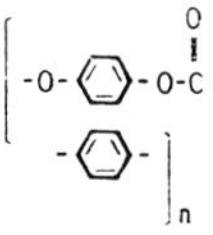
Additives	Stabilizer, pigment	Oxidation inhibitor, stabilizer, pigment	None	None	None
Color	Blue	Blue	Milky white	Milky white	Light brown
Specific gravity	1.43	0.91	1.77	2.77	1.30
Strength against stretching (kg/cm^2)	500-550	250	500-600	320	930
Elasticity (kg/cm^2)	2.7×10^4	1.5×10^4	1.4×10^4	—	4.0×10^4
Elongation (%)	50-150	400-600	200-300	280-300	150
Expansion const. (1/°C)	$6\text{-}8 \times 10^{-3}$	11×10^{-3}	12×10^{-3}	12×10^{-3}	5×10^{-3}
Heat conductivity (kcal/mh°C)	0.13	0.15-0.2	0.11	0.22	0.22
Applicable temp. limit (°C)	60	100	140	260	152

Motomura and Yabe (1991); Courtesy, Semiconductor Pure Water Conference chanical properties of these several polymers. The PEEK is characterized by a high tensile strength, 930 kg/cm^2, as compared to 500 to 600 kg/cm^2 for PVDF. It can be used at 300 psig at 316 °C (600 °F), even with sulfuric acid. Its elongation to break is reduced to 150%, compared to that of PTFE at 200% to 300%. More importantly, its maximum applicational temperature is 152 °C, marginally better than that of PVDF at 140 °C.

Piping of PVDF expands about 5 times as much as stainless steel, about 4 inches per 100 feet when heated to 80 °C from ambient temperatures.

Leaching of PVDF and PEEK

In their study, Motomura and Yabe (1991) found that both PVDF and PEEK leached TOC into water. However, the rate of leaching decreased with the increase in exposure times, an indication that the TOC present was of a finite amount, and not a product of polymeric degradation. Extraction increased with temperature from 25 to 80 °C (77 to 176 °F). The increase was less for the PEEK. The TOC derived from PVDF differed for different manufacturers. However, fluoride ions released from PVDF, while greater at the higher temperature, did not differ with different manufacturers. Actually, impurities released from both PVDF and PEEK were small, although the initial quantities realized from the PVDF seriously degraded high-purity water (Motomura and Yabe, 1991). The PEEK ought to leach less than PVDF. The latter is extruded at around 260 °C (500 °F), whereas PEEK is heated and processed at about 370 to 425 °C (700 to 800 °F). Higher temperatures are more likely to remove impurities by volatilization.

The degradation of high-purity water was measured as a function of its retention time in PVDF and PEEK piping, as determined in an experimental apparatus. When the temperature was elevated from 25 °C to 80 °C over a 10-minute retention interval, the degradation as determined by resistivity decrease

Table 11-5
Quality of High-Purity Water and Leach-Out Limits

Quality ng/L (ppt) (as total heavy metal)	*Leach-Out per Circulation ng/L(ppt)*	*Leach-Out Limit µg/m^2-day*	*Remarks*
100	10	75.1	Standard for 4Mbit DRAM
50	5	37.6	Standard for 16Mbit DRAM
10	1	7.5	Standard for 64Mbit DRAM
1	0.1	0.75	
0.1	0.01	0.075	Suggested by Dr. Ohmi
0.01	0.001	0.0075	

Leach-out per circulation = Quality of water x 100

Sugisawa et al. (1992); Courtesy, Semiconductor Pure Water and Chemicals Conference was 5 to 10 microohms-cm in the case of PVDF, but only 1 microohm-cm for PEEK piping. This was interpreted as meaning lower extractable levels for PEEK polymer (Motomura and Yabe, 1991).

While the results of the comparative extractables tests performed by Motomura and Yabe (1991) were undoubtedly correct, their implications to practical situations require consideration. The subject tests involved the imprisonment of a quantity of water in a sealed polymeric tube at an elevated temperature for a period of time. During that interval, the polymer containing the larger quantity of leachable TOC, or perhaps the TOC with the most rapid rate of leaching, conferred the larger quantity of TOC to the water. In actual applications, however, a quantity of water flowing through a polymeric pipe picks up TOC in proportion to the rate of TOC diffusing from the polymer. This depends upon time and temperature as well upon the diffusibility of the particular TOC species, and its concentration. Normally, such diffusions are slow. Therefore, the faster the rate of flow of water in the pipe, the less TOC will be picked up by a given volume of water per unit time.

In imprisonment testing there is no rate of flow. In practical situations there is such a consideration. Therefore, imprisonment tests may not reflect the situation inherent in practical applications. Thus Sixsmith (1991) calculated that if the water velocity in a pipe were 5 ft/sec, then the piping length would have to be 2,000 feet to match Motomura and Yabe's 10-minute imprisonment time. The drop in resistivity would have to go to 10 megohms-cm from the initial 19 megohms-cm to match the water quality of the imprisonment tests. In field installations involving 2,000- to 3,000-foot lengths of PVDF tubing, no such water quality deteriorations were noted (Sixsmith, 1991). The practical implications of the imprisonment test are thus questionable.

A translation of imprisonment extraction data to the conditions of practical usage was given by Sugisawa et al. (1992). These investigators explored the extraction of heavy metals from variously treated stainless steels at point-of-use locations. The surface area of the piping was 80 m^2 and its volume was 0.7 m^3. The water recirculation rate was 25 m^3/hr, and its retention time was 0.028 hours. The nominal size of the piping was 1/2 to 2 1/2 inches. As shown in Table 11-5, the water qualities required by the semicondustor industry for various line geometries (e.g., 4 M, 16 M, and 32 M-bit dynamic random access memory [DRAM]), permit distinctly different levels of heavy-metal content. The leach-out amount per circulation proved to be one-tenth of the permissible concentration, in parts per trillion (ppt) (nanograms/L). The leach-out limit per day, in micrograms/m^2/day, is thus well within the tolerable heavy-metal limits. Sugisawa et al. (1992) investigated electropolished stainless steel; electropolished and air-passivated stainless steel (Gold EP); and pickled, electropolished, air-passivated stainless steel (Gold EP White).

Temperature is also a factor. The imprisonment tests were conducted at room temperature and at 80 °C. At the elevated temperature, the degradations in water quality were greater. This could be the results of heightened diffusions, such as of ions and TOC. It may also reflect, however, enhanced diffusions permitted by the thermal disruptions of ordered polymeric segmental arrangements, if any, such as semicrystallinity. The thermal alteration of such polymeric architectural features would emphasize differences between accelerated imprisonment tests and the ambiences of practical applications. In this connection, it has been suggested that carbon dioxide diffusion through the pipe wall may account for some of the water quality deterioration observed in the imprisonment tests. Be that as it may, the effect of temperature upon polymeric morphology could particularly affect carbon dioxide permeation.

Static and accelerated tests have their utility. Caution must be used, however, in extrapolating their conclusions to the conditions prevalent in actual applications.

Additional Leaching Studies

In conjunction with the purity of the water conveyed by the piping, it should be pointed out that the stainless steels do rust, hence the concerns with passivation, with electropolishing (aside from its cosmetic contributions), and with the ongoing problem of rouging. Every material has its advantages and limitations. In pharmaceutical contexts, stainless steel has the advantage of already being in place in a conservative industry prudently cautious to change. Alternative polymeric materials may offer some advantages for piping and tank constructions.

Motomura and Yabe (1991) found that clean PVC pipe released chloride and calcium ions. Lead ions, derived from lead stabilizers against thermal dehydrochlorination, are known to be released from conventional PVC piping. Polypropylene piping was found to furnish sodium, calcium, and sulfate ions more rapidly at 80 °C than at 25 °C, these ions being the presumed derivatives of compounds introduced during the polymerization process. However, this ionic release decreased with subsequent extraction volumes.

Imbalzano and Kratzer (1986) reported from a study involving samples of piping composed, separately, of PFA, PVDF, and ECTFE (ethylene chlorotrifluoroethylene), each exposed at 100 °C for 9 weeks to water with 18-megohm-cm resistivity. At the end of the exposure period, longitudinally-split sections of each pipe were examined by electron spectroscopy for chemical analysis. No significant changes were detected for the PFA piping. Both the PVDF and ECTFE piping showed loss of fluorine (and chlorine), and each had acquired substituent oxygen atoms; the latter was a possible expression of oxidation by the oxygen present in the water.

According to Balazs, low quantities of fluoride ions can etch wafer surfaces in semiconductor settings. The release of fluoride ions from PVDF polymer in pharmaceutical high-purity waters ought to be less significant, however. The

USP 23 allows, in effect, a maximum of 2 ppm of chloride ions in compendial waters. The reported concentrations of fluoride ions are in ppb, probably a measure of the polymer's greater resistance to oxidative dehydrohalogenation.

Copolymers of polyvinylidene fluoride and hexafluoropropylene have been examined for their ability to provide adequate mechanical properties over wider applicational ranges. Holton (1993) investigated by neutron activation analysis (NAA) the extractables leached from such polymers. This technique, sensitive to parts per trillion for some elements, involves placement within the thermal neutron flux of a reactor core. The atoms thus irradiated may undergo nuclear transformations following thermal neutron captures. Radioactive nuclides are produced where decay emits gamma radiation characteristic of particular elements. Such measurements lead to quantification of the elements present. Neutron activation is nondestructive and is multi-elemental with few interferences.

Holton (1993) found that the modified PVDF resins tested were within the range of the PVDF homopolymers. This performance range did show fluoride ions to be potentially the highest extractable in high-purity water, greatly reduced, however, by a first washing of the resin. The extractable analysis showed the performance range capable of yielding water qualities of less than parts per billion of contaminants.

Other Piping Concerns

Yabe et al. (1989) found that fluoride ions were eluted from PVDF at 25 °C, and that the amount differed with different manufacturers of the polymer. At 80 °C, large quantities of the fluoride were eluted regardless of the manufacturer. The PFA polymer yielded fluoride ions roughly to the same extent as PVDF. These investigators claimed that PEEK, once ordinary surface contamination was removed, exhibited no elution of special ions. The TOC elution from piping materials gained at higher temperatures, though PFA and PEEK showed relatively low TOC elution valves. The PEEK was considered to be the most suitable piping material for constant use with 60 to 90 °C water.

Yabe et al. (1989) stated that pipes composed of PEEK most consistently had the smoothest inner surfaces exhibiting the fewest holes. Their statement that such smoothness helps to prevent bacterial attachment to any significant extent is, however, at variance with the findings of Costerton (1984B) and Mittelman (1985) (See "Surface Smoothness" in Chapter 2, page 92).

An important concern regarding all parts of water treatment systems, including the polymeric piping is thermal expansion. This is of special importance where hot-water systems are involved or where cyclical heating and cooling occur. An advantage of PEEK is its lesser expansion and contraction, almost like the stainless steels, at about one-third to one-tenth the amount of the fluoropolymers. A temperature rise of 100 degrees for a PEEK pipe occasions an expansion of somewhat less than 2 inches for a 100-foot length. A similar length of PVDF pipe will expand by 8 1/2 inches. Biofilms (or other coatings) are said to be more easily released from PVDF surfaces under such conditions because their rates of expansion will differ so from those of the polymer (Hanselka, 1991). Others disagree, seeing highly hydrated biofilms as accomodating dimensional alterations. Desirable where the shedding of biofilm may be involved, this expansion differential is a disadvantage when PVDF is being used as a cladding for less inert materials. The high thermal stability of PEEK commends it for high-temperature applications where no steady state obtains. Generally speaking, the higher thermal expansions and contractions of polymerics impose unwanted strains on their inner surfaces. Mechanical fatigue is a possible consequence.

A full compliment of pipes, valves, and connectors in various sizes should be available for whatever polymeric material is selected to build a distribution system. These are at present not available with PEEK.

By contrast, PVDF, whatever its limitations, is a widely used, dependable material of construction. Its limitations should not deter its use, and it should be employed within its proper modes and conditions of application.

Whatever their construction, the various pipes of a distribution system should be clearly labeled as to the contents they convey.

Rechen (1984) discussed piping materials and piping systems design. The physical and chemical properties of polymeric materials utilized in the construction of components for high-purity water were discussed by Hanselka (1987).

Comparative Piping Costs

There are three aspects to the cost of piping: the piping itself; putting it into place; and the fittings, valves, elbows, and various other joints that make it into a system.

Polyvinyl chloride piping is perhaps the least costly among the polymerics. The PVDF is approximately 6 times as expensive as PVC; PFA, about 10 times; and PEEK, about 26 times more in price, far more than stainless steel. Hango and Pettengill (1987) estimated that the installed cost of PVDF is usually 2.5 to 3 times the cost of PVC piping. They stated, however, that PVDF replacements can reduce contamination originating in the distribution system.

Stainless steel piping costs considerably more than PVDF, and stainless steel fittings, particularly polished, are far more costly than those of PVDF. The PVDF piping costs more to hang, however, and Manfredi (1991) held that PVDF piping installed can cost almost as much as stainless steel installed. Other estimates find PVDF to be less expensive by one-third. The discrepancy may lie in the pipe sizes being considered. Larger pipe diameters require more generous wall thicknesses for mechanical rigidity. The added mass increases the costs and often confines the polymeric piping to smaller-bore uses.

Since valves fabricated of PVDF are less expensive than those of stainless steel, small systems with much valving can advantageously be built of PVDF. Large systems may perhaps more economically be constructed of stainless steel. The plastic piping is easier to handle and can more easily be put up into a rack, but does require more supporting.

The joining mechanism may be a problem area for PVDF. The inner weld area can now be made crevice free by some craftsmen, but not by all. The experience and reputation of the PVDF pipe and system fabricator is important.

One considerable advantage of polymeric piping (except for organometallic-containing PVC) is that it does minimize sources for metallic impurities.

Housings and Vessels

Housings are intended to withstand working pressures by 2 to 2.5 times. The housings, as of filter cartridges, are tested hydrostatically to ensure an adequacy of tensile strength against bursting pressures. They are not, however, tested for creep, the phenomenon wherein, under maintained pressure loads over time, the material of construction (as of steel) stretches and undergoes elongation. The risk is that prolonged or additive creep may ultimately yield a vessel unable to withstand the tensile strength requirements of the burst pressures originally designed for.

ASME code vessels. The American Society of Mechanical Engineers (ASME) has a code that ensures that given vessels used for hazardous purposes, for example, the containment of hot 90% sulfuric acid, or filter holders/housings used in relatively dangerous operations, are built to design specifications that ensure safety (Perry and Chilton, 1973; Lawton, 1986).

In 1911, the Boiler and Pressure Vessel Code was established by the American Society of Engineers to specify rules for the design, construction, and selection of materials; and inspection of boilers and pressure vessels. Periodically, revisions and additions to the Code are made to incorporate new materials and current technologies. The American Society of Mechanical Engineers issues a Certificate of Authorization for fabrication of ASME Code pressure vessels after a rigorous review of fabrication facilities and quality control procedures.

"U" Stamp. The "U" Stamp symbol is applied to all filter housings over 5 ft^3 in volume and 250-psig design pressure, or 1.5 ft^3 in volume and 600-psig design pressure. An independent inspector is required to apply this symbol after witnessing fabrication and testing the filter housings. A "U" Stamp may be applied to any filter housing regardless of volume and design pressure.

"UM" Stamp. The "UM" Stamp symbol may be applied to filter housings that do not exceed the volume and pressure parameters required for a "U" Stamp. The

"UM" Stamp or Manufacturer's Stamp is limited to these parameters and may be applied to the filter housing by an authorized manufacturer's inspector.

Before fabrication of a Code vessel may begin, calculations, engineering drawings, bills of material, and process sheets must be presented for approval by an independent inspector. The inspector is employed by an independent insurance agency, and is authorized by the American Society of Mechanical Engineers to witness fabrication and testing of Code pressure vessels. The Code requires that only traceable, certified materials be used and that only highly trained and Code-certified welders fabricate the filter housings.

Upon completion, the pressure vessel is hydrostatically tested at 1 1/2 times the working pressure, and witnessed by the inspector. A Manufacturer's Data Report is filed containing all pertinent information on the filter housing's construction and testing. The Data Report is the official ASME record document and is signed by both the independent ASME inspector and the manufacturer's inspector. The report is submitted to the owner of the filter housing as a permanent record.

The code was established to preserve the safety of the general public and the workplace. Specifying as ASME Code pressure vessel ensures that specific, detailed records are kept and a certified level of quality is maintained.

Specifically, the code and the local governmental requirements will stipulate materials of construction, weld types and certification, design criteria, test parameters, and inspection procedures. The purpose of the code is to ensure safety in the operation of the vessel within the stated operating parameters. For instance, this may be ensured by using multiple securing methods for housing components (i.e., swing bolts versus a single securing method [e.g.., a single bolt in a V-band clamp]); 100% nondestructive pressure testing at a 1 1/2 times the rated pressure, and destructive burst testing of the design at 3 times the rated pressure or greater. Compliance with the ASME code results in lower insurance premiums for these hazardous undertakings.

Certain vessels are exempt from code jurisdictions; vessels with a volume of 120 gal (465 L) or less; vessels with an internal diameter not exceeding 6 inches (15.2 cm); vessels with an internal or external operating pressure not exceeding 15 psig (1 bar); and vessels under federal control.

Although ASME-coded vessels are not often required for filter holders/ housings in pharmaceutical applications, many of the criteria for design, raw materials, and testing should be considered when specifying housing requirements. It should be noted that ASME-code housings, usually multielement housings, are from 3 to 5 times the cost of conventional housings.

Rupture Discs

Rupture discs provide leak-tight seals in pressurized systems, unlike spring-loaded or other mechanical arrangements that may weep or leak. The ASME

for tanks that can withstand some pressure or vacuum differentials. When, however, they are required for tanks built for use at ambient pressures, they must be calibrated with some precision, and that renders them costly. The rupture of a rupture disk saves the tank against collapse. The tank contents, however, may become contaminated in the process, and sanitary rupture disks are very expensive. Rupture disks outfitted with automated alarms signaling their breakage are available

Relief valves are available. They open to redress pressure differential before closing again. They are not, however, of sanitary design, nor can they be calibrated with great precision (Manfredi, 1991).

Water storage tanks and the conveying pipes and pumps may be sanitized by 10% (or stronger) hydrogen peroxide (H_2O_2), prepared from 30% H_2O_2. The contact time may be 24 hours. In one such operation, the organisms count was reduced thereby from 200 to 300 cfu/100 mL down to 2 to 4 cfu/100mL. Live steam may also be used to effect sanitization. In this case, the tank should be permitted to cool gradually. A cold-water rinse may cause too sudden a condensation of the steam vapor within the tank, leading to tank collapse. The tank vent must, in any case, be sized for the proper rate of air passage.

Vacuum-rated tanks are common. They require walls of about 3/8-inch steel, are more difficult to fabricate, usually do not have as fine a finish, and are very expensive. However, rupture disks are often used in their manufacture.

Small chlorine or iodine residues are sometimes retained in storage tanks, particularly of RO water prior to mixed-bed installations. Typically, 0.2 to 0.4 ppm of chlorine or 0.4 to 1.0 ppm of iodine residuals are utilized. Ozone concentrations of 0.5 to 1.0 ppm are very efficient as residuals.

Mittelman (1987) stated that tank turnover rates of less than once per 48 hours will produce bacterial levels unless some continuous treatment is provided. It is indicated, therefore, that tanks not be oversized; and that their contents should continuously be heated or exposed to ozone residuals. Circulation through a UV light unit can be effective. Mittelman said that a 5,000-gallon storage tank would require a 3.5-gpm-capacity UV unit to manage a turnover rate of once per 24 hours. Recirculating systems are particularly suited to intermittent operations, being continually in a dynamic mode. Adequate mixing of tank contents is aided by the return pipe being plumbed to the tank top, withdrawal being from the bottom.

Storage tanks require using vent filters to equalize the tank pressure with the atmosphere when liquid is either added or withdrawn. If the filter becomes blocked (as by condensed moisture), withdrawal of liquid by way of a pump may cause an implosion of the tank. The use of hydrophobic vent filters facilitates the removal of condensed moisture, which would be tightly held by hydrophilic filter materials. Alternatively, the vent filter, of whatever composition, may be contained within a steam-jacketed or electrical-wire-traced housing whose temperature is maintained above the dew point of the air to preclude moisture condensation.

It is possible to dispense with vent filters by the use of a pressurized nitrogen gas blanket that will separate the tank contents from the outside environment and shield it from same. This will prevent the entrance of carbon dioxide into the tank, thus maintaining its contents at a high resistivity. The nitrogen gas can be obtained from cryogenic sources, and can be added to the nitrogen blanket automatically in response to pressure activated controls when liquid is withdrawn from the tank. The nitrogen gas is under a small pressure of from 2 to 10 inches of water (Sinha, 1991). As liquid is added to the tank, some nitrogen gas is displaced to atmosphere. The integrity of the nitrogen blanket remains intact.

Liquid-level sensing within the tank is either by way of sight tubes, or by electronic or acoustical devices. Liquid movement is by way of pumps or positive nitrogen gas pressure.

Fiberglass-Reinforced Plastic Water Storage Tanks

Stainless steel tanks are widely used to store compendial water in the pharmaceutical industry. The semiconductor industry, being ion-driven, largely eschews them (Hanselka, 1984). Even if the use of stainless steel were to become more widely accepted in the electronics industry, however, the expense of such tanks in the required sizes could be a deterrent. In pharmaceutical contexts, 10,000-gallon tanks are usually large enough. More capacious tanks of stainless steel capable of holding 40,000 to 50,000 gallons could be excessive in their cost. The electronics industry has traditionally used fiberglass-reinforced plastic (FRP) for large-volume storage. (In Europe these are called GRP tanks). Fiberglass confers structural strength to the plastic vessel. The polymers used are mostly isophthalates, usually cross-linked to 70% or 80% to confer rigidity.

Tanks present an enormous surface area for contact with the stored water; thus opportunities for leaching of the polymer components are very great. The tanks are commodity items, hardly optimized to ensure the maintenance of high-purity water standards. Consequently, the unpolymerized monomer, the remnants of the polymerization catalysts, and the end products of the catalysis are available to contaminate the contained water with TOC.

In any polymerization, as the quantity of polymer builds, the viscosity of the polymerization mix increases. This makes it progressively more difficult for the increasingly isolated, remaining monomer molecules to find one another for continuing polymerization. The result is that by the time the polymerization is judged to be "finished," a considerable portion of monomer, some 10% to 20%, may remain unconverted. The low molecular weight of the monomer makes possible its diffusion from within the polymer mass, slowed by the viscosity of the latter, into the water. Diffusion is a time- and temperature-dependent process. Leaching of TOC from the FRP can thus continue at a low rate over a considerable duration. When the polymerization of the FRP formulation is judged to be "finished" depends upon the tank's being able to be handled; upon the hardness and lack of tackiness of the outer surfaces. This is judged informally by a "knuckle" test, or somewhat more sophisticatedly by a Barcol hardness assay wherein the degree of penetration of a diamond point into the coating is measured under standard conditions. Either test reflects meaninglessly upon potential TOC contamination by diffusion from the FRP construction (Hanselka and Putzier, 1990).

Currently, FRP tank shells are faced internally by PVDF and other fluoropolymer liners. The assembly is artfully constructed around a collapsible mandrel that is withdrawn from the interior of the tank upon its completion. Manholes and the like are formed subsequently in accordance with appropriate design considerations. Some dozen or so workshops, scattered about the United States, are currently capable of such assemblages. The result, in essence, is a fluoropolymer tank relatively free of the problem of TOC leaching. Less expensive constructions are available composed of inner linings or facings of polyethylene, polypropylene, or even PVC. It should be noted that FRP compositions are not inert to ozone, and that the oxidative degradations of the polyolefinic materials by this reagent result in polymeric particulate matter being generated (Hanselka and Putzier, 1990).

Hanselka (1991) made this point:

> The details of proper material specification, fabrication, quality control, and shipping procedures will affect both the achieved purity levels and service life of the vessel. These details are often totally unaddressed after the decision to purchase this expensive vessel is made. Often these vessels can cost $100,000. Most of the manufacturers of dual laminate vessels build them for chemical resistance. If high purity is to be considered, critical items must be specified well in advance.
>
> For a long and ultrapure service life all of the following considerations should be followed. The liner must be virgin PVDF, or other fluoropolymer, extruded and calendered. The thickness should be one-eighth inch (3 mm). Since none of the fluoropolymers bond to anything a backing which is embedded in the thermoplastic fluoropolymer substrate must be carefully chosen. The backing should have a minimum peel strength of 100 in.-lbs./ in. and be a knit fiber of either acrylic or polyester. A high peel strength is needed to resist delamination. The fluoropolymer surface which will be exposed to the UPW [high-purity water] should have a clean plastic foil covering. The welding process must utilize nitrogen as a carrier and the weld rod must be of the same precise resin as the sheet. The sheet should be from 50-foot rolls and should be cut and welded such that the minimum number of welds are made. All liner welds must be backed by a conductive

material such that the welds can be tested for the life of the vessel. The FRP vessel must rigidly conform to ASTM D-3299 and ASTM D-4097-82. The resin should be of a high heat distortion type. Special care should be taken to ensure the stiffness of the vessel to minimize flexing of the liner. The vessel should have a false bottom sloped to drain. The bottom corners should have a large knuckle radius and the top should be domed. A top penetration should be provided for a nitrogen feeding relief valve. Be sure that the vessel has a 24-inch manway to facilitate entry. All penetrations should have conical gusseted flanges and the cut-outs must be retained for posterity." (Hanselka, 1991)

Considerations in Materials of Construction

Chemical imperviousness. Inertness to oxidative chemicals and to hydrolytic conditions are sought for materials of construction in order to secure freedom from property changes over long durations of service life. In semiconductor applications in particular, where exposures to aggressive chemicals occur, the chemical inertness of the fluorocarbons is depended upon. The fluorocarbons may be thought of as derivatives of polyethylene wherein fluorine atoms are substituted for the hydrogen atoms to yield the relative inertness of carbon-fluorine bonds for the carbon-hydrogen bonds that are susceptible to chemical degradations. The substitution of fluorine atoms for those of hydrogen can be carried to different extents. When all the hydrogens are replaced by fluorines, the material is called polytetrafluoroethylene (PTFE). Its structure is, perhaps, the archetype of polymeric chemical inertness. Less thoroughly fluorine-substituted polymers are less inert; nor need the inertness necessarily reflect the quantitative degree of substitution. Thus, polyvinylidene fluoride (PVDF) bears two fluorine atoms on one carbon of the two-carbon ethylene per unit. While the polymer is satisfactorily inert over broad-use conditions for extended periods of time, the juxtaposing of the two fluorine atoms on one carbon does tend to heighten their mutual liability. (See "Polyvinylidene fluoride" and "Other polymeric piping," earlier in this chapter.)

Regrettably, a number of different polymeric structures (Table 11-6) are commonly referred to as fluorocarbons. All do contain some fluorine atoms. But the number of such substituent atoms differ, and the chemical inertness of these materials differs as well. This is not always made evident; the term "fluorocarbon" can thus be misleading. Polyvinyl fluoride (PVF), reflecting substitution of one fluorine for only one of the four carbon-hydrogen bonds of polyethylene, is not nearly so inert as PTFE, where fluorines have replaced all of the four hydrogen atoms.

In general, the more highly fluorinated polymers have a greater regularity to their molecular architecture. This permits a closer approach of their chain segments. Degrees of crystallinity appear and manifest themselves as rigidity

Table 11-6
Structures, Trade Names, and Suppliers of Fluorocarbons

Fluorocarbon	*Structure*	*Typical Trade Names and Suppliers*
TFE (tetrafluoroethylene)	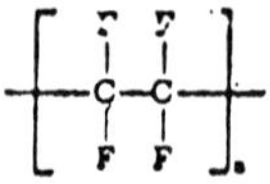	Teflon TFE (E.I. DuPont) Halon TFE (Allied Chemical)
FEP (fluorinated ethylene-propylene)	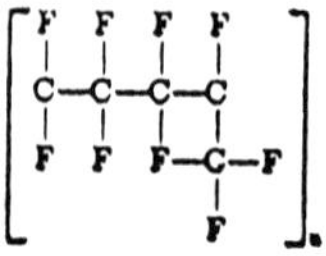	Teflon FEP (E.I. DuPont)
ETFE (ethylene-tetrafluoroethylene copolymer), copolymer of ethylene and TFE	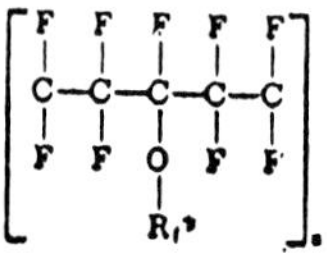	Tefzel (E.I. DuPont)
PFA (perfluoroalkoxy resin) CTFE (chlorotrifluoroethylene)	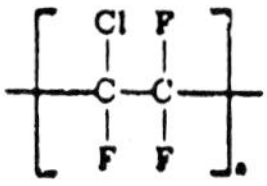	Teflon PFA (E.I. DuPont) Kel-F (3M) Halar E-CTFE (Allied Chemical)
ECTFE (ethylenechlorotrifluoroethylene copolymer), copolymer of ethylene and CTFE	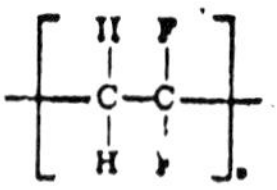	
PVDF (polyvinylidenefluoride)		Kynar (Elf Atochem Chemicals)
PVF (polyvinyl fluoride)	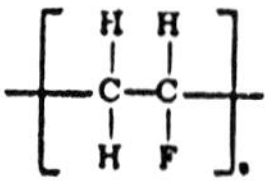	Tedlar (E.I. duPont)

Stronger, filled modifications exist, as do newer, more cold-flow-resistant grades. FEP fluorocarbon is quite similar to TFE in most properties except that its useful temperature is limited to about 400 °F. FEP is much more easily processed, and molded parts are possible with FEP that might not be possible with TFE.

and as a resistance to softening by heat. They are thus difficult to form into shapes where a polymeric flow and adaptability to fabrication are required. This leads to a use of more tractable fluorocarbons, albeit inevitably of a reduced inertness.

Seiler and Barber (1989) described a new family of flexible PVDFs. They are PVDFs made more amenable to shaping and forming by an admixture of PVDF with fluorocarbon monomers prior to being processed. In the process, the monomers become polymerized. The copolymer or blend of polymers (the article was not explicit) has a lower flexural modulus than PVDF, is less stiff, and has a lower deflection temperature. Its use was advocated by Seiler and Barber (1989) for piping and for other equipment construction. The mechanical properties of these modified PVDF materials were stated to meet those desired for DI water system applications. The point being made, however, is that a decrease in chemical inertness must inevitably accompany molecular modifications that result in mechanical property changes. These have not yet been assessed for the new flexible PVDFs.

Elastomers. Seals and gaskets require elastomeric materials for their construction. Hanselka et al. (1987) described a series of flexible polymers for such applications. Polyisoprene, natural rubber (NR), is stable over a fair pH range, but has a poor resistance to solvents. Neoprene (CR) has fair ozone and UV resistance, shows good abrasion resistance, withstands contact with oils, has a high tensile strength with good elongation, and is acceptable for ambient temperature DI systems. Nitrile rubber (NBR), being polar, is resistant to oils; but it does not withstand oxidizers well; and because of its polarity it is inferior in chemical and electrical resistance.

Ethylene-propylene rubbers (EPDM, EDM, EDT, EPR) generally have good resistances to solvents and acids and are even better in withstanding strong alkali. These rubbers (EPDM) are limited to applications at or below 100 °C, but are very abrasion-resistant. The ethylene propylene rubbers are used in general-duty applications and are suitable in DI water systems. Hypalon (CSM) resembles neoprene. It possesses good resistance to solvents, acids, bases, and even ozone. Properly conditioned, it can be used in DI water systems.

Fluorinated propylene rubber (FPM, Viton*) is about 50% fluorinated. It has good chemical resistance to chlorinated solvents (usually difficult to withstand) and to nonpolar solvents. Contrary to published but erroneous accounts, it is not suitable at high pHs. These cause its embrittlement. These fluorinated elastomeric materials have good resistances to ozone and to other oxidants. Having been compounded with metallic vulcanizers such as chromium salts, they must be carefully cleaned before being used in DI water systems. Fully fluorinated rubber (FFR, Kalrez*) exhibits an inertness to most reagents. It offers almost the same chemical and heat resistance as PTFE, and is very expensive.

*Registered DuPont trademarks.

Less resistant elastomerics are encapsulated within fluorocarbon polymer sheaths. In static applications they can be suitable. Under dynamic loading, however, the laminated structures perform less satisfactorily, as shear failures can occur. Additionally, the diffusive permeation of the protective sheath (e.g., by organic reagents, oxidizers, and solvents) is an almost inevitable function of time. Regrettably, PTFE, whether in gasket or sheath form, suffers from the phenomenon of cold flow. It inelastically distorts under pressure, losing its sealing function in the process. Despite such limitations, encapsulated O-rings and gaskets have their utility (Hanselka et al., 1987). Table 11-7 from Dunning and Hanselka (1989) compares various elastomeric materials in their resistance to 5% hydrogen peroxide, 5 ppm of chlorine, and 2 ppm of ozone. The FFR (Kalrez®) is the most resistant and the most costly.

System Appurtenances

A useful view of design factors pertinent to pharmaceutical water systems has ben presented by Collentro (1992, 1993). The author discussed system controls, heat exchangers, and distribution loop considerations. Collentro's observations concerning water systems and their components merit careful attention. Their critique is, however, outside the scope of this writing.

Heat exchangers. According to Section 212.76 of the GMP/LVP, "Heat exchangers other than the welded double-concentric-type or double tube-sheet type must employ a pressure differential and a means of monitoring the differential." The fluid requiring the better microbial quality, the WFI, is maintained at a higher pressure than the less pure cooling fluid. In the event of leaking from one compartment to the other, the greater pressure would force the WFI into the cooling fluid, thus preventing contamination of the WFI compartment and its contents. Gauges may be employed to attest to the positive pressure as from vapor compression stills, being on the clean fluid side.

In the case of single tube-sheet separating the WFI and cooling fluid compartments, a leak might not be noticed (as by the use of the conductivity

Table 11-7
Elastomer Resistance to Sanitization Agents

	Relative Cost	*5% Hydrogen Peroxide*	*Ozone (2 ppm)*	*Chlorine (5 ppm)*
EPDM	1	Excel.	Fair	Fair
CR(Neoprene)	1	Excel.	Fair	Fair
FPM(Viton)	10	Excel.	Good	Good
FFR(Kalrez)	200	Excel.	Excel.	Excel.

Dunning and Hanselka (1989); Courtesy, Semiconductor Pure Water Conference meters) when either Water for Injection or Purified Water is being cooled by deionized water (Figure 11-8).

Two chambers containing the WFI (or PW) and the cooling fluid, respectively, can each be bounded by a tube-sheet wall. Furthermore, the chambers can be separated from one another by an intervening space, so that leakage from one chamber cannot contaminate the other. Additionally, such leakage becomes evident as droplets within the separating space. Such a double tube-sheet heat chamber is represented by Figure 11-9.

Heat exchangers always convey the WFI on the tube side. Heat exchangers should be flushed frequently, at least weekly. Ultraviolet lamps and recirculating pumps both engender heat. Heat exchangers serve to ameliorate this condition.

In its "Guide To Inspections Of High Purity Water Systems" (FDA, 1993), the following remarks appear about heat exchangers:

> An FDA Inspectors Technical Guide with the subject of "Heat Exchangers to Avoid Contamination" discusses the design and potential problems associated with heat exchangers. The guide points out that there are two methods for preventing contamination by leakage. One is to provide gauges to constantly monitor pressure differentials to ensure that the higher pressure is always on the clean fluid side. The other is to utilize the double-tubesheet type of heat exchanger.
>
> In some systems, heat exchangers are utilized to cool water at use points. For the most part, cooling water is not circulated through them when not in use. In a few situations, pinholes formed in the tubing after they were drained (on the cooling water side) and not in use. It was determined that a small amount of moisture remaining in the tubes when combined with air caused a corrosion of the stainless steel tubes on the cooling water side. Thus, it is recommended that when not in use, heat exchangers not be drained of the cooling water.

Pumps. Pumps require being sized to meet peak demands and to maintain the minimum recycle flows. What is desired is a minimization of time between the final polishing and the points of use, to diminish the possibilities of water quality degradations. The belief is widespread that turbulent flows (with Reynolds numbers above 3,000, as usually obtained by linear flows of 2 to 3 ft/sec through 2-inch pipe or so) prevent or significantly impede biofilm formation. Untrue though that be, pumping is performed at rates designed to give the pipe-scouring actions of such flows. Turbulence will be helpful in tangential flow settings, however, to reduce concentration polarization.

Orwin and Gong (1986) stated that the following water flow velocities are recommended: main supply loop, 4 to 10 ft/sec; branch lines, 3 to 10 ft/sec; hookup lines, 1 to 2 ft/sec. These recommendations have no basis in theory. They do derive, however, from a good experience. The actual velocities selected will impact on both capital investments and operating costs. Higher velocities will usually mean smaller (diameter) pipe sizes. This translates to lower initial costs. However, as pressure drop increases as the square of the velocity, operating costs will be substantially higher (Orwin and Gong, 1986).

Both constant- and variable speed pumps are used. Variable-speed pumps are more versatile and are less prodigal of energy. Constant-speed pumps involve lower outlays for capital and maintenance. Also they require less space. They are, therefore, more frequently purchased. However, the flow and pressure output of a constant-speed pump varies with the changing water usage. The pump's efficiency and performance depends upon the demand for water. Pressure control valves are often used in conjunction with constant-speed pumps to establish a fixed pressure head.

Variable-speed pumps, albeit more costly, can be more energy-efficient in low-flow-demand situations. The versatility of variable-speed pumps permits the matching of the pumped flow to the user demand plus the minimum cycle flow. A scheme of variable-speed pumps and control valves permits operations at reduced speeds during low-flow periods. This cuts expenditures for pumping energy. The versatility of variable-speed pumps is especially valuable where the possibilities of facility expansion are to be considered. Overpressurizing the distribution system can be avoided, as can also excessive energy demands during periods of low water usage (McNutt et al., 1986).

In its "Guide To Inspections Of High Purity Water Systems" (FDA, 1993), the following remarks appear about heat exchangers:

If pumps are static and not continuously in operation, their reservoir can

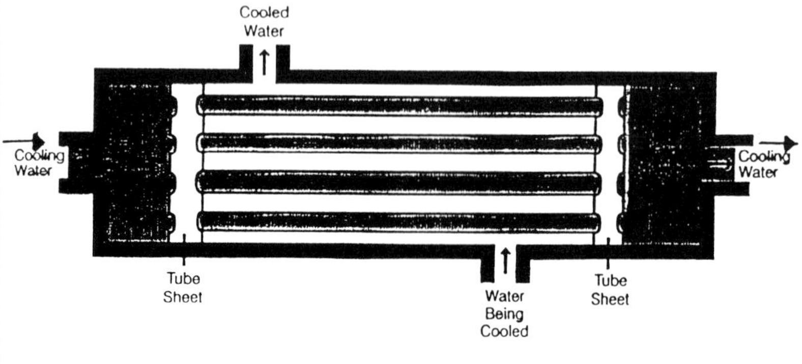

Figure 11-8. Single tube-sheet heat exchanger.

be a static area where water will lie. For example, in an inspection, it was noted that a firm had to install a drain from the low point in a pump housing. Pseudomonas sp. contamination was periodically found in their water system which was attributed in part to a pump which only periodically is operational.

Nickerson (1985) has treated on the subject of pump considerations of water systems. He advised that making a pump and energy requirement survey, although laborious and time-consuming, is worth the effort in terms of operating-expense savings and the knowledge gained of the water treatment system. A method for establishing pump requirements and of evaluating performance was set forth, as was also the means for calculating energy savings (Nickerson, 1985).

Most pumps are noisy. Some submersible pumps are not, but these are not used with pharmaceutical liquids. Industrial-style pumps are usually employed in preliminary or noncritical manufacturing steps.

Almost all larger pumps of 20 to 80 gpm are noisy enough to warrant being isolated in an equipment room, probably surrounded by an acoustic enclosure to accord with regulations regarding noise pollution. Pump manufacturers may characterize a pump as not exceeding a noise level of 85 decibels at a distance of 3 feet. However, that very pump mounted on a steel frame and having piping attached to it can still give a noise problem. There are many varieties of pumps, such as single-stage and multistage, that are very reliable for RO operations.

Centrifugal pumps are widely used in water systems. Generally they are noisy. Positive-displacement pumps are far less noisy, but are much more expensive because of their closer tolerances and the higher-quality steels required for their machining. For a 15-gpm delivery, a centrifugal pump may

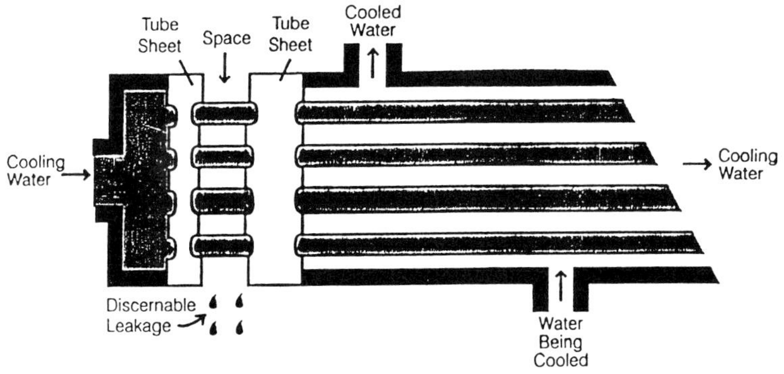

Figure 11-9. Double tube-sheet heat exchanger.
Meltzer (1991); Courtesy, Interpharm Press

cost about $800; a positive-displacement pump could cost about $3,000 and would be almost double in size. Sanitary pumps are available in either design, but are costly. Positive-gear pumps are not sanitary; those pumps that are have smooth transitioning lobes, precision machined, and operate at about 700 rpm. Centrifugal pumps, running at about 3,500 rpm, are inherently more noisy. The sanitary centrifugal pumps were designed for the dairy industry to deliver large volumes at low pressures, as in the emptying (or filling) of tank trucks.

Motivating volumes of water through long reaches of piping may require substantially higher pressures. In this region of performance the pumps are at low efficiencies, possibly 20% or lower. Their operation engenders heat and noise. In one example, water entering a loop at 21 °C (70 °F) attained 78 °C (172 °F) after being recirculated for 12 hours. The installation of chillers may be needed to protect heat-labile ingredients. Poor pumping efficiency results from a mismatch of the pump design to the application. The low number of high-pressure, low-volume centrifugal pumps demanded by the market has thus far rendered new pump designs uneconomical (Manfredi, 1991).

With reverse osmosis, the pressure needed for water permeation of the RO membrane must exceed the osmotic pressure of the feedwater, itself a product of its dissolved components. The higher the applied reverse pressure, the greater will be the rate of product water permeation.

Multistage centrifugal pumps are commonly used. Their advantage is their low rate of wear at the 3,450-rpm level normally used. Reverse osmosis systems involving low flowrates often rely on positive-displacement pumps. These suffer the disadvantages of high noise levels and, frequently, some vibration. High-speed centrifugal pumps operating at speeds of 10,000 rpm or more have been used for high-pressure feeds. Such pumps have noise levels approaching the maximum allowable by OSHA.

What is of importance is the awareness that all pumps generate particles by a wearing of their seals, rotors, and other moving parts. Improper pump operations may cause cavitation. This phenomenon is very productive of particles, and may in its severer manifestations actually destroy the pump. For this reason, pumps should be positioned sufficiently upstream so as to enable the filtrative removal of the particles that are produced.

Pumps do break down from time to time. It can, therefore, be useful to have standby pumps available for a more ready replacement.

System Balance

In designing a circulating water system, care must be taken to see that the system is properly balanced to provide water to the many users at acceptable levels of pressure and volumes. To achieve this, balancing valves and careful line sizing are required, together with the proper sizing of the circulating pumps. This is not easily achieved. Enough water volume must be provided to fill the entire system.

Beyond this, volume must be supplied for the demands at the points of use. This may be a bit tricky to balance when peak flows are factored in. After the removal at the points of use, the return loop will still have its volume and velocity requirements. A rough formula is based on the maximum water usage plus a 25% to 50% overage.

Large systems may need 40,000 gallons, plus excess for circulation. The pipe diameter is sized to deliver the water volume at velocities of 2, 3, or even 20 lineal ft/sec. Particularly at peak loads, however, the return loop will have less water to convey. The piping thus cannot be perfectly sized for all the possible circumstances. The supply line is the critical one, however, and its design requirements are paramount.

In a semiconductor facility, the maintenance of the operational pressures required by the fabricating (fab) equipment is a major consideration in designing the hydraulic system necessary to the storage and distribution of high-purity water. Also to be taken into account are the minimum, maximum, and average water usages, as well as storage for peak demands, equipment cleaning and regeneration, and emergency requirements. When coupled to considerations of space availability and building configuration, the calculations involved are complex enough to require computerized designs (Orwin and Gong, 1986). Operating pressures will be based upon the pressure needs of specific equipment; upon the differences in elevation between booster pumps and the points of use; and upon the need to compensate for frictional pressure losses, both within the distribution system and within the water treatment equipment (McNutt et al., 1986). The interrelationship among flow, velocity, and pressure means that the system design requires a holistic approach.

According to McNutt et al. (1986), the more modern facilities limit a feed loop to a maximum length of 600 feet from the polishing station to points of use. The objective is to minimize degradation of water quality. In such a design, the number of polishing stations is determined by the overall facility size, and by the fab divisions. Typically, there will exist one main loop from the control water treatment plant to the user areas. From this main loop will derive a number of user loops, each with its polishing station to ensure the water quality for use in the fab areas. Each user loop requires pressure and flow controls for its own regulation. Obviously, a close proximity of the control treatment facility to the user areas simplifies the distribution system and minimizes water quality decay. Where such an arrangement is not possible, more plentiful local polishing stations become mandated.

The use of water storage makes possible smaller-sized units, with advantages of lower capital and operating costs. However, the water quality tends to degrade with storage. A 1-megohm-cm-resistivity water may be stored for hours with no significant change. Water with an 18-megohm-cm resistivity, even under inert gas blanketing, may evince a drop in resistivity in less than an hour. Prudent engineering judgment must be invoked in the design and location of storage facilities. It would seem to be best to utilize water storage for peak demands. The operational facilities would be sized to run continuously on demand rather than to prepare makeup water for storage. Continuous operations reduce the bacterial proliferations that accompany shutdowns (McNutt et al., 1986). Storage tanks present hydraulic and microbial problems. Nevertheless, some designers prefer a multiplicity of tanks, made secure by the operational advantages that come with redundancies, especially the leeway to use one tank while servicing another.

Given equipment items may require specific levels of pressure for their proper operation. That pressure must be provided even to the points of use. McNutt et al. (1986) advocated the use of low pressures, about 30 psig for the main loop from the central purification system to the user loops. The pressure within the user loops is boosted to levels sufficient to compensate for the frictional losses suffered during distribution through the pipes and valves; to sustain the pressure levels needed at the points of use; and to supply the pressures required for the fab tools. The use of lower pressure levels where possible (within the main loop, for example) reduces the potential within the system for transient hydraulic surges, potentially equipment-damaging water hammers; and minimizes wear and tear. Booster pumps are then necessitated at the user loops, but this is to be preferred to the stresses and strains on the piping of the main loops caused by the high pressure (50 to 90 psig) required where booster pumps are not employed (McNutt et al., 1986).

Valves. Pressure control valves, pressure relief valves, and orifice plates are used to exercise pressure control and regulation. Valves are available in a multitude of designs and activations. A large distribution system can contain dozens of different valves and other pressure controls. Control valves are widely used because of the great flexibility they offer, being able to control fluctuating user demands in accordance with changing pressure requirements. To ensure the proper performance of the valve installations, they should be accompanied by suitable gauges. They should also be maintained properly to prevent excessive wear and corrosion.

Pressure relief valves are installed primarily to protect against pressure surges strong enough to rupture piping and equipment. Such transient pressure surges can occur when multiple outlets are closed simultaneously. The limited purpose of such relief valves is the protecting of equipment. They function too slowly, and usually require manual resetting, to be useful as a response to normal, variable pressure experiences. For such purposes, appropriate selection should be made from among the many other valve types available.

Many pharmaceutical processors set their own standards and specifications regarding valves, evaluating these on the basis of pilot plant studies. In the case of biotechnology applications, the compliance valve suitability in accord with

USP Biological Tests may be indicated. This is particularly so where the sensitivity of mammalian cell cultures may be involved.

Where the possibilities of corrosion are of concern, stainless steel valve bodies can be protected by claddings of elastomeric or polymeric materials. Alternatively, more-resistant compositions may be used. These can be made of titanium, Hastalloy B2., or of fluorocarbons such as PTFE, PVDF, or PFA.

In the actual valve constructions, care should be taken to make certain that the operating mechanisms can withstand sterilizing temperatures and pressures, and also the rigors of cleaning operations. Surfaces encountering the fluids being processed should be crevice-free and easily accessible to sterilizing steam, as well as to clean-in-place chemicals.

Carvell (1992) discussed the considerations important to valve selections pertinent to sterile or contained processes. He presented and critiqued various valve designs, and evaluated their several relevant features. He offered an appraisal of valves suitable for such sterile purposes, including surfaces finishes, materials of construction, and considerations of ease of cleaning and sterilization.

In the troubleshooting of water systems, it can be very helpful to be able to isolate individual treatment units by way of isolation waves.

Valve-caused microbial contamination. Ball valves are not considered capable of being sanitized. Their blank sides are shielded internally when the valve is open to the flow of liquids, whether sanitizing or other. It is, therefore, not possible to clean them thoroughly.

The FDA (1993) in its "Guide To Inspections Of High Purity Water Systems says the following regarding ball valves: "Also in this system were ball valves. These valves are not considered sanitary valves since the center of the valve can have water in it when the valve is closed. This is a stagnant pool of water that can harbor microorganisms."

At one biotechnology company where the limitations of ball valves are recognized, each ball valve is removed, disassembled, cleaned, and sterilized before being reassembled aseptically for reuse. This is done before every production batch, and at least once every 7 to 10 days.

Diaphragm valves are, however, generally considered to be sanitizable. Husted (1994) pointed out, nevertheless, that this is not strictly so. In the spaces wherein the elastic diaphragm sections are fixedly secured between the metal parts of such valves, there is room for microbial lodgements. Gressett and Korcyl (1994) stated that such occurrences may establish loci of organism contamination that may manifest themselves, misleadingly, as requiring more general and extensive sanitizations. They advised the periodic removal, disassembling, cleaning and steam autoclaving of diaphragm valves as a means of minimizing more general and arduous system sanitizations.

The Teflon facings of the elastomeric (usually Viton A) components of these valves, intended to protect against contamination and chemical attack, serve to invite biofilm deposition (Gressett and Korcyl, 1994). This focal source of microbial contamination is usually overlooked. It requires a specific localized address.

Orifice plates. Orifice plates, simple solid disks each with a sharp-edged hole in its center, are the simplest, least-expensive devices for pressure regulation. Their proper operation requires, however, the maintenance of an adequate back pressure while they pass a calculated flow volume. Insufficient flow may create an insufficient back pressure; excessive flow during periods of low user demand may create excessive back pressure. Orifice plates are useful in valve bypass situations, as when cleaning valves. Otherwise, they may be too inflexible to substitute for valves. They may be used reliably with systems having very stable demand requirements; large water uses may offer pressure levels that are too unstable for dependable operations (McNutt et al., 1986).

Hydraulic balancing. High-purity water distribution loops are dynamic systems. At any moment such a system will have a wide range of velocities for a given use demand. The velocities throughout the system are established by a hydraulic balancing of the entire system, reflecting the given configuration of the pipe arrangements. Changing pipe sizes in one area of the network, as to increase velocities, may thus decrease velocities in another area. A complete hydraulic balance of the entire system, usually achieved by computerized modeling, is required to establish the overall effects of alterations to the system. Changes should not be lightly undertaken. A proper hydraulic balance to the entire distribution system is highly to be desired. It is this that will ensure the needed velocities throughout the piping system, the pressure available at the use points, and the flow required for given demand conditions (Orwin and Gong, 1986).

The total daily consumption, the average use-volume, the peak usage, and the minimum circulation requirements all require accommodation in calculating the total volume of the system. To meet the circulation requirements, the distribution loop is designed first. The daily and peak loads are then allowed for.

Recirculating Distribution Systems

It is advised that the water pressure within the distribution system should be less than 10 bar (McWilliam, 1995). Otherwise, there may be difficulty in selecting a pump suitable for pharmaceutical water that can develop higher pressures while supplying a low positive suction head value. Also, the use of higher pressures will require heat-exchangers having higher pressure ratings, and will entail the costs of equipment capable of withstanding such elevated pressures.

The flow resistance of heat-exchangers makes for higher pressures. Where

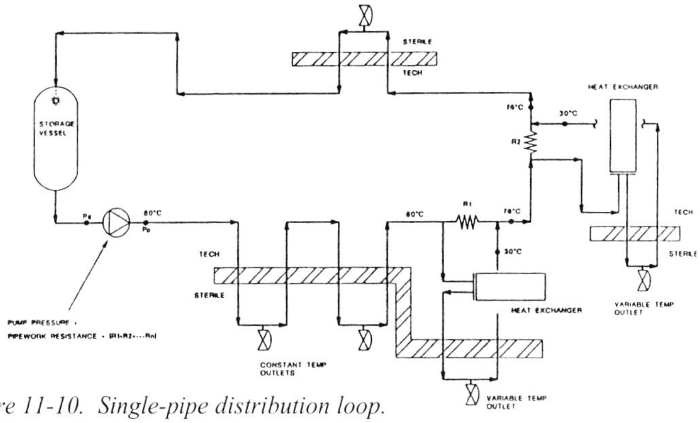

Figure 11-10. Single-pipe distribution loop.

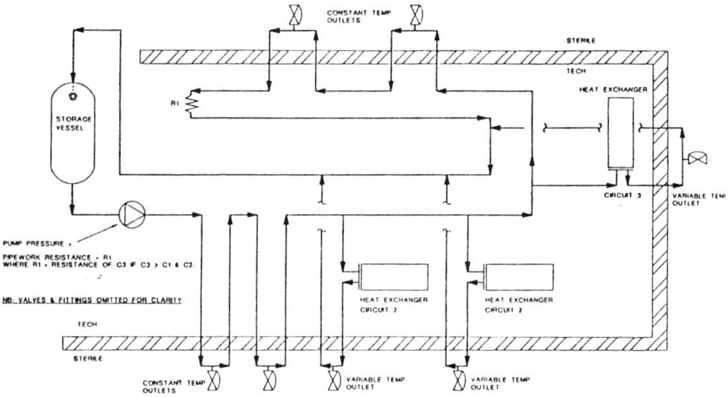

Figure 11-11. Double-pipe (flow/return) distribution loop.

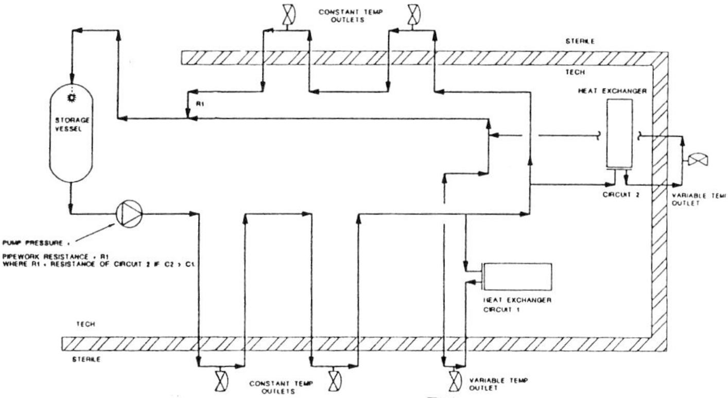

Figure 11-12. Double-pipe (flow/reverse return) distribution loop.

From McWilliam (1995); Courtesy, *Pharmaceutical Engineering.*

the number of heat-exchangers in a hot water loop is small, one or two, a single-pipe distribution system suffices; as it obviously does also in an ambient temperature loop that require no heat-exchangers. However, with a single-pipe loop, the flow resistances of the heat-exchangers have a cumulative effect on the system's pressure requirements. A single heat-exchanger subloop can have a minimum pressure drop of about 0.3 bar (McWilliam, 1995).

Where single-pipe distribution systems can be used they offer the advantage of an equal flowrate velocity throughout, as well as the requirement of the least amount of piping (Figure 11-10). However, they also necessitate flow-balancing devices, the use of which is complex. They also present the possibilities of higher pressure requirements. Double-pipe flow and return loops can accommodate multiple heat-exchangers without creating unduly high pressures. Providing for the easy regulation of flowrates, they do not require in-line flow-regulation devices. Also, they offer a potential for designing self-balancing loops, and a potential for smaller main-loop pipe sizes to be used (Figure 11-11). There are, of course, also disadvantages to double-pipe distribution loops. Greater quantities of pipework, as much as 100%, may be needed. A potential exists for high pressure differentials at heat-exchangers. Furthermore, the water velocity circulating within the loops is reduced; this is a concern for those who believe (erroneously) that biofilm minimization requires water velocities within the usual range of 1.5 to 2.0 meters per second. The effect of returning to the system water cooled by heat-exchangers present in double-pipe, flow/return loops is discussed by McWilliam (1995). Generally speaking, the water within the loop may fall below 80 °C. However, the heat-exchanger connections may be arranged to be downstream of the points-of-use, so that the utilized water is at its proper temperature.

A distribution arrangement system known as double-pipe, flow/reverse-return may be utilized (Figure 11-12). It offers the significant advantage of being self-balancing because of an equal pressure drop across all the heat-exchanger subloops. The shortcoming of this system lies in the greater quantity of piping involved in its double-pipe feature, and in the associated documentation and cost. The chief disadvantage of this distribution arrangement is that the main volume of water within the return pipes is that circulating within the heat-exchanger subloops. The diameter of the return pipe is, therefore, smaller and has a higher pressure drop per unit length. Consequently, the system pressure may be excessively high where many heat-exchangers may be present. However, in its equalization of pressure drops across each heat-exchanger subloop, this system eliminates the need for flow-regulation devices and their complexities.

Rate of Flow

A robust rate of water flow is prescribed. What is sought is an avoidance of quiescent zones adjacent to surfaces, for example, of pipes or tanks. Slow water velocities are seen as being productive of laminar flows. Turbulent flows are desired. The shear forces generated by water turbulence characterized by Reynolds numbers of above 3,000 are *hypothesized* as being less likely to permit organism surface attachments. Such flows may prevent nutrient concentration and thus minimize chemotactic bacterial movements in response to a chemical gradient. Laminar flows are characterized as having N_{Re} of less than 2,000 (Chapman et al., 1983a).

Reynolds numbers greater than 3,000 correspond to a water flow of at least 0.8 gal/min (3 L/min) in a 2-inch (5.0-cm) diameter pipe at water temperatures of 60 °F (15.6 °C) (Chapman et al., 1983b). In one application, a flow of 5.5 ft/sec is used in a 2-inch pipe, equivalent to 50 gpm and a Reynolds number of about 3,000 minimum. To achieve the turbulent flows that are sought, linear pipe velocities of up to 20 ft/sec are relied upon. Some semiconductor houses use 7, some 12 ft/sec, depending upon the pipe diameters. The average is around 12 ft/sec. Circulatory flows greater than 5 or so lineal feet per second involve a pumping penalty. More rapid circulation rates are advantageous, however, where heat exchangers are being used. The more rapid recirculation better maintains the temperature.

Nickerson (1985) and Riley (1983) recommended linear flow velocities of 5 to 10 ft/sec.

Fluid velocity may be calculated as follows:

$$\text{Velocity, ft/sec} = \frac{\text{flowrate, gpm} \times 144\ \text{in}^2/\text{ft}^2}{\Pi \times (0.5\ \text{pipe ID, in.})^2 \times 7.48\ \text{gal/ft}^3 \times 60\ \text{sec/min}} \qquad \text{Eq. 11-1}$$

Most systems are operated at Reynolds numbers in excess of 2,000 (Hanselka, 1991). Despite the greater shearing effects of higher Reynolds numbers, the liquid layers next to the pipe surfaces will always remain laminar (Pittner, 1988). It is these layers that define the biofilm of the sublaminar region. If instead of flows of 2 lineal ft/sec through a 3-inch pipe, the flow were to be 5 lineal ft/sec, some layers of biofilm might become sheared off to create floating or planktonic microbes. Yet several layers of biofilm would remain. Nevertheless, flow velocities are designed in the hope that they will prevent or remove biofilm formation. These expectations may well not be met, given the persistent formation of biofilm. Balazs (1988) has observed, however, very little such film formation on some waters at velocities above 2.5 ft/sec.

The maintenance of adequate flowrates and acceptable pressure drops with the avoidance of dead legs was treated by Bukay (1987) and Nickerson (1985). Dynamic pressure control valves are required to avoid unequal flows.

Dead Legs

Any unused section of pipe connected to another pipe or conduit through which water is flowing may contain, depending upon the venturi effect caused by the flowing water, relatively quiescent or stagnant quantities of water. This non-flowing water is of concern because of the higher planktonic organism counts found for such waters. (See page 98). Such unused sections of pie are called dead legs. The term has been extended to any container of nonflowing water during its period of stagnation, even if the stagnation is not continuous. Thus filter holders are sometimes characterized as dead-legs when containing water not in active flow. Transport into a dead-leg is not directly a function of recirculation velocity (Noble 1994).

The situation is further complicated when thermometer wells or probes are placed into the pipes. The presence of such physical insertions may be seen as creating channels whose dimensions may make for quiescent quantities of water within the pipe. Such conclusions come about not from any measurements of water flow or its absence, but because of ritualistic calculations of dimensions presumed automatically to restrict such flows.

The dimensions of a dead leg, the quiescence of the water, depends upon such factors as the relative pipe dimensions, the volumes of the water they contain, the rates of flow, and even the temperature; in short, upon the several factors governing the venturi effect in the pipe wherein the water is flowing, and the diffusional effects within the pool of nonflowing water in the dead leg. More than the pipe dimensions are involved. Nevertheless, a dead leg is defined as an unused section of pipe in a recirculation loop wherein the length exceeds by at least 6 times the diameter. More recently, design engineers have been concerned with ratios of 4 to 1 and even 3 to 1. In the conventional view, dead legs are seen as quiet havens where the organisms have time to attach themselves to the surfaces, usually nutrition-rich, to flourish and develop a biofilm undisturbed by scouring rates of water flow. Where water circulation is not part of the design, the entire system serves as an interim dead leg. Furthermore, the poorer circulation of water within a dead leg permits its contents to be at lower temperatures. The relatively quiescent water within a dead leg tends to be cooler, being passed less frequently through the heat exchanger. This too may encourage bacterial growth (Bukay, 1987).

The use of flush-diaphragm or sanitary valves is also important in eliminating the stagnant-water areas of dead legs. Point-of-use installations require special attention. The point of use must not match or exceed in its length the definition of a dead leg. Therefore, conveying and returning lines to the point of use should form a drop loop from the overhead mains. The point-of-use spout, appropriately short, descends from the lowest section of the conveying pipes. The short, fixed pipe from the distribution drop loop to the point of use should drain freely, to provide a physical break. It should be as vertical as possible to ensure the rapid drying of its inner surfaces. Prior to water being drawn at such a point of use, an adequate flushing of the dry pipe should be made.

The potential for dead legs usually occurs at valved branches. Special close welded branch valves have been devised that serve to eliminate or minimize such occurrences (McWilliam, 1995).

Periodic draining and flushing can be effective practices in maintaining microbial control of the system. In this connection, the pipes conveying the water ought to be inclined about 1/16 to 1/8 inch per running foot (0.15 to 0.31 cm per running 30 cm) to ensure thorough drainability. The FDA GMPs (1976) do not specify the pitch of the pipes, only that they drain completely. Installation verification should indicate how the pitch was measured; the horizontal reference points require being confirmed as to their levelness with each other.

Self-draining is particularly required where steam sterilizations are employed. Puddled water caused by steam condensation cannot exceed 100 °C in temperature (at atmospheric pressure). Attainment of 121 °C is needed for sterilizations, especially when Gram-positive spores may be present. The avoidance of collected water is ensured by the free drainage of pipes and hoses. To guarantee self-draining, McWilliam (1995) advises the pipework should be installed to a fall of at least 1:100.

There should be suitable air gaps at the drains. The terminus of the drain pipe should be at least 2 inches above the curb of the receiving drain pipe to prevent the possibility of backflow or back siphonage.

Documentary evidence regarding the efficacy of the periodic draining and flushing of pipes as a means of microbial management of the system is hard to come by. The practice seems to be unquestionably accepted. It seems intended for nonrecirculating, room-temperature, stored water. The practice is not followed with hot recirculating systems, which are self-sanitizing.

Given the widespread knowledge concerning the undesirability of dead legs, the frequency of their occurrence is a surprise. Most of those discovered by FDA investigators are seen not be be the results of poor design, but rather of accident. A vial-washing machine, for instance, may have been removed from a system. However, the pipe that led to it remains in place, forgotten to be removed. A 6 foot dead leg is the consequence.

Young et al (1994) treat on the subject of dead-leg sanitizations by saturated steam using sterilization-in-place techniques in conjunction with *Bacillus stearothermophilus* spores. These investigators found that the limiting factor, as in all steamings, is the displacement of air from the dead legs. Tubes 8.8 cm long with 0.4-cm i.d. could not be sterilized at 121 °C. As the diameter increases, sterilization becomes more easily achievable. The orientation of the dead leg is also an influencing factor; vertical positionings contribute to the frustration of steam sanitizations. To attain a 12-log reduction in the spore population, 75 minutes at 121 °C were required for dead legs 19.0 cm long with an i.d. of 1.7 cm in a vertical position; 167 minutes were needed for an 8.8-cm long tube 1.0 cm in diameter.

The data of Young et al. (1994) show that the length-to-diameter ratios do not provide a general guideline predictive of sterilizations.

FDA Observations Relative to Equipment

The FDA (1993) "Guide To Inspections Of High Purity Water Systems" has commented on several types of equipment:

> **Heat Exchangers**. One principal component of the still is the heat exchanger. Because of the similar ionic quality of distilled and deionized water, conductivity meters cannot be used to monitor microbiological quality. Positive pressure such as in vapor compression or double tubesheet design should be employed to prevent possible feedwater to distillate contamination in a leaky heat exchanger.
>
> An FDA Inspectors Technical Guide with the subject of "Heat Exchangers to Avoid Contamination" discusses the design and potential problems associated with heat exchangers. The guide points out that there are two methods for preventing contamination by leakage. One is to provide gauges to constantly monitor pressure differentials to ensure that the higher pressure is always on the clean fluid side. The other is to utilize the double-tubesheet type of heat exchanger.
>
> In some systems, heat exchangers are utilized to cool water at use points. For the most part, cooling water is not circulated through them when not in use. In a few situations, pinholes formed in the tubing after they were drained (on the cooling water side) and not in use. It was determined that a small amount of moisture remaining in the tubes when combined with air caused a corrosion of the stainless steel tubes on the cooling water side. Thus, it is recommended that when not in use, heat exchangers not be drained of the cooling water.
>
> **Holding Tank**. In hot systems, temperature is usually maintained by applying heat to a jacketed holding tank or by placing a heat exchanger in the line prior to an insulated holding tank.
>
> The one component of the holding tank that generates the most discussion is the vent filter. It is expected that there be some program for integrity testing this filter to assure that it is intact. Typically, filters are not jacketed to prevent condensate or water from blocking the hydrophobic vent filter. If this occurs (the vent filter becomes blocked), possibly either the filter will rupture or the tank will collapse. There are methods for integrity testing of vent filters in place.
>
> It is expected, therefore, that the vent filter be located in a position on the holding tank where it is readily accessible.

Just because a WFI system is relatively new and distillation is employed, it is not problem-free. In an inspection of a manufacturer of parenterals, a system fabricated in 1984 was observed. While the system may appear somewhat complex on the initial review, it was found to be relatively simple. The observations at the conclusion of the inspection of this manufacturer included, "Operational procedures for the Water for Injection system failed provide for periodic complete flushing or draining. The system was also open to the atmosphere and room environment. Compounding equipment consisted of non-sealed, open tanks with lids. The Water for Injection holding tank was also not sealed and was never sampled for endotoxins." Because of these and other comments, the firm recalled several products and discontinued operations.

Pumps. Pumps burn out and parts wear. Also, if pumps are static and not continuously in operation, their reservoir can be a static area where water will lie. For example, in an inspection, it was noted that a firm had to install a drain from the low point in a pump housing. Pseudomonas sp. contamination was periodically found in their water system which was attributed in part to a pump which only periodically is operational.

Piping. Piping in WFI systems usually consist of a high polished stainless steel. In a few cases, manufacturers have begun to utilize PVDF (polyvinylidene fluoride) piping. It is purported that this piping can tolerate heat with no extractables being leached. A major problem with PVDF tubing is that it requires considerable support. When this tubing is heated, it tends to sag and may stress the weld (fusion) connection and result in leakage. Additionally, initially at least, fluoride levels are high. This piping is of benefit in product delivery systems where low level metal contamination may accelerate the degradation of drug product, such as in the Biotech industry.

One common problem with piping is that of "dead-legs". The proposed LVP Regulations defined dead-legs as not having an unused portion greater in length than six diameters of the unused pipe measured from the axis of the pipe in use. It should be pointed out that this was developed for hot 75-80 °C circulating systems.

With colder systems (65-75 °C), any drops or unused portion of any length of piping has the potential for the formation of a biofilm and should be eliminated if possible or have special sanitizing procedures. There should be no threaded fittings in a pharmaceutical water system. All pipe joints must utilize sanitary fittings or be butt welded. Sanitary fittings will usually be used where the piping meets valves, tanks and other equipment that must be removed for maintenance or replacement. Therefore, the firm's procedures for sanitization, as well as the actual piping, should be reviewed and evaluated during the inspection.

A typical problem that occurs is the failure of operating procedures to preclude contamination of the system with non-sterile air remaining in a pipe after drainage.

A typical problem occurs when a washer or hose connection is flushed and then drained at the end of the operation. After draining, this valve (the second off of the system) is closed. If on the next day or start-up of the operation the primary valve off of the circulating system is opened, then the non-sterile air remaining in the pipe after drainage would contaminate the system. The solution is to provide for operational procedures that provide for opening the secondary valve before the primary valve to flush the pipe prior to use.

Materials Used in an Actual System

In connection with the foregoing, it may be of interest to refer to the WFI system at the Upjohn Company at Kalamazoo, Michigan, as described by Coates et al. (1983).

Stainless steel types 316 and 316L were selected as the materials of construction over 304 because of their greater resistance to pitting, crevice corrosion, and other forms of localized attack. The use of 316L was seen as minimizing carbide precipitation and its effects during welding; although when welded properly, both 316 and 316L were about equally resistant to corrosion. Certain components were fabricated of 316 stainless, however, simply because of excessive costs and time delays required for the same items fashioned of 316L.

All joints were of the sanitary clamp design or were machine welded, principally to provide better sanitizing and clean-in-place (CIP) capabilities. Machine welding was by an Astro-Arc automatic welder. The welds were not electropolished. A Certified Welder Inspector was employed to inspect all of the welds, using a borescope among other tools. Photographs were made of some of the welds for later routine inspections. Where removable joints were necessary (as for construction, inspection, and maintenance), sanitary design clamping using steam-resistant Viton gaskets was used.

Since one of the purposes of the Upjohn Company WFI design was to allow for CIP techniques, the stainless steel had imparted to it an electropolish finish. Preceding this was the necessary mechanical polishing. The 3A Sanitary Standards require a 150-grit finish as a minimum. The Upjohn Company practice imparted a 240-grit finish to all surfaces that would be wetted, except that all tubing and fittings received a 320-grit treatment. Electropolishing followed.

Clean-in-Place Techniques

The stainless steel alloys were used as materials of construction to secure inert surfaces for contact with the high-purity water and products. The smoothness of their surface finishes also promoted ease and thoroughness of cleaning to rid the equipment of product residues, impurities, and organisms. Inertness was also required against the sanitizing agents that would periodically be employed and against the cleaning procedure initially used after assembly and fabrication of the system.

One cleaning recommendation (like many procedures and protocols dealing with stainless steel equipment, its cleaning, and maintenance) came from the food industry, specifically from its dairy industry segment. This was the "3A Accepted Practices for Permanently Installed Sanitary Product-Pipelines and Cleaning Systems," (Serial No. 60500), which recommended that all interiors and weld areas of newly constructed installations be subjected to a circulation for a minimum of 30 minutes of a cleaning solution of from 0.5% to 1.0% alkalinity at 71 °C (160 °F). Following a postrinse adequate to remove all traces of the cleaning solution, a second circulation of an 0.5% to 1.0% nitric or phosphoric acid solution at 65 to 82 °C (150 to 180 °F) for at least 10 minutes was to be made, followed by an adequate rinse cycle.

Other cleaning devices and practices for stainless steel equipment have also been derived from the dairy industry. Two techniques used are known as cleaning in place and cleaning out of place. In the latter practice, fittings are removed from the main equipment assembly and washed in a parts washer using water forced by centrifugal pump at high velocity through nozzles. Details of one such cleaning device and its operation were described by Upjohn investigators, Grimes et al. (1977).

Grimes et al. (1977) also described a CIP system utilizable in conjunction with the main pieces of permanently installed equipment. It was an automated arrangement embodying a basic triclover design and utilizing a spray-ball low-pressure system that permitted reuse of the cleaning solution and prevented the air entrainment that could cause the momentary, incomplete emptying of tanks and other vessels. The interruption to tank emptying, however brief, resulted in impurities being entrained in the cleaning solution, then becoming deposited on the walls of the vessels.

High-speed spray nozzles that swivel while spraying cleaning solution within a tank are available, but were not used in the Upjohn study. The high-speed nozzle system cleans largely through an impinger action. In the low-pressure system actually used, a cascading action served to clean the lower portions of the vessel. The cleaning solution, like the subsequent rinse water, entered the tank by means of a spray-ball on a swivel connection that could be adjusted to fit tanks of seven different heights. The spray pattern served to cover all critical surfaces with the cleaning liquids it dispensed by way of a centrifugal force pump.

What was sought was a high flow at low pressure. An impinging action was not necessary. Rather, a cascading action was what is desired. A typical CIP program entailed the following:

1. A prerinse with RO-treated water, consisting of three bursts, each of a 1-minute duration (this removed a large portion of the soil load);
2. A continuous 30-minute wash with alkaline detergent at 82 °C (180 °F);
3. A 1-minute rinse with RO-treated water;
4. A 30-second rinse with a phosphoric acid solution;
5. A 2-minute rinse with RO water to remove the phosphoric acid residues; and
6. A final 1-minute rinse with deionized water.

Using this procedure, the Upjohn investigators (Grimes et al, 1977) found that the adjustment of the alkaline detergent concentration and of the duration of the rinse cycles sufficed to tailor this general procedure specifically to the removal of even recalcitrant products from their permanent stainless steel installations, and to bring the equipment to the requisite high degree of cleanliness for pharmaceutical productions.

Cleaning in place is particularly suited to electropolished surfaces, which may become marred by the use of a scrubbing brush. The trend in pharmaceutical contexts is toward automated cleaning and the use of spray-balls, perhaps manually operated, in conjunction with aqueous surfactant preparations. An advantage of cleaning in place is that it lends itself to shorter cleaning cycles.

Interestingly, in the semiconductor industry, where large quantities of high-purity rinse water are used, CIP cannot be used. There, because cold recirculating systems based on plastic piping are usually involved, the equipment must be assembled clean.

Corrosive Influences

The corrosion of metals involves electrochemical phenomena. At the anodic location, metal atoms lose electrons and enter the water (electrolyte) as cations. As a result of this chemical reaction, metal dissolves. The surrendered electrons, under the impetus of their potential, transfer through the metal to another site, which they enrich with their presence. This locale becomes, by definition, a cathode, to which cations in the solution migrate in their quest for electrons. A metal surface in contact with water will have a multitude of micro areas acting as anodes and cathodes. These areas may shift in location as the reaction products accumulate. Local corrosion effects can create pinholes; area shifts result in a generalized corrosion.

The practice of passivation is intended to shield against the corrosion of the austenitic stainless steels. To be considered are the stress-cracking manifestations of such corrosions that are of concern particularly in the high-temperature ambiences prevalent in the power industry. Corrosion can also take place at the more moderate temperature levels characteristic of pharmaceutical high-purity water systems.

Microbiologically induced corrosion is an entire field in itself (Costerton and Boivin, 1987) beyond the bounds of this present writing. Suffice is to say that by their utilization of oxygen, aerobic microbes create areas anodic to the metal and thus promotive of corrosion. Organisms may also produce corrosive metabolites. The complexities of biofilms allow corrosion-enhancing situations to develop (Costerton and Boivin, 1987). A 60-microvolt differential exists between the inner and outer regions of the glycocalyx, caused by the oxygen differential. This causes metallic corrosion. Oxygen penetration of the glycocalyx is diffusion-limited to about 2 mils. Mittelman for this reason preferred a nitrogen blanket in water storage tanks to repress organism growth.

Dissimilar metals constitute a serious and ongoing corrosive threat to stainless steel systems. Contaminants such as free iron become released into the aqueous stream, to be deposited upon surfaces where they can create galvanic cells that result in corrosion. Welds can easily be affected (Coleman and Evans, 1990). These investigators advised that gasketing materials may play an important role in corrosion, possibly through some impregnation with iron during their manufacture, or by creating oxygen-poor areas in the regions under the gaskets.

One of the intentions in using the TIG arc welding process of joining stainless steel sections, as of piping, is to minimize the oxidation of the metal. This is aided by the computer-directed welding that minimizes the metal area exposed to heat. Nevertheless, the welded area may come to exhibit "heat tint," a straw-colored (or even darker) boundary on the heat-affected zone. According to Coleman and Evans (1990), the heat-tinted areas are productive of rouging. They stated that passivation electropolishing of the heat-tinted area will not prevent the onset of rouging. Removal of the heat tint is not effected by nitric acid treatment. They advised a reducing treatment to convert oxides to metal, followed by a proprietary "mixed chelates" application of ammonium citrate potentiated by EDTA (in proportions not disclosed), using formulational methods being kept secret for patent purposes (Coleman, 1991). Passivation of the treated area completes the treatment. Rouging is thus eliminated. Strict orbital welding techniques in conjunction with a high-purity, inert-gas purge should suffice to avoid the formation of heat-tinted areas.■

CHAPTER 12

PHARMACEUTICAL WATER SYSTEMS

In a stipulation bearing upon the Food and Drug Administration for its enforcement, the *United States Pharmacopoeia 23* (1995) specifies the qualities required for compendial waters, and defines as well the manner of their preparation. Purified Water is prepared by ion exchange, reverse osmosis, and distillation, although the *USP 23* permits its manufacture by any "other suitable process." The preparation of Water for Injection, however, is permitted only by distillation or RO. The FDA requires that the employment of RO involve a two-pass, product-staged process. The preparation of WFI by RO is a rare practice in the United States and is forbidden by the *European Pharmacopoeia* only distillation being permitted. The *Japanese Pharmacopoeia* allows WFI preparation by distillation, RO, and ultrafiltration.

In addition to specifying the means of compendial water preparation, the FDA requires that the process be carried out in conformity with current good manufacturing practices, that it be validated as being productive of a water product of suitable quality, and that a standard operating procedure be devised for keeping the process and product ongoing at that quality level.

Good Manufacturing Practices

Under section 501 (a)(2)(B) of the Food Drug and Cosmetics Act (FD&C), a drug is deemed to be adulterated if it is not manufactured in accordance with current good manufacturing practice (CGMP). The FDA has promulgated regulations establishing minimum CGMP standards at 21 C.F.R. Parts 210 and 211. The CGMP requirements are intended to provide assurance that drugs are manufactured under systems and procedures such that the products will have the quality, purity, safety, identity, and strength that they are labeled or purported to possess.

These are more often referred to as Good Manufacturing Practices (GMP). The terms "CGMP" and "GMP" are interchangeable. (Both are used here to emphasize their equivalence.) A series of GMPs was proposed in 1972. Known as the "umbrella" GMPs, they deal with such subjects as personnel, records, and equipment. They compel, among other things, the proper operation of equipment. Finalized in 1978, they have the force of regulations. In the FDA view, validation of water system components and operation is mandated by the umbrella GMPs. A compendial water may be considered a component of a bulk drug and as such requires validation of its process of manufacture.

In 1976, the FDA proposed more specific GMPs for Large-Volume Parenterals (GMP/LVP). Intentions were that they would eventually be extended to Small-Volume Parenterals (SVP), those administered in quantities of less than 100 mL. The GMP/LVP were never finalized and were withdrawn in 1994. The proposed GMPs for LVPs, therefore, have no legal standing. Nevertheless, the FDA conducts its inspections in accordance with their teachings (21 CFR 212). Their application is justified on the basis of good manufacturing practice. Clearly, the concept of GMP requires elucidation.

One view holds that drug manufacturers are responsible for obeying regulations, but that otherwise they are free to meet, as they deem best, the drug standards set by the *USP 23* and enforced by the FDA. In this view, finalized GMPs constitute regulations; proposed GMPs never printed in the *Code of Federal Regulations* do not.

Another view can be taken, namely, that the GMPs are always evolving. In principle, they constitute the practices of a majority of the industry regarding a specific operation. The quality and operational level set by the majority automatically directs the remainder of the industry to conform. The GMPs then constitute a regulatory least-common-denominator of the industry's practices. As the industry itself strives to improve its operations, the GMPs and the standards they entail inevitably evolve further. Hence, the aptness of the word "current" in conjunction with the term GMPs; although commonly known more briefly as Good Manufacturing Practices, the operative strictures refer actually to Current Good Manufacturing Practices. Celeste (1995) characterizes the FDA view as follows:

> The CGMP regulations are very general in nature. They require manufactures to establish programs to maintain drug quality, but they generally leave the content of those programs to the discretion of the manufacturers. Thus, in many areas there are a number of different ways in which a manufacturer may comply. The regulations do require written standard operating procedures (SOPs) and production, control, and laboratory records (to which FDA has access under its inspection power).
>
> In many instances, FDA has provided informal guidance on CGMP issues, but these may not be the only way or even the best way of achieving compliance. Manufacturers will retain substantial discretion in determining what is appropriate to satisfy GMP standards. For example, the regulations require that manufacturing processes, analytical methods, and

> procedures be validated. They do not specify, however, how they should be validated. These procedures and others, such as sampling and analysis of the product, are left to the firm to decide. The appropriateness of the firm's decisions are reviewed by FDA during the course of the application review and establishment inspections.

At any time, GMP status is a matter of interpretation. The FDA headquarters staff adjusts its interpretations of what constitutes current GMPs mostly from the findings of its national and worldwide staffs of investigators, but also on the basis of the literature such as published papers, trade journals, and scientific reports. Although compilations of current GMPs are not made, efforts are underway at the FDA to develop a supportive data base.

As an evolving body of practices, GMP ought not and cannot be hobbled by being confined to exactly worded regulations. Indeed, in one view, a majority endorsement is a sufficient but not a necessary condition to recognize that a meritorious manufacturing practice is available and ought to be designated as a Good Manufacturing Practice. It is pointed out that media filling is now a recognized GMP for quantifying the contamination possibilities present in an aseptic filling operation. There was a time, however, when media-fill operations were not practiced routinely as part of GMP. Yet their now acknowledged value was inherent even then, although not then recognized. Was it wrong then for an FDA inspector to insist on the application of the media-fill technique to aseptic filling operations before it had attained "formal" GMP status?

One point of view holds that the pharmaceutical industry has the obligation to manufacture a product of requisite high quality, the attainment of which necessitates the use of sound technologies and reliable methods. To ensure the consistent production of such drugs may involve operations and procedures that are not specifically mandated by regulations and that are not (yet) widely practiced by the industry. Celeste (1995) has commented:

> By their nature, CGMP standards evolve over time. The law does not require, and FDA does not expect, manufacturers immediately to replace all of their equipment with potentially improved technologies. Rather, manufacturers may properly keep older equipment and facilities in use, saving new methods and materials, as appropriate, for new plants or production lines.

Interventions by officialdom are not always welcome. They may be seen as intrusions, and proffered advice may be burdensome. Inspectors from the FDA may, however, perceive an obligation untrammeled by legalisms. The FDA inspector, against the background of what is observed at a given site, must give it his or her best judgment. There is opportunity for error, and different inspectors can see matters differently.

Inspectors will list their critical observations, if any, on an inspectional observation document, FDA Form 483. These observations need not necessarily be correct. However, a copy of the 483 form is given by the inspector to the highest company executive at the facility. This may well be the plant manager. Thus, high company management becomes directly and immediately involved. Very often, pressure for rapid correction of a cited condition, whether it is an actual violation or not, is exerted by the management echelon in a preference to avoid confrontation. Indeed, the force of the form 483 is often just that, that the manufacturer comes to accommodate the inspector's judgment, whether justified or not, to avoid further involvements with officialdom (Chesney 1996).

The inspector's observations, listed on the 483 form, are just that. Their being cited does not establish violations of the law. These observations may or may not result in an adverse-findings letter. The decision of the FDA is made not by the investigatory branch but by compliance officers who must decide whether violations of regulations exist. This is in accord with the due process requirements of the law. As Celeste (1995) states it:

> FDA had broad authority under section 704 of the FD&C Act to inspect pharmaceutical manufacturing establishments, including all equipment, finished and in-process materials, and containers. For prescription drugs, this authority extends to "all things" in an establishment bearing on whether they may be a violation of the FD&C Act, including "records, files, papers, processes, controls, and facilities."
>
> FDA typically conducts inspections prior to approval of a new marketing application, after a recall or for other cause, and on a periodic (biennial) or other basis without cause. Following an inspection, the investigator usually leaves a report of his or her observations, the 'FDA 483.' It is agency policy and a requirement for investigators that an FDA-483 be provided if the investigator has any observations (in the case of pharmaceutical manufacturers, these would generally involve the current good manufacturing practice requirements). The FDA-483 represents the individual views of the investigator and not the position of the agency that there is a violative condition in the establishment. Few inspections of any magnitude will conclude without the issuance of an FDA-483.
>
> Although not required by FDA, it is customary industry practice for manufacturers to respond to an FDA-483 attempting to resolve any misunderstandings that may have led to a particular observation. The response should address all of the listed observations and should speak to whatever systems may be affected as a result of the inspection and how the deviations, if indeed they are such, will be corrected.

> Following an inspection, an investigator prepares a report known as an "Establishment Inspection Report" (EIR). In the normal course of the FDA reviewed at various management levels in the FDA district office. Ultimately, a decision is made by agency management as to the disposition of the report. In some cases, it may be referred to headquarters with a recommendation for appropriate legal action. If the district determines that no additional action is required, the EIR may be disposed of without any further action taking place.
>
> The agency has many enforcement tools at its disposal. Depending on FDA's assessment of the seriousness of the violation, the agency's action will vary.
>
> If agency management concludes that there is a serious violation, the agency often will issue a "Warning Letter" describing the violation and requiring that it be corrected. In cases meeting predetermined criteria (including for manufacturing violations), the district office may issue a warning letter on its own initiative. FDA may institute formal enforcement proceedings through the Justice Department. These include product seizures, injunctions against continued manufacturing or distribution, and criminal prosecution.

Obviously, in any contentions relating to the GMPs, gray areas of interpretation may exist. Reliance is therefore often placed on the opinions of experts in the relevant practices. *What is GMP* comes ultimately to be decided at FDA headquarters, subject to challenge and court review. At least philosophically, then, the final arbiter of what constitutes CGMP is the federal court system.

With regard to the proposed GMPs for LVPs, the FDA's position is that because the drug industry has already put many of the proposed actions into effect, the actions constitute Current Good Manufacturing Practices. As regards the remaining proposals, the FDA holds that the finalized umbrella GMPs are written broadly enough to warrant their extension to manufacturing practices in general.

What can be said regarding certain of the FDA's firmly held positions that do seem to overextend GMP? These views derive from FDA experiences, as gathered from FDA inspector observations. These observations have no regulatory status. They are only advisory, but they constitute strongly held FDA views. An example is the use of double-pass, product-staged reverse osmosis for the manufacture of WFI. *USP 23* states that RO may be used to prepare WFI. On the basis of long experience, however, the FDA believes that imperfections in RO devices, whether membranes or seals, occur commonly enough to render unlikely the consistent and dependable preparation of WFI by a single RO operation. It is therefore insisted upon by the FDA that two RO units in series, the second operating on the product water from the first, should be used if a successful validation is hoped for. The use of a single RO device is not enjoined. The FDA has no legal power to do so. However, its inspectors, aware of the history in the field, will be very critical in their examination of data supportive of validation claims made for a single RO unit. Manufacturers are entitled to try to prepare WFI using single RO units. (None apparently does so at present.) At the very least, an additional delay in achieving validation is to be expected, occasioned by the need to gather very convincing evidence persuasive to the FDA. Celeste (1995) has said the following:

> In addition to CGMP requirements, drugs generally must meet applicable standards established in the United States Pharmacopeia (USP). The USP includes monographs for drug substances and drug products, which typically set forth requirements for drug purity, identity, and the like. The USP also includes standards for water quality and other matters pertaining to drug manufacturing. Although the USP requirements are distinct from CGMP, compliance with the USP on a matter specifically covered by the compendium will usually be adequate to demonstrate compliance with CGMP with respect to the same matter. Manufacturers also must comply with any additional specifications established in the new drug applications or abbreviated new drug applications for their products.

GMPs Related to Water Systems

The Food and Drug Administration has established a number of GMPs that pertain to the preparation of pharmaceutical waters. Since their promulgation several have undergone modification in practice, as already discussed, a consequence of the FDA's ongoing and evolving understanding of what pharmaceutical water systems require.

210.3 Definitions.

(a) The following definitions of terms apply to Parts 210 through 229 of this chapter.

(b) The terms are as follows:

(3) "Component" means any ingredient intended for use in the manufacture of a drug product, including those that may not appear in such drug product.

(5) "Fiber" means any particle with a length of at least three times greater than its width.

(6) "Non-fiber-releasing filter" means any filter, which after any appropriate pretreatment such as washing or flushing, will not release fibers into the component or drug product that is being filtered. All filters composed of asbestos or glass fibers are deemed to be fiber-releasing filters.

(2) "Batch" means a specific quantity of a drug that has uniform character and quality, within specified limits, and is produced according to a single manufacturing order during the same cycle of manufacture.

(10) "Lot" means a batch, or a specific identified portion of a batch, having uniform character and quality within specified limits; or, in the case of a drug produced by continuous process, it is a specific identified amount produced in a unit of time or quantity in a manner that assures its having uniform character and quality within specified limits.

211.48 Plumbing.

(a) Potable water shall be supplied under continuous positive pressure in plumbing system free of defects that could contribute contamination to any drug product. Potable water shall meet the standards prescribed in the Public Health Service Drinking Water Standards set forth in a Subpart J of 42 CFR Part 72. Water not meeting such standards shall not be permitted in the plumbing system.

211.72 Filters.

(a) Filters used in the manufacture, processing, or packing of injectable drug products intended for human use shall not release fibers into such products. Fiber-releasing filters may not be used in the manufacture, processing, or packing of these drug products unless it is not possible to manufacture such drug products without the use of such a filter.

(b) If use of a fiber-releasing filter is necessary, an additional non-fiber-releasing filter of 0.22 micron maximum mean porosity (0.45 micron if the manufacturing conditions so dictate) shall subsequently be used to reduce the content of particles in the drug product. Use of an asbestos-containing filter, with or without subsequent use of a specific non-fiber-releasing filter, is permissible only upon submission of proof to the appropriate bureau of the Food and Drug Administration that use of a non-fiber-releasing filter will, or is likely to, compromise the safety or effectiveness of the drug product.

*212.3 Definitions.

(11) "Static Line" means any pipe containing liquid that is not emptied or circulated at least once every 24 hours.

Subpart B - Organization and Personnel

212.22 Responsibilities of quality control unit.

(a) The quality control unit shall have the responsibility and authority to test and accept or reject the design, engineering, and physical facilities of the plant, the equipment, and the manufacturing process and control procedures to be used in the manufacture, processing, packing, and holding of each large volume parenteral drug product. The quality control unit shall reject any such plant, equipment, process, or procedure if it does not comply with the provisions of this part or if, in the opinion of the quality control unit, it is not suitable or adequate to assure that the drug product has the characteristics it purports or is represented to possess.

(c) The quality control unit shall have the responsibility and authority to test and approve or reject any changes in previously approved plant, equipment, processes, procedures, and container-closures and delivery systems before

* Section 212 covers the proposed GMPs for LVPs. Officially withdrawn, it is used for guidance.

utilization in the manufacture, processing, packing and holding of a large volume parenteral drug product.

Subpart C - Buildings and Facilities
212.42 Design and construction features.

(c) There shall not be horizontal fixed pipes or conduits over exposed components, in-process materials, drug products, and drug product contact surfaces, including drug product containers and closures after the final rinse.

(d) In each physically separated area, pipes or conduits for air or liquids shall be identified as to their contents. Such identification shall be by name, color code, or other suitable means.

212.49 Water and other liquid-handling systems.

(a) Filters may not be used at any point in the water for manufacturing or final rinse piping system.

(b) Backflow of liquids shall be prevented at points of interconnection of different systems.

(c) Pipelines for the transmission of water for manufacturing or final rinse and other liquid components shall:

(1) Be constructed of welded stainless steel (nonrusting grade) equipped for sterilization with steam, except that sanitary stainless steel lines with fittings capable of disassembly may be immediately adjacent to the equipment or valves that must be removed from the lines for servicing and replacement.

(2) Be sloped to provide for complete draining.

(3) Not have an unused portion greater in length than six diameters of the unused pipe measured from the axis of the pipe in use.

212.67 Equipment cleaning and maintenance.
The following requirements shall be included in written procedures and cleaning schedules:

(a) All equipment and surfaces that contact components, in-process materials, drug products or drug product contact surfaces such as containers and closures shall be cleaned and rinsed with water meeting the quality requirements stated in 212.224.

(b) Immediately prior to such contact, equipment and surfaces specified in paragraph (a) of this section shall be given a final rinse with water meeting the quality requirements stated in 212.225.

(c) Steam used to sterilize liquid-handling systems or equipment shall be free of additives used for boiler control.

212.68 Equipment calibration.

(a) Procedures shall be written and followed designating schedules and assigning responsibility for testing or monitoring the performances or accuracy of automatic or continuously operating equipment, devices, apparatus, or mechanisms, such as, but not limited to, the following:

(1) Alarms and controls on sterilizing equipment.

(2) Temperature-recording devices on sterilizers.

(3) Pressure gauges.

(4) Mechanisms for maintaining sterilizing medium uniformity.

(5) Chain speed recorder.
(6) Heat exchanger pressure differential monitor.
(7) Mercury-in-glass thermometer.
(b) Written records of such calibrations, checks, examinations, or inspections shall be maintained, as specified in 212.183.

212.72 Filters.
(a) The integrity of all air filters shall be verified upon installation and maintained throughout use. A written testing program adequate to monitor integrity of filters shall be established and followed. Results shall be recorded and maintained as specified in 212.183.

212.76 Heat exchangers.
Heat exchangers, other than the welded double-concentric-tube type or double-tube sheet type, must employ a pressure differential and a means for monitoring the differential. The pressure differential shall be such that the fluid requiring a higher microbial quality shall be that with the greater pressure. Written records of the pressure differential monitoring shall be maintained as required in 212.183.

212.78 Air vents.
All stills and tanks holding liquid requiring microbial control shall have air vents with non-fiber-releasing sterilizable filters capable of preventing microbial contamination of the contents. *Such filters shall be designed and installed so that they do not become wet.* Filters shall be sterilized and installed separately. Tanks requiring air vents with filters include those holding water for manufacturing or final rinsing, water for cooling the drug product after sterilization, liquid components, and in-process solutions.

212.79 Pumps.
Pumps moving water for manufacturing or final rinsing, water for cooling the drug product after sterilization, and in-process or drug product solutions shall be designed to utilize water for injection as a lubricant for the seals.

212.100 Written procedures, deviations.
(b) Written procedures shall be established, and shall be followed. Such procedures shall:
(1) Ensure that all static lines are flushed prior to use. Such procedures shall require that flushing produce a turbulent flow for 5 minutes and that all valves on the line are opened and closed repeatedly to flush the valve interior.

212.82 Equipment cleaning and use log.
(a) Written records of the corrective action taken pursuant to 212.24 (a) and (c), and 212.225 (a) and (b), including validation of the effectiveness of the action, shall be maintained.
(b) Written records of equipment usage shall include documentation of the length of time the equipment was in use as indicated in 212.111.
c) Written records demonstrating a positive pressure differential, as described in and required by 212.76, shall be maintained.
(e) For filtration equipment, or devices, written records documenting the

installation, replacement, and sterilization (where appropriate) of filters such as those indicated in 212.72, 212.77 (b) and (c), 212.78, and 212.222 (a) shall be maintained.

212.183 Equipment calibration and monitoring records.
Written records of calibration and monitoring tests and readings performed shall be maintained *for at least 2 years* after the expiration date of each batch of drug product produced by the equipment.

(a) Calibration shall include:
(1) A description of the equipment.
(2) The date the equipment was purchased.
(3) The operating limits of the equipment.
(4) The date, time, and type of each test.
(5) The results of each test.
(6) The signature of each person performing a test.
(7) The date the equipment was installed.
(b) Monitoring records shall include:
(1) A description of the equipment.
(2) The date the equipment was installed.
(3) The date the equipment was last calibrated, if appropriate.
(4) The operating limits of the equipment.
(5) The date and time of the recording.
(6) The reading.
(7) The signature of each person performing the monitoring.
(c) Corrective measures employed to bring the equipment into compliance with its operating specifications shall be:
(1) Recorded in the appropriate equipment log.
(2) Noted in the calibration and/or monitoring record.
(3) Immediately followed by testing to assure that the corrective measures were adequate to restore the required operating characteristics.

212.188 Batch production and control records.
These records shall include the following information where appropriate:
(1) Verification that static lines were flushed prior to use according to established written procedures in 212.100 (b).

212.192 Production record review.
The review and approval of production and control records by the quality control unit shall extend to those records not directly related to the manufacture, processing, packing, or holding of a specific batch of large volume parenteral drug product but which have a bearing on the quality of batches being produced. Such indirectly related records shall include:

(a) Those dealing with equipment calibration or standardization.
(c) Those demonstrating the quality of water produced by various processing systems.
(d) Those demonstrating the quality of air produced by various systems.

212.190 Air and water monitoring records.
Written records of the air and water monitoring test results, readings, and corrective measures taken shall be maintained for at least 2 years after the expiration date of

each batch of drug product produced in the area being monitored or containing the water as a component.
The record shall include, at a minimum, the following information:

(a) Identity of the material being monitored.
(b) Each characteristic being monitored.
(c) Each specification limit.
(d) Each testing method used.
(e) Site sampled or monitored.
(f) The date and time of each monitoring or testing.
(g) The result of each test or monitoring reading.
(h) Batch number and expiration date of the drug product being processed in the area or equipment, or to which the component is being added at the time of monitoring or sampling.
(i) Corrective measures employed to bring the area, component or product into compliance with specifications.
(j) Retesting results to verify the adequacy of the corrective measures.

Subpart L - Air and Water Quality
212.220 General Requirements.

(a) Air or water as described in this part may not be used until the plant, processes, and procedures used in producing and distributing it have been tested and approved by the quality control unit as capable of consistently producing air or water meeting the requirements set forth in this subpart.
(b) In addition to the requirements of this subpart, air and water quality shall be monitored as specified in Subpart J.
(c) The results of all testing and data generated shall be recorded and maintained as required by 212.180.
(d) Procedures designating schedules, assigning responsibility, and describing in detail the action to be taken to assure that the systems produce and deliver air and water that conform to the requirements set fort in this subpart shall be written. Such procedures shall also specify the corrective action to be taken when testing reveals that the established standards are not being met. Records of corrective actions shall be maintained, as specified in 212.190.

212.223 Compressed air.
Compressed air used in manufacturing and processing operations, including the sterilization process, shall be:

(b) Supplied by an oil-free compressor and be free of oil and oil vapor unless vented directly to a noncontrolled environment area.
(c) Dehumidified to prevent condensation of water vapor in the pipes.

212.224 Water for cleaning or initial rinsing.
Water used to cleanse or initially rinse drug product contact surfaces such as containers, closures, and equipment shall:

(a) Meet the standards prescribed in the Public Health Service Drinking Water Standards set forth in Subpart J of 42 CFR Part 72;
(b) Be subjected to a process such as chlorination for control of microbial population;
(c) Contain not more than 50 microorganisms per 100 millimeters in three consecutive samples from the sampling site when tested by the method

specified in 212.225 (b) after neutralizing bactericidal agents, if present.

212.225 Water for manufacturing or final rinsing.
Water used as a component or as a final rinse for equipment or product contact surfaces shall:

(a) Conform to the specifications in the U.S.P for "Water for Injection"
(b) Contain not more than 10 microorganisms per 100 millimeters in three consecutive samples from the same site when samples of 250 millimeters or more are tested for total aerobic count by the plate method set forth in the Microbial Limit Tests in the current revision of the U.S.P. Alternate methodology may be used provided that data are available to demonstrate that the alternate method is equivalent to the official method. When the microbial quality falls below that specified in this section, use of such water shall cease, and corrective action shall be taken to clean and sterilize the system so that the water conforms to the limit.
(c) Be stored in a suitable vessel or system including a piping network for distribution to points of use:
(1) At a temperature of at least 80 °C under continuous circulation, or
(2) At ambient or lower temperatures for not longer than 24 hours, after which time such water shall be discarded to drain.

212.226 Water for drug product cooling.
Water used in the sterilizer as a drug product cooling medium shall:

(a) Be treated to eliminate microorganisms:
(b) Contain not more than one microorganism per 100 millimeters in three consecutive samples from the same sampling site when one liter or more are tested for total aerobic count by a membrane filtration method and placing each membrane filter on appropriate nutrient media after neutralizing any bactericidal agents present in the water samples.

212.227 Boiler feed water.
Feedwater for boilers supplying steam that contacts components, in-process materials, drug products, and drug product contact surfaces shall not contain volatile additives such as amines or hydrazines.

212.233 Water quality program design.

(a) Water quality monitoring shall include:
(1) Sampling and testing of water for manufacturing or final rinsing at least once a day. All sampling ports or points of use in the distribution system shall be sampled at least weekly.
(2) Sampling water for drug product cooling at a point just before entry into the sterilizer at least once each sterilizer cycle and testing by the method described in 212.226.
(3) Sampling and testing water for cleaning or initial rinsing at least once a week. All sampling ports or points of use in the distribution system shall be sampled at least monthly.
(b) Boiler feed water shall be sampled and tested periodically for the presence of volatile additives.
(c) If three consecutive samples of drug product cooling water exceed microbial limits, the sterilizer loads shall be rejected and shall not be reprocessed.

212.231 Monitoring of air and water quality.

(a) After the plant, equipment, manufacturing processes, and control procedures have been tested and approved by the quality control unit, there shall be performed in accordance with written procedures and schedules a sampling and testing program that is designed to monitor the microbial flora of the plant and its environment. The design of the sampling and testing program shall include monitoring of air and water quality in accordance with requirements set forth in this subpart and taking corrective action when such requirements are not met.

(b) If the results of any one sample of air or water exceed the quality limits specified in this subpart, more frequent sampling and testing shall be required to determine the need for corrective action.

(c) Representative colonies of microorganisms found by the monitoring required in this section shall be identified by genus. The colonies shall be quantified.

(d) Written records of all test findings and any resultant corrective measures taken shall be maintained, as specified in 212.190.

Some Actual Water Systems

It is to be expected that any presentation dealing with pharmaceutical water systems would set forth actual examples of such arrangements that already exist for water purification and manufacture. A study of such systems can be very informative as to the common principles and approaches that inhere in the pharmaceutical field. A word of caution is in order, however. Just because a system has been designed, installed, and is an apparently acceptable use does not mean that it is optimal, or that it should be emulated. The operational results of a given system may be successful despite certain of its features. If the present sharp focus on pharmaceutical water systems indicates anything, it is that often improvements in the present status can be derived from design optimizations. For this reason, hypothetical water systems are also presented for consideration, for the teachings they convey. There is much to be gained, of course, from an analysis of the many well-designed and -operated systems that already exist.

The correctness of a water treatment system cannot be fully gauged without an intimate knowledge of the quality of the feedwater, its constancy of composition, its peak loads and its long-term demands. These are seldom known in the cases listed. Nevertheless, an examination of existing pharmaceutical water systems can be rewarding.

Purified Water by ion exchange. Either RO or distillation is required for the preparation of WFI. Purified Water may be prepared more simply, however, by use of ion-exchanger reactions. Where nonsterile formulations are being compounded, methods based on deionization resins (DI resins) are accordingly employed.

First example. At one company, a preparer of nonsterile drugs, the incoming chlorinated water was passed through a carbon bed to remove the chlorine. It was then deionized using mixed-bed ion-exchange resins, then heated by heat exchanger and stored in a 3,000-gallon tank, from which it was continuously circulated while being maintained at 80 to 90 °C. Although ion exchange is not a method expected to yield low organism counts, storage of the demineralized water at 80 °C while undergoing circulation rendered it free of living Gram-negative organisms. It need not have been sterile, however. It could have contained the spores of spore-forming Gram-positives, which would have been absent from properly distilled waters. Moreover, such stored, hot Purified Water contains endotoxin. Above all, this PW could not be called sterile, not having been prepared specifically by a sterilizing process.

Second example. At another preparer of nonsterile drugs, municipal water chlorinated to about 1 ppm was filtered first through a 5-µm-rated depth filter and then through a 1-µm-rated depth filter before being conducted through a UV unit. The water was then flowed through a mixed bed of DI resins. Following passage through a second UV light unit, it was exposed to a pasteurizing heat treatment of 85 °C (185 °F) for 3 seconds. The water flowed at the rate of 75 gpm. It was drawn at the points of use at ambient temperature. The alert limit for this water was 25 cfu/mL; the action limit was 100 cfu/mL; and at 400 cfu/mL, the system was shut down. The water was assayed microbiologically every day at each of the five drops for total counts, specifically for coliforms, yeasts and molds, and pseudomonads. Traceability was to each of the five drops. The organism levels themselves were seen as being less important than their implications to proliferation, particularly in the presence of preservatives, in accordance with USP antimicrobial preservatives testing.

Third example. At this manufacturing establishment, unchlorinated well water was filtered through a 1-µm-rated depth filter before being passed through a carbon bed (previously installed in anticipation of a possible eventual use of chlorine). The water then passed through two mixed DI resin beds and then through a UV unit in such a manner and at such flowrates as to achieve the microbiological quality sought, as attested to by microbiological assays. (Normally, as shown by the FDA's experience, UV light treatment cannot be relied on consistently to kill more than 90% of the bacteria in the water.) Subsequent passage through a microporous filter served in this case to remove some live bacteria along with the dead. Before being batched, the water was heated at 80 °C for 30 minutes. The water quality as it issued from the membrane filter was so acceptable microbiologically that the heating step could have ultimately been dispensed with if so sanctioned by ongoing validation.

The filter served to remove dead organisms and other particles, and was insurance against bacterial passage. A 0.45-µm-rated membrane was used when the water was to be used to formulate preparations containing preservatives. When these were not employed, a 0.2-μm-rated microporous membrane was used, the more reliably to remove organisms.

Fourth example. At this establishment, water containing soluble silica was collected from numerous wells, each chlorinated at the well head. The water was led through sand and carbon beds, (maintained troublefree for at least 3 years by automated backwashing), and then into a train of three individual ion-exchange beds.

The three-bed deionization assembly consisted of a strongly acidic cation exchanger, followed by a weakly basic anion exchanger, followed by a strongly basic anion exchanger. No mixed bed was used. The resin beds were regenerated every other day at least. No brine rinses were required or used. The system routinely produced 50 gpm (189 liter per minute [Lpm]), and could serve a peak load of 100 gpm (378 Lpm).

The weakly basic anion exchanger sufficed to remove the conventional anions. The strongly basic anion exchanger served to remove the soluble silica as well as carbon dioxide. The use of a mixed bed was eschewed to avoid the troublesome manipulations associated with its regeneration.

Carbon dioxide had previously been removed by a vacuum degasifier. This technique, however, had been found to lead to organism contamination.

The water emanating from the deionizing train had a pH of 9 (possibly reflecting the minor residual sodium ion content common to twin-bed operations). Carbon dioxide gas was added through a filter at this point to redress the pH imbalance. The *USP* stipulation for Purified Water calls for a pH of 5 to 7. The product water here produced was pH 6.

The regenerants for the ion-exchange resins were stored in the form of 66 Baumé sulfuric acid and 50% sodium hydroxide. The concentration of the base regenerant was 4%. The acid was used in a staged 2% and 4% strength. The use initially of 2% sulfuric acid avoided precipitating calcium sulfate by avoiding concentrations of that salt in excess of its solubility product, and particularly in excess of its supersaturation limit. Finishing regeneration of the cation-exchange resin was with 4% sulfuric acid. Regeneration of the ion-exchange beds was performed about every 2 days—more precisely, after each 50,000 gallons (200,000 liters) of water. No organisms were said to be seen downstream of the DI beds.

Downstream from the ion-exchange beds, the water flowed through a battery of thirty 0.2-μm-rated (nominal) nylon cartridges within a single multicartridge holder. These filters at this position served to remove resin fines, but could also serve to retain organisms that might originate in the DI beds. The filter assembly had a capacity of 180 gpm. The Purified Water was stored in 10,000-gallon (40,000-liter) stainless steel tanks prior to conversion by distillation to WFI.

Fifth example. At another drug manufacturing facility, a municipally treated water with a low chlorine content was flowed through a roughing filter at a flow of 40 gpm (150 Lpm). The filter used was a 70-inch (24.9-cm) product bearing 2-µm (nominal)/10-µm (absolute) ratings. It was changed weekly.

Formerly the water exiting the filter was flowed through a carbon bed. This bed's use was eliminated, however, because it was found to give rise to endotoxins. The pretreated water then entered a twin-bed deionizer prior to permeating a mixed-bed DI unit. The capacity flow from the DI unit was nominally 40 gpm (150 Lpm), although peak loads of 75 gpm (265 Lpm) were accommodated.

The water emanating from the DI beds was said to have a resistivity of 18 megohm-cm. Bacterial counts were taken daily, specifically of *Pseudomonas,* endotoxin, and *E. coli.* The organism levels observed were said to be at 5 organisms/100 mL. Daily limulus amebocyte lysate (LAL) testing was performed also. There were no microbial problems.

The resin beds were regenerated weekly using hydrochloric acid and sodium hydroxide. The alkali was formerly secured in its near-saturation concentration of 50%. However, this caused handling problems in cold weather. A 25% caustic soda solution gave better results.

Sixth example. At a Pennsylvania pharmaceutical company preparing topical drugs, surface water containing 1.3 ppm of chlorine reached the plant through 36-inch mains. The water, of 7 to 8 grains hardness, was not softened. It flowed at a rate of 25 gpm through a sand and anthracite bed, through DI twin and mixed beds, and then through a resin trap. It could be recirculated at 18 gpm. Twin-bed regeneration was every 3 weeks, the mixed bed every 6 to 8 weeks.

Without prefiltration, the water was flowed through an ultrafilter and then through a UV light installation. The ultrafilter was sanitized twice weekly using 50 ppm of sodium hypochlorite (NaOCl) for a 30-minute interval. Membrane filters of 0.2-µm-ratings were utilized at the points of use. Elimination of these filters was planned for fear that their upkeep would create maintenance lapses. No storage tank was used. Its absence necessitated shutdowns, however, when the pipes were being sanitized by use of 200 ppm of NaOCl resident for 15 hours. This was done every 3 months.

Permitting the 1.3 ppm of chlorine to enter the mixed beds generated amines in the water. The resin was designed to withstand 0.5 ppm of chlorine.

Seventh example. In the preparation of Purified Water at a northern New Jersey pharmaceutical plant, city water was first led through a sand bed. The bed was regenerated weekly or whenever the pressure drop across it exceeded 15 psig. It then flowed through an organic-removal bed consisting of layers of carbon and anion-exchange resins supported by stone. The resins were regenerated weekly using 9 gallons of hydrochloric acid and 11 gallons of caustic. The water then flowed through 5-μm-rated (nominal) string-wound polypropylene filters arranged in two parallel rows. Their purpose was to remove iron and silica colloidal particles. The water was then led through an UV installation into a storage tank of 1,000-gallon capacity. The contents of this tank were recirculated at the rate of 80 gpm (4,800 gallons per hour [gph]). Turnover was thus between 4 and 5 times per hour. From the storage tank, the water was flowed through mixed beds in parallel, using a sanitary Triclover pump. The deionized water was stored in a 2,000-gallon tank. Water of 1-megohm-cm resistivity would have been acceptable. The water actually produced was of a higher quality, being of 8-megohm-cm resistivity. It was analyzed daily using *USP* tests such as those for chloride and pH.

Eighth example. At a pharmaceutical plant in eastern Pennsylvania, well water was put through a string-wound filter, and then through twin DI beds followed by a mixed bed. The well water was chlorinated only as daily microbiological assays revealed the need (very occasionally). The added chlorine was not removed from the water, which flowed into the DI resin beds. The deionized water was used in the preparation of solid dosage forms, or it was distilled into WFI by a Finn-Aqua still. Production was 1,000 gpd. To enable its use, the distilled water was cooled in a heat exchanger, the temperature being measured by calibrated thermometers at the point of use. The water was tested daily at the points of use for organisms and endotoxin. System sanitation was performed every 6 months unless the microbiological data indicated the need for a more frequent operation.

Filters were not used in the water loop, but one was placed just before the bottle washer. Filters used with pharmaceutical preparations are preflushed in keeping with their manufacturer's specification. Their compatibility is assessed by use of the bubble-point integrity test; a constancy of values is sought after a 24-hour soak in the drug preparation.

Ninth example. A pharmaceutical Purified Water system consisted of a chlorinated raw feedwater being pretreated (including coagulation and softening) with activated carbon to remove the chlorine, followed by reverse osmosis. Water drawn from the RO storage tank was then pumped through a UV radiation area prior to flowing through a mixed-bed DI unit. Downstream of the mixed bed the water permeated a 0.2-μm-rated microporous membrane filter followed by an ultrafilter. One disadvantage as seen in using the ultrafilter was that its reject steam represented expensively treated water going to waste. An advantage was the fineness of the ultrafilter's filtrative action.

Tenth Example. A chlorinated feedwater from a potable water source is led through a purification train consisting of a carbon bed and two mixed ion-exchange beds in series. The exiting water is passed through a 1-µm-rated filter followed by an ultraviolet unit. The piping is of 316-L stainless steel. The water thus processed is stored in a 316-L stainless storage tank that is rated from 30 psig to cull vacuum. It is capable of sustaining direct steam sterilizations. However, it is actually sanitized by hot water. The stored water is recirculated by passage through a 3- to 5-µm-rated filter, and then through the carbon filter and the rest of the purification train.

Water is withdrawn from the storage tank into the loop by way of a 316 steel pump having a capacity of 50 lpm. The loop containing a 3 to 5 um-rated filter supports six points of use outfitted with diaphragm valves. The water pumped from the storage tank has a recirculating return that contains a heat-exchanger. This enables the periodic heat sanitization of the storage tank and loop. The loop is also outfitted with a cooler. A three-way diverter valve makes possible minimization of the heating and cooling loads.

The design permits continuous hot water storage. It also allows cold water use during the day, and hot water sanitizations during the night. This furnishes a versatility to any hot water sanitization regimen that may be defined in the validation exercise.

Purified Water by RO. Purified Water is also prepared by way of reverse osmosis. At Schering Plough (Farrington, 1984), municipal water, originating from deep artesian wells and therefore rather constant in composition, was pretreated by first being flowed through a deep-bed sand filter containing manganese dioxide (MnO_2), and greensand. The MnO_2 was intended to oxidize soluble ferrous and manganous ions to their higher valence states wherein they would precipitate as their hydrated oxides. The deep-bed (sand) filters removed these precipitates plus rust particles and corrosion-induced entities arising from the old cast-iron pipes used to distribute the Memphis (Tennessee) city water. The incoming water had an elevated level of iron and manganese and contained particles, many of which were smaller than 0.5 µm. The sand filter was capable of removing particles 80 to 300 µm in size. Retention of the smaller particles was effected by a bank of 1-µm-rated prefilters, followed by a second array of 0.45-µm-rated prefilters. It usually required about a month of operations to clog the prefilter system, as evidenced by elevation in differential pressure. The sand beds themselves need not clog before completion of 3 months or so of usage. They were cleansed by an automatic backflush system.

The Memphis municipal water was of such suitable quality (see Table 12-1) that after the above treatment it was directly led to RO. The RO units were of cellulose triacetate compositions. There was therefore no need to remove the chlorine (of concentrations 0.5 to 1.5 ppm [mg/L]) as added by the municipal potable water treatment. (Cellulose triacetate, unlike polyamide, withstands oxidative degradations by chlorine.) Indeed, part of the dissolved chlorine permeated the RO membrane, helping to keep both its downstream surfaces and the permeating waters under bacteriostatic control. The presence of the chlorine was otherwise ignored.

The Schering Plough RO units were of several sizes. The first production unit consisted of two 35-gpm-rated arrays that could be used singly or in tandem to give double-pass RO. This system's rated capacity of 70 gpm could, however, process up to 100 gpm. Usually, the RO units were operated singly on a daily rotational basis. The RO arrangement included a pressure-actuated switch that placed both units into operation when the line pressure dropped; and came with automated conductivity, pH, pressure, and temperature sensors, in addition to a silt density index meter. Performance logs were maintained, and entries were made several times per day. Such careful operation led to the anticipation and avoidance of problems, so that this RO operation essentially proved to be troublefree.

The water distribution system consisted of a circulating loop without a reservoir or storage tank, hence avoiding the cost and problems associated therewith. It was an on-demand operation satisfactory for a use-rate of approximately 30 gpm. The circulation loop connected back to reenter the feedwater flowing to the treatment unit, or it could be directed to drain. The loop was composed of 316L stainless steel machine-welded tubing with valves and ports necessary to prevent backflow and to enable the introduction of sanitizing agents and steam and the withdrawal of water samples. An initial eight points of use were included, although only two or three were expected to be drawn from simultaneously. Overall, the distribution system had a volume of 50 to 100 gpm.

Sampling by quality control (QC) personnel was made daily at the extremes of the distribution loop, at the points of entering and leaving the RO unit, and at the points of use. Conductivity and pH were measured and organism counts made. Endotoxin, not of concern to nonsterile drugs, was not monitored here. Full chemical analysis was done periodically. The microbiological action limits were set at 100 cfu/mL, with alert limits at 10 cfu/mL or at the presence of any Gram-negative organisms. On a routine basis, using the techniques published in *Standard Methods of Chemical Analysis* 17th Edition, the RO units were found to produce organism counts of less than 1 cfu/mL, and no Gram-negative microbes. Although the product water was not tested for endotoxin, its low bacterial count and the customary absence of Gram-negative organisms led to the presumption that the Schering Plough water purification system, operating on Memphis municipal quality potable water, could be capable of furnishing WFI water. In the actual event, the water so produced was used as Purified Water.

The Schering Plough purification system did not use double-pass RO. It was composed of three banks of RO units. The permeate from the first was employed as product water. The reject was fed into the second RO bank, and the reject from

Table 12-1
Impurity Levels of Memphis City Water

Impurity	*Range mg/L (ppm)*	*EPA Max mg/L*	USP XX *mg/L*
Chlorine	0.5-1.5	NA	NA
Iron (mg/L)	0.02-0.12	NA	NA
Manganese	0.00-0.03	NA	NA
Fluoride	0.91-1.01	1.4-2.5 (Depends on temp.)	NA
pH	7.0-7.3	NA	5.0-7.0
Alkalinity ($CaCO_3$)	32.0-90.0	NA	NA
Hardness ($CaCO_3$)	27.0-80.3	NA	NA
Calcium	18.0-46.3	NA	Passes test (4.0)
Magnesium	9.0-34.0	NA	NA
Sodium	6.5-9.3	NA	NA
Potassium	0.6-21.2	NA	NA
Sulfate	0.4-6.8	NA	Passes test (1.0)*
Chloride	3.2-8.1	10	Passes test (0.5)*
Nitrate	0.3-0.8	NA	NA
Phosphate	0.5-2.0	NA	NA
Dissolved solids	54.0-127.0	NA	NA
Silica	10.0-17.6	NA	NA
Color (unit: PCS)	<5	NA	NA
Turbidity (NTU)	0.04-0.08	NA	NA
Specific conductance micromhos at 25 °C	91.0-192.0	NA	NA
Aluminum	0.01-0.05	NA	NA
Arsenic	<0.005	0.05	NA
Barium	<0.1	1.00	NA
Cadmium	<0.001	0.010	NA
Chromium	<0.001	0.05	NA
Copper	0.01-0.06	NA	NA
Cyanide	<0.01	NA	NA
Detergents (MBAS)	0.00	NA	NA
Lead	<0.005	0.05	NA
Mercury	0.000	0.002	NA
Selenium	<0.005	0.01	NA
Silver	<0.001	0.05	NA
Zinc	0.01-0.12	NA	NA
Total solids	NA	NA	0.001% (10.0)*
Ammonia	NA	NA	Passes test (0.3)*
Carbon dioxide	NA	NA	Passes test (5.0)*
Heavy metals	NA	NA	Passes test (1.0)*
Oxidizable substances	NA	NA	Passes test (0.8)*
Bacteriological purity	EPA STDS	Coliform limit	Action limit OK 100 cfu/ml

*Calculated from *USP XX* procedure
NA: not addressed
Farrington (1984); Courtesy, Non-Prescription Drug Manufacturers Association

that into the third bank. That reject was discarded to drain. The three permeate streams were blended to produce the desired Purified Water. The overall water recovery was about 65%. The recovery efficiency, a matter of economic importance, could be increased by the use of higher differential pressures. However, higher transmembrane pressures would have decreased the RO rejection activity and the permeate quality. The usual differential pressure was at 400 psig.

At one point of use, water from the distribution loop was heated to 90 °C by passage through a heat exchanger. This water was usually tested for endotoxin, and generally *but not consistently* found to be free of endotoxin. (Since RO membranes should be capable of removing endotoxin, a dual-pass product-staged RO arrangement could, in keeping with FDA views, be capable of being validated to produce WFI.)

The site specificity of water purification merits being emphasized. The source water quality has an enormous influence on the ability of the purification train to handle it. Additionally, the capacity of the purification system requires being married to the volume requirements of the usage. The same purification system operating on lower quality water might not suffice. Larger-volume demands or excessive peak demands could also have deleterious effects on the water quality produced. The teaching of the Schering Plough experience was not that RO treatment can inevitably be depended on to prepare WFI or Purified Water, but rather that RO treatment properly operated and maintained and utilizing source water of a suitable quality will yield product water suitable for compendial usage, presumably even WFI.

Benedek and Johnston (1988) compared RO and ion exchange for their use in pharmaceutical water preparation. The principal application was the treatment of feedwaters to prepare them for distillation. These authors stated that single-pass RO did not produce a water as low in total dissolved solids as eventuated from twin DI resin beds. However, this was not extremely important for water intended for distillation, given the elevated TDS levels in the feedwater. The RO-treated water sufficed for use in the still. Benedek and Johnston (1988) also compared a double-pass RO system to ion exchange followed by ultrafiltration polishing. For lower TDS waters, the ion-exchange alternative was more economical. However, for higher TDS levels, both capital and operating costs became lower for the double-pass RO system. An added advantage was that operation of the RO utilized a single, compact, automated technology; whereas the ion-exchange and ultrafiltration manipulation involved different operational and maintenance protocols. (Additionally the use of double-pass RO should in itself suffice to prepare WFI.)

Purified Water by two-pass RO. Existing double-pass RO systems described in the literature have been applied to semiconductor usage and have often focused on the difficult-to-attain elimination of silica. The requirements of compendial pharmaceutical water purifications are different. The semiconductor applications have taught, however, that the use of dual-pass systems may usefully simplify pretreatment protocols to make possible the elimination of multimedia deep beds, the avoidance of bicarbonate removal by acidification and degassing, and the removal of organics without the use of carbon beds or subsequent use of mixed beds (with their implications to organism recontamination). Indeed, the use of double-pass RO for Purified Water preparation logically suggests itself for source waters of more complex compositions and of less constant character (surface waters, for instance).

With double-pass RO, the need for prior deionization and multimedia filtration becomes eliminated, along with the chemical regeneration costs. Of course, water softening may be entailed. Though such installations are in successful operation, the application is still novel.

There is some difference of opinion concerning how much more a two-pass system costs than a single-pass mode. Estimates vary from 60% to 100%, clouded by different views of the ancillaries such as instrumentation and valves that are needed, and of the degree of sophistication that is necessary. The second unit must, of course, be sized to provide the necessary volume. Operating on comparatively pure water, the second stage can provide a 90% recovery; the first stage, probably the conventional 75%. Two sets of instruments will be required. A product-staged double-pass RO system providing 100 gpd may cost around $3,000; one furnishing 50 gpm could cost $50,000. Some savings result because a double-pass system requires no ion-exchange demineralizers. Also, the multimedia deep beds in advance of the ion-exchange units are also dispensed with.

A simpler west coast system utilizes city water. It is filtered through backwashable steel screen filter units, followed by either of two sand beds in parallel. Each of the sand beds leads to an activated carbon bed. This arrangement enables the use of one train of sand bed and carbon bed to be in operation while its parallel counterpart is being renewed or replaced.

The pretreated water is fed through a series of five 1 μm-rated depth filters to a reverse osmosis installation for conversion to the desired Purified Water.

Contemplated future changes in the system may involve replacement of the sand beds by ultrafiltration units. Some additional filtrative protection for the ultrafilter is foreseen. The use of a steel "edge" backflushable filter device will be considered. A booster pump upstream of the ultrafilter will also likely be necessitated.

A biotechnical operation in New England offers an example of Purified Water manufacture utilizing two-pass, product-staged reverse osmosis based on cellulose acetate membranes. A municipally treated water is led through roughing filters to a softening bed. The softening operation removes barium and strontium along with more conventional hardness elements. The softened water is flowed through the activated carbon bed whose primary purpose is to remove chlorine from the water. During this process some portion of the water's TOC is also removed. The carbon bed is sanitized weekly using steam supplied by a clean steam generator.

The softened and dechlorinated water is pumped through a two-pass, product-staged cellulose acetate RO unit for purification into Purified Water. The water thus prepared is stored in a 50,000-gallon stainless steel tank at 15 ± 3 °C. The water is recirculated at the same temperature through a loop from which points of use derive.

The alert limit set for the operation is at a microbial count of 30 cfu/mL. The action limit is set at 50 cfu/mL. The microbiological sample drawn is 100 mL in volume.

The chemical and microbiological analyses performed in connection with the validation of one Purified Water system were as follows:

The chemical constituents of the water were checked at different points along the system to see how their levels accorded with the corresponding stipulations in the USP. The entities tested for were conductivity, hardness, pH, chlorine content, and TOC.

Hardness, in this system removed by ion-exchange, was assayed in an assessment of its scaling effect if RO were to be used. By the same token, silica might have been measured for its scaling effect upon RO and for its potential deposition upon still surfaces. The water issuing from properly operated stills should be at pH 7. The range of pH 5 to 7 is accepted because ambient carbon dioxide, the acid anhydride of carbonic water, rapidly equilibrates with water to yield lower equilibrium pH values. The solubility of CO_2 from the air manifests itself on distilled water within minutes. Where ion-exchange is used to prepare Purified Water, particularly twin-bed installations, sodium-ion leakage manifests itself as water alkalinity, pHs above 7, often incorrectly ascribed as being caused by an imperfect removal of alkali regenerant from the anion-exchange resin.

Simultaneous with the chemical analyses, microbiological assays were performed at various test sites along the water purification chain. Plate counts were made for total heterotropic contents using tryptone soy agar (TSA) of double strength as a bacterial culture over a 48-hour incubation at 35 °C. Gram-negatives were counted, enteric species were assayed using McConkey's medium, and *P. aeruginosa* was also assayed for; total coliform counts (TCC), were assayed per 100 mL aliquots.

The chemical assays were performed on the incoming water, after the carbon bed, after the mixed DI bed, after the ozonator but before entering the storage tanks, after the storage tanks upon the ozone-destructed effluent, and at the point of use midway along the distribution loop, the point at the furthest distance from the storage tanks.

The microbiological assays were performed after the carbon bed, after each mixed DI bed but before the ozonation, after the ozonation but before the storage tanks, and after the storage tanks following the ozone removal, at each of the six points of use, and just before the water is returned to the storage tanks.

Six weeks were devoted to prospective validation, during which period the water was not used for compounding. The validation involved assaying three times weekly, and each point of use was assayed each time a lot was made using water from that point of use. The test interval was reduced during the next 6 months, and again after 9 months of operation. The loop, initially assayed thrice weekly, now undergoes weekly testing; except that each point of use receives testing every time it is used. Each POU is tested once per week. a microbiological goal for the Purified Water is that fewer than 5% of the samples should show heterotropic plate counts of greater than 100 cfu/ml. The action limit is set at 100 cfu/ml. An absence of Gram-negative organisms is also sought. Typically, fewer than 10 cfu/ml are found after the ozone treatment.

Purified Water by distillation. Jackman and Sneed (1990) described a Purified Water system based on vapor-compression type distillation. The common belief is that energy costs associated with the employment of a still makes the practice uneconomical as compared with reverse osmosis or ion exchange. Jackman and Sneed (1990) provided an economic and reliability study whose conclusion was the opposite, except for large water systems in excess of 500,000 gpd. They cited a greater reliability as characterizing still operations, and suggested adoption particularly in specialized applications.

Jackman and Sneed (1990) utilized a municipally treated potable water supply with a composition as shown in Table 12-2. The system had a capacity of 1,600 gph of Purified Water. The incoming water was dechlorinated using a carbon bed, to avoid corrosion of the still. The passage of carbon fines was restrained by use of a 5-μm (nominal) cartridge filter. Sodium cycle softening was depended upon to remove hardness (calcium and magnesium ions), to prevent scaling of the still with concomitant loss of still capacity. The depth of the carbon bed exceeded the 30 inches generally recommended. It thus served, at least in part, to remove organic contaminants from the water. The softener was sized with a capacity of 210 kilograins. It contained 7 ft^3 of resin, and required regeneration approximately daily, consuming about 100 pounds of salt in the process. Both the carbon and softener vessels were of 316 stainless steel, enabling their periodic sanitization by hot water (90 to 95 °C) for periods of from 30 to 60 minutes, preceded and followed by brief (15-minute) backwashes. The softened water was stored in a fiberglass holding tank, from which it was fed to the still. Distillate (part of which was directed to the sanitation line) was produced at 90 to 95 °C. The suitability of the distilled water to be designated as

Purified Water is shown by its analysis (see Table 12-3). It was characterized by a maximum microbial count of 10 cfu/mL, and was free of lactose-fermenting organisms, and of yeasts and molds (Jackman and Sneed, 1990).

Proposed Purified Water Systems

Zoccolante (1989) proposed a series of Purified Water preparation systems of progressively more sophisticated and costly devices intended to accommodate more challenging feedwater characteristics or to produce effluents of more demanding qualities. Zoccolante's cost figures of 1989 are now out of date. However, their relative levels, from one system to another, are still approximately accurate. Their inclusion here may therefore be instructive.

Of the nine systems proposed by Zoccolante (1989), the most typical of a *USP* water system design was his System 1 (see Figure 12-1). In this proposal, a basic deionization system, the depth and carbon pretreatment are followed by a two-bed demineralizer, which for *USP* water systems is the most frequent means of bulk ion removal. A mixed-bed demineralizer follows in order to bring the two-bed's normally alkaline effluent into the pH range of 5 to 7 and to bring the water's ionic content below *USP* requirements.

All of System 1 would be under continuous flow. For bacterial control of

Table 12-2
Supply Water Analysis

Impurity	*Quantity*
Total dissolved solids	185 ppm
Suspended solids	0.3 ppm
Temperature	43.8 °F
Turbidity	<0.1 NTU
Bicarbonate alkalinity (as $CaCO_3$)	104 ppm
Carbonate alkalinity (as $CaCO_3$)	0.0 ppm]
Calcium	36.0 ppm
Chlorides	10.2 ppm
Fluorides	1.12 ppm
Iron	0.01 ppm
Noncarbonate hardness (as $CaCO_3$)	30.0 ppm
Total hardness (as $CaCO_3$)	134 ppm
Magnesium	12.7 ppm
Nitrates	0.62 ppm
pH	7.48
Phosphates	<0.02 ppm
Potassium	1.1 ppm
Sodium	4.9 ppm
Silica	4.0 ppm
Sulfates	27.1 ppm
Residual chlorine	0.5-0.7 ppm

Jackman and Sneed (1990); Courtesy, *Ultrapure Water* journal pretreatment, a flow switch senses when the demand from makeup water is low, and starts a pump to recirculate water through pretreatment filters and the UV sterilizer. Another pump continuously recirculates the demineralized water throughout the distribution network and back to the upstream side of the two-bed demineralizer. The ultraviolet irradiated water is recirculated through the carbon bed. If UV is not used, the organism content in the effluent of the carbon bed can be reduced by backwashing countercurrent with chlorinated water.

System 1, with a projected capital cost in 1989 of $100,000, would not be state-of-the-art technology, but it would provide reasonable bacterial control. For a location with moderate feedwater organic levels and high usages, this type of system works quite well.

The proposal for System 2 (see Figure 12-2) adds hot storage and distribution (at 65 to 80 °C) to the basic components used in System 1. Hot storage would need to be in a 5,000-gallon 316L stainless steel tank meeting ASME code. It would have a hydrophobic vent filter, and level controls for makeup and for protection of the two distribution pumps (one in service and one for standby).

System 2's 1989 capital cost of $220,000 indicates that its hot distribution system would cost more than its basic deionization system. Such a distribution

Table 12-3
Product Water Composition

Parameter	*Measurement*
Color	Colorless
Odor	Odorless
Appearance	Clear
Specific resistance	1.0 megohm-cm
pH	5.0-7.0
Chloride	0.5 ppm max
Sulfate	0.5 ppm max
Ammonia	0.3 ppm max
Calcium	0.5 ppm max
Carbon dioxide	4.0 ppm max
Total heavy metals	0.5 ppm max
Iron	0.1 ppm max
Copper	0.01 ppm max
Chromium	0.01 ppm max
Cobalt	0.1 ppm max
Manganese	0.1 ppm max
Nickel	0.1 ppm max
Oxidizable substances	Meets test in monograph
Total solids	≤1 ppm
Microbiology	≤1 fecal coliform/100 mL: 10 cfu/mL; free from lactose-fermenting organisms, yeasts, and molds

Jackman and Sneed (1990); Courtesy, *Ultrapure Water* journal system, properly designed, is an expensive but also an absolute way to provide bacterial control, a feature in which much interest has been expressed at technical conferences. This system relies upon ion exchange, not upon carbon, to remove TOC.

Zoccolante's System 3 (see Figure 12-3) supplements the basic deionization of System 1 with bacterial control by ozone. Generated from air, the ozone would be continuously applied to the water in a 5,000-gallon storage tank of 316 stainless steel. Two distribution pumps (one in standby) pass the water through an ozone-destruct ultraviolet unit. Variants of this system are much used for Purified Water preparation. The presence of ozone in the storage tank obviates the use of a nitrogen blanket.

Daily, during periods of no production, the UV unit would be turned off to allow the ozone to sanitize the whole system. This procedure seeks to minimize or prevent the accumulation of biofilm, and can usually be accomplished in 30 minutes per day, although it can be allowed to continue as long as is practical.

Bacteria counts of zero to 5 cfu/mL could consistently be expected from System 3, and its bacterial control is therefore not as absolute as that of System 2. In cases where bacteria counts of zero were expected at all times, or where trace residual ozone might impact on final products, System 2 would be preferred over System 3. Where ambient water temperature was needed at all use points, however, System 3 would in many cases be preferred.

Because the storage tank for System 3 operates at ambient temperature, it would not need insulation or steam jacketing; and because it operates at atmospheric pressure, it would not need to meet ASME code. Thus the storage

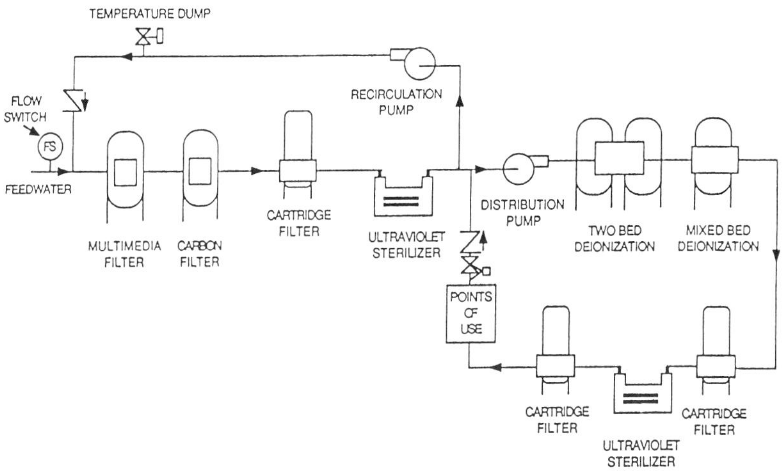

Figure 12-1. System 1, deionization.
Zoccolante (1989); Courtesy, Continental Penfield Liquid Treatment Systems

tank for this system would be a lower capital cost than the one for the hot water distribution system. The operating costs would also be lower, reflecting the lesser costs of producing ozone as compared to the energy costs for a hot system. The 1989 cost for System 3 was estimated at \$190,000.

System 4 (see Figure 12-4) is the last of Zoccolante's proposals that would use deionization as a basic system, and it adds ultrafiltration as a final component for polishing. The ultrafilter is capable of keeping the bacterial count relatively low, by rejecting a quantitative amount of microorganisms such as bacteria and viruses. It would also reduce the quantity of dissolved organics in the product water.

Heat and ozone affect the choice and therefore the cost of the materials of the distribution piping downstream; but UF product water, which is no more corrosive than its feedwater, does not. On the other hand, chemicals would be needed to sanitize System 4's distribution piping. This and the continuous 5% waste stream from the ultrafilter are major disadvantages, although the 5% blowdown does have the benefit of causing the makeup to the system to run continuously.

With a 1989 capital cost of \$145,000 (which includes an automated UF with cleaning system), System 4 would start out costing less than Systems 2 or 3. Operationally, it should cost less than the hot-distribution System 2, but more than the ozonated System 3. Bacterial counts would not be as low as those for

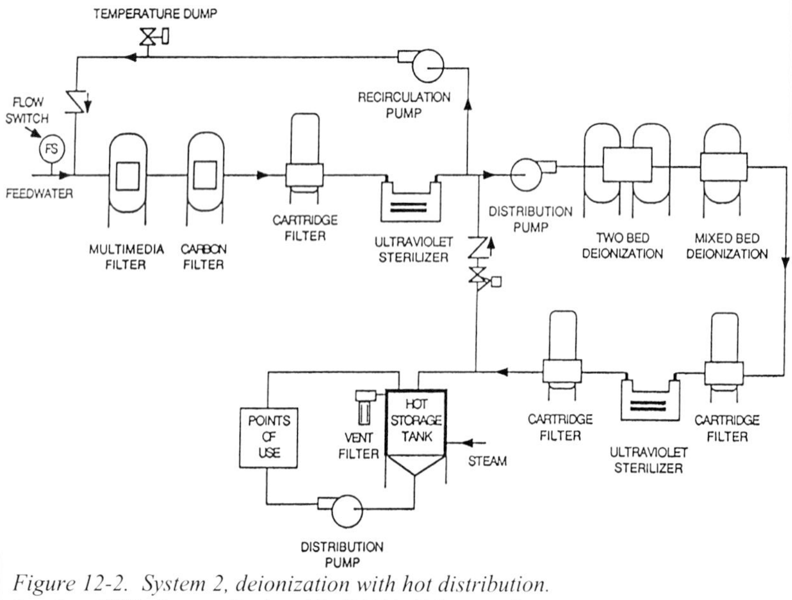

Figure 12-2. System 2, deionization with hot distribution.
Zoccolante (1989); Courtesy, Continental Penfield Liquid Treatment Systems

Systems 2 or 3, but would be better than those for System 1, and would show consistent good counts for a reasonable capital expenditure.

Zoccolante's proposed Systems 5 through 9 use reverse osmosis for primary demineralization in place of the ion-exchange resin beds used for Systems 1 to 4. System 5's pretreatment system (see Figure 12-5) calls for depth and carbon filtration, and a water softener that eliminates the need for acid feed to the RO. When the RO unit is not in operation, the pretreated water is to recirculate through an in-line UV sterilizer that keeps bacterial counts down in the dechlorinated feedwater to the RO.

The RO unit itself would use thin-film composite membranes that are not chlorine-resistant but that do allow the lowest consumption of energy, the longest membrane life, and the highest organic rejection. The unit would be sized to deliver 20 gpm to a 10,000-gallon fiberglass storage tank, which would allow for a 50-gpm consumption rate for extended periods. A continuously recirculating distribution polishing system would include service demineralizers that are regenerated off-site, and 5-µm cartridge filtration, another UV sterilizer, and 2-µm final filters.

The RO system that is the basis of System 5 would have a product water approaching a resistivity of 18.3 megohm-cm, a theoretical limit. The high organic rejection of the RO membranes would give a low TOC count. Since the membranes would reject nearly all of the incoming colloids, the use of submicron

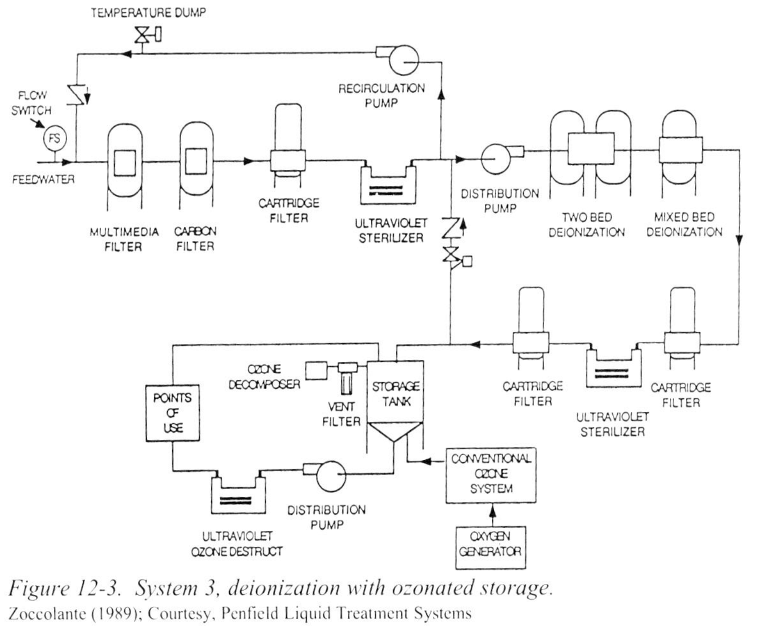

Figure 12-3. System 3, deionization with ozonated storage.
Zoccolante (1989); Courtesy, Penfield Liquid Treatment Systems

final filters would be very practical, as they could be expected to last a year or more. Redundancy of the final filter housings would allow their weekly sanitization, as with hydrogen peroxide, thus preventing the proliferation of bacterial colonies on filter surfaces. (This technique has been used extensively in electronic applications.)

Because the salt used for the pretreatment softener in System 5 does not present hazardous handling problems, and because the polishing service demineralizers avoid the problem of on-site regeneration, a primary advantage of System 5 would be the lack of chemical handling problems. Additionally, the pretreatment by the RO system allows the service demineralizers to be quite economical.

In order to have their best bacterial control, RO units need to operate for 12 hours or more per day. To achieve this, however, an increased flowrate and adequate cold water storage are required. These increase system cost and RO idle time, giving System 5 its primary disadvantage.

The capital cost of System 5 (in 1989) was estimated at \$165,000. This is 65% greater than System 1's cost. The capital costs of a single-train demineralizer-based system such as System 1 tend to be lower than those of an RO-based system such as System 5, whereas the costs of a dual-train demineralizer system would be comparable to the RO.

Where the Purified Water is stored at room temperature it is kept under a nitrogen blanket in a break tank. This tank separates the rest of the system from its polishing loop. A check valve could be used to isolate the polishing loop, but Zoccolante (1989) finds such valves less reliable than the certainty of break tanks

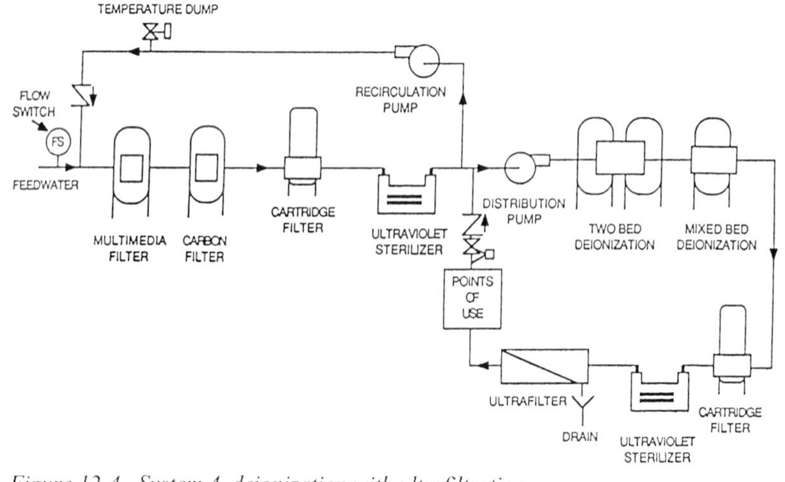

Figure 12-4. System 4, deionization with ultrafiltration.
Zoccolante (1989); Courtesy, Penfield Liquid Treatment Systems

in avoiding contamination at the points of use.

Tank protection can come in the form of blanketing by medical-grade nitrogen controlled by the regulation of a pressure switch. Pressurized tanks can be protected by blow-patches.

The design for System 6 (see Figure 12-6) adds hot storage and distribution to System 5. Because RO's production rate is low, 10,000 gallons of storage would be needed. The considerable expense of a 10,000-gallon 316L stainless steel, ASME-coded storage tank is avoided by using a 5,000-gallon tank of the same type for hot storage; and earlier in the process using a 5,000-gallon fiberglass tank for cold storage of the RO product water. Even so, the 1989 capital cost of $275,000 for System 6 would make it the most expensive of Zoccolante's nine suggested systems. This price tag would, however, pay for production of water with very, very high resistivity and absolute bacterial control, and do it without chemical handling.

An ozonated storage and distribution system is added to a modified RO system for the design of System 7 (see Figure 12-7). As would be done in System 3's DI/ozone system, ozone is produced conventionally from air, added to the 316L storage tank, and then removed by ozone-destruct UV light. As with System 3 also, the whole system could be sanitized intermittently by turning off the UV unit.

For Zoccolante's other RO systems, the polishing DI/UV/filtration is part of the continuous distribution flow. For System 7, it is sized for the 20-gpm makeup

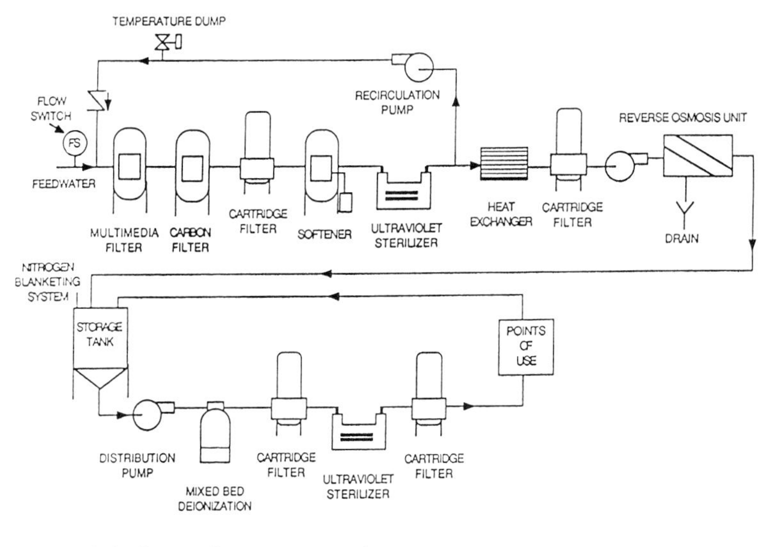

Figure 12-5. System 5, reverse osmosis.
Zoccolante (1989); Courtesy, Continental Penfield Liquid Treatment Systems

rate. When water is not needed for makeup demand for the storage tank, it runs on bypass recirculation from the tank to keep the purity level up.

In 1989, the capital cost of System 7 would have been $240,000, slightly lower than that of System 6. As with System 2 (DI/hot distribution) and System 3 (DI/ozonation), with heat comes the greater capital and operating expense, but also the ultimate in bacterial control. The good bacterial control by the ozonated systems would come at a reasonable expense.

While the conventional production of ozone is from air, another method, the MEMBREL system, produces it from demineralized water. This water must be highly demineralized so that it does not foul the catalytic membrane cell used by the process. The ozone unit's feedwater, rather than being the RO product water, should come from after the mixed-bed demineralizers. Since the ozone is produced from a split stream, it is immediately dissolved in water. The typical ozone concentration required to be generated for a conventional system is 0.3 to 0.5 ppm, whereas for a MEMBREL system, the ozone is effective at approximately 0.1 ppm, it all being dissolved as generated in water. Compared to air-derived ozone, this unit causes few safety concerns.

Except that it uses the MEMBREL ozone production, System 8 (see Figure 12-8) is similar to System 7, continuously adding the ozone to the storage tank and removing it with in-line UV before the DI polishing system. When ozone sanitization of the distribution piping is needed, it is provided by a bypass around the polishing components.

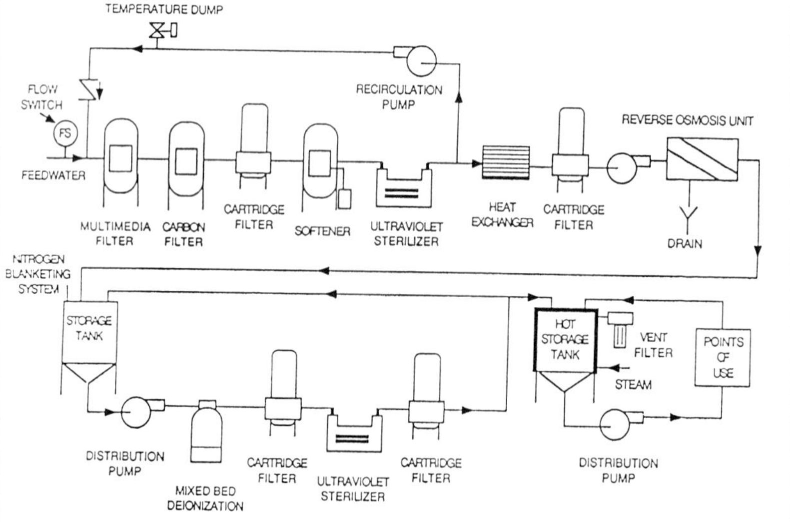

Figure 12-6. System 6, reverse osmosis with hot distribution.
Zoccolante (1989); Courtesy, ContinentalPenfield Liquid Treatment Systems

Because of the higher cost of the MEMBREL system, and a larger polishing system (sized for a full 50-gpm distribution flowrate), System 8's 1989 capital cost came to \$265,000. The larger polishing system means that all water would be continuously repurified before point of use. Although this would not be necessary for most USP applications, it could be useful for a biotech application requiring water of high resistivity.

The last of Zoccolante's proposals, System 9 (see Figure 12-9), is based on a product-staged RO system, which can produce USP Purified Water with a resistivity of 1 to 5 megohm-cm from most feedwater sources. This is lower than the typical resistivities for Systems 1 through 8, and would give this system a lower margin for error or media degradation. It is the only one of Zoccolante's proposals that does not call for a demineralizer, regenerable or otherwise.

The two passes through RO membranes would keep this system low in dissolved organics and microorganisms, as would the conventional ozone system used in the distribution system. No acid or caustic handling would be needed, nor an outside demineralizer regeneration service, and maintenance requirements for this system are relatively low. The RO-quality feedwater to the second pass is basically free of suspended solids, and quite low in organics, so this pass needs very little attention. System 9 would consistently provide high-quality water, at a 1989 capital cost of \$250,000.

None of the capital costs given for Zoccolante's proposed systems have taken

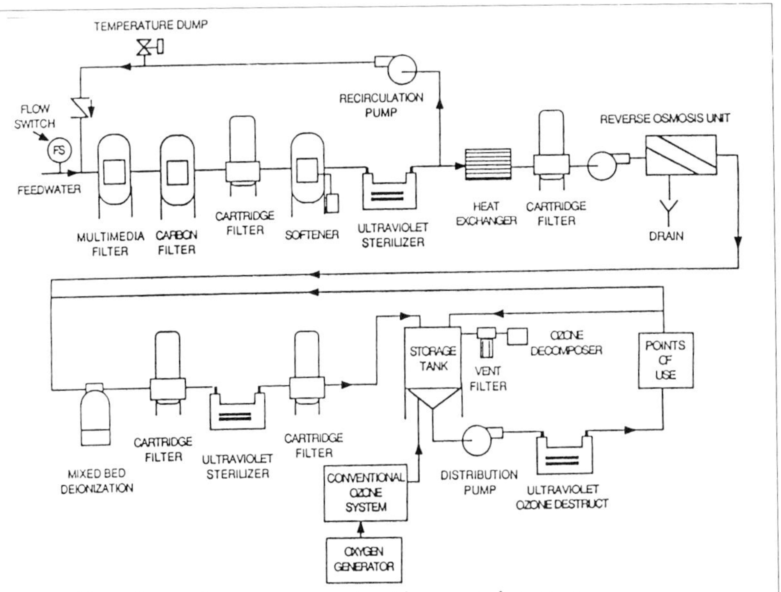

Figure 12-7. System 7, reverse osmosis with ozonated storage.
Zoccolante (1989); Courtesy, Continental Penfield Liquid Treatment Systems

the costs of a sanitary 316L distribution piping system into account, although pipe insulation for 1,000 feet of 2-inch distribution piping was included for those systems using hot distribution.

The ionic quality of all nine of Zoccolante's systems would be far above the requirements for USP Purified Water. The choices among them would usually be based on a single overriding need on the part of the user. The systems differ as to costs (both capital and operating), bacterial control, and the need for chemical handling. For greatest bacterial control or minimum maintenance, one of the more comprehensive systems would usually be chosen, whereas a simpler system would be selected when the main concern was capital expense. To be successful, however, any of the systems described above would need to be properly installed, and maintained by well-trained operators.

Studies of WFI by Dual-Pass RO

An 8-month pilot study involving RO module application for Water for Injection production was reported from the Upjohn Co. (Juberg et al., 1977). The study simulated the operational conditions of a production setting.

Well water was chlorinated with 3 ppm of chlorine at the well head. A 10-µm-rated depth-type filter was used to free the water of iron and particulate matter. Filtration through an active carbon bed was then used to remove the chlorine, whose presence would have degraded the aromatic polyamide constituting the

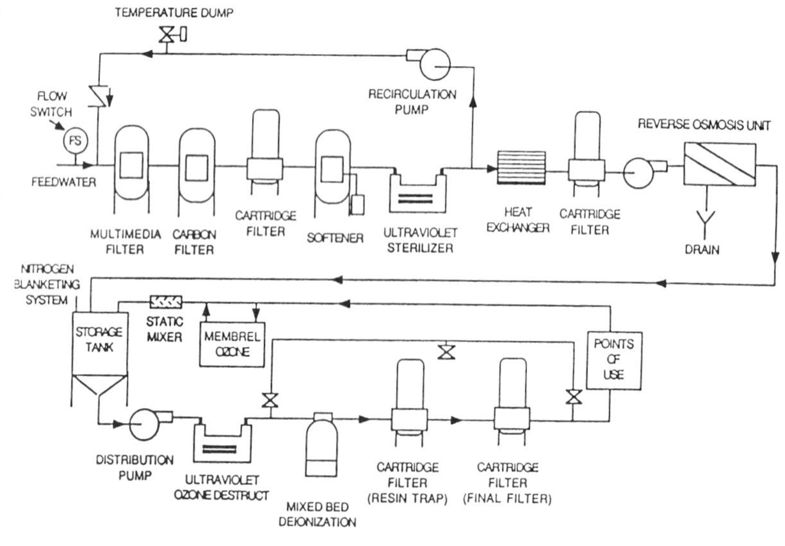

Figure 12-8. System 8, reverse osmosis with MEMBREL ozone.
Zoccolante (1989); Courtesy, Continental Penfield Liquid Treatment Systems

RO module to be used. Two water softeners, sized to the RO unit capacities, served to protect the RO devices against scaling during use.

Removal of the chlorine prior to the softening operation exposed the softening media to poorer bacterial controls and posed to the RO units a heightened organism challenge that would necessitate their more frequent cleaning and sanitization. It had been planned that upon translation of the pilot plant to full production scale, chlorine removal would be made after the softening units, at the last instance before the RO devices, so that the umbrella of the chlorine presence against bacteria could be prolonged as long as possible.

Two DuPont hollow-fiber Permasep modules were employed to perform the RO function. Particulate matter was removed from chlorine-free, softened feedwater by 5-μm filtration to avoid plugging the RO modules. A multistage centrifugal pump was used to feed this water at 400 psig (28 bar) to the first of the RO units. This first-stage Permasep unit was 4 inches by 28 inches (10 cm by 70 cm). Its operation was at the 50% recovery level and the waste was discarded. The permeate was repressurized to 400 psig and fed to the second RO unit, a 4-inch by 24-inch (10-cm by 61-cm) Permasep unit. The second-stage unit was operated at 75% recovery. Wastewater from the second stage was not dumped, but was recycled as feed to the first-stage pump. The permeate water from the second stage was collected as product water. This system produced 1 to 1.5 gpm (4 to 6 Lpm) of final product water. The RO process operation

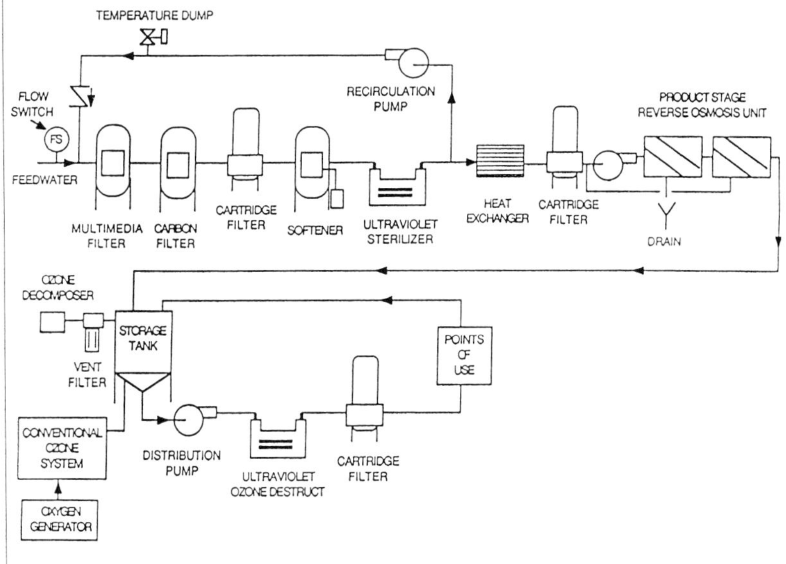

Figure 12-9. System 9, product-staged reverse osmosis with ozonated storage.
Zoccolante (1989); Courtesy, Continental Penfield Liquid Treatment Systems

removed 99.6% of the total ion content present in the raw water at a recovery rate of 43%.

The above mode of product staging the two RO, results in high overall total dissolved solids reduction and ionic rejection because all of the product is subjected to successive treatment by two RO units. The disadvantage of the product-staging arrangements is that its lower recovery rate requires a higher consumption of softened feedwater. Repressurization of the water at the second stage involves energy cost considerations. The product water produced, however, is of very high quality.

Evaluation of the operation was in accord with a simulated operational schedule. Data gathered on inlet water fouling and hardness, water temperature, pressure, and rate of flow demonstrated the operational constancy of the RO operation. Over the duration of the 45-day test period, the total ionic reduction was on the order of 99.6%. The water produced fully met the chemical quality requirements of USP Water for Injection. Microbiological water assays were made using 0.45-µm-rated membranes incubated 48 hours at 37 °C on glucose extract agar. While the RO feedwater organism content averaged 10^3 organisms per 100 milliliters (10^3/100 mL), twice-weekly disinfections of the RO units served consistently to keep the organism counts of the product water at less than 10/100 mL the standard of acceptability.

Pyrogen testing by the rabbit test showed the feedwaters to be pyrogenic on a majority of the days tested. The product water was always found to be nonpyrogenic. Test results by LAL demonstrated a greater than 1 log titer reduction of bacterial endotoxins across the RO units.

Sanitization of the RO membranes was achieved by a 2% solution of formaldehyde circulated through the RO modules for 1 hour, followed by an 18-hour holding period. This disinfected the pumps and piping as well as the RO units. The sanitizing solution was mixed in a stainless steel tank. Pretested RO feedwater was used to prevent scale formation on the membrane. On a preventive maintenance schedule, sanitization was routinely performed once every 2 weeks. Washing the formaldehyde sanitizing solution from the equipment with water prepared the RO units for further use.

The system as actually built, however, came to rely on distillation rather than on RO. The use of Permasep D-9 RO units necessitated critical attention to prefiltration to avoid irreversible plugging. This proved too labor-intensive and costly in terms of prefilters; nor were the periodic replacement costs for the RO unit insignificant. Perhaps most important, the FDA was not happy with the testing of pooled permeates. Pooling of permeates could dilute and serve to mask a problem in an individual permeate. Individual testing was therefore required.

In another example, an orthopedic implant and medical device manufacturer utilized dual-pass, product-staged RO to produce WFI quality water. The source water came from a 100-foot-deep, 6-inch well and was pumped to the surface at a maximum 85 gpm. The water was first pumped into a series of four bladder tanks, the purpose of which was to smooth out the pressure pulse of the pump and to store a sufficient amount of water to allow the pump to cycle on and off periodically. Deep-well water was used because of its consistent quality and temperature compared with available city water. The well water did contain colloidal iron. It was not chlorinated.

The water passed through a multilayer particulate filter that served to remove or reduce the total suspended solids. The deep-bed filtered water was then softened by the action of twin out-of-phase sodium cycle ion exchangers. The softened water was piped some 200 feet through two parallel 5-μm-rated prefilters made of spun-bonded polypropylene. These were replaced weekly or when the pressure differential across the filters became elevated to 10 psig.

The prefiltered water was subjected to the action of a thin-film composite RO unit of polyamide as the water was unchlorinated, it could enter the RO directly. This unit's main purpose was to remove silica and other total dissolved solids from the water. The permeate then flowed through two UV lights (lamps cleansed daily with wipers) and then became feedwater for the dual-pass RO with polysulfone membranes. The product water from the dual-pass RO circulated at ambient temperature through a loop to points of use, and what was not used continued through the loop to be rejoined as feedwater between the RO and the UV light.

The reject water from both RO units ran to drain to help dissipate heat. Total permeate recovery was roughly 50%, and product water production ran continuously at the rate of 10 gpm. The system was sanitized weekly with 1-to-20 dilution of commercial bleach solution (original concentration of 5.25% sodium hypochlorite) to RO permeate, over a contacting time of 30 minutes. This was followed by a water rinse sufficient to remove any sanitizing agents to below levels detectable by colorimetric moniotoring for oxidizing chlorine. The sanitization frequency was routine and prophylactic, being motivated by concerns of biofilm formation, especially on the downside of the RO membrane.

The organism count of the source water at the well head was high (200,000 to 500,000 cfu/mL as determined by total plate count). The permeate from the dual-pass RO arrangement seldom exceeded and was usually well below 10 cfu/100 mL directly after the membrane, and seldom exceeded 50 cfu/100 mL in the distribution loop.

During the 21-day period devoted to the initial validation phase, the water was tested daily for its organisms, endotoxin, and chemical composition through the entire process, starting at the well head and ending at the points of use. Subsequently, and until more information could be compiled, pyrogen testing was performed every morning, while microbiological and chemical testing was carried out 3 times per week. Organism counts were usually under 10 cfu/100 mL, and the endotoxin level was seldom within detectable limits. When endotoxin was measurable, its source was sought and the system was sanitized.

Although the company's application did not require WFI quality, the dual-pass RO product water thus manufactured consistently met WFI microbial and endotoxin quality levels.

Montgomery and Bradley (1985) described in detail the equipment and operational requirements of one such double-pass system to produce water with 4- to 8-megohm-cm resistivity to feed stills of 7,000-gpd capacity. In such arrangements it is usual to treat the reject water from a second stage with twin-bed ion exchangers, and to reintroduce it into the first stage. The reject water as it emerges from the second stage may be passed through organic removers as, for example, reticulated non-ion-exchange resin beads, before it is deionized. It may also be warmed to about 27 °C (80 °F) before being treated and reintroduced into the first RO stage. The untreated water, usually at about 7 °C (45 °F), may first also be heated to 27 °C because the heated water permeates RO membranes far better than does cold water. A 10% recirculation of the recovered water is maintained through the two RO units in order to prevent fouling of the membranes. To prevent scale formation, where this is likely, the feedwater is usually kept on the acid side and/or is softened.

In yet another example, a formulator of antibiotic injectables utilized dual-pass RO to prepare WFI. Chlorinated municipally-treated water entered the facility at varying pressures, sometimes as high as 80 psig. A booster pump raised it to 120 psig to create a flow of 80 gpm. The pressure-regulated water flowed through a 10-μm (nominal) rated string-wound prefilter to remove suspended solids, and then through a carbon bed that was changed at 6-month intervals, and then through a twin-bed ion exchanger followed by a mixed bed. The latter was relied upon to adjust the pH to near-neutral. (Such a practice is usually necessitated to overcome sodium ion leakage from the cation-exchange column of a twin-bed system). Actually, there were two parallel arrangements of carbon: twin beds and mixed beds. These alternated in their operation and standby postures. Replacements (for regeneration) of the ion-exchange beds were on a service basis, as alerted by resistivity readings and the water-use history. The beds serviced 18,000 gallons between replacements.

The water exiting the ion-exchange beds was prefiltered through a 5-μm nominally rated cartridge prior to passing into a spiral-wound polysulfone ultrafilter. The ultrafilter consisted of eighteen cartridges having a total effective area of 900 ft^2 and a rating of 10,000 daltons. The water flow into the ultrafilter was 40 gpm. The 25-gpm permeate, at ambient temperature, was directed to a dual-pass, product-staged RO arrangement. The RO membranes were of cellulose acetate, and each RO unit consisted of a bank of four spiral-wound tubes of 4-inch diameters containing six elements per tube.

To the 25 gpm forthcoming from the ultrafilter was added about 21.5 gpm of the first-stage reject plus about 3.5 gpm of the second-stage reject. This total of about 50 gpm fed the first-stage RO. The product water from the first stage was produced at 20 gpm. Of the reject, 21.5 gpm was recirculated; 9.5 gpm went to drain. The 20-gpm product water from the first RO fed the second RO unit to produce 17 gpm of product water (plus 3.5 of reject, which was recirculated to the first-stage feed). Overall, the recovery was approximately 70%.

The RO dual-pass assembly usually operated for about 16 hours. It, as well as the ultrafiltration unit, could be shut down periodically for up to 2 months. When not in use, the filters, both UF and RO, were stored in 1% formaldehyde solution after the reagent was recirculated for 20 minutes. Prior to the resumption of operations, the formaldehyde was washed out, as evidenced by resistivity measurements and by a colorimetric control testing involving Formalert test kits.

The ultrafilter and the ROs were sanitized with 4% peracetic acid over a 20-minute period of flow and recirculation every 10 days. After three such sanitizations, a treatment was made with a 1% solution of formaldehyde at a flow of about 15 gpm for 4 hours. The sanitizing solution was drained from the system by way of the storage tanks and distribution piping so that all water-encountering surfaces were contacted by the sanitizer. Complete removal of the sanitizing reagents (whether 4% peracetic acid, 1% formaldehyde, or both) was confirmed by resistivity measurements, by a colorimetric test for formaldehyde, and by performance of the USP oxidizable substances test with potassium permanganate.

So treated, the RO units lasted for 2 to 3 years, as assessed by their salt rejection ability. The ultrafilter required only one replacement in 6 years. (It could be speculated that the somewhat abbreviated RO service life could have been occasioned by the low pH of the peracetic acid sanitizer causing hydrolysis of the cellulose acetate membrane).

Upon exiting the dual-RO unit, the water passed through a heat exchanger where it was heated to 80 °C. It was stored at this temperature in each of two stainless steel jacketed tanks of 6,000-liter capacity under constant circulation. The batched water was to be used within a 6-day period. Each tank was given a batch number and was analyzed for its electrical resistivity and for its endotoxin content when filled. The endotoxin specifications were 0.25 EU/mL or less. Weekly microbiological assays were performed, but for information only; no organism specifications applied. In any case, there was a uniform freedom from microbes as determined by total plate counts. Daily water usage was sometimes as high as 18,000 liters.

The WFI was dispensed from its tanks through a once-through, dead-leg-free pipe of about 200 feet in length leading to points of use. A preflush of 150 to 170 liters was made over a 3-minute period prior to utilization of the water. The water was tested daily with LAL kits at the points of use, and weekly for total plate counts.

The water thus prepared by dual-pass RO and stored at 80 °C under circulation conformed to WFI quality stipulations, including those pertaining to endotoxin content. Having this quality, and having been prepared in conformity with *USP* and FDA requirements, it constituted WFI.

The dual-pass RO arrangement is well suited to the production of high-purity waters such as are of interest for pharmaceutical purposes where the ultimate in electrical resistivity is not the concern.

Water for Injection by Distillation

Case A. Coates et al. (1983) described, for the Upjohn Co.'s WFI, procedures that were distinct in four aspects from more conventional WFI processes. First, WFI for product and rinsing purposes were separately maintained. The second difference was that the system, although designed for higher or lower temperatures, was validated for storage and circulation at 60 °C, although actually maintained at 65 °C. This departure from the recommended 80 °C level proposed in the GMP for LVPs reduced the likelihood for corrosion, was less degradative to elastomeric components, and had implications for the safety of personnel. The third distinct point to the Upjohn process was that the WFI was stored under a positive nitrogen pressure of 3 psig (0.21 kg/cm^2). Nitrogen gas filtered through PTFE membranes was chosen to minimize corrosion of the storage tank, particularly at the liquid level line. There was some concern, however, that serious oxygen depletion could make difficult the restoration of passive oxide coatings to stainless steel surfaces. The fourth point of distinction was that the WFI cooled at the point-of-use stations but not used was not discarded, but was reheated and returned to the system.

Multiple-effect stills. In the Upjohn Co. WFI system, the water previously purified to the Purified Water USP storage was led to one of two six-effect Finn-Aqua stills. Movement was by Triclover pump with a Chesterton No. 241 double mechanical seal type that utilized Water for Injection as the lubrication and barrier fluids. The valves were of the highly electropolished ITT Grinnell diaphragm type, or Triclover throttling plug valves, and the seals were Chesterton No. 241 types, as detailed in the paper describing this Upjohn system (Coates et al., 1983). Each of the two six-effect Finn-Aqua 2000-H-6 stills had a capacity of 1,000 gph. The Water for Injection from each of these stills was collected in an atmospheric pressure surge tank protected by a vent filter. The distilled water was then moved by a Triclover centrifugal pump through a single-pass shell-and-tube double-tube sheet cooler manufactured by Beaverle Morris Co. The Water for Injection was cooled thereby from 95 °C to 65 °C. A loop carried the cooled water to the storage tanks, its temperature maintained at 65 °C by a Triclover concentric tube-type heat exchanger. The 65 °C Water for Injection was stored in each of two 5,000-gallon tanks and in each of two 10,000-gallon tanks.

Storage tanks. The WFI in the 10,000-gallon (37,850-liter) storage tanks was for rinsing, and that in the two 5,000-gallon (18,925-liter) tanks was intended for product formulation and for the rinsing of utensils and tanks utilized in the manufacturing areas. Water for Injection for product and rinsing were thus separately maintained. All the tanks were unjacketed, of 316L stainless steel manufactured by Dairy Craft Industries (DCI) of St. Cloud, MN. The two 5,000-gallon tanks were batched under a series of double-valve shutoffs and fitted with their own internal recirculation.

The two 10,000-gallon tanks for WFI for final rinsing were on continuous flow; some 25,000 gallons (94,650 liters) of WFI were used daily for rinsing. This WFI was generated in response to water level controls in the tanks. The storage tanks were not pressure rated and were protected by Teflon rupture disks. They were kept under nitrogen gas blankets at 3 psig (0.21 kg/cm^2), supplied through a 0.2-µm-rated silicone-treated nylon cartridge. The positive pressure militated against unfiltered air entering through a leaking gasket. A split-range pressure controller permitted nitrogen gas to be admitted and the tank vent to be closed when the pressure fell, as when water was withdrawn from the tank. When the tank was filled and the pressure rose, the vent was opened and the valve admitting nitrogen was shut. When the pressure was steady at 3 psig (0.21 kg/cm^2), both the nitrogen valve and the vent were closed. Twice weekly, each tank was cleared of its water content and was given a 1-minute flushing by means of spray-balls using 65 °C Water for Injection.

The hydrophobic vent filters were sterilized with live steam from a clean-steam generator operating on WFI. They were integrity-tested upon installation and removal, and their replacement was on a yearly schedule.

The hot water loop emanating from and returning to the tanks was maintained at 65 °C, although validated at 60 °C. The Johns-Manville CeraWool insulation so maintained the heat level of the product water that there was no need to use an existing in-line heater. Pumping was by a No. 218 Triclover pump utilizing a WFI seal. Frictional heat from the pumped circulation helped to maintain the 65 °C level for the water. A central panel monitored the entire operation, including some 28 temperature-sensing points. Thermocouple printouts were automatically made periodically, but any untoward temperature deviation was printed out within 30 seconds of its occurrence. All of the system piping was color-coded.

Water quality. The batched water in the two 5,000-gallon WFI product storage tanks, after being assayed, was controlled for release by the Quality Control Department, to be used in preparing products by Production. The nonbatched WFI in the two 10,000-gallon tanks was initially analyzed daily using the complete, appropriate USP test battery. After that, the contents of these tanks underwent such analyses weekly, a change in practice instituted and supported upon proper documentation. However, pyrogen and microbiological testing continued to be rigorously performed daily. In addition, points of use and sample ports were randomly tested at 1- or 2-week intervals, never more than 2 weeks. Testing results by LAL were usually zero.

Points of use. At each of four manufacturing areas and at one sink there were point-of-use stations. These consisted of a drop loop with controls and indicators. The desired water temperature was dialed, actuating the operation of a heat exchanger through which water was supplied. Reaching of the desired temperature was signaled by a green light, and only then could the production operator open the point-of-use valve. It required from 60 to 90 seconds for the water to cool from 65 to 25 °C. Should the dispensed water temperature be above 44 °C, a level considered capable of inducing burns, a red light indicator was also activated. No water began to flow until the dialed temperature was reached. Another dial indicated the actual water temperature at all times, even as it cooled. At the end of the desired water flow, the pipe from the drop loop drained free. Upon subsequent flow resumption, a momentary drain of water served to preflush the pipe. The cooled water returning from the drop loop was reheated to 65 °C by a second heat exchanger prior to rejoining the main loop. The water at the points of use was checked regularly for its conformity to WFI standards. A Royco particle counter was used to ascertain that internal company limits concerning particles larger than 10 μm were adhered to.

Observations. The Upjohn Co.'s WFI met the GMP requirements in exemplary fashion. That it did so while differing notably from other systems demonstrated that there are many possible means of WFI production. What is fundamentally involved is the devising, validating, and maintenance of a suitable system. The particular components and their arrangements within the system provide leeway in choice.

Case B. The system in Case B used well water, and included carbon bed, twin DI beds, mixed DI bed, and a vapor compression still. Water drawn from wells, the company's own and those belonging to the North Wales Water Authority, PA, was treated with chlorine. Retaining its residual chlorine along with a hardness of 200 ppm, the water was permeated through a Calgon carbon bed serviced by that company. The carbon bed did not utilize downstream filters to restrain its fines, if any.

The deionizer consisted of two dual-bed systems followed by one mixed bed. The dual-bed system had a capacity of 496,000 grains per regeneration and a flowrate of 63 gpm (238.5 Lpm). The effluent quality averaged 5 μmhos of conductivity. The mixed-bed system had a capacity of 140,000 grains per regeneration and a flowrate of 63 gpm. The deionizers were manufactured by

Hydromax Corporation of Milwaukee, WI.

Vapor compression stills. The deionizer delivered treated water (with a resistivity of approximately 1 megohm-cm) to two MECO vapor compression stills, each rated at 1,750 gph (6,625 Lph). Normally, one unit was capable of supplying the water demands, with the second unit available to handle peak demands and to serve in a standby posture.

The stills were the vapor compression type manufactured by the Mechanical Equipment Company, New Orleans, LA. The quality of the distilled water was of less than 1 microsiemens (μS) of conductivity. Each unit was driven by a 100-horsepower motor, with steam consumption of approximately 1,935 pounds per hour at 40 to 100 psig.

Storage tanks. The stills delivered hot water with a purity of 1 microsiemens conductivity to each of three 22,000-gallon (83,275-liter) stainless steel storage tanks. These tanks were not pressure vessels and were therefore equipped with rupture disks. The water in these tanks was continuously maintained at 82 °C (180 °F) by use of a steam-heated coil on the outside of the tank. The tanks were type 316L stainless steel with a 180-grit finish inside. They were approximately 30 feet (915 cm) high and 13 feet (397 cm) in diameter and were insulated with chloride-free fiberglass. The insulation was covered by a type of 304 stainless steel outer jacket. One of these three storage tanks was dedicated to supplying water to a manufacturing area in a separate building. This was also a heated recirculating system with supply and return lines.

All of the surfaces that came in contact with the distilled water were of 316L stainless steel, either electropolished or passivated with nitric acid. For future tank installation, both an electropolish finish and passivation, as with nitric acid, might be resorted to. (Anxiety over corrosion attends any system for handling highly purified water.) Some minor rouging in this installation was occasionally noticed on pump and flowmeter surfaces. It was attributed to the inevitable metallurgical problems that accompany the welding of stainless steels. Welding was done mainly by automated machine using the tungsten arc inert gas process. Welds were regularly inspected and in some cases were cut out of the system for closer examination.

Distilled water to sterile manufacturing. There was a second system that supplied distilled water specifically to the sterile manufacturing area. This system comprised three 300-gallon (1,136-liter) stainless steel tanks. The vapor compression stills supplied the water. These tanks were also of 316L stainless steel, with provision for continuously maintaining water at 82 °C by use of a steam coil. Triclover sanitary pumps delivered this water to the sterile manufacturing users.

These tanks were not batched. Their contents were routinely monitored daily for organisms and pyrogenicity. The organism count was rather consistent, routinely not exceeding 1/100 to 2/100 mL. The sampling ports were equipped with rubber diaphragm valves, and the sampling protocol involved a flushing of the port prior to securing the sample.

Cherry Burrell Co. or Triclover brand sanitary centrifugal pumps delivered the hot water to the points of use. The hot water was continuously circulated, going back to the tank by a return line. The criterion for the rate of recirculation was the maintenance of the water temperature at 82 °C. Dumping of the water was hence unnecessary.

Tank vents. The 22,000-gallon tanks were vented through a 0.45-μm-rated sanitary filter. The vent was heated by low-pressure steam to prevent blockage of the filter by condensed water (with consequent risk of tank collapse upon withdrawal of its contents). Vent filter heating was also seen as militating against organism growth in the filter, thus ensuring an inviolate tank sterility. The vent filters were replaced every 6 months. The integrity of the vent filter and of its installation were assessed by a pressure-hold test.

An alternative to the use of tank vents that was considered and rejected was the use of nitrogen gas pressure. The use of a nitrogen gas blanket would have required continuous monitoring.

Cooling of water at point of use. Certain point-of-use stations required cold water. The securing of same from the circulating hot water system without impairing its purity or breaching its integrity was ingeniously although not uniquely accomplished.

At a signal from a floor switch, a timer was started that, after a delay, opened the water supply and permitted flow into a heat exchanger, and then into a dispensing pipe at a maximum flow of 3 gpm (11.4 Lpm). The water temperature was reduced from 90 °C (194 °F) to 21 °C (70 °F), while the temperature of the cooling water rose from 9 °C (48 °F) to 16 °C (60 °F). The water was able to fill the dispensing pipe because the floor switch simultaneously closed an air vent to that pipe. The air vent was protected by a sterilizable filter assembly. Subsequent release of the flow switch closed the distilled water dispensing pipe and, after a time delay, opened the air vent to drain the point-of-use dispensing system.

Sanitization. The history of consistent high water quality demonstrated the lack of need for periodic chemical sanitization of this system. In any case, given the enormous weight of metal in the system, steaming would have been eschewed as excessively giving rise to large amounts of condensation. Validation of the system was conferred by the documented long-term evidence that the system operated as designed to give water of the proper purity.

Case C. The system in Case C used municipal water, and included DI beds, mixed DI beds, ultrafiltration, vapor compression still, and a four-effect still. Chlorinated municipal water was put through a sand filter and then run through a granulated Darco activated carbon filter. Both sand and carbon filters were backflushed twice a week.

The water then entered individual DI beds, from which it emerged with a minimum resistivity of 100,000 ohm-cm, prior to treatment in a mixed DI bed that yielded a minimum resistivity of 1,000,000 ohm-cm (1 megohm-cm). A small continuous circulation of some 3 to 5 gpm (11.4 to 19 Lpm) was maintained through the DI resin beds.

The emerging water was tested weekly for bacteria, for pyrogens by the LAL method, and continuously for conductivity, although the last was not a consideration. No problems were encountered, and the organism count never attained the maximum allowable limit.

The DI resin beds were manually regenerated two or three times per week using hydrochloric acid and a high grade of sodium hydroxide. The flow capacity of this system, which had a redundant counterpart, was 35 gpm (133.5 Lpm).

Ultrafiltration treatment. The deionized water was stored in two 1,000-gallon (3,785-liter) tanks, from which it entered a 10-cartridge ultrafiltration unit set up to deliver 2 to 3 gpm (7.6 to 11.4 Lpm) per cartridge. The stored water was continually recirculated at 3 gpm through the UF unit. (Maximum pressure was 25 psig [1.7 bar]; maximum operating temperature was 45 °C).

This system was sanitized weekly for a 2-hour duration by the use of 2 quarts (1.9 liters) of 30% hydrogen peroxide diluted with 40 gallons (150 liters) of filtered water. Hydrogen peroxide was selected as the sanitizing agent because its use offered freedom from concern regarding residuals. The UF was expected to last 3 to 5 years. There were no problems even after that time.

Distillation and storage. The water pretreated by ultrafiltration was then fed to each of two AquaChem vapor compression stills, modified in-house for intermittent operation; and also to one MECO vapor compression still. The distilled water, stored in each of three 1,500-gallon (5,678-liter) jacketed storage tanks with ultrasonic level controls, was maintained at 82 to 85 °C (180 to 185 °F). It was pumped by Triclover pumps through the hot circulation loop, which was maintained at 77 °C (170 °F) as a lower limit. The hot loop flow capacity was 35 gpm. The water in these tanks, intended as Purified Water, was not batched; it was on demand. The suitability of its quality was tested weekly. Steam-jacketed vent filters were used, heated to 108 °C (227 °F) by 5-psig steam.

Possible changes. Plans were made to use a heat exchanger to bring the caustic backwash to 43 °C (110 °F) to help remove silica from the mixed bed. That temperature would give the mixed resin bed the 45% swell required for the proper positioning of its two separate resin layers, necessary to economical regeneration. A heat exchanger would also be used to bring the water that goes through the sand filters to the UF unit to a range of 21 to 24 °C (70 to 75 °F) to give better control to the necessary flowrates.

Some of the water from the hot-distribution loop in this facility was cooled to 48.9 °C (120 °F) for washing. Some was also used in the preparation of oral liquids. A third portion was further distilled.

Multiple-effect still. From the three 1,500-gallon storage tanks, the hot loop fed 82 °C (180 °F) water through a pump to a Vaponics four-effect still. This still yielded water with a resistivity of 6 to 15 megohm-cm. Usually the value was 12 megohm-cm.

This further-distilled water was stored in each of two jacketed 1,000-gallon tanks equipped with filters within jacketed vents. These tanks could be steamed, using clean steam from the first effect of the Vaponics still. There was no need to dump water from these tanks because they were maintained at 82 °C. These tanks were batched, and WFI from the batched system was kept padlocked and under QC approval. It was released only following complete chemical and microbiological assay (Blackmer, 1984). The batched water was used to manufacture parenteral and ophthalmic solutions and for the final rinsing of medical device components. Validation of this system consisted of successfully replicating and documenting three successive runs leading to water of suitable quality.

The return and supply loop from the batched tanks was state-of-the-art, interior electropolished 316L stainless. Electroarc welding was used, and sanitary fittings were employed. The longest run of piping, about 175 feet (53.4 m), was from the tank to the end of the line. Two Beaverle and Morris double-tube-sheet 316L stainless steel heat exchangers were included. A compressed air segment of the system in Case C used a purification system to dry and clean the air.

Case D. The system in Case D used municipal water, and included sand bed, 1.0-µm bag strainer, 0.4-µm-rated polypropylene filter membrane, mixed DI beds, and a six-effect still. Municipal water originating from creeks was led serially through anthracite and sand filters at a flowrate of 100 gpm (380 Lpm). These were redundant beds to retain particles larger than 10 µm in size. The filters were backwashed routinely on a 60-hour cycle. From the sand filters, the water flowed into a 1-µm bag filter followed by a 0.4-µm-rated polypropylene cartridge filter.

Following the prefiltration, the water flowed through mixed beds of deionizing resins, which were on a 30-hour automatic regeneration cycle. The mixed beds required no saline flush to rid them of organics. After the mixed-bed units, to remove resin fines, the water encountered polypropylene filters of 0.4-μm rating, with seven 10-inch (24.9-cm) cartridges in each of two housings.

Multiple-effect still. The deionized water was next fed into a six-effect Finn-Aqua still. It was called pyrogen-free distilled water, not WFI, because at this point it was not batched. The operational temperature was 80 °C (176 °F) ± 5 °C.

Storage tanks. The distilled water was stored in each of two 5,000-gallon (18,925-liter) tanks whose sterilization was accomplished by clean steam drawn from the first stage of the still. The main distribution loop consisted of three sections, each utilizing Triclover sanitary pumps operating at 55 psig (3.7 bar) and with a flow capacity of 110 gpm (416 Lpm), or 6,600 gph (25,000 Lph). Each of two sections of the main loop contained two 600-gallon storage tanks wherein the pyrogen-free distilled water was batched, becoming WFI.

The 600-gallon (2,275-liter) storage tanks, as well as all the piping in each of the different department loops, were steam-sterilized by clean steam from each of three clean-steam generators.

All tanks, of 316L stainless steel, were each welded with one continuous seal. They were full-vacuum rated and fitted with vent filters. The tanks were sterilized monthly following inspection. Tanks vents were changed at that time.

Ultrasonic level detectors, previously employed, were found not to be reliable at 80 °C, although probably suitable at 65 °C. A capacitance-type level detector was satisfactorily utilized instead. The small tanks also had redundant float controls. There were regenerative turbine pumps on each tank to circulate its contents. Texas Instrument PI-5 microprocessors controlled the storage tanks, as well as Kay-Digi 3 printouts (every 15 minutes) for the logbooks.

The 600-gallon storage tanks were located adjacent to formulation areas. There was a total of 12,400 gallons (47,000 liters) of tank storage. The usage was from 18,000 to 22,000 gallons (68,000 to 83,250 liters) per day. There was therefore no need for dumping, but when there was an excess of water it was used as rinsewater.

Vent filters and ancillaries. The vent housings were jacketed and maintained at 100 °C (212 °F) to keep the filters from wetting out because of water vapor condensation. Two or three pounds of steam pressure were used in jacketing. The vent filters were 20-inch (49.8-cm), 0.2-μm-rated PTFE cartridges. They were changed every month, and integrity-tested using aqueous isopropanol 60% volume-to-volume ratio for the bubble pointing.

Liquid flow control was managed by the use of Triclover pumps located on the holding tanks and by means of the orifices positioned throughout the system. The Triclover pumps, in conjunction with upstream and downstream shutoff valves, served to keep the water going in one direction without the use of check valves, which are considered to have dubious sanitary qualities. The upstream and downstream shutoff valves also were used to boost the line pressures to 55 psig (4.7 bar).

The system was all of 316L stainless, welded with an automatic welding machine. The welds were mechanically polished, with some electropolishing. There was about 1 mile of piping, of 1.5-inch (3.81-cm) diameter. The longest run of pipe was 1,400 feet (427 m), from the Triclover pump to the farthest reach of the system. The system sloped to drain pumps, and the valves were all Teflon diaphragm valves. The flow was controlled by limiting orifices.

Product water. The system boasted remote control stations and electronically controlled trickle-steam-bathed sampling ports. Each loop was sampled every day along with one of the two 5,000-gallon tanks. The four WFI tanks were sampled as used. The system used step-down piping so that samples to 500 mL could be drawn. The points of use gave water cooled by means of timers and cooling jackets where needed. Conductivity (actually measured as resistivity, its reciprocal) was an index of freedom from ionic entities and was usually at the 7- to 9-megohm-cm level. Pyrogenicity was absent. On the basis of such analytical findings, it was anticipated that sanitization would be required only at 6- or 12-month intervals, if then.

Case E: room-temperature storage. Room-temperature storage and distribution of distilled water has at least two advantages over a high-temperature system. The cooler water is less corrosive, and the energy costs are less. The cooler water is less discouraging to bacterial growth, however, and special safeguards are required for low-temperature arrangements. In the Abbott system (Brown, 1982), level sensors in each of two large storage tanks commanded water from the still. Each storage tank was equipped with a hydrophobic vent filter, so placed as to avoid being wetted. All tank bottoms were sloped. Each of the storage tanks fed (by way of pumps) other, smaller tanks throughout the system. These secondary low-use-point tanks were isolated from the main tanks by air breaks and overflows to prevent back-siphoning. An absence of cross-connections prevented cross-contamination. Each tank was equipped with its own microbial-retentive vent filter.

The piping used throughout avoided threaded connections, utilizing only flanges and steam-resistant Viton or Teflon gaskets or welded joints. There were no dead-legs and all piping was sloped at least 1/16 or 1/18 inches per foot (0.15 to 0.31 cm per running 30 cm) to provide free and complete drainage. The overflows and steam traps were so piped as to promote drainage and avoid wetting of the vent filters. When tank overflow did occur, a divert valve closed the line to the vent filter and opened the drain. When the storage tanks were sterilized by steaming, the vent filters were also steamed. A downstream trap permitted drainage of the steam condensate.

All the instrumentation fitted to the system had sanitary connections and sensors. The heat exchangers were of a double-tube sheet type or the concentric double-pipe design. Maintenance of the system at room temperature made it necessary to drain it every 24 hours. Periodically, the entire arrangement was steamed at 121 °C for a 2-hour period. Thermocouples placed even in remote areas of the system ensured that this time/temperature regimen was met. During the steaming, all valves and drains were open to permit unimpeded passage of the steam and hot condensate, so that the entire system was steam sterilized.

Case F. According to Abshire (1982), the Alcon Laboratories of Fort Worth, TX, utilized a five-effect still to produce WFI. The source water to the still had previously been subjected to activated charcoal filtration followed by a two-bed deionizer using a strongly basic anion exchanger. The WFI was batched in each of two 4,500-gallon (17,635-liter) storage tanks, each representing a day's use, and each used alternately while the other was being filled. The stored WFI was maintained at about 70 °C while being circulated through a closed loop to 22 points of use. A heat exchanger cooled the water at formulation points of use. The WFI thus prepared was used as product water as well as for the final rinsing of surfaces (bottles, vials, and filling machines) that were to encounter product.

The WFI met the USP stipulations for that type of water. It was validated to exhibit a resistivity of not less than 150,000 megohm-cm; a total aerobic organism count of not more than 10 organisms/250 mL (as determined by three consecutive samples from the same site) using a membrane filtration procedure; a negative coliform count (determined at 20 use points and at the storage tanks); and negative LAL pyrogen tests.

The release criteria for the batched WFI was an absence of coliforms, a total aerobic count not to exceed 50 organisms/250 mL, and no more than 0.25 EU/mL of endotoxin. The aerobic organism counts were determined daily at each of two major use stations. In actuality, coliforms were never detected; and the total aerobic count, usually zero, never exceeded 3 in any sample of 250 mL. The suitability of the WFI thus prepared was amply demonstrated.

Case G. What was notable about the Astra WFI installation at Westborough, MA, was that it was *not* a batched system (Del Ciello, 1982). Distilled water from a Finn-Aqua model 3000-H-6 still was produced at a top capacity of 1,500 gph (5,678 Lph). It was discharged into a 10,000-gallon (37,850-liter) storage tank (at approximately 85 °C), provided that the water conductivity did not exceed a set maximum level. If the stipulated water conductivity was not attained, an alarm was sounded and the water was dumped to drain. The bottom of the tank was steam-jacketed to maintain the temperature of the contents. The storage tank was equipped with high- and low-level switches that governed the operation of the still.

Two recirculation loops and a once-through loop constituted the distribution system from the 10,000-gallon storage tank. Tests ensured the WFI quality of the stored water. The conducting tubing was of unpolished 316L stainless steel. Joint welding was by way of an automated tube welder, carefully supervised, each weld documented, sample welds retained, and a certain proportion examined by X-ray, all in accord with a strict protocol. All the pipe lines were sloped a minimum of 1/16 inches per foot (0.16 cm per 30 cm). There were no dead legs. Water movement was by means of Triclover pumps. Ultrasonic flowmeters were used. The glycerin-filled pressure gauges all had sanitary connections. The flanged connections utilized Viton gaskets, and were all of the standard sanitary type. The valves were of the diaphragm type, whether manual or automatic, utilizing either PTFE or Viton gaskets. Thermal wells were used to contain all thermocouples.

The flows of the two recirculating loops were balanced by means of restrictive orifices. As a safety consideration, the once-through loop provided cooled WFI, by means of an in-line heat exchanger, to areas of personnel contact. This nonrecirculating loop was flushed with hot WFI every several hours as a sanitizing procedure. One recirculation loop provided hot WFI for closure and glass washing. Excess water was recycled. The other recirculation loop supplied WFI to the solution preparation area. Plate-type heat exchangers, in-line, cooled the WFI to 10 °C upon demand. Each loop temperature and flowrate was monitored by thermocouples and ultrasonic flowmeters. Alarms signaled out-of-specification levels.

The Astra WFI system was rigorously validated as supplying WFI as designed prior to being brought on-stream officially, and continued to operate satisfactorily in accordance with its design and requirements.

Case H. The system in Case H used municipal water and included cation-exchanger carbon bed, twin-bed DI resins, mixed-bed DI resins, and distillation. The initial cation-exchange unit before the carbon bed was for the purpose of generating an acidic water, by substituting hydrogen ions in the exchange reaction to promote chlorine adsorption by the carbon. From the coke bed, the acidic water flowed through a twin-bed DI resin system that underwent appropriate regeneration with sodium hydroxide/hydrochloric acid after every passage of 25,000 gallons (94,625 liters) of water. The mixed bed was not regenerated, but was exchanged for a new mixed bed on a service basis.

The water was distilled by a 15-year-old Amsco still of great reliability. Its capacity of 20 gph (75 Lph) was used to furnish 200 gallons (750 liters) of product water per day. The product water was tested daily for organisms, pyrogens, and electrical resistivity. The latter value was usually around 2 megohm-cm. If its reading fell below 0.25 megohm-cm, the product water was dumped to drain.

Storage and distribution. The constant feed of WFI product water was stored in two 500-gallon (18,925-liter) linked tanks of passivated 316L stainless steel. The storage tanks were equipped with heated jackets that maintained their contents at 88 to 93 °C (190 to 200 °F). These tanks were supplied with vent filters in the form of 142-mm 0.2-μm-rated hydrophobic disk membranes. The vent filters were bubble-point tested before installation and upon their removal in accordance with their 3-month scheduled replacement cycle. The storage tanks were inspected and preventively sanitized during unscheduled shutdown intervals.

The water was circulated through the insulated, heated loop of 1 1/2-inch (3.79-cm) 316L stainless steel tubing, assembled by automated tungsten arc welding under argon gas. (Each weld was numbered and its complete inner circumference photographed.) The water was moved by a Reliance Motor Triclover pump. The insulated loop was equipped with sanitary fittings. Its interior surfaces were electropolished to remove the metal folding caused by prior 180-grit mechanical polishing. One-inch (2.54-cm) diameter 316L stainless steel drops terminated at points of use in silicone rubber hoses that were autoclaved nightly. The water, used hot at 88 to 90 °C (190 to 200 °F), was first tested by LAL assay.

Expansion. An increase in WFI production capacity was achieved by installation of a four-effect Stilmas-Milano still to yield 600 gpd (2,271 Lpd). The water thus produced was stored in a 2,000-gallon (7,570-liter) 316L stainless steel tank from Letch equipped with vent filters and a hot recirculation loop.

Ancillary equipment. Teflon-faced valves were seen as objectionable because Teflon takes a cold set; it manifests cold flow under pressure, thus relieving the pressure and the close dimensional fits that are desired concomitances. Stainless steel ball valves were preferred.

The air used was first filtered through sintered stainless steel filters at 8 psig (0.56 kg/cm^2), and then through 0.2-μm-rated membrane disks.

Strunck tunnel. The resin-deionized water was used for two purposes. For the first, it was converted into steam in a clean-steam generator in the first stage of the still, and was then condensed and redistilled in the successive stages of the still to emerge as distilled Water for Injection. The second purpose of the generated clean steam was to serve the autoclave, a Metromatic vial washer, and a Strunck washer. The latter was steam-sterilized in conjunction with a Strunck Tunnel that could process 300 ampuoles per minute, drawing on WFI to final-rinse the glassware before automatic depyrogenation at 320 °C.

The WFI was used in the final rinse. This water was then filtered, first through a 0.45-μm-rated membrane used as a prefilter and then through a 0.2-μm-rated membrane final filter for initial rinses.

Case I. The system in Case I used well water, and included twin DI beds, mixed bed, UV treatment, and a five-effect still. The well water, which contained a colloidal silica-iron complex, but to which no chlorine had been added, was filtered through a 5-μm-rated polypropylene prefilter with a replacement frequency of once per month. The emerging water was microbiologically monitored weekly using a Millipore Total Count Water Tester. The acceptable limit was 100 organisms (per milliliter). From the polypropylene prefilter, the water flowed through individual DI beds and then through a mixed DI bed. The deionizing resins were automatically regenerated every 8 to 9 days. The mixed bed was on a 24-hour-service exchange basis.

Ultraviolet treatment. The water from the DI beds flowed through a UV unit from which it usually emerged with an organism count of about 5/mL. The maximum acceptable level was 25 organisms/mL. Following the UV treatment, the water was passed through another 5-μm-rated polypropylene prefilter whose purpose was to serve as a resin-fines scavenger. Here the water was again tested for organisms, the acceptable upper limit being 10/mL. This polypropylene filter was changed once every 2 weeks. Microbiological testing was performed once per week.

In this section of the process, PVC piping was used, along with Valex centrifugal pumps equipped with Lincoln motors. Otherwise the piping was all 316L stainless joined by sanitary clamps. This portion of the system did not required sanitizing over the 18-month period of its existence. Were sanitation necessary, sodium hypochlorite solution, Haline, would have been used.

Multiple-effect still. Downstream from the resin-fines scavenging filter, the water entered a 40-gallon (150-liter) surge tank with a float. The tank served to supply the five-effect Finn-Aqua 300H_5 still that was used. The still had a maximum capacity of 115 gph (435 Lph) at 116 psig (7.7 bar) steam pressure. The surge tank was sanitized with sodium hypochlorite solution that was injected after the UV stage, then was pumped into the tank, and then discarded to the drain.

Storage and distribution. Clean steam from the still was used to sanitize the Water for Injection tank and the distribution loop, which was fitted with 5-μm-rated thick Teflon 293-mm filters.

The 1,000-gallon (3,785-liter) storage tank, made by the Letch Co., was composed of 316L stainless steel. It was lagged so that the heat of the water entering from the still was conserved. Although insulated, the tank was not heated. When the circulated water fell below 65 °C (149 °F), it was dumped. The tank was equipped with vent filters (20-inch, 0.2-μm-rated polyvinylidene fluoride cartridges). On the basis of microbiological monitoring, the tank was sterilized using steam for 1 hour. The vent cartridges were steamed in place for

30 minutes.

Filters were not utilized at points of use. The pipe nipples were sanitized with sodium hypochlorite solution and flushed before water was taken for microbial sampling. Anderson sanitary gauges were used throughout the system.

Case J. The system in Case J used municipal water, and included water softening, carbon bed, twin DI beds, mixed DI bed, vapor compression still, and batched Water for Injection. Water from a municipal source, itself dependent on a river, was utilized without additional chlorination. This water underwent a softening process and was then filtered through a carbon bed to remove the residual chlorine. The water then entered twin-bed deionizers, from which it flowed through a mixed DI resin bed.

Vapor compression stills and storage. The deionized water was used to feed two AquaChem vapor compression stills. The distilled water was batched and maintained at 80 °C throughout its circulating/distribution loop. A total of 66,000 gallons (250,000 liters) of Water for Injection was batched within three 316L stainless steel storage tanks. The stored water was tested for organisms and pyrogens with the customary battery of USP tests for Water for Injection.

The storage tanks were outfitted with PTFE vent cartridges, and sterilized with 15-psig (1-bar) steam flowed into them through these vent filters. The 80 °C water was used to perform hot water sanitizations, to provide final rinse water, and to supply Water for Injection for formulations after being cooled in a heat exchanger to about 40 °C.

Case K. The system in Case K used municipal water, and included a vapor compression still and batched Water for Injection. One parenteral plant, in an unusual setting, received municipal water derived principally from snow melts. The ionic content was so low, 2 ppm of sodium, for instance, that deionization by resins or RO was not practiced. The water was fed directly to a vapor compression still, and emerged to be batched in two 10,000-gallon (37,850-liter) 316L stainless steel storage tanks. It was kept circulating at temperatures between 60 to 80 °C. The water was analyzed for organisms, with zero said to be the usual level. A particle count and LAL testing for pyrogens were performed.

On the basis of the particle count test, and not by casual decision, the main circulating loop contained a filter designed to remove the particles that as a consequence of ordinary wear and tear on the system had become suspended in the batched Water for Injection. This loop filter was sterilized and integrity-tested when first installed.

The WFI storage tanks were equipped with microporous 0.2-μm-rated PTFE vent filters. These were integrity-tested upon installment, and replaced according to a regular maintenance schedule. Air was filtered through a 0.45-µm-rated mixed esters of cellulose membranes. Compressed air was dried by chilling to dew point of -30 °C, and and also filtered. Air filtration was at the points of use.

What was singular about this installation was the use of a filter in the circulation loop, a practice generally considered to be contravened by the once-proposed GMP for LVPs. This filter fulfilled its designed purpose of removing particulate matter from the Water for Injection. Its documented efficacy and established maintenance program served as its validation.

Case L. A manufacturer of deionized water intended for use in diagnostic analytical procedures produced 2,000 to 3,000 gallons (7,570 to 11,355 liters) per month for distribution in 1-gallon jugs. The water, of a low mineral content, originated in deep wells. It was chlorinated and led through a 1-µm-rated string-wound cartridge to remove suspended solids. Prior to undergoing resin deionization, the water was freed of chlorine by passage through an active carbon bed, which was replaced after every 60,000 gallons (227,000 liters) of water had passed. The dechlorinated water was subjected to the deionization action of a three-bed system composed of strongly acidic cation-exchange resin, strongly basic anion-exchange resin, and mixed resins, in that order. The resin beds, their impending exhaustion signaled by a warning light, were replaced on a service basis.

Exiting the DI resin beds, the water was filtered through a 0.2-µm-rated microporous membrane before being stored in a 2,000-gallon (7,570-liter) stainless steel tank. The product water underwent recirculation at the rate of 15 to 20 gpm (57 to 76 Lpm) during its storage, moved by an Eastern Industries cast-iron pump (brass wears very quickly). Sanitization of the system did not proved necessary.

The product water conformed to internal company standards of 10-megohm-cm resistivity and organism counts of fewer than 10 cfu/mL, the same as National Council Clinical Laboratory Standards (NCCLS). At bottling, the water was filtered through a presterilized 0.2-µm-rated disposable capsule filter, and was stabilized by the addition of sodium azide or thimerisoll (Merthiolate) preservatives in the jug.

Of note was the supplying and regeneration of deionization resin facilities on a service basis. This practice is more expensive, per volume of deionized water, than a central DI resin system, but offers advantages to small-volume users.

Case M. This was an older system utilizing chlorinated municipal water that was lead through a periodically backflushed coke bed, and then through twin DI resin beds involving a weakly basic anion exchanger. No mixed-bed operation was involved. The deionized water was tested at three periodic intervals each day. Its pH varied between 6 and 9, usually on the acidic side. Regeneration of the resin beds was performed upon evidence of chloride ion breakthrough, an occurrence usually after some 60,000 gallons (227,000 liters) of water had been processed, at the rate of approximately 20,000 to 25,000 gpd (76,000 to 95,000 Lpd). (An FDA letter specifically warned that bed regeneration was to be based on organism levels [Michels, 1981]).

The deionized water was fed to an AquaChem compression still. The distilled product water was batched at 85 °C in each of five 5,000-gallon (19,000-liter) 316L stainless steel tanks. The product water was tested for endotoxins, organisms, and heavy metal content.

The product water storage facility, lagged to preserve its heat but otherwise unheated, had no recirculation loop. It was a dead-end distribution system, drained every 24 hours. Before its contents were utilized, LAL endotoxin testing was performed at five different points. Any single failure would have called for a repeat of the LAL testing. Confirmation of a positive test would have resulted in a dumping of the water from that storage tank. (Such endotoxin failures were not experienced, however.) Before product water was drawn from the distribution pipe, a 5-minute flush was performed.

Case N. The high-purity water system designed for the Steris Laboratories in Phoenix, AZ, was described by Cutler and Nykanen (1988). It was proposed to deal with the Phoenix city water supply, but also to be able to accommodate Colorado River water, whose chief challenge would be high mineral content. The feedwater characteristics are shown in Table 12-4. Sodium could reach a level of 277 ppm; chlorides, 445 ppm; silica, 28 ppm; and TDS, 1,270 ppm. The hardness could attain 450 ppm (as $CaCO_3$); the alkalinity, 296 ppm (as $CaCO_3$); and sulfates, 151 ppm. The TOC level could reach 28 ppm; calcium, 117 ppm; and magnesium, 44 ppm. Barium was also present, to 0.08 ppm, and the presence of strontium was assumed.

The Steris water purification system is sketched in Figure 12-10. It involved water softening by duplex sodium cation exchangers. Brine regeneration of the resin was used. The softened feedwater downflowed through a multimedia filter whose backwash was sequenced automatically for off-peak intervals. The service flowrate was 28 gpm and was ensured by the use of a feedwater pressurization system composed of a 500-gallon surge tank and 316 stainless steel single-stage sanitary centrifugal pumps. Chlorine and TOC removal was obtained by use of an activated carbon bed. The shell was noncorrodible, permitting sanitization by steam. The carbon bed was also backwashed periodically to lessen its compaction and the attendant rise in the pressure drop, as well as to remove foulants. The service flowrate continued at 24 gpm.

At this point three additions of chemicals were made to the water. Iodine from a saturated aqueous solution of iodine was added for microbial control. Sodium hexametaphosphate was added as an antiscalant to prevent scale formation upon the RO membrane subsequently used. Finally, sulfuric acid was added to adjust the original feedwater pH of 8.4 to the level required for cellulose acetate. The RO service flowrate at this point was still 24 gpm.

Prefiltration for the RO operation was furnished by a 5-µm-rated (nominal) cartridge filter. The RO unit itself was a cellulose acetate membrane, multistaged and arranged for two-pass separation. Each pass yielded a 50% recovery to give an overall recovery of 75%; the 50% reject water from the second pass was recycled as water to be processed by the first RO unit. The RO product water was reduced in its TDS content by at least 90%. This minimized the ionic load on the downstream ion-exchange units and reduced the frequency of their regenerations. The carbon dioxide liberated from the feedwaters by their acidification permeated the cellulose acetate membrane, and was removed after the RO unit by way of a vacuum degasifier. The degasified water was passed through an UV sanitization unit into a RO permeate storage tank. The service flowrate was 14 gpm.

The permeate storage tank was a fiberglass-fabricated tank of 11,500-gallon capacity. The stored water was used for bed backwashing, for regeneration and rinsing of the deionizers, and as feedwater for the downstream ion-exchange units. The stored water was continuously recirculated through the deionizer by way of an UV light sanitization unit to maintain microbial control. The storage tank was vented using a HEPA filter.

Deionization following purification by RO was accomplished by use of dual downflow mixed beds containing strongly acidic and strongly basic resins. A single-stage 316 stainless steel sanitary centrifugal pump continuously recirculated deionized water through a UV unit and back to the DI bed whenever the deionizer was off-line. The deionized water, used to feed the distillation facility, had a resistivity of 10 to 12 megohm-cm. When not flowing to the stills, the

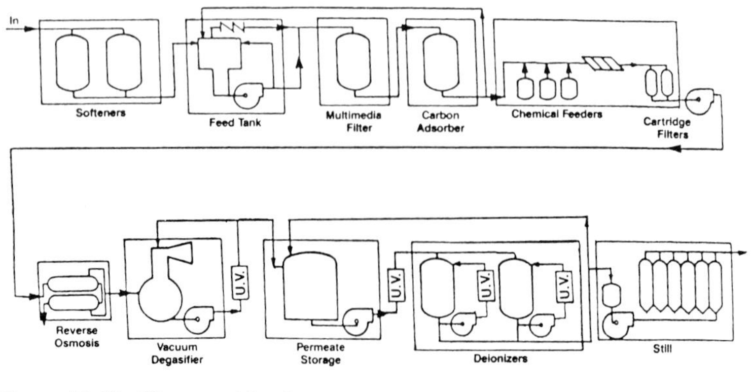

Figure 12-10. Water purification system.
Cutler and Nykanen, (1988); Courtesy, *Pharmaceutical Engineering*

deionized water recirculated to the permeate storage tank to maintain a constant flow through the ion-exchange beds. The service flowrate could be 30 gpm. Daily, automated regeneration of the beds was practiced. Hydrochloric acid and sodium hydroxide were used, stored in polyethylene tanks and introduced by metering pumps. The waste solutions were fed to a limestone-neutralization tank prior to release to the city sewer system.

The distillation system was a Stilmas six-effect unit composed of 316L electropolished stainless steel. It could produce 1,000 gph of WFI quality having a resistivity of at least 2 megohm-cm. The blowdown rate to waste was less than 10%. The distilled water was directed to the hot distilled water storage and distribution, or to batched WFI storage and distribution. The hot distilled water was used for rinsing; although repeatedly tested to hold it to WFI standards, it was not used in formulations. The batched WFI was used for that purpose.

Cutler and Nykanen (1988) described in detail the design of the Steris hot water storage and distribution system:

The hot, deionized water (HDW) is stored in a 12,500-gallon alloy 316L

Table 12-4
Water Supply Characteristics

Water Quality Parameter	*Design Concentrations (mg/L)*		
	Min.	*Avg.*	*Max.*
Arsenic (As)	< 0.001		0.01
Barium (Ba)	<0.01		0.08
Calcium (Ca)	18	42	117
Chromium (Cr)	<0.001		0.047
Copper (Cu)	<0.01		0.07
Iron (Fe)	<0.01	0.01	0.08
Lead (Pb)	<0.001		0.002
Magnesium (Mg)	6	21	44
Potassium (K)	1.8	2.7	5.1
Silver (Ag)	<0.001		0.008
Sodium (Na)	14	59	277
Strontium (Sr)		Unknown	
Zinc (Zn)	<0.01		0.19
Chlorides (Cl)	7	96	445
Fluorides (F)	0.21	0.32	0.87
Nitrates (NO_3)	<0.01	7.3	53
Silica (SiO_2)	3.9	13	28
Sulfate (SO_4)	8	53	151
TOC (C)	1	7	28
TDS	141	400	1,270
Chlorine (Cl_2)		Variable	
Alkalinity (as $CaCO_3$)	82	120	296
Hardness (as $CaCO_3$)	72	191	450
Temperature range (°F)	67	78	89
pH range	7.4	7.9	8.4

Cutler and Nykanen (1988); Courtesy, *Pharmaceutical Engineering* stainless steel tank supplied by Mueller. This vessel is pressure rated at 50 psig, full-vacuum rated, of horizontal design with a sloping bottom to ensure drainability, dual jacketed, insulated, and sanitary fitted, including a sterile vent filter. The dual jackets allow for both steam heating and chilled water to maintain desired storage temperatures. Generally, due to the tendency of the system to gain heat from mechanical heat generated by the recirculating pumping system, chilled water cooling is routinely required to prevent the HDW water from reaching the boiling point. This system has been validated at a storage and recirculation temperature of 60 °C and will be routinely operated at between 65-70 °C. The tank includes instrumentation for the continuous measurement and routine recording of temperature, water level and pressure differential across the sterile vent filter. The 0.2 micrometer sterile vent filter is also steam jacketed to prevent condensation of water vapor within the filter element. The tank is designed for pure steam sanitization and is equipped with a discharge to drain system using an automatic cold water mixing device to prevent high temperature damage to the process of wastewater system. [See Figure 12-11].

Duplex HDW alloy 316L stainless steel, single stage sanitary, centrifugal pumps were installed to maintain recirculation in the HDW storage tank and the supply loop providing HDW water to various use points throughout the plant. These Triclover pumps were supplied by Ladish and are WFI-type units fitted with Chesterton Model 241 double mechanical seals with carbon-tungsten carbide seal faces and are flushed with HDW water. Pump casings are drainable through sanitary diaphragm valves and are installed with a discharge angle of 45 degrees from the vertical to assure that all air is displaced from the pump casings. A full tank of HDW water is recirculated at least once each hour to ensure dynamic control of stratification and the potential for biological instability due to inadequate temperature within the storage system. In normal operation, one of the pumps is run, with the second on stand-by status. A ported check valve is installed at the discharge of each pump which allows a 7 gpm flow of HDW back through the stand-by pump to prevent a deadleg. To minimize pressure drop in the pump suction lines, which could allow the HDW water to boil and/or create cavitation at the pump inlets, large diameter (6-inch) 316L turbine was used with specially modified eccentric reducers to adapt the available 6-inch pipe-size valves.

The WFI was stored in two 1,500-gallon 316L stainless steel tanks of the same construction just described. As the contents from one tank were being used, the other tank was being filled. The water volume in the tanks was recirculated at least four times per hour. Sufficiently sized single-stage centrifugal pumps were used, of the construction described by Cutler and Nykanen (1988). As with the HDW system, the WFI piping and pumps were completely drainable and were free of dead legs. Back pressure was maintained by the use of ported spray bars installed at the return to each tank. The tank contents were used alternately. Since water quality was maintained under storage conditions, the contents of each or of both tanks were available for use at any time and over any interval.

Water For Injection distribution was managed by diverting the flow from the recirculation pump into the distribution header wherein it was cooled by a chilled-water heat exchanger. Since the WFI distribution, as distinct from its storage and recirculation system, was not maintained in circulation at high temperature, it was steam-sanitized daily from the water cooler to each use point. Monitoring and control of the WFI storage distribution systems were carefully performed and documented.

The Steris facility utilized header and pipe diameters designed to maintain recirculation flows and pressures at all major use points. Thus a 4-inch supply header was selected to furnish a total flow requirement of 383 gpm, allowing for peak demand. The corresponding water velocity in the supply header was a maximum of 10 feet per second. The maximum velocity in the return header was 4 feet per second. The supply header was a 4-inch-diameter pipe, and the return header had a diameter of 3 inches.

Case O. At a New England facility, municipally treated water is led through a succession of three sand beds in series to each of two parallel treatment lines. In each line there is a multimedia bed, followed by an activated carbon bed, succeeded by a cation-exchange column preceding an anion-exchanger. This is followed by a filter whose purpose is to retain resin fines. Upon emerging from this pretreatment train, the water is led through an ultraviolet zone before being

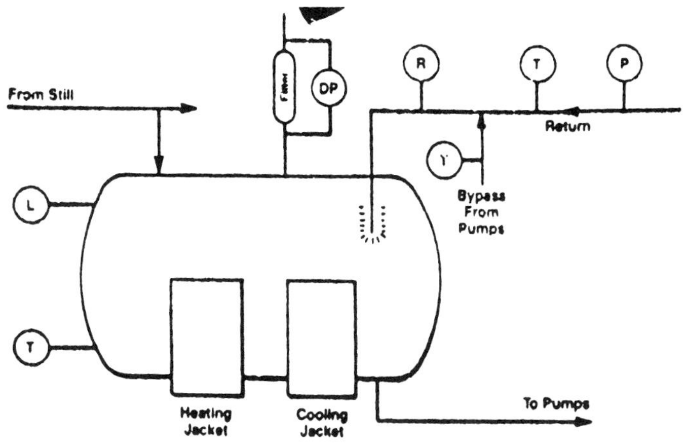

Figure 12-11. Distilled water storage system.

fed to a vapor compression still, from whence it enters a 2,000-gallon storage tank to be held under recirculation at 85 °C.

The WFI in the heated storage tank is circulated through a heat exchanger where it is cooled to 40 °C. The water in this portion of the tempered loop is available for withdrawal at the points of use. The water still circulating in that loop is then reheated in a heat exchanger to 85 °C before it reenters the storage tank on its recirculatory journey.

Plant steam furnishes heat to the appropriate heat exchanger, and also supplies heat to the vapor compression still, and to the clean-steam generator. The WFI from the hot storage tank is also utilized in feeding the clean-steam generator.

Case P. One interesting water purification system is used in conjunction with the preparation of pharmaceutical solids. Its pretreatment section is older, and consists largely of PVC piping and a PVC storage tank for RO permeate. Incoming municipally treated water is led to a water softener by way of a 10-μm depth filter. Following the water softening, the water is dechlorinated using an activated carbon bed. It is then pumped through a polyamide RO unit. The permeate is stored in a PVC tank of 500-L capacity, equipped with a vent filter.

Attached to the RO storage tank is a new section of the water purification system consisting of a stainless steel polishing loop. The loop contains a mixed ion-exchange bed, which may be isolated by being bypassed. The water enters the DI bed through a 0.45-μm-rated cartridge filter, and exits through a 0.2-μm-rated cartridge filter. Water is withdrawn from this polishing loop to be stored in a 1,000 L stainless steel tank outfitted with a vent filter. The stored water is withdrawn by pumps to pass through a heat exchanger that brings it to 38 °C. The heated water is passed through parallel arrangements of 0.2-μm-rated membrane cartridges into two courses of pipe from each of which six points of use depend. The pipe continues in loop fashion, returning to the 1,000-L storage tank. All the piping of this newer section of this system is of stainless steel.

The latter part of the system, with the exception of the mixed bed, is periodically sanitized using water at 85 °C for a period of 4 hours.■

CHAPTER 13

VALIDATION OF THE PHARMACEUTICAL WATER SYSTEM*

Definition of Validation

The validation of water systems for pharmaceutical applications encompasses system design qualifications, and attention to the regulatory requirements and the necessary documentation thereof. Among the system design considerations are the decision points for choosing among alternative purification units and their proper operations. These considerations include materials of construction, system sanitizations, and clearing of foulants. The engineering requirements for water volume and flow balancing include definitions of pumps and pipe sizes. There are also documentary, microbiological, regulatory, and unit process operational considerations relating to the validation issue.

This chapter levels itself to the nonengineering aspects of water system validation. It describes the validation exercise in terms of what is required to demonstrate, by documented experimental effort, the confirmation of the purported actions of the individual water purification units constituting pharmaceutical water systems. In keeping with the concept of process validation, the validation of each unit operation of a water system will, in sum, establish the validation of the total system.

The validation exercise, however, is infinitely more than the demonstration that each individual purification unit performs as designed and intended. The intention of the validation effort is to establish that the system as a whole functions consistently, when operated in accordance with the standard operating procedures (SOPs) defined for that purpose, to produce water of the quality required for the given pharmaceutical application. The adequacy of the relevant SOPs is supported by documented data that the system does consistently produce water of the specified quality. Consistency becomes validated over so long a span of time as to encompass seasonal feedwater changes; and as to define the

*This chapter intends a stand-alone presentation of the validation requirements. Some repetition of previous sections is, therefore, necessitated for an unbroken flow of logic.

renewals, refurbishings, and replacements necessary to ensure prolonged system operations.

Validation

There are many different definitions of validation. An FDA definition enunciated in 1987 stated: "Validation is the attaining and documenting of sufficient evidence to give reasonable assurance, given the current state of science, that the process under consideration does, and/or will do, what it purports to do."

A less eloquent but very serviceable definition was given in the FDA Guidelines on Sterile Drug Products by Aseptic Processing (June 1987): "Establishing documented evidence which provides a high degree of assurance that a specific process will consistently produce a product meeting its predetermined specifications and quality attributes."

In essence, validation seeks answers to two questions. Does the process or device do what it is intended to do? If so, for how long does it do it? As regards water systems, Artiss (1986) defined validation as ensuring that the particular system will consistently produce water of predictable quality when operated in the prescribed manner.

The FDA requires validation of each of the manufacturing processes whereby drugs or drug components are prepared. Each step or piece of equipment utilized in the process must be demonstrated and documented to be performing the function that it is purported to do. As a consequence of such demonstrated suitability, the entire process (the total assemblage of each proven component and operation) will, by inexorable logic, have ensured its ability to fulfill its intended function. In the case of a water system, frequent testing before and after each purification stage will attest to its purported operation. The test frequency will be such as to span time durations wherein expected variations can occur. Thus, there will be revealed whether each purification unit operates properly, unaffected by the variations that may occur over time. Such intense and frequent testing will serve to validate each unit and ultimately the entire process as operating dependably and consistently.

Process Validation

The FDA wished to place dependency upon process validation. This is an exercise wherein the proper performance of each stage in a chain of manipulations and/or devices serves to ensure the logical and desired outcome of the entire operation. Analyses serve only, though importantly, to confirm the continuing appropriateness of the validation. Process validation is therefore said to be "building quality in," as distinct from a sole reliance on end-product testing analysis. The latter could be said to serve as a procedure of culling the good from the bad as produced by the same process. What is desired is an assurance that the process produces only the "good."

The FDA is correct in its insistence upon process validation. It requires, as has been said, that the process consistently and reliably produce only acceptable product, in contrast to a reliance upon analysis to differentiate between "good" and "bad." Since analyses are relied upon in either instances, in both the validation and in assessing the product, it may be asked why analysis can be depended upon in one case but not in the other. A subtlety is involved here. It arises from the nature of the hypothetical proposition in scientific logic: If A, then B. Confirming the antecedent A confirms the consequence B. However, confirming the consequence B does not confirm the antecedent A. If the process, A, is valid, then the product water, B, will be suitable. But finding through analysis that B, the product, is acceptable does not establish that the process is validly dependable. In this instance B may be confirmed for some reason other than A. Therefore, analysis of the product water alone cannot be used to establish the validity of the process in producing only acceptable product. Process validation itself is required.

The FDA requires, as has been said, validation of each of the manufacturing processes whereby drugs or drug components are prepared. Each step or piece of equipment utilized in the process must be demonstrated and documented to be performing the function that it is supposed to do.

Another View of Validation

Consider the undertaking by a pharmaceutical company to plan, construct, equip, and operate a compendial water manufacturing facility. Having been given the assignment to do so, the individuals and groups responsible would be expected by management to report periodically on the progress being made and on the status of the undertaking.

Declaratory statements in the periodic reports would be illustrated and confirmed by relevant data obtained using reliable, and hence calibrated, instruments. The system design necessary consistently to produce water of the required quality in sufficient peak and total quantities would be decided upon. The correct constructions and dependable functioning of installed units would be checked and substantiated. Proof would be offered that the system designs, their constructions, and their safe operations were on target. Pertinent documents relating to safety, drawings and descriptions of equipment, operational protocols, and sampling and testing procedures would all be collected and retained.

The reports and documented presentations would be intended to demonstrate to management by way of data that the assignment was being carried out correctly. Ultimately, the successful completion of the task would be attested to in a final report. The claims of an operationally functional water purification system, dependable over long durations, would be supported by an adequacy of appropriate data and documentation. Consistency in the stipulated quality of the product water over prolonged periods of time would be the proof of the attained

eliminated or becomes tolerable. For example, the presence of certain types of total organic carbon in the feedwaters may serve prematurely to foul an RO purification unit. The use of an activated carbon bed in a pretreatment mode to remove all or some of the TOC by absorption can prolong the life of the RO to an extent that is operationally practical. It bears notice that the definition of what is "practical" in water purification contexts has an economic component. Water purification exercises are not simply technical practices; they are technico-economic undertakings.

The practice of pretreatments is an essential part of the pharmaceutical water purification operation, particularly so when the composition of the source water is so sufficiently variable over short-term intervals as to threaten periodically to overwhelm the principal purification unit. In such cases, outsized pretreatment units may be necessitated. The proper matching of pretreatment arrangements to whatever principal purification operations are employed (e.g., ion exchange, reverse osmosis, distillation) becomes defined in establishing the standard operating procedure for the water purification system.

Since the pretreatment unit operations may greatly influence the principal purification results, they require being validated along with the principal units.

Specific impurities: *Total suspended solids*. It is necessary to reduce or remove suspended and colloidal matter from the feedwaters entering any of the principal purification units. Ion-exchange beds, in addition to their demineralizing functions, serve as deep-bed filters. They are composed of a packed volume and depth of resin beads, generally between 16 and 50 mesh size, although the range of 20 to 40 mesh is often preferred. They accumulate particulate matter within their interstices precisely in the manner of deep-bed filters. The accumulated particulate material, the suspended matter present in the feedwater, causes elevated pressure differentials within the ion-exchange beds. This occurrence slows the flow of water, may foul macroreticulated resin beads, and may otherwise offer spatial interferences that will detract from the intended ion-exchange function.

In the case of reverse osmosis operations, suspended matter will foul by blockage areas of the RO membrane, effectively removing the affected area from useful contributions. Unlike the ion-exchange beds, reverse osmosis devices will retain colloids, further interfering with the RO ion-removal function.

The accumulation of suspended matter in the still-pot of distillers interferes with the designed heat-transfer effects and increases the likelihood of particle entrainment in the vapor. It is this very occurrence that is the object of the blowdowns, largely automatic, that are part of still operations.

To forestall the fouling occasioned by suspended matter, such materials are removed by the use of sand filters and/or multimedia deep-bed filters in a pretreatment step. Colloid removal is accomplished by the use of coagulation and flocculation, usually by the addition of alum or polyelectrolyte. (Such treatment is usually standard in potable water preparations.)

The colloidal content and nature of a water should be known, particularly if the water will be fed to an RO unit and especially if hollow-fiber RO units with their more easily blocked small bores are involved. The silt density index test, however fallible, provides such information. Feedwaters exhibiting SDIs in excess of values of 5 for spiral-wound ROs and of 3 or less for hollow-fiber units require coagulation and flocculation pretreatment.

Scale-forming elements. In Tables 13-2 and 13-3, analyses are cited for parameters such as pH, calcium, magnesium, alkalinity, sulfate, and silica. These are entities that in certain concentrations and combinations will produce precipitates and deposits that will interfere with distillation and RO unit operations.

A chief concern is the hardness elements. Calcium ions combine with sulfate ions to form insoluble calcium sulfate deposits. The avoidance of such scale formation is particularly to be sought in RO operations. Calcium carbonate can also be deposited as interfering scale, and its formation from soluble calcium bicarbonate is a consequence of a shift in the pH of the water to the alkaline side. The Langelier Solubility Index provides a measure of a water's tendency to form calcium carbonate scale, and indicates the pH adjustment towards the acidic necessary to avoid such formation (Nalco, 1988).

Because the precipitation of salts of leveled solubility reflects the solubility products of such entities, the concentrations of the relevant ions should be made known through analyses. The total dissolved solids content of a feedwater should, therefore, be quantitated.

Table 13-2
City Water Analysis
Sanger, CA

Calcium	32.5 mg/L as $CaCO_3$
Magnesium	79.1 mg/L as $CaCO_3$
Sodium	58.7 mg/L as $CaCO_3$
Potassium	5.1 mg/L as $CaCO_3$
Alkalinity	111.0 mg/L as $CaCO_3$
Sulfate	25.9 mg/L as $CaCO_3$
Chloride	38.5 mg/L as $CaCO_3$
TDS	175.4 mg/L as $CaCO_3$
Conductivity	334.0 mg/L as $CaCO_3$
Silica	31.7 mg/L as SiO_2
pH	7.4
Carbon dioxide	8.0 mg/L as CO_2

Comb and Fulford (1991); Courtesy, Ultrapure Water Expo '91 East

Table 13-3
Design Spec and Contaminant Characterization Procedures

Charcterization Parameter	*Specification*	*Limit*	*Analytical Procedures*
Resistivity	18.0 mΩ-cm		Thornton
Dissolved oxygen	< 75.0 ppb		Orbisphere
Bacteria	< 1 cfu/100mL		ASTM F60-68
SEM bacteria	8/L	8 ± 10	SEM
TOC	<10 ppb	10 ppb	Anatel A100
Silicon	< 5 ppb	5 ppb	Hach, Colormetric (molybdosilicate)
Chloride	< 0.2 ppb	0.5 ppb	Ion chromatography
Sodium	< 0.2 ppb	0.2 ppb	ICP/MS
Calcium	< 1 ppb	1.0 ppb	ICP/MS
Potassium	< 3.0 ppb	3.0 ppb	ICP/MS
Lithium	< 1 ppb	1.0 ppb	ICP/MS
Nitrate/nitrite	< 0.1 ppb	0.5 ppb	Ion chromatography
Sulfate	< 0.3 ppb	0.3 ppb	Ion chromatography
Phosphate	< 0.2 ppb	0.5 ppb	Ion chromatography
Iron	< 0.1 ppb	1.0 ppb	ICP/MS
Copper	< 0.1 ppb	0.1 ppb	ICP/MS
Aluminum	< 0.5 ppb	0.5 ppb	ICP/MS
Nickel	< 0.1 ppb	1.0 ppb	ICP/MS
Chromium	< 0.1 ppb	0.1 ppb	ICP/MS
Zinc	< 1 ppb	1.0 ppb	ICP/MS
Magnesium	< 0.5 ppb	0.5 ppb	ICP/MS
Lead	< 1 ppb	1.0 ppb	ICP/MS
Particles:			
5.0 μm	< 1/L	0 ± 120	Particle Monitoring Systems (PMS) laser-based particle counter
2.0 μm	< 1/L	0 ± 120	Particle Monitoring Systems (PMS) laser-based particle counter
.5 μm	< 1/L	0 ± 120	SEM
.2 μm	< 1/L	0 ± 120	SEM
>.1 μm	< 10/L	10 ± 117	SEM
Temperature	70° F		Temperature probe
Pressure	55 psig		Pressure gauge

Martyak et al. (1991 A and B); Courtesy, *Microcontamination*

The formation of scale and deposits of other compositions is also possible; calcium fluoride, voluminous magnesium hydroxide, and silica deposits are among them. Appropriate pH management, and the use of antiscalants, some promotive of calcium sulfate supersaturation, can be effective in preventing scale. The subject of fouling of reverse osmosis membranes, as by scale formation, is discussed in Chapter 9.

The most effective way of avoiding scale formation caused by the bivalent alkaline earth elements that represent permanent water hardness, and the bicarbonate ion that defines temporary hardness, is to rely upon a water-softening operation. Usually, ion-exchange resins in their sodium form are utilized to remove calcium, magnesium, barium, and strontium. The latter two elements, if not removed in the water-softening pretreatment, can so irrevocably combine with cation-exchange resins as to impair, by defying regeneration, the capacity of these resins. Alternatively, the deposition of insoluble barium sulfate scale and, to a somewhat lesser extent, strontium sulfate upon an RO membrane will prove recalcitrant in the extreme to removal. Therefore, barium and strontium should be analyzed for, and if present their removal in the water-softening step should be affirmed.

Water softening will also serve to remove soluble iron and manganese. These elements are commonly removed in a separate pretreatment step involving their oxidation, whether by chlorine or greensand zeolite, followed by the filtrative removal of the insoluble oxidized product, usually by deep sand beds or by multimedia deep beds. Where smaller quantities of iron and/or manganese are involved, their removal by way of cation-exchange resins may be more economical.

The temporary water hardness caused by bicarbonate ions is eliminated by the addition of acid to lower the pHs below 4.4. This converts the bicarbonate to water and carbon dioxide, the latter being removed from the system by way of a degasification or decarbonation unit. Such acidification becomes necessary when RO units are composed of cellulose acetate, in order to minimize the hydrolysis of that polymer. Bicarbonate ions are also eliminated as such by being rejected by polyamide RO units at pHs above 8 or 8.5. Care must, however, be taken not to expose the polyamide RO to the ruinous effects of chlorine.

The alkalinity of a water is described as the sum of its titratable bases. It is a measure chiefly of the bicarbonate, carbonate, and hydroxide ions present (there being a pH-dependent equilibrium among carbon dioxide, bicarbonate, and carbonate). The strength of the bicarbonate concentration can be measured by titrating a water with acid to bring it to a methyl orange end point of approximately 4.4.

Soluble silica can be removed from the waters being purified by the use of strongly basic ion exchange or by rejection in the RO operation. Soluble silica should not be permitted to enter stills, although in certain successful water purification operations it is actually permitted to do so. Curiously, soluble silica is not removed in any pretreatment step. None has been designed for that purpose, unless strongly basic cation exchange is considered.

TOC. In formal terms, TOC means *total organic carbon*. As such it is a misnomer. At most, it signifies total *oxidizable* carbon as defined by an automated TOC analyzer. There are several such TOC instruments, each with different oxidizing capabilities. The definition of TOC may vary among them since organic compounds have each their own susceptibility to oxidation, and very little is known about the TOC constituents of any water. The readings of the various TOC instruments will be standardized by the use of reference compounds (WQC/PMA, 1993c). These present developments are an improvement over the USP's traditional "Oxidizable Substances Test," an analysis noteworthy for its insensitivity (see page 27).

There is no universal way of removing TOC from waters; it depends upon the specific nature of the organics involved. Some organic compounds cannot be removed with an assured efficiency. Largely, adsorption of TOC to activated carbon granules is relied upon. The flowrates involved in such an exercise are low, about 1 gpm/ft^3 of carbon. By contrast, the removal of chlorine by activated carbon is possible at double or triple these flowrates. The adsorptive process for organics is slow. Organics, with some notable low-molecular-weight exceptions such as phenols, acetic acid, and alcohols, are rejected by RO membranes. Ultrafiltration can also be used to retain organic compounds. Some still designs incorporate the means oxidatively to destroy organic materials in the still pots.

Ion-exchange resins are also relied upon to remove TOC. Organic molecules containing carboxylic acid moieties, usually the consequences of oxidative alterations, can be removed by anion exchange. Advantage can be taken of this fact to subject the TOC to oxidation by ozone, ultraviolet light, or hydrogen peroxide, or by various combinations of these agencies. The resulting oxidized TOC, bearing carboxylic acid groups that normally characterize one stage of the TOC oxidative degradation chain, is then amenable to removal by anion exchange. The trihalomethanes that are themselves the end products of organic matter oxidized by chlorine are exceedingly difficult to remove from water by any means; especially so chloroform. Adsorption to activated carbon has only an indifferent success. Loosely mirroring an increase in molecular size, TOC can increasingly be removed by adsorption to ion-exchange resin beads because of the large surface areas these present. The danger is, however, that the beads may become excessively fouled thereby, compromising their intended function of ion-exchange. Therefore, sacrificial resin beds are sometimes used in a pretreatment mode to achieve TOC removal.

Microorganisms are perhaps the most insidious of the impurities present in source waters. Other impurities, once removed, remain removed; but organisms, even when removed to the state of sterility, can reinvade the water and multiply to significant populations. Organisms and their derivative pyrogenic lipopolysaccharides, the bacterial endotoxins, require levelation in their concentrations in waters intended for parenteral pharmaceutical applications.

Once freed of microorganisms to the specified acceptable degree, the pharmaceutical water, whether Purified Water or Water for Injection, needs to be so maintained during its storage and transfer, to the same degree of microbiological and bacterial endotoxin purity.

Ionic constituents. The chemical impurities whose presence and quantitation are the subjects of source water analyses are almost all ionic in nature. Calcium, magnesium, barium, strontium, sodium, and potassium are all present as cations. The pH measurement reveals the concentration of the hydrogen ion (more properly, hydronium ion), also cationic; or, at its higher values, of the hydroxyl anion. Sulfate, nitrate, and chloride are anions. Carbon dioxide, the acid-anhydride of carbonic acid, relates to the existence of bicarbonate or carbonate ions. These latter two anions, along with the hydroxyl ions, also anionic, constitute the water alkalinity. Ammonia is the basic-anhydride of ammonium hydroxide. Added to water, it yields hydroxyl ions through the feeble dissociation of ammonium hydroxide into ammonium cations and hydroxyl anions.

Ion-exchange practices and/or reverse osmosis processes are the principal purification methods relied upon to remove these ionic impurities. Distillation is the other well-established purification method commonly used for this purpose. (Certain electrically motivated techniques may also be used to effect deionizations or demineralizations. Their use, although small, is on the increase. Chief among these is an electrodeionization process called *Continuous Deionization* by its manufacturer.) However, distillation does not suffice for the removal of carbon dioxide or of other volatile impurities having significant water solubilities and which, in consequence, may remain to some degree in the condensed distillate.

System Design Considerations

The purification unit processes. As the concept of process validation has it, if each unit process of a water purification system is demonstrated and documented to be operating as designed and expected, then the sum of those units processes, the total system, must, of necessity, be dependable in its production of the water quality proper for its intended purpose.

The design of water systems being quite site-specific, it is difficult to generalize concerning the unit process components of a "typical" system. Broadly speaking, however, pharmaceutical water purification arrangements could generally involve the following:

- A chlorination unit to supply the means of controlling the organism content of the feedwater.
- A sand or multimedia bed to remove suspended solids down to 10 to 40 μm in size.
- A water softener to remove scale-forming ions. These are principally the divalent cations that can yield insoluble sulfate, carbonate, hydroxide, or fluoride salts whose preemption of ion-exchange sites, whose blockage of RO or other membrane areas, or whose scaling of stills would interfere with water purification activities. Where the alkalinity content of the water would so indicate, the presence of bicarbonate would have to be taken into account, lest its generation of carbon dioxide unfavorably influence the pH of the product water.
- An activated carbon bed to remove chlorine and TOC. The presence of TOC in the water could result in the choice of anion-exchange resin traps to remove it. Otherwise the water could be flowed directly into activated carbon beds for the same purpose, but more especially to remove the chlorine that had previously been added. The chlorine could also be removed by the addition of chemical reducing agents.

  The removal of volatile TOCs, and particularly of the trihalomethanes, could well depend upon the use of vacuum degasifiers.
- The above pretreatment steps having been accomplished, some principal means for deionizing the water would next be selected. This would call for the use of ion exchange, of reverse osmosis, or of combinations of the two. Where RO is used, it should be in the two-pass product-staged mode. Particularly in parenteral water manufacturing contexts, distillation is usually the principal purification unit process used.

A decision to use RO would involve a selection of the membrane type. The use of cellulose acetate RO, often selected in pharmaceutical contexts, would entail acidification to about pH 5.5 to 6 and, where bicarbonate is present, carbon dioxide removal. This would involve the employment of degasification equipment.

- In addition to the above, a number of accouterments could be utilized, such as ozone, ultraviolet units, filters of various sorts and ratings, and chemical additions of antiscalants or of the acids or alkalies necessary to pH adjustments.

Chlorination. Because organisms, particularly the Gram-negative varieties native to aqueous habitats, can proliferate in water, their control is sought early on. Municipally treated waters generally arrive chlorinated, or containing a given concentration of some biostat, generally chloramine. Otherwise, the source water is chlorinated as soon as it is acquired by the pharmaceutical plant. Usually, the chlorine content of the feedwater is adjusted to a residual of 0.5 to 2 ppm. On occasion, higher concentrations are used, such as 2 to 6 ppm when there is concern regarding *Legionella pneumophila* (Muraca et al., 1990). Whatever chlorine level is selected, its concentration is maintained at that level to compensate for the quantity expended on chlorine-oxidizable substances present in the water. Where sand beds are employed to remove suspended matter, they are often periodically sanitized by being subjected to the "superchlorination" of 5 to 10 ppm of chlorine for from 1.5 to 20 minutes.

The purpose for introducing chlorine into the water may be to eliminate live organisms completely, or to regulate them to a particular count. It is important to define with some exactness the goal intended to be achieved by the chlorination, as that objective has significance in the operational qualification step of the validation process.

The protective chlorine umbrella is maintained over the water for as long as possible as it is being processed; usually through the water-softening pretreatment. Eventually, however, the chlorine must be removed lest its oxidizing action cause harm to certain of the water purification units downstream. Polyamide RO membranes are ruinously susceptible to chlorine; stainless steel stills are corroded thereby, and even by the chloride ion that is a product of chlorine in water, as shown in Equation 13-1:

$$Cl_2 + H_2O \longrightarrow HOCl + H^+ + Cl^- \qquad \text{Eq. 13-1}$$

Ion-exchange resins are also oxidatively degraded by chlorine. They suffer a loss of capacity and generate TOC (Hoffman et al., 1987). Nevertheless, it is not unusual for the chlorine to be removed by permitting it entry into the ion-exchange beds. Whether this action is wise or not depends upon how much TOC generation and how much ion-exchange degradation is tolerable. If the ion-exchange unit has a polishing function, chlorine should not be allowed to contact the resin, as the negative consequences of the resin degradations would be excessive.

Chlorine removal is normally accomplished by its adsorption to and reaction with activated carbon. Carbon beds have been used successfully for this purpose for almost 30 years in at least one pharmaceutical company. However, the proper maintenance of carbon beds is often seen to be onerous. Moreover, all too commonly, the carbon bed construction, usually in the interests of economy, does not permit its sanitization by hot water or steam. The result is that the carbon bed can then serve as a focal point of organism contamination. Chlorine is, therefore, in some 30% of all instances, removed by chemical injection, usually of sodium bisulfite or metabisulfite, into the water. The chlorine undergoes destruction, its oxidizing power neutralized by reaction with the reducing agent.

Chloride ions are a product of this chemical reaction. Their subsequent removal is necessitated.

Ozone is a more efficient biocide than is chlorine. It is more rapid in its killing action and is more effective against a wider variety of microbes, including viruses. Its action against *E. coli* is 3,125 times as rapid as that of chlorine (Meltzer and Rice, 1987). Indeed, no microorganisms seem immune to its -cidal effects.

Additionally, ozone offers the tremendous advantage of being removable in seconds by the destructive action of 254-nm ultraviolet radiation. Unlike the removal of chlorine, the elimination of ozone requires no difficult-to-maintain carbon beds, chemical injections, or prolonged effort. In quantitative terms, 90,000 microrads/cm^2/sec of UV light energy are required to eliminate completely 1 ppm of ozone. An ample dosage of UV radiation for ozone destruction can be supplied to waters moving at 40% the velocity used when the germicidal effects of ultraviolet light is sought. For example, if a flowrate of 60 gpm is set to achieve germicidal effects, then a flowrate of 24 gpm should be used to attain ozone destruction. Ozone concentrations of less than 1 ppm can be removed at even higher flowrates.

Different concentrations of ozone over different contact times are variously used to eliminate viruses, spores, and bacteria. Residual ozone levels of 0.4 mg/L have been maintained for 8 to 12 minutes for the primary disinfection of potable water supplies; 0.2 to 0.5 mg/L concentrations have been relied upon over a 10-minute contact time where spore populations are involved; and 0.01 to 1.0 mg/L amounts of ozone have been employed over 5-minute durations for the destruction of counts of 106 to 107 cfu/mL of vegetative organisms (Meltzer, 1993).

Ultraviolet radiation. Ultraviolet wavelengths have germicidal effects. They produce photochemical reactions involving biomolecules in organisms. The resulting molecular alterations inhibit the growth of microorganisms, and in higher doses will kill them. The germicidal effectiveness of UV radiation depends upon its wavelength, and different organisms show different sensitivities to various parts of the UV spectrum. Table 13-4 shows the data for UV resistance to 100-microwatt (μW)/cm^2 intensities for selected organism strains. Figure 13-1 illustrates the roughly Gaussian germicidal action curve whereby germicidal effectiveness is plotted against wavelength.

Disinfection action depends not only upon the UV emission spectrum, but also upon the radiation intensity, the duration of the organism exposure, the sensitivity of the organism involved, and the UV transmission of the medium that suspends the organism. Suspended matter will reflect and block UV transmission, but even optically clear solutions may contain entities such as certain hydrocarbons, sugars, colored materials, and iron or manganese salts that can adsorb UV emissions and so prevent their reaching the suspended organism. Moreover, UV lamps do not have standard outputs, change in their radiation qualities over time, and are subject to fouling during their use.

For all these reasons, the performance of a UV installation is hardly a constant exercise; the variables require assessment and attention. Ultraviolet radiation is, therefore, not considered an absolute method of killing organisms. In particular, the radiation exposure time is an expression of the water flow velocity and of the geometry of the radiation chamber. These, in addition to the quantity of energy delivered by the UV lamp, are the determinants of the effectiveness of the UV installation. It is the UV dosage reaching the organism that is the real consideration. It is expressed as the product of the radiation intensity and the exposure time, in terms of microwatt-seconds per square centimeter ($\mu Ws/cm^2$). The control of the several factors governing the performance of the UV operation must be assured in its validation exercise.

The oxidation of TOC by ultraviolet light, particularly of the 185-nm wavelength, proceeds through the agency of free hydroxyl radicals. These become generated by the action of the ultraviolet radiation on the water molecules. The action is heightened by the presence of hydrogen peroxide, and

Table 13-4
Approximate Dose Values for 1 Survival Ratio of 0.1 DE Various Microorganisms at 253.7 nm

Bacteria	*Dose*	*Bacteria*	*Dose*
Bacillus anthracis	45	Pseudomonas aeruginosa	55
B. megaterium (veg)	11	*P. fluorescens*	35
B. megaterium (spores)	27	*Salmonella enteritidis*	40
B. parathyphosus	32	*S.typhosa*-Typhoid fever	22
B. subtilus	70	*S. paratyphi*-Enteric fever	32
(spores)	120	*S.typhimurium*	80
Micrococcus luteus	197	*Sarcina lutea*	197
Serratia marcescens	24	*Serratia marcescens*	24
Clostridium tetani	130	*Shigela dysenteriae*	
Corynebact diphtheriae	34	dysentry form	22
Eberthelia typhosa	21	*Shigela flexneri*	
Escherichia coli	30	dysentery form	17
Leptospira Sp-		*Shigela paradysenteriae*	17
infectious jaundice	32	*Spirillum rubrum*	44
Micrococcus candidus	61	*Staphylococcus albus*	18
Micrococcus piltonencis	81	*Staphylococcus aureus*	26
Micrococcus sphaeroides	100	*Streptococcus hemolyticus*	22
Mycobacterium tuberculosis	62	*Streptococcus lactis*	62
Neisseria catarrhalis	44	*Streptococcus viridans*	20
Phytomonas tumefaciens	44	*Mycobacterium tuberculi*	100
Proteus vulgaris	26	*Virbio comma* cholera	34

Meulemans (1986); Courtesy, International Ozone Association

by the synergistic effects of ozone (Glaze et al., 1987). The oxidative alteration of the TOC, as previously stated, culminates with the appearance of carboxylic acid groups at one stage of the oxidation chain reaction. The presence of these permits the removal of the altered TOC by anion exchange.

Multimedia deep beds. The use of deep-bed sand filters and of multimedia deep-bed filters for the removal of suspended matter has already been alluded to. Silica sand is commonly used in sand bed constructions (Ogedengbe, 1984). Such beds acquire nominal porosities of 10 to 40 μm; newer beds have lower porosities. The size of the sand grains determines the packing densities. Suspended-matter retention takes place in the top 6 inches or so of the bed. The remaining depth of the bed serves to regulate the flow of water through the bed. At moderate rates of flow (4 to 16 gpm/ft^2 for rapid sand beds, 2 to 3 gpm/ft^2 for slow sand beds), the flow volumes are defined by the extent of bed surface. Actual flows will depend upon the silt density index of the feedwater. Pre-RO sand beds require flows as low as 1 gpm/ft^2 to ensure the sufficient removal of the suspended particles.

In the construction of a sand bed, the sand grains stirred into the water will settle, in response to Stokes' law, in such a fashion as to segregate progressively the particles with the smallest sizes in the top layers. The smallest particles are hydraulically floated to the top where they form the densest layer. The result is a deep-bed filter with the finer pores upstream and the coarser pores downstream.

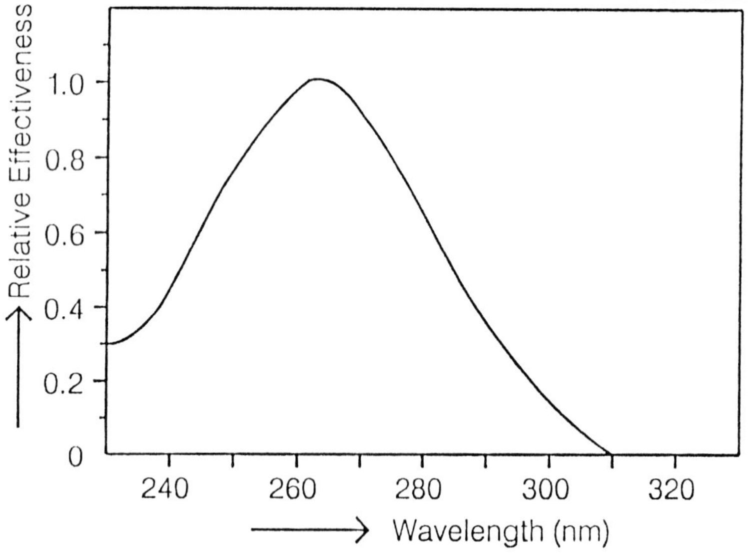

Figure 13-1. Germicidal action curve in the UV region of the energy spectrum.
Meulemans (1986); Courtesy, International Ozone Association

In consequence, the filtration performed by the bed occurs largely in its top layers.

If, however, different granular media are mixed, for instance sand, anthracite, and garnet rock, then the formation of the bed will be comprised of three strata. Anthracite, the least dense with a relative density of 1.5, would form the top layer, the silica sand having a density of 2.5 would constitute the intermediary layer, and the garnet with a relative density 3.5 to 4.5 would constitute the bottom layer. Such a multimedia bed would perform filtrations at three levels. If in addition the succeeding two denser layers were ground progressively finer, they would pack closer to give the multistructure an overall funnel-shaped morphology conducive to accepting higher particulate loadings (Figure 13-2).

The factors to control in multimedia bed construction are the densities of the granules and the fineness of their size. Interestingly, a multimedia bed construction of five layers, consisting of five different sizes of silica sand, has been reported.

The accumulation of suspended matter by the deep-bed filters occasions a progressive buildup of differential pressure leading eventually to an unacceptably low rate of water flow. Usually at the development of about 15 psi of differential pressure the bed is backwashed to a "quicksand" consistency to rid it of its accumulated matter. It is then allowed to drain and resettle into its original configuration for reuse.

In the operation of the deep-bed filter, its standard operating procedure becomes developed. This SOP describes the manipulations and operational protocols necessary to secure the proper deep-bed performance, including the backwash exercise, and the sanitization by chlorine (previously mentioned). During the validation of the deep-bed operation, the adequacy of the SOP becomes attested to by trial.

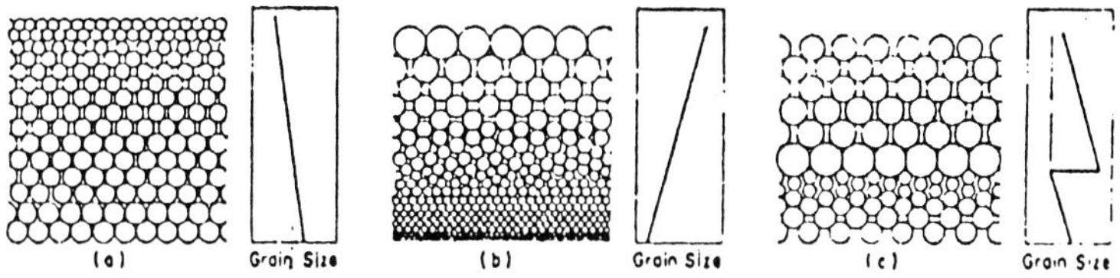

Figure 13-2. Cross sections of representative filter particle gradations. Diagram (a) represents a single media bed such as a rapid sand filter. The bottom half of a filter of this type does little or no work. Diagram (b) represents an ideal filter uniformly graded from coarse to fine from top to bottom. Diagram (c) represents a dual-media bed, with coarse coal above fine sand, which approaches the goal of the ideal filter.

Courtesy, American Water Works Association.

Carbon bed operation. One example of a successful carbon bed operation may serve to focus what can be a diverse and sometimes contradictory experience. A pharmaceutical company has for some three decades been using a carbon bed downstream from sand beds, and separated from downstream ion-exchange beds by filters. The carbon tank or shell is 6 feet high and 54 inches in diameter, and contains about 50% of freeboard. The normal effluent rate is about 120 gpm. The beds are backwashed twice daily, largely to cleanse them of iron deposits. The backwash is at the rate of 200 to 250 gpm.

Microbial assays are performed on alternating days, thrice weekly. Microbial alert levels are set at 600 to 700 cfu/mL. The action level is 1,000 cfu/mL for 3 consecutive days on the cold-water system, ascertained as total heterotrophic plate counts. This action level invokes hot (65°C) water sanitization. The heated water is flushed into the bed and is then trickled to a total volume of 500 to 1,000 gallons in an overnight operation during a weekend. Carbon fines are removed from new beds by an upward flush (backwash), barely vigorous enough to overflow the fines to drain. This backflow fines removal is done overnight.

The successful operation of the carbon bed is ascribed to its continuous recirculative flow from its inception. The flow, through a 1- to 1½-inch line capable of delivering about 30 gpm, is at a minimum of from 25 to 40 gpm (approximately 10 to 2 gpm/ft^2) regardless of whether water is being supplied to the downstream ion-exchange beds or not. The return loop to the carbon bed is by way of the preceding sand beds. In summary, the three elements of this carbon bed's maintenance are continuous recirculation, twice-daily automated backwashes, and weekly sanitizing with 65 °C hot water.

The water softener. The brine makeup tank may itself serve as a haven for organism proliferation. To minimize this possibility, the brine should be maintained in a clean area under closed conditions, at a saturated concentration, agitated (preferably by recirculation), and should periodically be prepared fresh.

It is good practice to use two softeners that are out of phase by design, so that one is being regenerated while one is operative. To avoid organism growth, softeners not in use should be kept in recharged condition with 26% brine, ready to be flushed free of the brine and thus made water-operative on signal. The addition of calcium hypochlorite pellets to the salt supply helps to keep the latter sanitized. Also, wherever possible, hot-water sanitization of the water softener should be performed at 65 to 90°C. The cation-exchange resins survive heating at 90°C.

Water contaminated with organisms derived from the water-softening operation will inoculate the ion exchangers that follow in sequence. For this reason, use is made of ultraviolet light units and of organism-retaining filters to minimize such possibilities.

Principal unit purification processes. As stated, generalized pretreatment design would consist of chlorination of the source water; the removal of iron, manganese, and suspended matter by coagulation and flocculation and/or deep-bed filtration; water softening; and the removal of TOC followed by elimination of the chlorine from the treated water. Each of these pretreatment steps will require documented experimental verification or validation to make certain it conforms to the operational SOPs devised for it, and to ensure that its purported action is indeed attained.

The pretreated water is then ready for purification by any or all of the principal processing units.

Ion exchange. Ion-exchange resins are polyelectrolytes immobilized by the cross-linking of their large organic moieties.

The cation-exchange resin has as its functional group anchored sulfonic acid substituents whose mobile hydrogen ions (actually hydronium [H_3O^+]) can exchange with other cations. The law of mass action as modified by specific ion selectivities governs these exchanges. The result is an uptake of cations by the spatially fixed resin, and a release of hydrogen ions in exchange.

The anion-exchange resins, of which (like the cation-exchange resins) there are several types, utilize spatially fixed quaternary amine groups associated with mobile hydroxyl ions. As anions are acquired by the anion exchangers, hydroxyl ions are liberated. The released hydrogen and hydroxyl ions interact to form water, largely undissociated into ions.

The overall effect of cations and anions being removed from solution is one of demineralization, or of deionization. This is the very purpose of the ion-exchange purification unit. The chemical reactions whereby ion-exchange resins function and are regenerated are depicted in Figures 13-3 and 13-4.

It is part of designing the ion-exchange procedure to elucidate the operational protocol whose practice, formalized in an SOP, will ensure the degree and quality of the deionization being sought. In the validation exercise, documented proof of adherence to that SOP and verification of its expected results will be investigated.

Ion-exchange beds may also be employed for the removal of TOC. If that be the case, the extent of such intended TOC reduction must be examined as part of the validation of the ion-exchange unit process.

Strongly basic ion-exchange resins are required to remove weakly acidic entities such as silica. The regeneration of these resins requires the action of heated (50 to 60°C, usually no higher) sodium hydroxide. However, the carbon-nitrogen bond that is a feature of the quaternary amine group is thermolabile. Upon being heated it ruptures in a reaction called the Hofmann degradation. In fact, these resins are unstable enough to lose some of their capacity even at room temperature. The Type I strongly basic resin will give rise to a few ppb of trimethylamine, the fishy smell of which is objectionable. Type II resins undergo the Hofmann degradation to release ethanol or acetaldehyde, of more pleasant odor. Accordingly, it is the Type II strongly basic resin that is more widely used in pharmaceutical contexts.

Organisms can thrive in ion-exchange beds whose moist interiors contain an abundance of nitrogenous, carbonaceous, and other nutrients. The sanitization of these beds is difficult, the applicability of heat being leveled because of the thermal lability of the strongly basic anion-exchange resins. The best means of sanitizing the ion-exchange beds is by way of regenerating the resins, since organisms are not resistant to the alkali or to the mineral acids (hydrochloric acid or sulfuric acid) used in the regeneration process.

There is a history of organisms released from ion-exchange beds having contaminated Povidone Iodine preparations (Berkelman et al., 1984). The FDA has accordingly warned that pharmaceutical water processors should regenerate their ion-exchange beds as a means of sanitizing them, not on an engineering basis that reflects loss of exchange capacity, but at frequencies dictated by the microbiological counts emanating from the ion-exchange beds (Michels, 1981). This being so, it becomes necessary for pharmaceutical water preparers periodically to assay microbiologically the waters issuing from the ion-exchange columns to detect departures from the trend lines. Such departures would signal the need for action to keep the organism counts under control.

The SOP for operating the ion-exchange columns would come to define the frequency of such regenerations. The validation exercise for the ion-exchange process unit would include documented evidence of conformity with the SOP protocols and of the results achieved thereby.

The *United States Pharmacopoeia 23* in its monograph section permits the use of ion exchange or, indeed, any suitable unit process for preparing Purified

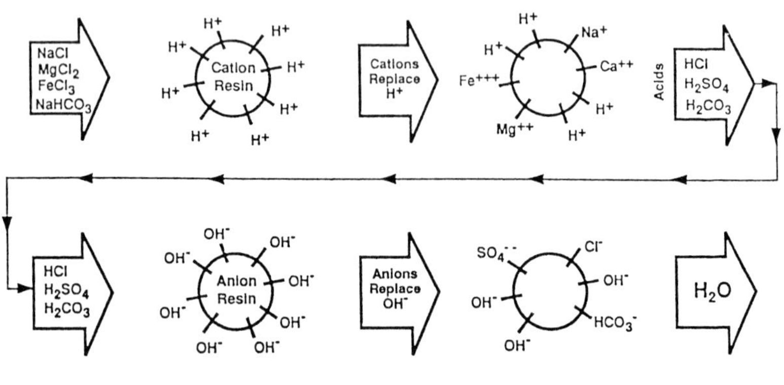

Figure 13-3. Deionization process.
Courtesy, Gary Zoccolante, U.S. Filter Corp.

Water, that substance being directed to the compounding of noninjectables. However, ion-exchange is interdicted for Water for Injection (WFI) manufacture because the organism counts released from the resin beds would likely be excessive for application to injectable preparations by the USP. Distillation or reverse osmosis is currently required for WFI preparation in the United States. The Japanese Pharmacopoeia permits the use of ultrafiltration as well. European authorities permit WFI to be prepared only by distillation.

Reverse osmosis. The *USP 23* sanctions the use of RO along with distillation for the preparation of Water for Injection. It may, of course, also be utilized for the

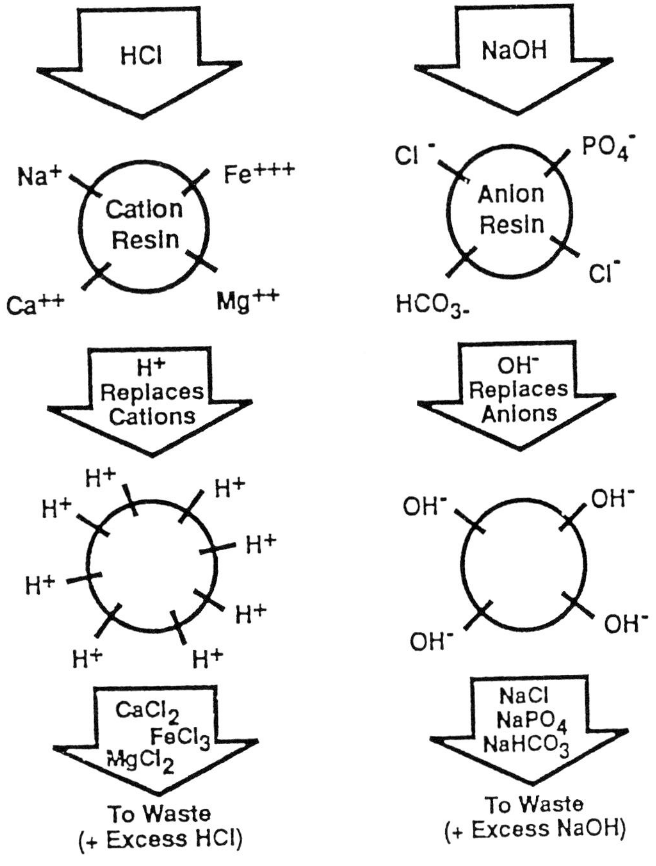

Figure 13-4. Deionizer regeneration.
Courtesy, Gary Zoccolante, U.S. Filter Corp.

preparation of Purified Water. However, the FDA insists that if reverse osmosis is used for the preparation of WFI, it must be in the form of a two-pass, product-staged arrangement. In such a disposition the product water that is effluent from the first RO unit is used as feedwater for the RO unit that follows.

Even in their solid or glassy state, long-chain polymeric molecules, in their normally coiled configurations, contain intersegmental spaces. These are present in all polymeric materials, and provide separating distances among the different segments of the long polymer chains. At temperatures above absolute zero, these spaces continually undergo dynamic alterations.

These intersegmental spaces are peculiar in their dimensions to each given polymer structure. Some polymeric materials, notably the cellulose esters and some polyamides, are characterized by intersegmental spaces having dimensions that permit permeation by water molecules, connected as these are to one another by hydrogen bonding. However, these intersegmental distances are too small to permit the passage of hydrated ions, ions whose small crystallographic dimensions are made overlarge by their skirts of waters of hydration. Such polymeric entities, prepared in very thin-film form to minimize resistance to flow, can be utilized to permit the passage of water under applied pressures. They will discriminate, however, against permeation by hydrated ions. (In addition, some solubility effects are involved.) It is this activity that characterizes the utility of RO membranes in their demineralizing operations.

There are at least three different types of RO membranes available in the field. The oldest type is composed of cellulose acetate. Reverse osmosis units based on polyamide membranes are newer and have the advantage of exhibiting better rejection qualities. However, the polyamide RO membrane is subject to catastrophic ruination by chlorine. A third available RO membrane type is composed of polysulfonated polysulfone. Its virtue is that it is impervious to the degradative action of chlorine; but it is little used.

Cellulose acetate is also oxidatively affected by chlorine, but at an acceptably slower rate. What is desirable is that the cellulose acetate RO membrane passes chlorine. In doing so it provides protection for the RO permeate against microbial contamination. The chlorine is removed subsequently, usually by chemical (bisulfite) addition. The polyamide RO, although superior in its rejection powers, cannot do this. As a result, in pharmaceutical settings where freedom from organism contamination is a leading consideration, cellulose acetate RO units are often preferentially employed.

Cellulose acetate RO units have their own levelations, however. The polymer undergoes hydrolysis at all pH levels, but minimally at pH 4.5. Its practical use dictates, therefore, that it be employed at acidic pHs. Usually, a pH range of 5.5 to 6 is used; cellulose acetate rejects best at pH 6, as measured on mixed ions. However, if bicarbonate is present in the feedwaters, carbon dioxide will be released from them. The passage of the carbon dioxide through the cellulose acetate membrane will impart an unacceptably low pH to the product water. To avoid this, the generated carbon dioxide will require being removed by a decarbonator, usually a forced-air degasifier. These devices risk exposing the waters to air-entrained organisms. By contrast, polyamide RO membrane rejects bicarbonate ions at pH 8.5. Acidification and its consequences are avoided.

Distillation. Stills vaporize water. This permits the separation of water from its nonvolatile impurities. The water vapor is then condensed, allowing its separation from volatile impurities. Unfortunately, the need for stills to furnish large volumes of distillate involves high heat inputs that provide opportunities for vapor entrainment of droplets. A consequence is the carryover of impurities. This is addressed by still design and by the proper operation of the still to avoid such occurrences. This proper operation becomes defined in the development of the SOP suitable to the distilling exercise. The validation of the still operation must, therefore, involve documented experimental evidence that the SOP protocols appropriate for the still were adhered to. Still design is also concerned with minimizing the heating costs by optimization of vaporizing and condensing functions.

Still manufacturers will specify the purity of the feedwaters considered suitable for their stills. Evidence is, therefore, to be provided attesting to conformity with these requirements. One of the chief concerns in still operations is the possibility of the carryover of endotoxins from the feedwaters. Still operations, like those of all the unit purification processes, are not absolute in their performance. Rather, they can be depended upon to provide log reductions of impurities. Still manufacturers, for whatever reasons, not necessarily imposed by still design, may be reluctant to guarantee more than a three- or four-log reduction in endotoxin, although better results can be obtained (Saari et al., 1977). The FDA requires, therefore, that the endotoxin content of the still feedwaters not attain concentrations whose management by distillation cannot be ensured. It is common, therefore, for the intended feedwater to be treated with ultrafilters or with charge-modified microporous filters to eliminate or reduce the endotoxin content.

Whatever quality parameters are set in the relevant SOPs for the still feedwaters and for the operational manipulations of the still must, as part of the validation exercise, prevail in practice.

Testing and GMPs

Microbiological validation. It is the FDA whose views must be accorded with in performing the microbiological aspects of the validation process. It should be emphasized, however, that the pharmaceutical water processor is responsible for ascertaining that the validation exercise is sufficient and proper for his purposes. Complying with FDA regulations, advises, and guidelines should lead to reassuring results. However, if despite the FDA's "approval" (or lack of disapproval) the "validated" system does not prove suitable for drug processing, the responsibility is that of the pharmaceutical manufacturer. The FDA imprimatur confers no immunity for the drug processor against untoward consequences.

Munson (1993) divides the validation exercise into three phases:

In phase 1, daily water samples are taken downstream from each unit in the treatment system and from each point-of-use in the holding/distribution system to assess the chemical and microbiological quality of the water. The data from the daily samples taken over a one month period should be used to develop SOPs, appropriate maintenance and cleaning protocols, and analytical schedules for each unit in the system.

Daily sampling is continued in phase 2 for another month. During this phase the water system is operated according to the protocols and schedules developed during phase 1. The data from this phase are used to confirm that the operating and maintenance protocols and schedules are adequate and that the system can consistently produce water meeting its specifications. The data can also be used as the base line data for trend analysis of the system (Singer 1994).

At the end of phase 2 the sampling schedule changes to that of routine monitoring. Chemical testing of pharmaceutical water systems should be performed at least weekly. Microbial testing of Water For Injection systems should be daily, with each point-of-use being sampled at least weekly. For Purified Water systems microbial testing should be performed on each point-of-use at least weekly.

Phase 3 of the validation program consists of reviewing the routine of monitoring data for at least 6 to 10 months. This time period will demonstrate that the operating protocols are adequate to handle variations in the quality, both chemically and microbially, of the incoming feed water. At the end of phase 3, if all data indicate that the water system when operated according to its SOP consistently produces water that meets its specifications, the water system can be considered validated.

The validation program described is only a suggestion. It should not be interpreted as the only acceptable program that FDA will accept. Each water system, including the validation data and program, will be judged on its own merit.

The water generated during the validation phases 2 and 3 can be used to manufacture drug products. You do not have to wait for a whole year before you can use the water."

Microbiological levels. The bacterial endotoxin content of Water for Injection is set by *USP 23* at the 0.25-EU/mL level. The microbiological content of Purified Water is not to exceed 100 cfu/mL; and that of Water for Injection is not to exceed 10 cfu/100 mL. These, however, are not rejection limits but are rather action levels (FDA, July 1993; USP, 1995). The organism action level for Water for Injection permits little room for maneuver.

The Purified Water action level is, however, amenable to modification, depending upon the use to which it is put. When the Purified Water is designed for antacid preparation, the level may need to be reduced, depending upon the drug manufacturing process. For example, if heat is involved, the level need not be as low. This is necessitated by the ease with which organisms grow at the alkaline pHs of such preparations, where preservatives are generally ineffective. A lower level would reduce the risk caused by the potential for organism growth in the product. Oral medications might be permitted higher counts than otic, nasal, or topical wound preparations. (Ophthalmics are to be sterile.) Where one water system is depended upon in the preparation of several products, the action level should be set in accordance with the needs of the product offering the highest risk for microbial growth. Room is thus left for individual judgments as regards the action levels for Purified Water, depending upon its ultimate use.

Munson (1993), as spokesperson for FDA, advises as follows:

> Failure to meet these action levels does not mean automatic rejection of products. As the definition indicates, action levels are points which signal a drift from normal operating conditions and which require action on the part of the firm. When these levels are exceeded you should conduct an investigation designed to determine why the action level is being exceeded. Then identify and implement the corrective action needed to restore the system to normal operation. You should also recheck products made prior to the corrective action to determine if the contamination has affected the quality of the product. You should increase your sampling rate for a period after the corrective action is implemented to insure that the system has returned to a state of control. This also does not mean that if you get a count of 110 CFU per mL for your Purified Water that you must shut down the system during the investigation.
>
> Because microbial test results are already two to five days old you should not wait for two consecutive samples to exceed the action level before you perform an investigation. This is when control charts or trend analysis can be a very useful tool. If the organism(s) isolated do not represent a potential problem and the historical profile of the system indicates that this single result is unusual and not part of an upward trend, then the follow-up action may simply consist of re-sampling or stepping up the rate of sampling for a short period so that a more accurate determination of whether the system is out of control or not can be made. The important thing is to document what follow-up action you took and that the problem was corrected. No documentation means no follow-up action and no correction.

Testing for specific organisms. The types of organisms present in the Purified Water must be considered. Previously the FDA had advised that no pseudomonads should be present in the water system. That is not the present FDA position (Munson, 1993). *Pseudomonas* species do not have to be monitored for, unless such organisms represent potential hazards to the product. The burden for knowing whether that situation exists, as well as the consequences attendant upon it, devolves upon the drug manufacturer. It is the responsibility of the drug manufacturers to learn and know the situation as regards their products. It has been known that the presence of *P. aeruginosa* in topicals can produce infections in people with abraded skin or wounds. Therefore, the presence of these pseudomonads in waters used for topicals is objectionable. The general situation is that water systems are required to be free of particular organisms only if they represent pathogens or potential pathogens in the products being produced (i.e., when their presence in the drug preparation poses a potential health hazard during use as directed). The relevant knowledge is the responsibility of the drug preparer.

As stated, the number of microbes restricted in the compendial waters by the alert and action levels is attended by a prohibition against objectionable organisms. The presence of opportunistic pathogens needs also to be considered, however. These may be pathogenic when applied to patients with compromised immunities, a situation not known in advance to the drug preparer, who is, nevertheless, liable for untoward consequences. It may be prudent, therefore, to maintain even Purified Water under self-sanitizing storage, as at 80 °C or in the presence of ozone. The use of a sterile Purified Water could eliminate the presence of undesirable organisms from the drug preparation. This would minimize dependency on preservatives whose action is sometimes uncertain.

Viable nonculturable bacteria. The possible presence of viable but nonculturable bacteria is being increasingly recognized. The question is whether their presence has disease-causing implications. The general belief is that they do not pose significant threats to health. The practical meaning of their potential presence seems minimal.

Microbiological assay methods. There is by no means unanimity regarding how the microbiological assays are to be performed. There are different views concerning the methods, (such as direct count or pour plate), the nutrient media to be employed, the incubation times, and the incubation temperatures.

Recommendations on this subject by the Water Quality Committee of the Pharmaceutical Research and Manufacturing Association are as follows (WQC/PMA 1992a, 1993b, 1994):

Purified Water: POUR PLATE METHOD
Minimum sample - 1.0 mL
Plate count agar
Minimum 48 hours incubation at 30 °C to 35 °C

Water for Injection: MEMBRANE FILTRATION METHOD
Filtration using 0.45-μm porosity filter
Minimum sample - 100 mL
Plate count agar
Minimum 48 hours incubation at 30 °C to 35 °C

It should be remembered, however, that the responsibility for selecting or even for devising culturing techniques suitable for revealing organism types that may be present in a particular water is that of the pharmaceutical processor.

FDA does not have any significant problems with these proposals except that the sample size for water injection should be 250 to 300 mL to obtain a more accurate determination of the microbial count. We also know that these methods are not the only methods that can be used and they may not work for all water systems across the country. It is simply a starting point. If you use this method and still have product failures, then you will still have to develop a method appropriate for your water system (Munson, 1993).

It should be noted that there is no one method that will detect all possible organisms present in the water. The method chosen should adequately characterize the predominant organisms present. The most important aspect of the monitoring is to look for changes in the numbers and types of microorganisms that are present.

Alert and action levels. It is intended that pharmaceutical water manufacturers set and utilize alert and action levels to guard their WFI and Purified Water from exceeding the specified microbial levels. (PMA 1984). In this exercise, the alert levels indicate that a process may have drifted from its normal operating condition. It provides a warning. The action level signals such a departure from the normal range that investigative and corrective actions require being instituted.

It is helpful and prudent for the waters being prepared to attain normally an even greater purity than that stipulated. For example, consider a Purified Water with an action level set at 100 cfu/mL, but which is normally purified to better than that amount, for example to 50 cfu/mL. If a periodic analysis indicated a level of 70 cfu/mL, the water system operators would become alerted to check the accuracy of that finding by promptly repeating the analysis. Were the recount to affirm the higher level, action could be undertaken promptly to learn the cause of the excursion and to implement the remedial steps that should be taken to bring the system back into control.

The numerical values for alert and action levels are often set rather arbitrarily. It is desirable that they be set on a statistical basis. Trend analysis is used to interpret what the microbiological data signify by way of standard deviations. In some cases the levels are established as multiples of the standard deviation from the normal, namely, 2 times the standard deviation or sigma for the alert level, and 3 times the standard deviation for the action level. On this basis, the alert level accounts for 95% of the data, and the action level covers 99%. A 1% outside the action level is considered normal. Exceeding this level is unusual and requires attention. There is also room for ambiguity in how the alert levels are responded to. The alert level may be addressed by the retesting of samples to make sure the higher numbers are real. The alert response may, in addition, include corrective actions in advance of those to be taken when the action level is reached.

The water processor is expected to set his own alert and action levels. The FDA inspectors will insist, however, that the records show that these are respected and adhered to in practice, and will insist that the USP action levels are Good Manufacturing Practices at this time. Action levels above those suggested by the USP will have to be justified.

Conductivity measurements and pH. The standards of chemical acceptability for Purified Water and Water for Injection are shown in Table 13-1, as translated and quantified from the relevant analytical procedures described in *USP 23* (FDA, July 1993; USP, 1995). A single conductivity measurement in conjunction with pH values will be substituted for the total of the specific measurements for chloride, sulfate, ammonia, calcium, and carbon dioxide.

This becomes possible because the several relevant impurities are all ionic, or ion-producing; and therefore find reflection in electrical conductivity measurements (or in the reciprocal function, electrical resistivity). The electrical conductivity value read for a water will be ascribed to the ions having the specific lowest conductivity. This approach will maximize the presumed concentration of these ions. This will have the prudent effect of ensuring that the ionic concentrations within the water do not exceed their stipulated levels.

Different ions have different conductivity values at different pHs and temperatures. Conductivity curves modeled on the chloride and ammonium ions overlap. The chloride ions have the lower leveling conductivities from pH 5.0 to 6.2, the ammonium ions from 6.3 to 7.0; the pharmaceutical waters have acceptable pHs in the range of 5.0 to 7.0. Temperature, as stated, also has an effect upon the equilibrium concentrations and upon the specific conductance of each ionic species.

Testing the suitability of the product water will be possible at each of three stages. Stage 1 will be assayed by on-line conductivity tests, a situation presumably free of the influences of carbon dioxide and its ionic pH and conductivity consequences. The temperature of the water will also be read directly, not compensated for. Comparisons will then be made of the conductivity/temperature values with those presented in an official table of acceptable levels. The conductivity at the temperature value equal to or less than the measured temperature will define the acceptable level.

If the conductivity is equal to or less than that tabulated value, the water quality will be acceptable. If it is greater, a Stage 2 determination will be made to see whether the higher conductivity is occasioned by the presence of carbon dioxide. In the Stage 2 assay, the water is stirred vigorously at 25 ± 1 °C to permit its complete equilibration with the atmospheric carbon dioxide. The attainment of equilibrations is measured by the leveling off of the periodically determined change in conductivity. When the net alteration becomes less than 0.1 μS/cm per 5 minutes, the sample conductivity will be recorded. If it is no greater than 2.1 μS/cm, the water will be deemed to be acceptable. If the conductivity value is greater, the possible influence of pH will be ascertained in a Stage 3 assay.

Saturated potassium chloride will be added to the sample examined in the Stage 2, to enable its pH to be measured. Reference will be made to a predetermined pH/conductivity requirements table to find the acceptable conductivity level at the measured pH level. Unless either the conductivity of the water is greater than the acceptable level, or the pH is outside the range of 5.0 to 7.0, the water quality is judged to be proper. (Table 1-14, see page 24).

By the same token, if at either of the earlier stages of testing the conductivity is found to be acceptable, then the pH, of necessity, must be within its proper range. Indeed, the original role of pH was to level the concentration of ions not otherwise specifically identified. Therefore, the specific requirement to determine directly the pH of the water would seem to be redundant where the conductivity is suitable. Nevertheless, pH measurements will be required.

TOC measurements. It will be made permissible to utilize TOC measurements as a substitute for the USP potassium permanganate oxidizable substances test. The acceptability standard will be set at 500 ppb.

The TOC measuring devices available in the marketplace differ significantly in their abilities to detect (by oxidation and its consequences) organic molecules of varying complexities. There is a desire not to exclude from consideration any TOC monitor capable of measuring the presence of organic molecules likely to be found in pharmaceutical waters. A suitable reference compound must, therefore, be defined. Several have been proposed. The criteria were water solubility, nonionicity, nonvolatility, and a sufficiently molecular complexity to be difficult for some TOC instrument technologies to accommodate. A choice was made from among 1,4-benzoquinone, a-naphthylresorcinol, and o-octyl-β-D-glucopyranoside, based on a widespread laboratory evaluation.

The reference compound selected for the instrument suitability test was 1,4-

benzoquinone. It has the useful properties of being a powder at room temperature, readily available in pure form, relatively safe to handle, and well defined chemically. In the multilaboratory testing exercise, its average recovery was the lowest among the organic compounds examined. Its use as the standard for the TOC suitability test therefore suggests that it offers the greatest challenge to oxidation. This presents a prudent choice to the subject of TOC determinations.

For the TOC instruments to be acceptable, the 1,4-benzoquinone recovery is to be within the test levels of 80% to 115%. Sucrose serves as the TOC test standard.

Source-water testing. It is required that the pharmaceutical waters be prepared using sources of drinking-water quality as defined by the U.S. EPA, or comparable European Unior or Japanese regulations (*USP 23, Fifth Supplement*). When the feedwaters are of municipally-treated origins, certification of the quality can be obtained by the drug producer from the municipal authorities, perhaps on a quarterly basis. Where unprocessed source waters are used, or when the pharmaceutical processor undertakes to do the testing to establish in-house EPA certification, then the full panoply of EPA potable water analyses, including testing for pesticides possibly present, should be carried out. An annual performance of such analyses should suffice. Yearly spot checks, including pesticide analyses, should also be made by users of municipal waters to see how well the levels found match those reported by the municipal suppliers.

GMPs Related to Water Systems

The Food and Drug Administration has established a number of Good Manufacturing Practices that pertain to the preparation of pharmaceutical waters. Since their promulgation, several have undergone modification in practice, a consequence of the FDA's ongoing and evolving understanding of what pharmaceutical water systems require. Those that are particularly pertinent to water systems are here set forth.

Operational Qualification of Purification Units

Specific unit process validations. A separate assessment is needed for the operation of each individual purification unit part of the Operational Validation procedure, soon to be discussed. The system having been correctly designed and installed, how is it to be validated? A number of questions must be answered in the validation exercise:

- What component or unit of the system is being addressed?
- What is its function?
- What is the measure of its performance?

- What are its normal maintenance requirements?
- What additional maintenance may occasionally need to be performed?
- When are sanitizations to be carried out?
- What sanitization method is to be utilized?

Consider, for example, the purification unit that is the carbon bed. Its chief purpose is to dechlorinate the water. Secondarily, it may be relied upon to reduce the TOC load. To assess the performance of its purported function, one would measure the chlorine content of both the incoming and effluent waters. One could do likewise for the reduction of TOC, using an on-line TOC monitor. What would be the measure of the carbon bed's performance? In the case of dechlorination, complete chlorine removal would be expected. Therefore, the effluent water should contain zero chlorine! The performance standard for the reduction of TOC could be set variously. It could, for instance, be judged against a goal of less than 1 ppm, or the target could be a reduction to 50% of the original TOC burden. Use whatever seems appropriate.

The next step would be to list and carry out the normal maintenance needs. For instance, consider the backwashing, bumping (to eliminate channeling), and rinsing. Shall it be performed (as a multimedia bed would be) on the basis of pressure-drop, or in response to a diminution in TOC uptake: in other words, in accordance with the achievement of a measured value? Alternatively, maintenance could be instituted on a time basis, such as daily. The time basis can be set experientially against an historically measured value, or in keeping with a prophylactic philosophy.

Are there occasionally additional maintenance protocols that must be invoked? The replacement of the carbon bed is an example.

When is the carbon bed sanitization to be accomplished? Shall it be in response to specific levels of organisms in the effluent water, or periodically on a time basis? How is the sanitization to be performed: by hot water, by steam?

Safety protocols require being observed. In the design of the water purification system for every purification unit; the installation of test ports, isolation valves, and pressure gauges should be made and protocols for microbiological and chemical assays are to be provided for. All performed operations and the data they generate will require being analyzed, documented, and countersigned.

Chlorination unit. Chlorine is usually added to a water supply to a residual concentration of 0.5 to 2 ppm. Municipally treated waters drawn into a pharmaceutical plant probably reflect such a treatment. However, municipally treated waters may, for a variety of reasons, also fall short in their chlorine content. It is, therefore, best to analyze the incoming waters for their actual chlorine content and to adjust as necessary.

The targeted chlorine concentration is measured by way of a chlorine monitor. The automated chlorine analyzer is responsive to the concentration present in the water. Chlorine being an oxidant, its concentration can also be determined by way of an oxidation-reduction potential (ORP) analyzer. This type of instrument senses the oxidizing status of the water. In effect, then, it assays the chlorine concentration that is present. It is used in conjunction with a metering device that permits a proportioned addition of chlorine as necessary to maintain a preset concentration. Figure 13-5 illustrates an instrument that simultaneously displays pH, ORP, and temperature measurements. Amperometric titrations also serve to analyze for chlorine. Figure 13-6 illustrates a Hach Company amperometric titrator.

The purpose of the chlorine treatment being the addition of chlorine, the validation of its function is obtained from comparisons of the before and after chlorine concentrations. This includes demonstration that the requisite chlorine concentration is being maintained.

The biocidal efficacy of the chlorine treatment is usually assumed. However, its validation can be confirmed by microbiological assays of the feedwater, before and after chlorination.

Deep-bed filter. For the water exiting the media beds, the free-chlorine content should be held at 0.1 to 1 ppm, to be measured weekly. The corresponding microbiological levels, to be assessed weekly, should not exceed 100 cfu/mL. The bed sanitizations are commonly performed once or twice yearly using 200-ppm sodium hypochlorite solutions. Generally, the beds are functional for a 5-year period.

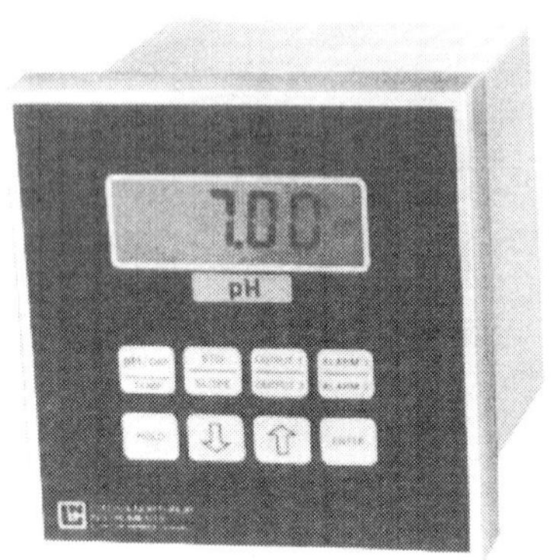

Figure 13-5. Simultaneous pH, temperature, and oxidation-reduction potential analyzer.
Courtesy, Leeds & Northrup

The deep-bed filters, of whatever construction, generally require flowrates of between 5 and 15 gpm/ft^2, depending upon the application. When they accumulate enough particulate matter to boost their pressure differential to about 15 psi (1 bar), they are backflushed in a maintenance operation.

The function of the deep-bed filters is to remove suspended matter. Validation of their performance is obtained by comparing the suspended-solids contents of the before and after filtered waters. It usually suffices, however, to measure the proper flows by way of flowmeters, and to arrange for timely automated backflushes in response to pressure buildups in the beds.

Backwash operations in this context, as also for any deep bed, can be assessed using a backwash turbidimeter. One such Hach Company instrument is shown in Figure 13-7. The operational principle of such a device is depicted by Figure 13-8.

Softening operations. Because organisms may proliferate in the water-softening unit, the chlorine content of the feedwater is usually not removed until after the water is softened. Indeed, a free-chlorine residue is advised. On the other hand, the water-softening resin will undergo degradation by the oxidizing action of the chlorine. Some choose, therefore, to remove the chlorine before the water enters the softener.

Periodic sanitizations of the water softener should be performed using water at 80 °C (176 °F) over a 2-hour contact period. The validation exercise should define the frequency of sanitization. The water-softening resin should last for about 3 years. Prior analyses should have revealed whether barium, strontium, iron, or manganese are among the more conventional elements present.

The water softener's function in reducing or removing hardness can then readily be validated by comparison with the analytical results shown for the water emerging from the softener.

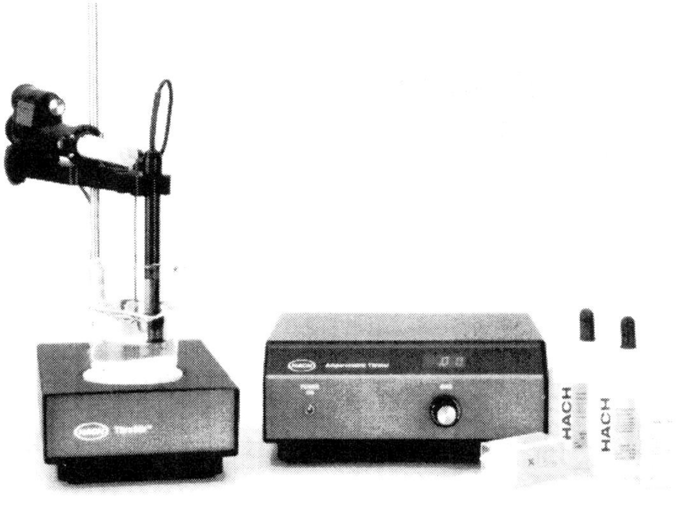

Figure 13-6. Amperometric titrator.
Courtesy, Hach Company

The water-softening ion-exchange resin needs periodically to be regenerated by brine. Organism growth is possible in the salt solution. Periodic microbial assays should be used to establish a sanitizing schedule. Also, the validation exercise should define the frequency of the resin regeneration, as indicated by a drop in the softening efficiency as measured by water-hardness element concentrations. Having this point defined as a function of time or gallonage permits the regeneration to be accomplished automatically. Ultimately, the resin used in the water softener will need to be replaced. The need for this activity will be signaled by a decrease in the regenerability of the resin. A Hach Company hardness monitor is pictured in Figure 13-9. A two-cell softening monitor is shown in Figure 13-10.

Instruments are available for securing the analytical data necessary for validation. A Leeds & Northrup data sheet (1989) states the following:

> Many softeners are regenerated based on time or totalized water flow. However, this is a predictive technique with no feedback and does not take into account any variation in water supply hardness. The most sensitive method would be to monitor the hardness of treated water, but continuous instrumentation for this is costly and maintenance intensive. A more economical method is to monitor conductivity ratio across the softener. Sodium is typically more conductive than the hardness minerals it replaces so higher conductivity at the outlet is to be expected. As the ratio approaches 1, hardness ions are breaking through and regeneration is needed. A low ratio alarm can trigger this.

In addition, conductivity can be used to monitor and control the concentration of the regenerating brine, usually in a 10% strength, to provide more consistent regeneration.

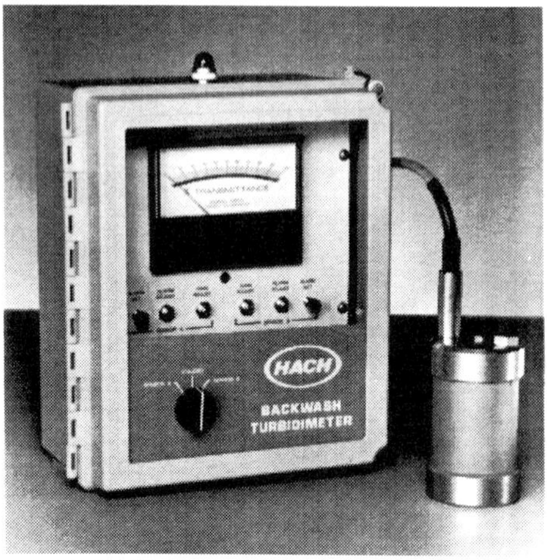

Figure 13-7. Backwash turbidometer.
Courtesy, Hach Company

Carbon beds. The actions to be taken in the validation of carbon beds have already been considered. Briefly, their ability to remove chlorine should be affirmed by an analysis of their effluent water. The chlorine content should be zero. As already stated, the chlorine can be analyzed for in a number of ways.

The backwashing, bumping, and rinsing procedures normal to carbon bed maintenance should be implemented daily. Recirculation of the water is indicated.

The sanitization of the carbon beds should be performed in accordance with the standard operating procedures developed during the prevalidation stage of the process. Eventual replacement of the activated carbon should be made in keeping with the requirements as defined in the SOP. Sanitizations using water at 80 °C (176 °F) for at least 2 hours should be performed as dictated by the validation exercise.

Reverse osmosis operation. The proper way to validate the operation of the RO units depends upon their intended functions in the purification system. Their purpose in 99% of RO usages is to reduce the ionic content of the treated waters. Single-pass ROs are usually expected to reduce the ionic concentrations by greater than 95%. Reductions of greater than 99%, as measured daily, are usually the goals of two-pass systems.

Depending upon the qualities of the feedwaters, two-pass, product-staged RO operations may be needed to yield waters that have acceptable chloride ion levels. If the feedwater contains 400 to 500 ppm of chloride, and the single-pass RO gives a 5% leakage, the two-pass, product-staged RO becomes mandatory.

Whether the performance of the RO function is as purported can be gauged by measuring the salt rejection of the single RO unit. Instrumentation determines the conductivity of the influent and effluent streams and displays the results in terms of salt rejections. For the two-pass units, where the ionic reduction is

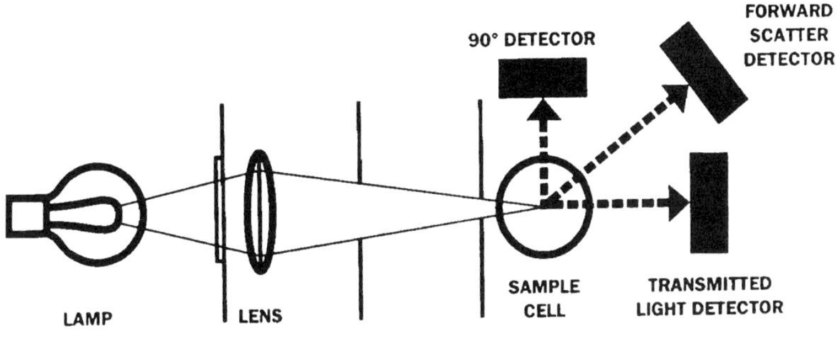

Figure 13-8. Schematics of Hach backwash turbidometer.
Courtesy, Hach Company

expected to attain some 99%, the performance is judged by the direct measurement of the effluent water's resistivity. The RO operation should also reduce the colloidal and endotoxin loads of the water.

For the RO function or that of ion-exchange, conductivity-resistivity measuring instruments are used. One such analyzer is shown in Figure 13-11. Another, which displays RO percentage rejections, is illustrated by Figure 13-12. A relevant display panel is presented in Figure 13-13.

Another function planned for the RO may be the removal, to whatever expected or designed extent, of TOC. Depending upon the source water, the TOC reduction can be 80% to 90%. Rarely will the TOC reductions be at the optimum of 99%. The validation of the TOC reduction function by the RO can be assessed by the use of TOC monitors. Usually, one is mounted on-line at the RO outlet. However, the analyses can be performed using grab samples in conjunction with off-line TOC analyzers.

Reverse osmosis is also used to remove bacteria and bacterial endotoxins. The validation of those functions to the levels designed can be assayed using suitable microbiological analytical techniques and limulus amebocyte lysate testing. The purported removal or bacteria-diminishing actions can be the 10 cfu/100 mL required for WFI, the 100 cfu/mL desired for Purified Water, or any other designed-for standard, as determined weekly.

In some instances, albeit rarely, the second RO of the two-pass arrangement

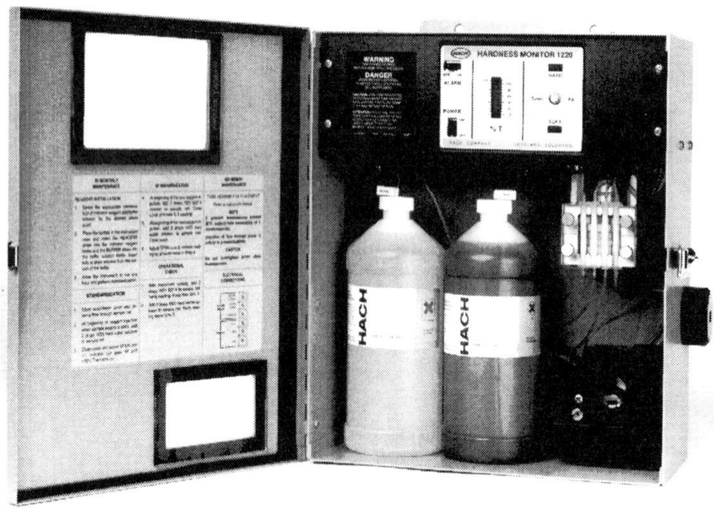

Figure 13-9. Hardness monitor.
Courtesy, Hach Company

is assigned the sole function of assuring the removal of organisms and bacterial endotoxin. Ionic removal is not involved. That has presumably been accomplished adequately by the first of the two ROs. In these instances the validation of the operation can be determined by suitable assays of the product water. The water exiting the second RO unit should have resistivities in excess of 300,000 ohms-cm as measured daily.

The normal maintenance of the RO operation should include the automatic inspection of the O-rings. Damaged O-rings can cause the reject water to mix with the clean permeate water. Cleaning of the RO should be undertaken upon a 25% increase in differential pressure, upon a loss of flow by as much as 10%, or when the rejection decreases by 1% (Zoccolante, 1995).

Commercial cleaners may gainfully be employed. Unless the foulants are known, some degree of trial and error will be involved. Sanitizations are to be performed periodically. A discussion of suitable sanitizers for RO membranes is presented in Chapter 2; cleaning agents are discussed in Chapter 9.

Purveyors of RO devices usually stipulate the feedwater quality that is required to be used with their units. The specifications may reflect the quality desired for the effluent product water. Such considerations as pH; hardness; total dissolved solids; operational temperatures; and levels on copper, aluminum, and iron are numerically defined. The metals should be analyzed for at least quarterly. A conservative estimate of RO service life would be 3 years.

The RO operation should require pretesting to ensure the presence of feedwaters with silt density index levels of 5 or less. Testing should be performed weekly. Prefiltration should be employed to achieve this SDI level. The microbial content of the RO feedwaters should not exceed 500 cfu/mL, as

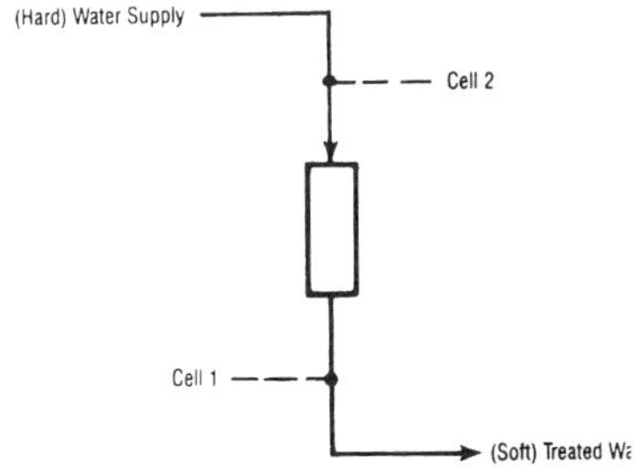

Figure 13-10. Two-cell softener monitoring.
Courtesy, Leeds & Northrup

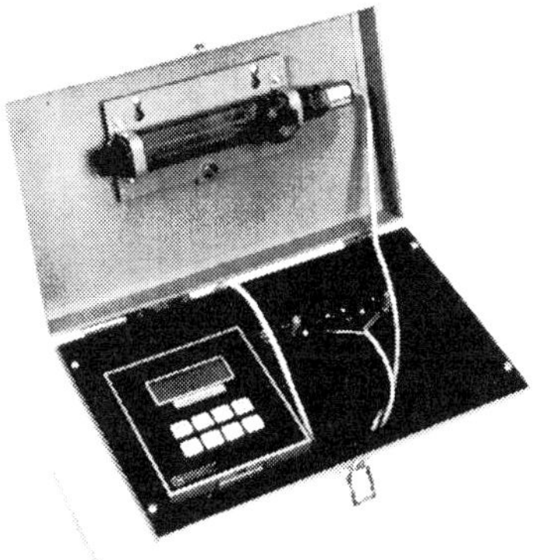

Figure 13-11. Conductivity-resistivity analyzer.
Courtesy, Leeds & Northrup

assayed weekly. Sanitizations should make use of 1% peracetic acid solutions, and should be conducted in accordance with the results of the validation exercise, usually about 4 times per year. Recirculation through the RO unit should be practiced to help control the organism counts.

Ion-exchange operations. The performance of ion-exchange units of whatever construction, including twin beds and mixed beds, depends upon two considerations: bed capacity and the onset of ion leakage. Therefore, in the validation of the ion-exchange operation, these two items require assessment. The ion-exchange capacity must be determined in establishing the operational SOP so that regeneration can be undertaken in timely fashion. The exhaustion of capacity is defined by the onset of ion leakage. For the cation exchanger, the first ion to break through is the sodium ion. For the anion-exchange bed, it is silica that first manifests leakage. Therefore the measurement of these ions in the influent and effluent waters will provide evidence, to be documented, that the ion exchangers are doing what they are purported to do. Sodium ions can be measured using electrodes specific for sodium ions. Ion-specific electrodes are expensive and they require periodic maintenance, but they are very useful. Silica can be analyzed for colorimetrically using an on-line silica analyzer.

More generally, information concerning ion leakages can be obtained from conductivity measurements, because increasing ionic concentrations yield higher electrical conductivities. Conductivities are the easiest of these assays to perform. Although the least specific, they may suffice. The baseline conductivity should be measured as an indication of conductivity. After the bed is regenerated, it is washed down until its effluent waters show a flat conductivity area. This continues until ion breakthrough manifests itself. The flat area is the

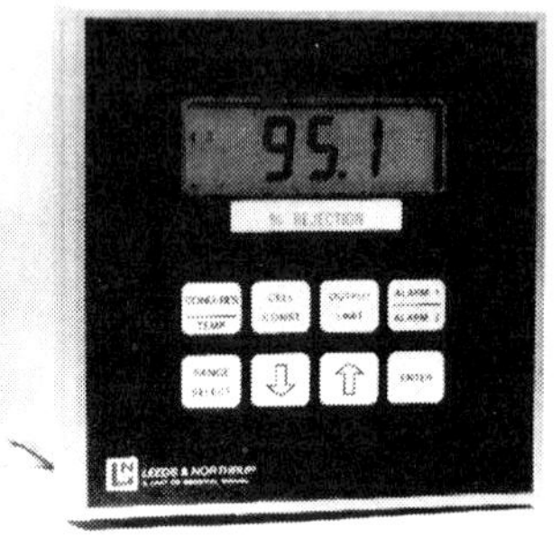

Figure 13-12. Two-cell conductivity analyzer displaying percentage of rejection by RO.
Courtesy, Leeds & Northrup

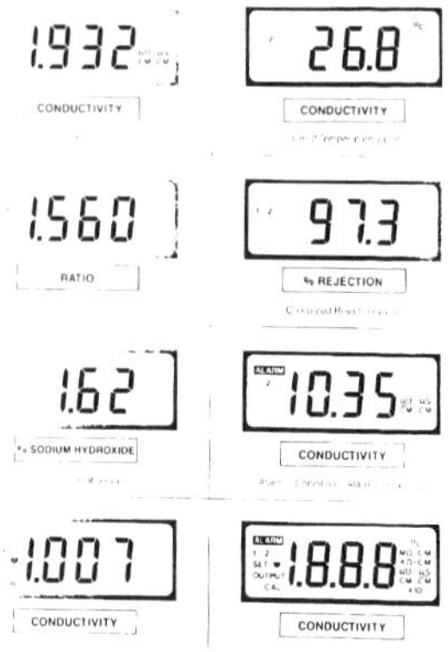

Figure 13-13. Typical instrument display messages.
Courtesy, Leeds & Northrup

baseline conductivity. Conductivity measurements can be taken every 6 hours or so in the search for early manifestations of ion leakage.

There are several purveyors of relevant instruments. Figure 13-14 illustrates a portable conductivity and TDS meter. Figure 13-15 shows a photograph of a silica analyzer. The general usefulness of two-cell conductivity analyzers is made evident in Figure 13-16.

While the essentials of the ion-exchange operation involve the analyses just indicated, other tests can usefully be conducted as well. The chlorine content of the water where such is permitted entry into the beds can be measured, as by amperometric titrations on the incoming and outgoing waters. It would be most helpful to have periodic microbiological assays performed on the waters flowing out of the ion-exchange unit. Indeed, the FDA requires that the ion-exchange beds be sanitized whenever the effluent organism counts depart from the normal trend lines. This can be accomplished by regeneration of the beds. Also, since ion-exchange beds can serve to reduce TOC, where such action is part of the system design, TOC analyses should be conducted to make sure that the purported performance is realized.

Implementation of the SOP should be keyed to the flow diagram of the system. Which way the water is flowing, to where, and which valves should be opened or closed should clearly be indicated during every step of the ion exchange and the ion-exchange regeneration process.

The standard maintenance procedure dealing with ion-exchange bed upkeep should have its own analytical protocols necessary to the regeneration step. Safety procedures will direct the proper handling, use, and disposal of the regenerant chemicals. Measuring instruments should be kept in proper calibration. How to perform such calibrations should be specified.

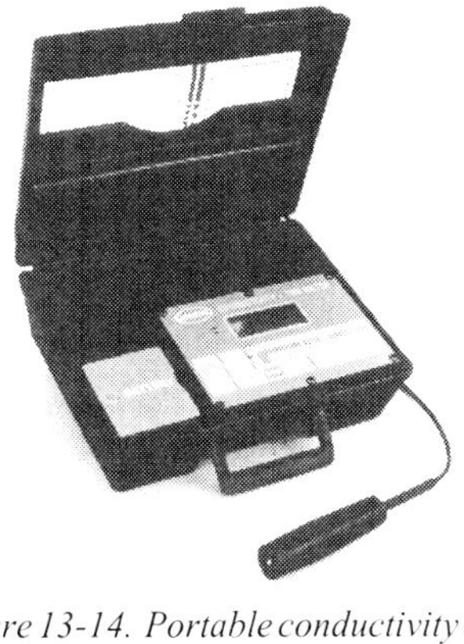

Figure 13-14. Portable conductivity and TDS meter.
Courtesy, Hach Company

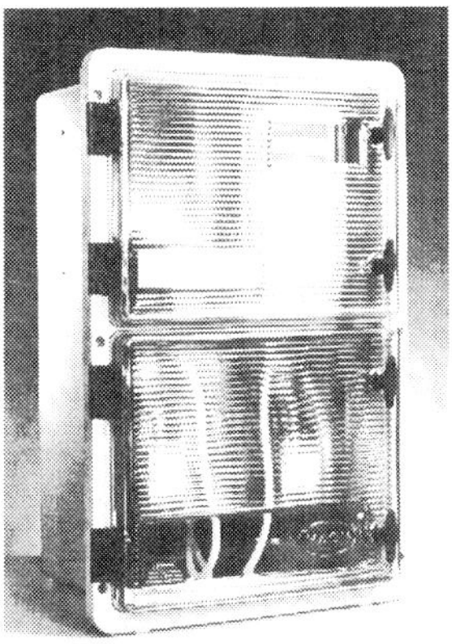

Figure 13-15. Silica analyzer.
Courtesy, Hach Company

The resins themselves should receive at least yearly examinations to determine their moisture content or uptake (a measure of their cross-link deterioration), and to determine the wholeness of the beads. While twin ion-exchange units can tolerate less than an 80% portion of fragmented or split beads, the mixed-bed resins become more difficult to separate at that level of fragmentation. Additionally, the cation-exchange beads may be soaked in dilute hydrochloric acid to obtain a slow elution of iron. Other bead examinations may be conducted as well.

Sanitizations of the DI resins should be attempted using 70 °C (160 °F) water. (The upper temperature levels are defined by the thermal lability of the anion-exchange resins.) This should be performed weekly. Recirculation through the bed should be part of the design. The water exiting the bed should have resistivities greater than 10 megohms-cm. The bacterial counts should preferably be under 50 cfu/mL, as determined on a weekly basis. The mixed-bed life-to-renewal depends, of course, upon the feedwater quality, but is usually 3 months or so.

In particular, the characterization of the product water should be an ongoing activity. Signed daily logs of the various operations are kept. The data should be tracked, and trend lines drawn frequently.

Distillation. The proper action of a still depends upon the use of water of a requisite purity coupled with its being operated in accord with the experimentally

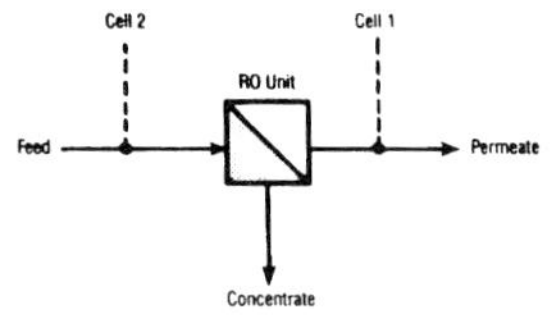

leverse osmosis efficiency is monitored by comparing inlet nd outlet conductivity (or TDS). Automatic calculations of 'ercent Rejection or Percent Passage are provided. emperature readout assists with normalized performance omparisons. For seawater desalination the wide range nalyzers are used. For more information, see Application)ata Sheet C2 2217-ADS.

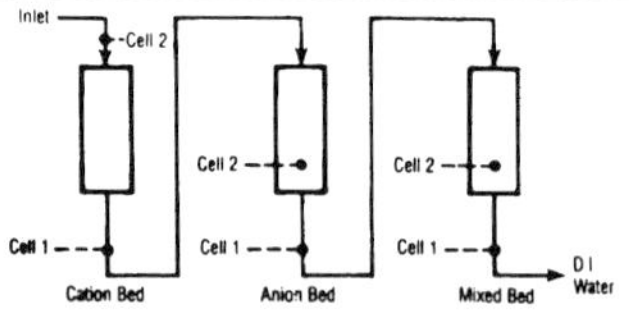

Ion exchange operations can achieve especially precise control using the conductivity ratio of two points with each bed. Ratio measurement accounts for feedwater variations when the upstream point is measured at the cation bed inlet. With the upstream point in the bed as shown for following stages, it can identify exhaustion before breakthrough. Concentration ranges of diluted acid and caustic used for regeneration are also available. For more information, see Application Data Sheet C2 2216-ADS.

Conductivity/Resistivity/TDS difference using redun-lant cells on critical processes can provide a valuable liagnostic capability. If the difference in measurements exeeds the alarm point, an operator is summoned for correcve action. Monitoring may be switched to the alternate cell luring maintenance. A different kind of diagnostic can be proided by a precision check resistor in place of one cell to give ontinuous analyzer checking at one value.

Another use of conductivity difference in water treatment ; to assure chemical delivery. The treatment chemical is in-ected into the process line between the cells. An increase in onductivity, regardless of background changes, can indicate 'roper treatment. For more information, see Application Data heet C2 2218-ADS.

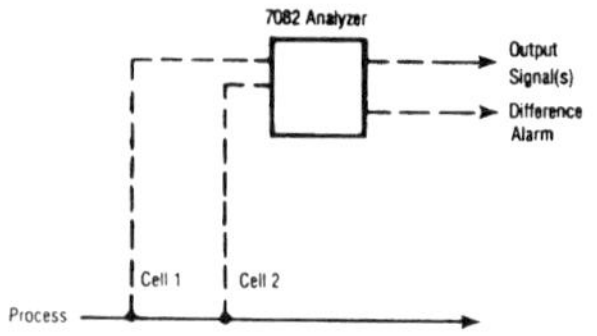

Figure 13-16. Versatility of two-cell conductivity analyzers.
Courtesy, Leeds & Northrup

defined SOP conditions sufficient to avoid impurity carryover by vapor entrainment. Some still manufacturers argue, therefore, that the validation of the still operation, given the proper feedwater quality, entails no more than the certainty that the established SOP is being adhered to. By the same token, using feedwater of the requisite quality, the SOP necessary to proper still operation can be defined by the still manufacturer in his factory.

Distillation is not an absolute method of effecting bacterial endotoxin removal; instead, a certain log reduction is accomplished, depending upon the still, but more especially upon the mode of its operation. What is required, therefore, is to ascertain by LAL analysis that the feedwater to the still is sufficiently low in endotoxin content to ensure that the product water emanating from the still will not exceed 0.25 EU/mL, or whatever standard is set for the operation. To validate that this purported goal is reached, LAL testing of the distilled water is required.

While distillation operation almost invariably will include the use of an on-line conductivity meter, it should be emphasized that readings from that meter do not reflect on the presence or absence of microbes or of bacterial endotoxins in the water. In any case, where the waters are as pure as they should be on both entering and exiting the still, their electrical resistivities (the reciprocal of conductivity) should show no difference.

The distilling process is often the last unit process in the water purification train. Its feedwater is, therefore, usually very pure. Indeed, Kuhlman (1995) advocates that multieffect stills use feedwaters of 1-megohm-cm resistivity and that they be free of chlorine and chloride ions; that they contain not more that 1 ppm of silica; and that they contain no amines, for these have volatilities so like that of water as to be inseparable by distillation. No TOC content is specified. Water of that purity can be utilized at the still factory in order to develop the SOPs necessary to define its proper operational conditions before the still is shipped. These SOP will preclude misting, flooding of the still, and corrosive and scaling influences. The observance of the defined SOPs in the water pretreatment would, in this view, constitute the validation of the distilling process. This approach to the validation of the still operation is not at all prevalent in the industry. It is expected that validation of the still operation will be performed in the pharmaceutical water production setting.

There is a competition among the various still manufacturers regarding the most suitable type of still. It is more costly to prepare purer feedwaters. Thus, an advantage of the vapor compression still may be its operation on softened water, as against the need for 1-megohm-cm feedwater for the multieffect stills. This is said to be possible because of the vapor compression still's lower operation temperature. It is fair to add, however, that the marketing of such stills may sometimes be advanced competitively on the basis that less pure, and therefore less expensive, waters are adequate for their operation.

The question raised is whether less pure feedwaters do not eventually manifest operational and/or maintenance problems. The purity of the feedwater may define the frequency at which periodic cleanings and descalings will be required. (Blowdowns are now continuous in most stills). The validation requirements in such cases can only be set forth in accordance with the particular operation and the purity of its feedwater.

The distilled water should be free of organisms. This condition can be validated by employing microbiological assays. Even were the still, in a down condition, to acquire organisms and spores, then in its operation (while being brought up to temperature and maintained for 2 hours or so at the elevated temperature before product water is collected), these foreign entities should become killed or removed by flushing. The microbiological testing of the stored distilled water should be performed routinely.

Ozone. The validation of the ozone operation involves the regulation of the production of the gas, and of its introduction into the water by way of a contactor. The control of these two activities governs the concentration of the ozone in the water, as measured by an ozone analyzer. The almost universal application of ozone is for the destruction of organisms, (although it can serve also oxidatively to degrade TOC). It would seem, therefore, that the validation of its function would entail microbiological work. Yet, so certain is the destructive action of ozone on microbes that the expected end is often assumed, provided that the ozone concentration sought is assured by measurement. Confirmatory microbiological analysis should be performed.

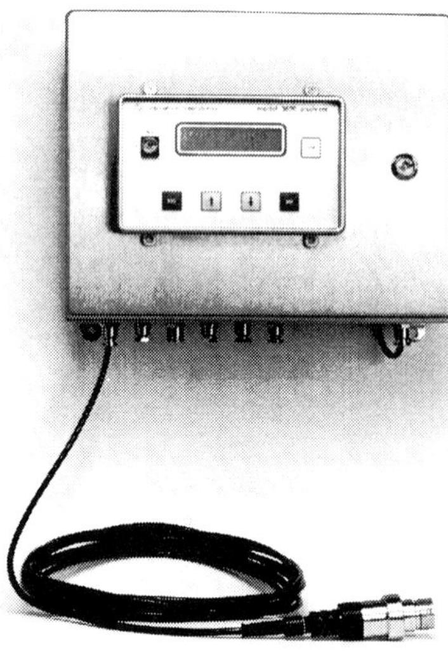

Figure 13-17. Ozone analyzer.
Courtesy Orbisphere.

Ozone can be prepared by corona discharge using oxygen, or air as the source of oxygen. Although the latter is sometimes done for economy's sake, complications are caused by the presence of humidity. Moreover, the nitrogen of the air generates oxides of nitrogen. These give rise to acidic components with unacceptable consequences to the pH of the water. Therefore the generation of ozone from air is seldom, if ever, used in the pharmaceutical industry.

When the ozone is electrolytically prepared, as by the Membrel process, no gas flow is involved. The monitoring of the ozone concentration and its maintenance at a given level are then straightforward. When ozone is prepared from oxygen (e.g., as fed by a swing generator) the purity of the oxygen can be ascertained by analysis. When this is held constant, a constant ozone concentration is ensured by the measurement of three factors: the gas pressure, the gas flowrate, and the electric current being supplied to the ozone cell. The ozone production can be varied by changing the current. Keeping the ozone concentration constant may require adjustments to the current. This can be signaled and controlled by a dissolved-ozone monitor. Changes in the purity of the feedwater may lead to different rates of ozone consumption. It is this that may cause variations in the residual ozone concentration. Therefore, the cleaner the water the better.

An on-line analyzer can be used to measure the ozone concentration. Analog signals can be used to provide continuous recordings of the ozone concentration.

Where the water is very clean, one can relate the ozone function to the residual ozone concentration. When, however, the water contains entities that can foul the analytical probe, that relationship becomes uncertain. One way of addressing the problem is to feed enough ozone to make sure that a residual is present in the off-gases, and to relate that ozone concentration to the function sought.

On-line ozone analyzers or monitors can operate in a number of ways. In clear water systems, double-beam ultraviolet spectroscopy is very satisfactory. Alternatively, amperometric determinations can be made using probes that are shielded against fouling by membranes selective for ozone penetration. A third method for analyzing for the ozone concentration is to sparge the sample with nitrogen gas to strip the ozone into the gas phase wherein it can be detected by means such as spectroscopy. Wet chemistry involving colorimetry based on dye loss can serve as an analytical backup method. Figure 13-17 depicts a residual-ozone analyzer.

In some biotechnology operations, where the drug product is extremely costly, the possible degradative effects of ozone concentrations even below detectable levels may raise concerns and insecurities. In one such operation, in an ultraconservative approach to the removal of ozone, an eastern pharmaceutical manufacturer employs two ozone-destruct units in series. The reading of zero ozone by the ozone monitor is not totally relied upon. Therefore, the compatibility of the processed water with the product is monitored very carefully.

Ultraviolet installations. The validation of the UV light units consists of two distinct activities. In the first, the UV lamp manufacturers seek to make constant and sufficient the wavelength and radiation outputs of the UV lamps. In the second, the user has the obligation to ascertain that the SOPs defined experimentally to ensure proper UV action are conformed with in practice.

It is necessary that the UV radiation be supplied in its proper dosage. The UV lamp outputs, initially high, decrease during the first 2 days or so of use. Some

UV lamp suppliers, therefore, recalibrate their lamps after 100 hours of use, when the output decline had leveled off to a relatively constant value. Continuous-intensity meters based on recordings of the voltage across the lamp are available. Lamp-out alerts are available; unsatisfactory lamps send a signal indicating same. A fixture is available whereby each individual lamp, as from a multilamp arrangement, upon removal from the unit, can be inserted into a test device to have its intensity measured.

The ultimate validation of the UV unit devolves upon the user. The user must be depended upon to ensure that the water being treated is sufficiently free of radiation-attenuating particles, as by turbidity measurements; and of UV-adsorbing entities, as by chemical analysis, in accord with the SOP established for the UV operation.

By the use of test ports, water samples can be withdrawn to assess whether the purported organism reductions expected from the UV instrument were actually attained. Before and after the water is treated by the UV light, microbiological analyses are central to the validation effort.

The UV devices are not absolute in their killing of organisms. Their contribution to the water purification system could be the reduction of the microbial content by 1, 2, or 3 logs, or to some particular level, say 100 cfu/mL. The validation of their designed action could then be had by appropriate microbiological testing.

The normal maintenance of the ultraviolet lamps would entail periodic replacements, perhaps at yearly intervals, or whenever the need to do so is indicated by the on-line intensity meters whose presence is required. The periodic wiping of the sleeves to remove radiation-attenuating film also requires periodic performance in keeping with the SOP experimentally defined for this purpose.

The validation methodologies appropriate to other units, devices, and portions of the water purification system should by now be apparent. The validation consists of answering such questions as to why the arrangement is present in the system, what its purported function is, and whether the performance standard set for it is being met. The operational concerns relevant to other appurtenances, such as chemical additions, iron and manganese removal, and their maintenance, should be forthcoming from the technical information available on these subjects.

Filter validations. The subject of filter validation is one of complexity caused in no small part by the lack of agreement among filter manufacturers regarding the proper way to conduct integrity testing. It is certain that filters require being integrity-tested periodically, particularly upon being newly installed, and also on some fixed schedule of a frequency that should be keyed to the potentials for problems. Microporous filters are traditionally replaced, not cleaned and reused.

Filter changeouts are to be justified by pertinent data.

An exception is made regarding filter refurbishing and reuse in the case of air filters whose use, even over prolonged periods, leaves their capacities so little impaired that their frequent replacement, however justifiable on the grounds of avoiding cross-contamination, would be judged economically wasteful. In these instances, however, it is necessary periodically to retest them for their integrity. This is most conveniently done on-line, as by use of the water intrusion test method.

It is questionable whether RO units or ultrafilters can be integrity-tested, at least in any way practical to their reuse. They cannot be integrity-tested as regards their retention of microbes. Ultrafilters may have as their function the reduction of microbial counts, of particle numbers, and of bacterial endotoxin levels. Their performances and validations can be judged accordingly. Ultrafilters should be cleaned and sanitized on a monthly schedule, the latter using a 1% or so solution of peracetic acid to keep the cfu/mL level at or below 10. This should be ascertained by weekly microbiological analyses.

Considerations for the cleaning, refurbishing, and replacing of membranes of these types are to be defined, as also their periodic sanitizations. Careful inspection of O-rings for possible replacement should be made. This should be done at every installation of a filter.

However, as regards the validation of specific filter functions, there need be no doubts. Analytical measurements are made, upstream of the filter and down, to gauge whether the filter has performed to the standard set for it. Bacterial endotoxin elimination can be assessed by LAL testing; organism reductions or sterilizations involve microbiological investigations; and the retention of sand, carbon, and resin fines, to the degree designed for, can be validated by the use of particle counters.

Flowrates, pressures, temperatures. The various deep beds, such as those constructed of multimedia, activated carbon particles, resin beds, and depth filters, will have been sized to yield particular flowrates in conjunction with their purification activities. Whether these intended functions are indeed achieved may depend upon adequate flowrates as defined in the operational SOP. These, in turn, are consequences of specific pressure levels and bed dimensions. Too-rapid flows may detract from exchange or adsorptive efficiencies. Too diminutive a flowrate may cause channeling and other improper water distribution problems within the bed, and the overloading of localized areas.

All of the unit operations require certain permissible ranges of flowrates in order to be effective. This includes water softening, ultraviolet effects, and ozone applications, in addition to those of the deep-bed varieties. Certainly, ion exchange and reverse osmosis require given flowrates for optimal performances. Temperature is also often of significant influence in a given unit process, particularly for reverse osmosis. However these operational factors are defined in the SOPs that govern the purification operations, their proper observance forms part of the validation operation.

Therefore, the validation exercise, aided by testing equipment such as flowmeters, pressure gauges, and thermometers, must ascertain that the flows, pressures, and temperatures defined as necessary in the SOPs are indeed adhered to in the actual operation. Figure 13-18 illustrates the use of analytical measurements in pharmaceutical water treatment.

Municipally treated feedwater. It may not be amiss to say a word about the water supply coming into the plant. It is generally considered advantageous to be able to use a water that comes from a municipally treated source. After all, it has already been brought to potable water quality, as is necessitated for the starting waters of all pharmaceutical water manufacture. No doubt that is the case in most situations.

It is, however, possible in some instances that problems inhere in the municipally treated waters. Such sources may contain quantities of aluminum ions from excessive alum treatments that, health implications aside, may contribute to the fouling of RO membranes. Iron fouling may come about where ferric chloride is used as the coagulating agent in place of alum. The very use of chlorine, in conjunction with TOC, can create the difficult-to-remove trihalomethanes; and efforts to avoid that situation by the neutralization of the chlorine with ammonia lead to the generation of the chloramines that, their bactericidal properties aside, are objectionable in their own right. In such instances, the municipal water supply is not an unmixed blessing. Perhaps most important of all, as has already been alluded to, where the municipal water source changes in its quality over relatively brief periods of time, validation can be a problem.

For operational systems, Zoccolante (1995) recommends that the feedwater be tested weekly for its chlorine content, to be maintained at 0.1 to 1 ppm, enough to keep the organism levels at lower than 100 cfu/ml; and that the microbiological testing also be performed weekly. Conductivity measurements carried out weekly should give values not exceeding 1,000 μS/cm. The pH range should be from 6 to 8 as determined weekly. Monthly examinations should be made for TOC, (to be kept under 3 ppm), and for the silt density index (to be kept under 6 to 20). A full analysis of the feedwaters should simultaneously be made to ascertain that their quality accords with the EPA guidelines for drinking water.

Batched water supplies. The use of batched water supplies is often considered advantageous. The water thus isolated in its storage can be characterized as fully as desired by pertinent analyses. The likelihood of its undergoing chemical change is remote. Its microbiological stability is less assured, depending upon the duration of the storage; but is subject to control, particularly where high temperature retentions or containment under ozone are involved. In essence, batched water can offer the security of a well-defined ingredient. Its promise is the constancy of its composition. The batching process, therefore, more easily lends itself to validations. By contrast, a system under continuous flow is not really defined by its characterization at any given point. The changes it may undergo are less certain to be detected and plotted with confidence.

Batch-style operations are expensive in terms of capital outlay and they are, therefore, justified only where the certainty of the batch water identity is required to ensure and protect a high product value. Batching operations are also demanding of careful design, in order to eliminate dead legs and to guarantee batch integrity. Where large volumes of water are involved, as for both rinse and product water, batching may involve storage in several very large tanks. These can be very expensive. At this point, continuous-flow systems become advantageous.

In continuous-operation designs, the necessary quantity of water is automatically maintained in the supply tank by the ongoing water production units. Artiss (1986) asserts that the piping requirements for continuous operation are simpler, and are less likely to introduce dead legs. Overall, the continuous-flow requirements prove less costly in terms of capital expenditures. In the need to try to keep constant the quality of an ever-flowing (and possibly ever-changing) water product, a greater reliance must, however, be placed on sophisticated purification units. By the same token, the insurance of system predictability and

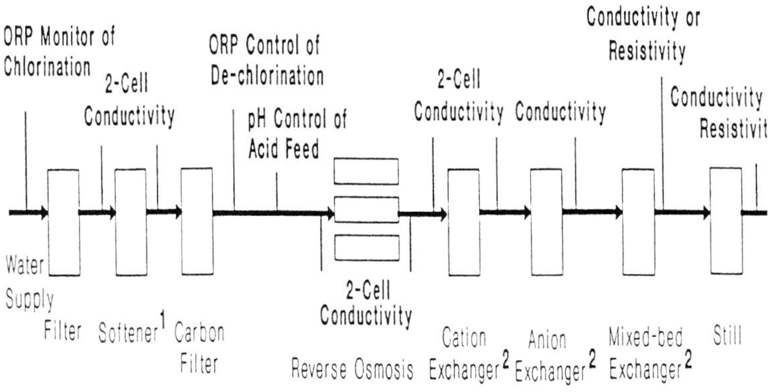

Figure 13-18. Analytical measurements for pharmaceutical water treatment. Stages are shown as examples only — a real system uses selected components depending on the type of water supply and the requirements of the treated water.

[1]Softener regeneration brine concentration is measured directly by wide-range conductivity.
[2]Deionizer regeneration acid and base concentrations are measured directly by wide-range conductivity.

of water quality constancy is more difficult to validate.

The Validation Exercise and Its Documentation

Documentation and information. As part of the validation requirements, a documentation and information master file will come to be established. It will include a full description of the system, specifying its acceptable ranges and levels. It will contain schematics of the electrical, mechanical, and water flow details. This will enable subsequent verification of the proper installation of the several purification units, of the control devices, of the safety and alarm systems, and of the provisions for instrument calibrations.

The documentation will list the activities necessary to the consistent production of the stipulated grade of pharmaceutical water. Perhaps the most important of these will the standard operating procedures that set forth in detail the measures required for the dependable production of waters of requisite quality. A subset of the SOPs that will come to be developed will be the standard maintenance procedures (SMPs) for the given water purification system. They will detail the replacements, regenerations, renewals, sanitizations, and maintenance operations that are necessary to extend the system's reliability. Another subset of the SOPs will set forth the procedures relative to sampling, testing, and equipment calibration. Documentation of all that is entailed is an important part of the validation exercise. It is the adherence to the pharmaceutical company's policy regarding validation, as set forth in the SOPs and their allied protocols and as revealed by the documented data and the conclusions drawn, that the FDA inspectors will investigate.

The documentation gathered during the validation process can be very substantial. Its management and control require considerable effort at organization. Included will be enumerations of equipment, instruments, material, and computer hardware, to name a few of the necessary lists. Angellucci (1995) offers the appended lists common to the concerns of validation documentation (Appendix A through G). The subjects covered range from critical instrument checklists to specifications involving flowrates and pipe diameters. Although not necessarily typical, some examples derived from pages of SOPs, SMPs, standard cleaning procedures, and system descriptions are presented in Tables 13-5 and 13-6. Each of the qualification steps, soon to be discussed, will variously include such items as equipment receipt verifications, installation verifications, calibration and instrument checks, and change-control related documents. The documentation will also include those items associated with vendor audits.

There are architectural and engineering firms and other consultant services that on the basis of long experience are competent to deal with the designing of plants and systems and with assembling and organizing the documentation in the form of validation control files. They and the equipment manufacturers can be counted upon to be helpful in collecting the information that should constitute the necessary documents for the Validation Plan. Inevitably, however, that file will bear the imprint of the individual water processor and must importantly reflect the operational knowledge gained from that company's particular proceeding.

Documentation is a Good Manufacturing Practices requirement. Extensive records are to be kept as a check on procedures. They constitute a paper trail of information demonstrating process control. This permits auditing of a company's practices.

The documentation aspect of the validation process is extremely important. A very large proportion of the FDA investigation is involved with the documentation. Documentations of the operations and of the results obtained are the only evidence that these activities have been performed. They are, therefore, the focus of FDA auditors during an inspection. Documentation enables an after-the-fact review of the validation process. Such retrospective examinations of the data permit an FDA auditor to judge the appropriateness of the procedures and of the conclusions reached. To enable this to be done, the raw recorded data and the written conclusions drawn by the system operators must be available in clear documented form for the FDA to examine.

Keer (1995) summarizes the documentation needs as follows:

Documentation of a water system is a continuous exercise that starts at the very beginning of the project and ends when the facility is closed. A systematic approach to the task will yield the proper documentation to give the Owner and Regulatory Authorities the confidence in the system's control. The Owner's objective is to meet all regulatory requirements in a cost effective manner. The regulatory agencies want to ensure there is no compromise or adulteration of products. Full and organized documentation satisfy the inspector's concern with minimal interruption to a facility's operation and at a small relative cost.

Tables 13-7 and 13-8 present Keer's views of certain basic design documentation desired, and of submittal documents to be supplied in conjunction with design operations.

The documentation requirements, as set forth by Artiss (1986) include the written validation procedures and protocols necessary for the dependable long-term operation of the water system, the written authorized approval of these, the written validation reports, and the relevant physical report forms.

It is possible, however, to be critical of certain current practices relevant to validation documentation. One authority states, "Some in the pharmaceutical industry believe that validation is a paper chase, that it is a costly endeavor providing little quality or value to the product or process." Indeed, the gathered documented information sometimes seems to have less bearing on controlling and maintaining quality processes than on recording serial numbers and pipe finishes. Validation involves more than documentation, whether as protocols or as checklists. Validation is intended to be a process whereby a company

Table 13-5
Validation Document--DI Water System

VALIDATION DOCUMENT			
Pharma-Renfrew Co. Parenterals Division Arlington, Virginia		Approved May 1, 1995	Section 9
Title: **Performance Qualification of the Deionized Water System** *Study Number:* 009 *Date Prepared:* April 15, 1995		Effective May 1, 1995	Page 8 of 82
Name-Title-Date	Name-Title-Date Countersigned	Name-Title-Date Quality Assurance	

9 PROCEDURE

SAFETY - Plant safety rules shall be strictly observed to prevent the possibility of injury, in particular all procedures contained in any appropriate Pharma Renfrew chemical handling instructions and Material Safety Data Sheet (MSDS).

9.1 General

The DI water produced and circulated throughout the facility will be tested for conformance to the acceptance criteria listed in this document. The initial, intense validation testing will consist of frequent sampling of water at various stages of the pretreatment and intermediate treatment process and sampling of each point use and sample port in all the loops at least twice a week for a five week period.

The pretreatment system is defined as the portion of the process from the incoming water through the Reverse Osmosis stage. The intermediate treatment system is defined as the process from the RO treated water feed to each loop through the final filters of the individual loops. Testing in these portions of the process is designed to determine proper performance of the elements of the pretreatment and intermediate treatment systems.

The testing program for the loops is designed to insure that the loop can maintain the requisite quality of water throughout the loop in a regular and consistent manner.

The testing program is defined in the *Sampling/Testing Schedules* below. All tests shall be conducted using the appropriate EPA or USP methodology, where such methodology exists. Acceptance criteria for each test is described in Section 18 of this document. Laboratory results of the testing will be appended to this document and entered on the Water Test Logs. (Attachment M)

9.2 Sampling Procedure

9.2.1 Prepare the required number of containers necessary for the scheduled water samples, insuring that each sample container is identified with the date, time, location, type of test(s) required, and person taking the sample.

9.2.2 For microbial samples, spray the port with a 70% isopropanol solution.

9.2.3 For microbial samples, wear latex gloves when handling sample containers.

9.2.4 For microbial samples, attach a length of sterile tubing to the port, if possible. In all cases, flush the port being sampled to drain for at least 3 minutes.

9.2.5 Collect the required quantity in the container insure the container is properly identified, and remove to testing laboratory.

Table 13-5
Validation Document--DI Water System (cont.)

VALIDATION DOCUMENT			
Pharma-Renfrew Co. Parenterals Division Arlington, Virginia *Title:* **Performance Qualification of the Deionized Water System** *Study Number:* 009 *Date Prepared:* April 15, 1995		Approved May 1, 1995 Effective May 1, 1995	Section 9 Page 9 of 82
Name-Title-Date	Name-Title-Date Countersigned	Name-Title-Date Quality Assurance	

9.3 Sampling Plan

9.3.1 Pretreatment
The pretreatment system will be sampled and tested as follows:

9.3.1.1 Feedwater from sample port, SP-01 will be sampled and tested for conformance to EPS drinking water standards once every two weeks.

9.3.1.2 Water from sample port, SP-02, after the Multimedia Filter, G-1, will be sampled and tested twice each week for particulate content.

9.3.1.3 Water from sample port, SP-03, after the Carbon Filter, G-2 will be sampled and tested twice each week for residual chlorine.

9.3.1.4 Water from sample port, SP-04, after the Softener, G-3, will be sampled and tested twice each week for residual hardness expressed as $CaC0_3$.

9.3.1.5 Water from sample port, SP-05, after the Reverse Osmosis, G-4, will be sampled and tested twice each week for microbial and chemical levels.

9.3.2 Manufacturing Intermediate Treatment
The Manufacturing intermediate treatment system will be sampled and tested as follows:

9.3.2.1 Feedwater to the Manufacturing intermediate treatment, sample port will be sampled and tested twice each week for microbial and chemical levels.

9.3.2.2 Water from the mixed bed bank, sample port, SP-06, will be sampled and tested twice each week for microbial and chemical levels, and resistivity/conductivity.

9.3.2.3 Loop supply to the Manufacturing loop, sample port, SP-07, will be sampled and tested twice each week for microbial and chemical levels.

9.3.3 R&D Facility Intermediate Treatment
The R&D Facility intermediate treatment system will be sampled and tested as follows:

9.3.3.1 Feedwater to the R&D Facility intermediate treatment, sample port, SP-08, will be sampled and tested twice each week for microbial and chemical levels.

Table 13-6
Standard Cleaning Procedure

STANDARD CLEANING PROCEDURE		
Agate-Biopharm-Arlington, Inc.	Procedure Number 001-064-10-14	Page of Pages 12 of 18
	Supersedes None Previous	Date Approved May 1, 1995
	Department Maintenance - Sub 2	Date Effective May 1, 1995

STANDARD CLEANING PROCEDURE FOR THE CARBON BED STEAMING IN PLACE

Name - Title - Date	Name - Title - Date	Quality Assurance (Name - Title - Date)

PURPOSE

The purpose of this document is to define the Standard Steaming in Place Cleaning Procedure for the carbon bed.

8. SCOPE

- Schedule
- Steam-In-Place

9. RESPONSIBILITY

It is the responsibility of the Maintenance - Sub 2 group to properly implement this Standard Cleaning Procedure.

10. PROCEDURE

A. Schedule.

1. This Standard Cleaning Procedure is to be performed at seven day intervals.

B. Steam-In-Place Procedure.

CAUTION: Before initiating this procedure, ensure the purified water storage tank is at a level of 0% or greater and the reverse osmosis unit is not operating. Turn off the reverse osmosis unit at Control Panel, EP-001-1

CAUTION: Record all necessary information on the Carbon Column SIP Log 6B6.

CAUTION: Ensure the Clean Steam Generator is operating as per Standard Operating Procedure for the Clean Steam Generator SOP 40-A,B, and C-1.

CAUTION: Signal the Carbon Bed to be hot, by hanging red tag.

1. Turn off Soft Water/Reverse Osmosis Recirculation Pump P-74-A at the local BB6 switch. Close discharge valve V-10-10B.

2. Open the following valves:

V-10-12-B (Softener feed to Deaerator)

Table 13-6
Standard Cleaning Procedure (cont.)

STANDARD CLEANING PROCEDURE FOR CARBON BED STEAMING IN PLACE	Procedure Number	Date Approved	Page of Page
	001-064-10-14	May 1, 1995	13 of 18

10. PROCEDURE (Cont'd)

B. Steam-In-Place Protocol (Cont.)

3. Close the following valves:
V-10-13 (Carbon Bed to Reverse Osmosis System), V-10-14 (Carbon Bed to Deaerator), (Softener to Carbon Bed).

4. Open vent valve 10-15 and valve V-12-2A and then drain valve V-10-18

Allow the carbon bed to drain completely.

5. Close valves V-10-15, V-10-18 and V-12-2A

6. Open valve V-10-20 to drain Soft Water Inlet Pipe. Close V-10-20 after drained.

7. Open the steam condensate valve V-10-23. Cautiously open the carbon bed clean steam supply valve V-10-26. Allow low pressure steam to enter the carbon bed. Monitor the carbon bed temperature at and the inlet steam pressure at PI-C-100 and PI-C-160.

NOTE: Steam pressure should not exceed 18 PSIG as indicated at PU-C-100. Manually regulate steam pressure at drain valve V-10-15.

8. When TI-A-01 reaches 65°C, close inlet steam valve V-10-26. Close V-10-15. The carbon bed should continue to heat to a temperature of 95 -115°C.

MAINTAIN THE CARBON BED AT >99°c FOR AT LEAST TWO HOURS.

CAUTION: **The carbon bed temperature must not exceed 120°C.**

9. Record the pressure at PI-C-100 and PI-C-160 and temperature at TI-A-01 every 30 minutes.

10. Connect a hose from the Clean Steam Line at valve V-10-201 to the R.O. Feed Line at valve V-10-167. Verify V-10-43 is closed and open V-10-32. (Both valves located on the R.O. skid) Open valves V-10-33 and V-10-34 located on the 5 micron filter housing. Open V-10-17-A.

11. After the required two-hour hold time, open the following valves: V-10-15, V-10-18. Open V-10-168 for five minutes. This will allow the carbon bed to cool before initiating the required backwash.

12. Monitor the temperature of the carbon bed at TI-A-01. When the temperature is 38° or lower, the backwash must be instituted. Refer to Standard Cleaning Procedure for the carbon column.

demonstrates and documents a mastery of its operations.

Meshnick (1995) has useful observations concerning general documentation procedures:
First, there should be a short discussion of how records and documents should be assembled and the data should be certified by the technicians.

One of the goals of the validation documents is to provide evidence of when, how, and by whom the work was performed, and a precise record of what results were obtained. In other words, what protocol procedures were intended to be done, what actions were actually performed, and why there is a difference (if there is): What results were obtained and what raw data support the results? To accomplish this documentation, it is a good practice to keep an accurate chronology of a project, and to follow standard GMP procedures for recording and counter signing of data. For example, the original recordings of data, even handwritten notes or calculations, should be kept, initialed and dated by the technician performing the work. Work should be recorded in ink, not pencil. Corrections to this information should be made by drawing a single line through the incorrect entry, and the correction dated and initialed. This information must be maintained as part of the final report.

Hand written notes and drawings are acceptable, but must be legible and signed. An investigator may request to see your original data, and typewritten observations were obviously not taken in the field. If a typewritten transcription of the observations is used, the final copy should be checked against the original to guarantee against transcription errors. Do not complete all the checks at the end of the day, or when the report is completed. Initial what you have verified, at the time you verify the work.

It is common practice, and regularly cited in audits, that criteria for tests are too general and not specific enough for the tests being performed. Statements such as "Ensure that the system is installed according to manufacturers specifications..." may sound sufficient, but these do not provide the specifics necessary to judge the effectiveness of the test. Make your statements clear, concise, and easily tested. Avoid broad and sweeping terms such as "performs as intended" or "surface appearances are good". Subjective, general evaluations such as these cannot be proven, and are not supportive of a qualified condition.

Validation steps. A sequence of steps is involved in the validation of the pharmaceutical water system. The definition and design of the total system, and hence of its constituting purification units or modules, comes first. The Design Qualifications of each separate unit are ascertained, to be succeeded by the Installation Qualification wherein the correct linking of the several purification units is made. Each of the linked modules is tested and challenged in an Operational Qualification that demonstrates its and the system's operational capability. The long-term suitability of the system's functioning, the establishing of its dependable reproducibility is attested to in the Performance or Process Qualification step that follows. Traditionally, these steps are identified as Design Qualification (DQ), Installation Qualification (IQ), Operational Qualification (OQ), and Process Qualification (PQ). Some groups add a Performance Qualification prior to the Process Qualification; others call the Process Qualification the Validation.

However performed, it is required that there be a logical progression of one qualification to another. For example, it is inappropriate to pursue a Process Qualification before completion of an Installation or Operational Qualification. If the system has not been properly installed and verified to operate over the

Table 13-7
Conceptual Design Documentation

	Document	*Preparation*	*Input*
1	Raw water sample	Operations	Design
2	Product water quality	Operations	Design, validation
3	Facility operation	Operations	Design, construction
4	Quantity	Operations	Design
5	Diversity	Operations	Design
6	Pressure/temperature	Operations	Design
7	Microbial control	Design	Operations, validation
8	Purification technology	Design	Operations, validation
9	Monitoring requirements	Validation	Corporate, design
10	Documentation for validation	Validation	Corporate, design
11	Design codes & standards	Corporate	Validation, operations, design
12	CGMPs	Validation	Design, operations
13	Budget	Corporate	Design, construction
14	Schedule	Corporate	Design, construction, validation
15	Environmental/safety	Operations	Design, corporate
16	Control philosophy	Operations	Design, validation, corporate
17	PFD/preliminary P&ID	Design	Operations, validation
18	General SOO	Design	Operations, validation
19	Symbols & abbreviations	Design	Operations, corporate
20	General equipment layout	Design	Operations
21	Calibration requirements	Validation	Design, contractor
22	Mechanical space limits	Operations	Design, construction
23	Documentation submittals	Validation	Design
24	Weld inspection requirements	Validation	Design, corporate
25	Installation requirements	Design	Validation, operations
26	Construction plan	Construction	Design, operations
27	Approved vendors	Design	Validation, operations
28	Bid package division	Design	Corporate, construction
29	Control philosophy/hierarchy	Operations	Design, corporate
30	General pipe routing	Design	Operations, construction
31	Materials of construction	Design	Operations, contractor
32	Cost estimate	Design	Corporate, operations
33	Calculations	Design	Operations, validation
34	Location of sample ports	Validation	Operations, corporate, design
35	Design review & approval	Corporate	Design, operations

required range of conditions, then water testing of the system PQ is not warranted. The final validated condition is a sum total of the preceding qualifications.

Control of the system's reliable operation is again required to be demonstrated following the implementation of alterations and changes that may be instituted from time to time. The question to be answered is whether the changes involved are substantive enough to significantly alter the quality of the product water. If so, revalidation is required. Change controls should indicate who made the decision, on what basis, and should amply justify that decision.

Validation sequence: *Design qualifications.* The design of the equipment constituting the water purification system obviously comes first. It derives from the requirements of the water purification process. With a pharmaceutical water system, this generally means that the quality of the water will minimally meet

Table 13-8
Detail Design Documents

	Document	*Preparation*	*Input*
36*	P&ID	Design	Validation, operations
37	Instrument loop diagrams	Design	Contractor, operations
38	Equipment data sheets	Design	Contractor, operations
39	Instrument data sheets	Design	Contractor, operations
40	Control panel face layout	Design	Contractor, operations
41	Control screen presentations	Design	Contractor, operations
42	Sequence of operation	Design	Contractor, operations
43	Pipe routing plans	Design	Contractor, operations
44	Pipe isometrics	Design	Contractor, operations
45	Skid pipe arrangement	Design	Contractor, operations
46	Junction box wiring	Design	Contractor, operations
47	Construction plan	Construction	Contractor, operations, design
48	Instrument/equipment/valve tag numbers	Design	Contractor, operations
49	Instrument list	Supplier	Design, operations
50	Equipment tag numbers	Operations	Design, supplier, validation
51	Valve tag numbers	Operations	Design, supplier, validation
52	Pressure-test procedure	Design	Contractor, operations
53	Flushing/cleaning procedure	Design	Contractor, operations
54	Passivation procedure	Design	Contractor, operations
55	Sanitization/sterile procedures	Design	Contractor, operations, validation
56	Software documentation	Design	Contractor, operations
57	Detailed specifications	Design	Validation, operations
58	Approval of specifications	Corporate	Validation, operations
59	Bid review report	Design	Operations, corporate

*The numbering in this table continues the document listing begun in Tables A and B of the first article in this series (1).

either USP Purified Water or Water for Injection specifications, depending on its usage. It is the design documents that set the standards and goals of the hardware.

Next, there should be a definition of the process capacities, such as the total volume needed per hour or day; the average consumption; the peak demand requirements; the reserve capacity; the minimum circulation needs; and whether elevated temperature storage is necessary. In other words, somewhere early on in the project, someone should write a functional definition of the project or process, so there is a clear understanding of how the system must perform. This document, after it has been approved by the responsible groups, becomes the basis of the system design.

The succeeding procedures and reports will then document how the manufacturing system was designed to address these requirements. This link between the intended purpose and the final design of the system is important. Too often, the qualification process begins with the system after it has been purchased, and there is no clear statement of user requirements. The enduser is ultimately required to provide the criteria to judge the system. Do not leave these to the system manufacturer or fabricator; what is important is not that a system meets an equipment manufacturer's specifications, but that what the vendor has provided meets the process requirements of the water preparer.

This functional definition is a valuable document for describing the system during an inspection, upgrading, or repair of the system; and especially for controlling the validated condition of the water system as part of a change-control procedure.

This functional design basis is easily included for new construction, but it is not so simple to obtain or develop with existing water systems. Still, some description of the construction and design of the system must be committed to paper for an existing water system. This is important for future reference, especially to individuals who may not have been involved with the validation, but who may have to redesign and revalidate at a later date. It is especially useful to someone who may have to explain the design and validation during an inspection 5 years later. It is difficult to defend a report or procedure without a clear statement of the design basis and functional goals.

There are, regretfully, no meaningful design or construction standards presently used for water production in the drug industry. All too often, the information and recommendations forthcoming from equipment suppliers must be relied upon. These are necessarily leveled to their own expertise and are not always objective.

The critical considerations of operational suitability, microbial control, and adherence to regulatory needs should first be set forth. The engineering design should then be formulated to meet these needs. Therefore the Design Qualification should, from the onset, include the participation of all appropriate groups, such as engineering design, production operations, quality assurance, and analytical services. The need for a team approach is necessitated by the complexity of the undertaking. Materials selection, equipment suitability, operational controls, construction techniques, cleaning and sanitization procedures, component compatibility, preventive maintenance, sterilization programs, sampling, and regulatory requirements are all involved. It is essential that an adequate address to all these considerations be "designed into the system." Where an insufficiency of guidance from other disciplines is involved, "add-ons" usually eventuate in an effort to correct an inadequate system design.

Indeed, the appropriate group to consider the design qualifications can usefully be expanded to include the eventual users, representatives of technology development services, informational systems facilities, and system analysts, as well as consultants and vendors. Inclusion of the vendors will facilitate the vendor/user relationship, enabling vendors to better serve user needs.

Even before the validation exercise begins, a description and print of the entire system, from start to finish, must be available. This should also make plain the location of the sampling ports. This will set forth the process and equipment design, of which the purpose is the achievement of consistent product water specifications.

The Design Qualification will list the activities necessary to the consistent production of the stipulated grade of water. It will contain a full description of the system, specifying its acceptable operating ranges and levels. It will supply full schematics of the electrical, mechanical, and water flows for subsequent verification of their proper installation. It will identify the specific purification units, the various control devices, and the safety and alarm systems. It will also provide for the calibration of critical instruments. The Design Qualification will also set the microbial action and alert levels, will specify sampling plans and ports for chemical and microbial testing, will stipulate sanitizing methods, and will define procedures for the analysis and plotting of data.

Artiss (1978) stated that the basic design package should include the following:

1. Flow schematics for the proposed water system showing all of the instrumentation, controls and valves necessary to operate, monitor, and sterilize the system. All major valves and components should be numbered for reference.

2. A complete description of the features and function of the system. This is of critical importance to enable production and quality assurance personnel, who may be unfamiliar with engineering terminology, to fully understand the manner in which the system is to be designed, built, operated, monitored, and sterilized.

3. Detailed specifications for the equipment to be used for water treatment and

pretreatment.

4. Detailed specifications for all other system components such as storage tanks, heat exchangers, pumps, valves, and piping components.

5. Detailed specifications for sanitary system controls and a description of their operation.

6. Specifications for construction techniques to be employed where quality is of critical importance. These techniques should be suitable for exacting sanitary applications.

7. Procedures for cleaning the system, both after construction and on a routine basis.

8. Preliminary SOP's for operating, sampling, and sterilization. These procedures will be cross referenced to the valve and component numbers on the system schematics.

9. Preliminary SOP's for filter replacement, integrity testing, and maintenance.

10. Preliminary sampling procedures to monitor both water quality and the operation of the equipment.

11. Preliminary system certification procedures.

12. Preliminary preventive maintenance procedures.

The design package should be as complete as possible to enable all disciplines involved to understand what the final system will entail.

Validation plan. As stated above, the functional definition is often included as part of a Validation Plan. This document is not a requirement of the FDA, but it has become almost an industry standard. The FDA will perform an in-depth evaluation of the validation data because without a Validation Plan a firm is more likely to overlook some required activity. It is a good idea to include such a document as part of the validation, as it sets the overall goals and levels that will be followed during the validation, and can be referred to throughout the project, but especially much later, well after the study has been completed. As a reference document, the plan permits a reviewer immediately to understand the scope of the validation, and to ensure that all parts of the system are validated.

The Validation Plan will set forth the facility organization responsible for the activity. It will define the responsibilities; make plain the available resources and scheduling; and specify the tools, techniques, and methodologies to be employed in the task (Johnson, 1993).

The Validation Plan should contain all the information relevant to the water system. It will be a repository for the basic design information, drawings, specifications, procedures and protocols. It will state the reasons for equipment selection, for cleaning and sanitization frequencies, and for component replacements and renewals. It will contain the records for equipment modification and of procedural alterations. It will have the equipment and filter logs, and any recertification data. In short, it will constitute the major reference file for the entire water production system. As such it will serve internal investigatory purposes, and will form the basis for outside regulatory reviews. It is, therefore, critical that the Validation Plan be carefully controlled as part of a change-control or overall quality system.

The Validation Plan may also have its counterpart as a Validation File or Master File. (The term *Master File* should not be confused with the various Master Files made use of by the FDA.) Meshnick (1995) sees a difference between a Master File and the Validation Plan. The Master File is readily accessible. It is under a liberal control, permitting easy modification of the change-control system. It is readily available to personnel such as maintenance and the engineering staff without the strict control accorded the Validation Plan. In consequence, the Master File may too often be in an incomplete status: Drawings may be on an engineer's desk, manuals may vanish. The Master File is a useful concept, but can too often be out of control. By contrast, the Validation Plan or the Master File for the Validated System must be strictly controlled, as by the manager of the change-control activities or by someone with QC or GMP responsibility.

The Validation Plan is used to set the levels of the validation: to define the scope of the project, the systems included and not included in the qualifications, and what the project will attempt to prove. For example, if the project includes the use of deionized water to feed a clean-steam generator, the Validation Plan would define which components would be involved in the preparation of such a water; what general quality attributes each purification unit would be expected to achieve; and the length of time the system will undergo sampling and at what frequency. Issues involving choices should be addressed in the Validation Plan, including the reasons for the choices. It must be made apparent why the selected decisions are appropriate. The Validation Plan must be consistent with the company QC policies, and with previous projects.

Such a Validation Plan will be much appreciated when the validation is reviewed at a later date, as in response to an out-of-tolerance condition, in a quality audit setting, or during performance of a revalidation.

Installation qualification. The Installation Qualification is usually the first validation document that is prepared. It will consist of a System Description followed by a Procedures Section. Before the operational characteristics of the system can be investigated, the proper installation and assembly of the various items of equipment require verification. This follows a careful check that each piece of equipment ordered and received is identical to that stipulated in the system design. All the critical features of the several items and their installation must conform to the written and approved specifications. As sagely advised by Artiss (1978): "Consideration should be given to conducting an inspection of the equipment before it is shipped from the supplier. Features of operational function and compliance with specifications can be verified and any deviations can be corrected without incurring the cost and time delay of reshipment."

The Installation Qualification ascertains that all of the unit components are installed as per specifications and according to the design drawings. It provides a construction verification in that the established specifications have been complied with. This also involves instrument connections. Included in this operation are such items as a review of Process and Instrumentation Drawings (P&ID) and isometric representations, verification of materials of construction, examination and documentation of welds, inspections for dead legs and for correct pipe slopes, and verification of stainless steel passivation. The Installation Qualification confirms the "as built" drawings, and ensures the suitability of the completed system. The absence of leaks, which may provide pathways for invading organisms, can be ensured by vacuum testing, or by the use of pressurized air or water.

As stated in the FDA Guidelines (1987), "This phase of validation includes examination of equipment design; determination of calibrations, maintenance, and adjustment requirements; and identifying critical equipment features that could affect the process and product. Information obtained from these studies should be used to establish written procedures covering equipment calibration, maintenance, monitoring, and control."

The first step in the Installation Qualification should be a detailed description of the water purification system. This will constitute the System Description.

This is to be followed by a Procedure Section, setting forth a plan on how to proceed in performing what is specifically required. The protocol should define the procedures to be performed, the documents to be assembled, and the items to be checked and verified. The plan thus set forth is to be approved before the qualification work begins. Subsequent changes may become indicated. These will require being quantified, recorded, and approved in the final report.

The Installation Qualification Procedures are generally in the form of check sheets that verify components or details critical to the validated condition of the equipment. Confirmation of design items such as materials of construction, surface finishes, weld mapping and inspection documents, major equipment inventories (such as pumps, filters, UV lights, and control valves), process instrument lists, and utility connections (including drains) define the system as installed.

In developing these IQ check sheets, individual components must first be identified, as in the System Description or in a comprehensive equipment listing. Vital characteristics, necessary to the proper operation of the components, are included, along with the specific criteria that must be met. Spaces must be provided for the verification of each item with the date and the initials of the individual checking.

A requirement of validation is that there be specific acceptance criteria, set prior to beginning the qualification. The raw data gathered as part of the verification must be included as part of the final report, along with a description of the procedures used during the check. There should especially be space provided for any actions or corrections taken to address out-of-specification results.

These check sheets should be prepared with the intent of being taken into the field and completed as the work is performed. If raw data are recorded on separate sheets, these must be included with the completed checklists.

Process and Instrumentation Drawings (P&IDs) are ideal documents for providing a clear description of where critical instrumentation and major system components are located. "As built" construction drawings showing features such as actual measured piping layouts, filter locations, sampling stations, an absence of dead legs, and pipe pitches are necessary as verification of how these critical items are installed. A common practice is to initial the drawings along with the date as a component is verified. Any notes or comments regarding the verification should be recorded right on the drawing, or attached and referenced.

Areas that are often overlooked during Installation Qualification are items that are generally contracted to service groups. Cleaning and passivation documents, especially the procedures, types, and concentrations of acids and neutralizers and also the pH results of the various rinses are often neglected. Request these items beforehand, and make sure they are signed and dated by the technicians performing the work. This is especially important for documents such as weld certifications, where quality procedures are sometimes lax. Make sure the welders will document the welds as they are made, not at the end of the day or the end of the project. The purpose of the inspections and verification is to insure careful, precise welds.

The actual construction techniques used for system installation should be carefully monitored to ensure compliance with the written specifications.

The Installation Qualification should be well documented with regard to its flow of logic. This can prove critical to change control, serving as a basis upon which subsequent changes to the water purification system can be explained and justified.

Instruments and controls. Items that fall between the Installation Qualification and the Operational Qualification are the instrumentation and control systems. These two groups contain issues that could be included in either or both qualifications.

The first step in qualifying instruments and controls is to make a list of all system instruments. This must be available for inclusion as part of the Installation Qualification. Such a comprehensive list should be available as part of the P&ID. At this point, determinations must be made to class each instrument as either critical or noncritical to the process.

Critical instrumentation (needed for direct process control and monitoring/recording) will require periodic calibration under CFR21, section 211.68 and 211.160 of the GMPs. These calibrations must be traceable to a recognized standards organization such as the National Institute for Standards and Technology (NIST). Critical instruments include such items as temperature-controlling resistance temperature detectors (RTDs), tank-level sensors, resistivity meters and controls, chart recorders that provide documents for monitoring records, and flowmeters used to control resin bed regeneration. Procedures must be available for the calibration of these instruments, including the method of calibration, the range and accuracy of the instruments, and an appropriate schedule for performing these calibrations. Records of the results of these calibrations must be kept in order to comply with the GMPs. Instrument identification numbers and a sticker indicating date of calibration and the date of next calibration must be clearly visible on all critical instruments.

Noncritical instruments, such as instrument air regulator gauges, or redundant pressure or temperature instruments, do not need rigorous calibration schedules. Noncritical instruments must still be identified, however, and logged into a calibration program. There must be a clear identification on such an instrument that it is not used for process control.

Instruments and controls require careful installation and identification. Generally, on new systems, the instruments should be left uninstalled until the majority of the heavy construction has been completed. Wiring, instrument air lines and supplies, and transmitters can be checked and verified for proper installation, but instrument calibration and tuning of controls should be left for the end of the construction process. For this reason, some companies like to postpone these installations and include these functions in the Operational Qualifications.

Calibration of instrumentation can be performed either at the end of the Installation Qualification, and recorded as part of the IQ; or at the beginning of the Operational Qualification. Either way, before operational testing is begun, all system instruments must be verified as calibrated.

When completed, this information is included not only as part of the qualification package, but also as the company's Metrology, or Instrumentation Program. This ongoing program is to ensure that the controls and recordings from the system will continuously be accurate and reliable. In it are documented calibration procedures, schedules, calibration results, and responses to out-of-specification calibrations.

Operational qualification. The installation of the equipment assemblage having been verified as being correct, it becomes possible to undertake the Operational Qualification of the system. The system should be carefully cleaned and all construction debris removed to minimize any chance of contamination or corrosion. Passivation should follow the cleaning. Verification of passivation should then be made. Cleaning and passivation should be the last steps of the IQ or alternatively, the first steps of the Operational Qualification. Once the cleaning and passivation have been completed, the equipment should be started up and carefully checked for proper operation. The purpose is to demonstrate that each component of the system functions throughout all the anticipated operating ranges. The Operational or Equipment Qualification of the water purification system assumes that there are defined acceptable product specifications.

The specific considerations involved in the Operational Qualifications of the various purification units have been detailed in this chapter.

Operational Qualification verifies the capability of the processing equipment to perform satisfactorily within operational levels. Considerations of feedwater quality, system capacity, temperature controls, and flowrates are involved in the Operational Qualification of the water purification process. It involves an examination of the equipment design to identify features critical to the process and product. The goal of the Operational Qualification is to evaluate the levels of control within which the validated system is expected to perform. One seeks information to evaluate changes to the operation. The focus is on defining the critical items and practices. Alarm conditions for utilities such as low steam pressure or instrument air; diverter conditions resulting from low condensate resistivity; differential pressure levels, high or low; all are just several examples of events that should be confirmed as functioning correctly.

In this operation, reliance solely upon information from the equipment supplier is inappropriate. However, the manuals relating to each piece of equipment are parts of the documentation. The calibration needs are determined for each unit. A review is made of the maintenance and adjustment procedures. Post-repair and calibration requirements are stipulated in advance to avoid confusion following emergency repairs. An emphasis is placed on the avoidance of improper product quality caused by the use of incorrect parts and/or procedures. Documented procedures are developed regarding the maintenance, adjustment, calibration, monitoring, and control of the equipment involved. The support systems, such as the instrument calibration programs, are addressed.

The protocol should begin with an introduction and then a description section, this time describing the operations of the system. This will entail repeating what may already have been written previously. Meshnick (1995) has the following to say regarding repeated material or references thereto:

Some may think that it is much easier to simply add references to reports, allowing the reader to access procedures or design information from other protocols or SOP's. While there is no set format as to how to reference other documents, this should be carefully considered, since this practice guides a reviewer into other documents that may not be the focus of his interest, and will generally confuse the audit. If it is an item specific to the Qualification, then include it. Better to repeat the information at the point required, than trek over the entire paper trail. Also, it is important that any documents which are subject to updating and revision, such as general procedures or protocols, be included or referred to as the official revision number in effect when the study was conducted.

Subsequent to writing the Operational Qualification requirements and procedures, the specific acceptance criteria are to be set forth. It is by way of these that the system's results will be judged. The specifying of the acceptance criteria is key to the protocol development effort. It defines the bounds within which the system is to be controlled. What are required are acceptance criteria that, while they challenge the system, are appropriate to the system's operation. Exaggerated standards are unnecessary. However, the criteria that are set must adequately assure the proper product-water quality. The system's specifications should be precisely defined and adequate for its operation.

As Artiss (1978) cautions, "A sufficient number of cycles of operation, batch changeover and sterilization should be conducted to ensure that the design objectives have been satisfied as far as the Operational Qualifications of each purification unit are concerned. The preliminary procedures for operation and sterilization should be reviewed and modified as necessary to suit the physical configuration of the completed installation."

The Operational Qualification provides a functional testing of the system components. The Operational Qualification of each purification unit leads to the Performance Qualification of the system as a whole.

Performance Qualification. The purpose of the Performance Qualification is to provide rigorous testing to demonstrate the effectiveness and reproducibility of the total integrated process. This results in a documentation of the system's consistent performance as designed and operated. The system's setpoints, control sequences, and operating parameters are probed. All the acceptance criteria are to be met under the worst-case process conditions. Where failures occur, they should be identified and corrected. Tests should be rerun to vouch for the elimination of the causes of failure. Consistency of acceptable product water quality is sought. Documentation of every operation involved in securing same is necessitated.

The performance verification ensures the suitability of the system's function. The proper operation of the system's equipment and controls should lead to a repeatability in the system's characteristics, and in the product it produces. This is established by repeated start-ups and shutdowns, simulating manual, automated, and emergency conditions. In the process of so doing, operational SOPs are confirmed and protocols for operations are finalized. The goal is to achieve the production of a dependable product in a continuous mode. A procedural verification of the written SOPs is sought. The levels of the product quality are explored by sampling and by the analytical testing, chiefly of its electrical resistivity, its TOC content, and its bacterial and endotoxin levels. Long-term trends and evaluation are explored. The general strategy of how the process is challenged should be a part of the Validation Plan, and the PQ protocol should elaborate on the specifics of the program.

As will be seen, the customary plan of the PQ would include an intensive pattern of sampling for a relatively short time, 1 or 2 months, while the system is operated under normal conditions. As much information as possible concerning operating conditions should be gathered during this phase. Some firms attempt to challenge the system to the levels of the operating ranges during this testing, while others run the system as close to the center of the operating ranges as possible. Both have their merits; however, challenging the levels may have detrimental effects to the study, such as random failures; and certainly presents difficulties in determining which combination of variables would represent the most appropriate challenges. Thus, it is easier to run under conditions that represent the normal system. The water produced by the system may be used, provided this intensive period of investigation so indicates.

After the intensive monitoring phase has been successfully completed, the system should undergo a long-term evaluation, for perhaps a year or more. The system is considered qualified based upon the data from the first phase of monitoring; but because of time-dependent effects, such as the variability of feedwater supply, the effects of wear or deterioration of components such as UV lights, and the ability of organisms to adapt to harsh conditions, longer-term evaluation is appropriate before a system is considered validated.

The developed program should be described in the Validation Plan, and detailed in the Process Qualification protocol. If a two-phase (or longer) program is implemented, the data review and summary reports must be approved when each phase is completed. Do not wait until the end of an extended monitoring program before determining the validated condition of the system, especially if the water is being used.

A smoothly operating water system may undergo departures for reasons other than alterations in its water supply. Time-dependent changes are involved. These are to be elucidated, defined, and documented. Given purification units such as ion-exchange beds may become exhausted; RO membranes will come to require cleaning; tanks and pipes may need sanitizations. In general, the devices and accouterments constituting the system will periodically require such maintenance-related activities as replenishment, refurbishing, cleaning, sanitization, replacements, and renewals of different kinds. Furthermore, the various items will require attention on different time schedules. The necessary system documentation will, therefore, also include a body of information relating to the proper maintenance of each piece of equipment. Much of this will be forthcoming from the equipment suppliers and may, indeed, constitute stipulations connected with their guarantees of equipment performance. The relevant documentation composes the standard maintenance procedures necessary to the system's correct handling.

On a timeline basis, the Installation Qualification and Operational Qualification of the system are performed parallel to the installation of the purification and ancillary equipment and to the preparation of the product water (Figure 13-19). This leads to the commissioning of the system, and to the qualification of its performance. As will be seen, the validation exercise can be divided into three phases. On the timeline basis, the system's start-up overlaps both the Operational Qualification and the prospective performance phase of the validation. The system's performance parallels the concurrent and retrospective phases. Another view of the overall purification process is shown in Figure 13-20. A review of the entire operation should be performed at least annually to ensure the ongoing appropriateness of the product water and operational specifications; and the system must be revalidated after any significant system design, mechanical, or operational change.

Qualification/validation final reports. Once the validation has been planned, the design documented, the procedures written and then executed, and the data collected, the last and the most important step of the process is the evaluation and reporting of the study.

Meshnick (1995) advises as follows:

The final report is your opportunity to focus the study. It is where you describe what the data means. Take this opportunity. Results are not self explanatory. The report should include a section that summarizes the raw data: in tables, figures and drawings, graphs, or other means. Review, explain and finally, conclude what the data support, based upon the acceptance criteria in the protocol. The review section should specifically review each point in the protocol acceptance criteria, and state whether the criteria were met. Then, based upon this review, the conclusion section should state whether the system is considered qualified or validated. In any event, do not just present the raw data in the report, or fail to make a conclusion. Do not allow the reviewer to judge the data alone, since he may not come to the same conclusions as you did. In a properly formatted and concluded report, there may still be disagreements, but at least there is a clear stand as to what the data mean. Without this, there is an open invitation to a differing view.

The final report must be written as an adjunct to the individual protocols, relating the observations recorded during the study, to the procedures and acceptance criteria in the protocol. Most often, the procedure employed during an audit review, is to begin with the protocol and perform a step-by-step comparison with the report. It is critical that the protocol be followed, and that deviations be documented and justified. Often, when the procedure is being implemented, it becomes obvious that it cannot be performed as planned, or a better procedure becomes apparent. At this point some groups feel a protocol rewrite is needed, with the resulting effort for circulating the documents for review and approvals.

Deviations from an approved protocol require being dealt with carefully. They must be the exception, and not the rule. Consider what effect deviations have on the protocol and the Validation Plan. If the protocol is substantially changed by the deviations, then a rewrite is in order. Even major excursions from the protocol can be addressed in a deviations section of the report, provided they are justified and approved by authorized individuals. But consider the consequences. Lost or destroyed information, failures to follow SOP's, and other faux pas may indicate to investigators an insufficiency in the required technique.

It will also indicate that the personnel developing the protocols are inadequately trained in this area.

The validation phases. In the United States there are several organizations that seek to define the activities appropriate to pharmaceutical water system validations. These are the Pharmaceutical Research and Manufacturing Association (PhRMA) (formerly the PMA), whose Water Quality Committee is advising the United States Pharmacopoeial Convention on the subject; the USP itself, free to accept or reject the proffered advice; and the FDA. The views of these three organizations are largely congruent, but not identical, on all validation matters. None has dealt deeply with the specifics of particular unit purification process validation requirements. All see water system validation as consisting of a series of consecutive stages.

The validation exercise has been characterized as consisting of a prospective phase, a concurrent validation phase, and a retrospective phase. According to spokespersons for the FDA, in the prospective phase of the validation, daily samples are to be assayed for their chemical and microbiological quality at each unit of the water purification system and at each point of use. This is to be done for a minimum period of 1 month. The data obtained during this first period is used to develop the SOPs and confirm that they, the operational SOPs, are adequate.

During the second period of a month or so, the concurrent validation phase, the same frequency of testing is to be observed. The resulting data serve to establish the short-term consistency of the water system when it is operated according to the SOPs developed in the prospective phase. In essence, the two 4-week periods constitute the Performance Qualification.

The long-term effects are yet to be explored. These will be investigated during the remainder of the year in the third phase, the retrospective validation step. During this phase, microbiological testing of the WFI systems should be performed daily, with each point of use being tested at least weekly. For Purified Water systems, each point of use should also be tested weekly. It is to be emphasized that the analytical numbers are not to serve as pass/fail values but as alert and action levels. Their utility is to establish trend lines. The *USP 23* (1995) chapter on the subject agrees that this 1-year period should normally suffice for the validation exercise.

Even when there are many points of use, each requires being tested at least once per week. This is so regardless of whether water for drug formulation is drawn from that particular point of use or not. The condition of each point of use, part of the overall water system, reflects upon the status of the system in general.

As Cooper (1994) points out, however, assumptions are inherent in accepting this duration of 1 year. Is it sufficiently long to disclose all the possible alterations in the source water supply, seasonal and otherwise? Will the second year's characteristics mimic those of the first? The systems are dynamic; they do change. Cooper correctly observes, "The application of the term 'validation' to this ever-changing situation surely adds a new and dubious dimension to the mystique of the validation concept." It must be concluded that the parameters of the water purification system may continue to change and that an ongoing, continual monitoring of the system is necessitated.

Underlying the setting of the time period for the initial phase of the validation is the assumption that the constancy of the feedwater composition is such that its management in the purification process can be defined and described in an SOP within a period of 1 month or so. But a source water, particularly when processed by a municipality using mixes from different origins, may alter in character even on a daily basis.

One American biotechnology company depends upon a municipal source that in answer to its own urgencies may, upon very short notice, mix well waters with river waters containing large quantities of TOC of unknown compositions derived from industrial sources and farm runoffs. This particular source water changes often with dramatic frequency and suddenness. The system is made manageable only by the use of pretreatment purification units sufficiently exaggerated in size and scope so as to handle peak contamination loads. More than a few months were required to define an acceptable SOP for this water purification system, and intensive ongoing daily monitoring is involved to ensure that the developed SOP really suffices from day to day, the source water being of such inconstant quality.

The three-phase validation scheme is intended for new systems. It is the one proposed by the FDA. However, that agency is prepared to accept other validation approaches. Some companies perform validations consisting only of the concurrent phase, a practice wherein the process is evaluated simultaneously with manufacture of the product water. In this approach, individual batches may be used even before the entire validation has been completed. Such concurrent validations entail much risk and may result in rejection of finished product.

Historical data may solely be relied upon to establish a retrospective validation in instances where the water has been produced for many years by a process that remains unchanged. This applies to old systems undergoing validation. In such cases, it is required that documented evidence firmly establish that there is a significant ongoing experience reflecting a constancy of practice. This signifies the existence of a rugged system productive of consistent performance.

As stated in the FDA "Guideline on General Principles of Process Validation" (1985), "In some cases a product may have been on the market without sufficient pre-market process validation. In these cases, it may be possible to validate, in some measure, the adequacy of the process by examination of accumulated test data on the product and records of the manufacturing procedures used." The objective of retrospective validation is to demonstrate that the water purification process has performed satisfactorily and consistently over time. Such documented evidence can serve to ensure that the specific process will consistently produce water of the same quality in the future.

Sampling program. The defining of suitable protocols for sampling and testing and a rigid adherence to the scheduling are all part of the validation program. As Artiss (1978) stated, "A carefully controlled sampling program is of paramount importance. The sampling technique must be carefully defined and followed so that the results accurately reflect the conditions that exist. The procedures must be so specific as to eliminate human variability and ensure that accurate results are obtained at all times. The sampling program should be designed to monitor

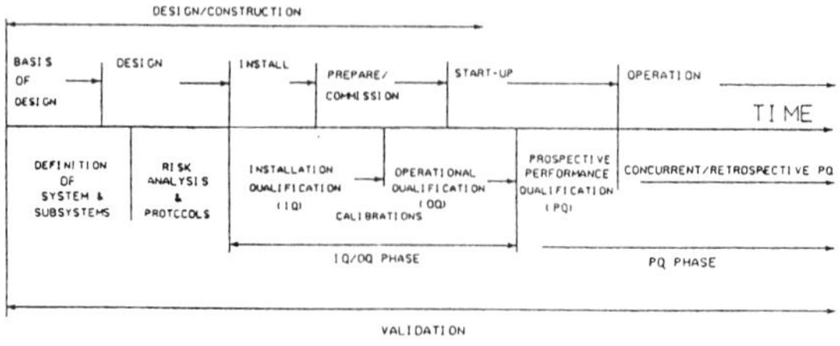

"*Updating Requirements for Pharmaceutical Grades of Water: Validation and Technology Selection*
Water Quality Committee - Pharmaceutical Manufacturers Association
Pharmacopeial Forum, Volume 19, No. 6
Copyright The USP Convention, Inc.
Permission granted"

Figure 13-19. The validation timeline.
WQC/PMA (1993a); Courtesy, the USP Convention, Inc.

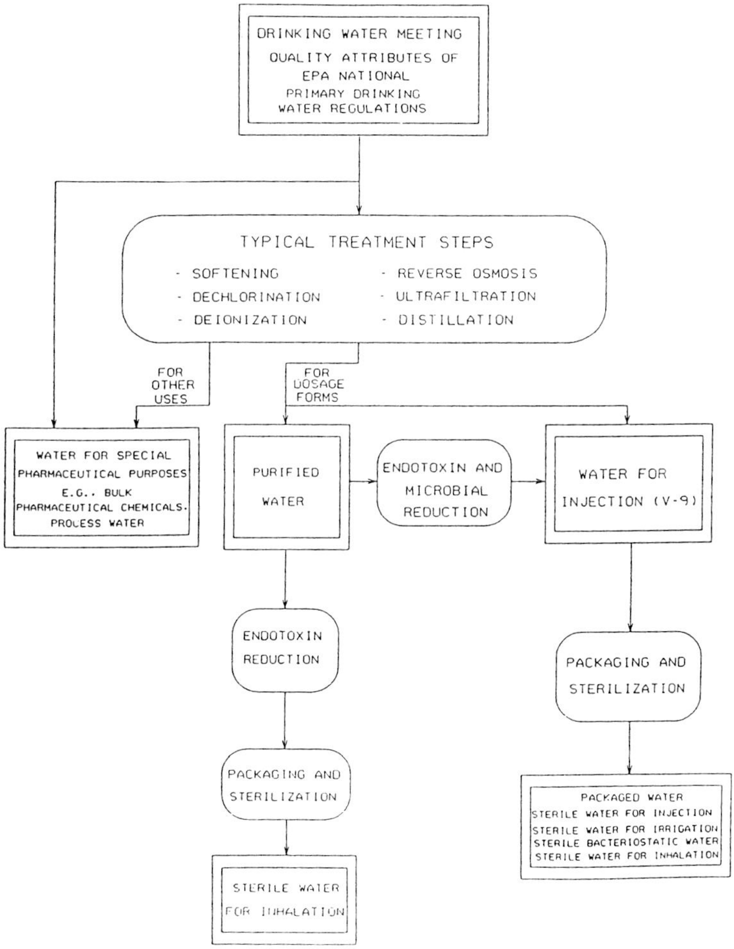

Figure 13-20. Water for pharmaceutical purposes.
Artiss (1986); Courtesy, Parenteral Drug Association

the equipment operation and preventive maintenance procedures as well as to determine the chemical and microbial quality of the water." His more recent addition is succinct, "The sampling procedure must be concisely written and then adhered to absolutely to ensure that there is no variability caused by different personnel or procedures."

The positions of the sampling valves or sampling points should be evident on the drawings of the system layout. Ideally, sampling ports should be installed before and after each purification unit, and before and after storage tanks. All the sampling valves should be of the same kind. Each valve should be numbered or otherwise unambiguously identified. The valves should be of small inside dimensions. This will permit their prompt, full opening and their flushing under high velocity to ensure the removal of organisms presumed to be contaminating the downstream side of the valve. In the distribution system, samples should be taken at the points of use, unless the water system is hard-piped to a piece of equipment. Sampling should reflect worst case conditions. Samples should not be taken immediately after sanitizations.

A description of the actual manner in which the samples are taken, sample size, containers to be used, method of identifying sample with sampling location and time, equipment employed, points to be sampled, time frames for analysis to be initiated, and disposition/approval of sample results should be indicated.

Inherent in sampling is the assumption that the sample is representative of the entire bulk of the water being characterized. Care should be taken not to vitiate that assumption. Artiss (1986) wisely points out that point-of-use samples should be drawn using the hose or pipe employed in delivering the water for manufacturing or rinsing. In this way contamination problems possibly inherent in that pipe or hose will become reflected in the microbiological assay results.

Tables 13-9, 13-10 and 13-11, (Artiss, 1986) illustrate a disposition of sampling sites, the water components being tested for, and the frequency of the testing; and offer certain relevant comments. It is precisely such sampling schemes that are required as part of the water system validation.

Cleaning and sanitizations. The water lines, sampling points, unused legs, and hoses off of water transmission lines should be periodically cleaned, sanitized, or sterilized; and flushed. If sanitization of the water system is performed using hot water, such sanitization must be validated. A protocol, record of time and temperature, adequate raw data, formal review, and an evaluation of the final report should be prepared.

If sanitization is performed using a chemical agent (e.g., peracetic acid, hydrogen peroxide, formalin, or antimicrobial agent) or plant steam, a routine analysis for chemical residues should follow sanitization. Residues should be eliminated by subsequent flushing and residual analysis should be performed. Pertinent details regarding sanitizations are presented in Chapter 2. Documentation consisting of formal logs should be kept of these activities. A record of sanitization, equipment replacement, and maintenance is required.

Post-Validation and Audits

The validation in its several phases having been completed, the water system requires periodic examination and testing as long as it remains in use.

Change-control is a serious issue. Have alterations, additions, or deletions been made to the system? Have operational changes been made? What are the risk implications of such alterations? Are the drawings of the system kept up to date? Periodic checks should be made to see that this is so. If changes are made to the system by the substitution, for instance, of a pump, was the same or a

Table 13-9
Sampling Program for Raw Water and Deionizer

Location	*Component*	*Frequency*		*Comments*
Sample Point		*Validation*	*Operation*	
Raw water (potable)	Microbial	Daily	Daily	Review together to determine contact time
	Cl_2 residual	Daily	Daily	
	Chemical TDS*	Daily	Weekly	Fast, low cost test
	Full chemical**	Weekly	6 months	
	pH	--	--	Depends on equipment use
Sand filter	Microbial	Daily	Daily	
	Cl_2 residual	Daily	Weekly	
Carbon filter	Microbial	Daily	Daily	
	Cl_2 residual	Daily	Daily	
Deionization equipment***	Conductivity	Daily	Daily	
	C12 residual	Daily	Daily	
	Total solids USP	Daily	Daily	Depends on use of this water
	Microbial	Daily	Daily	
	Pyrogen	Daily	Daily	Depends on use of this water
	Silica-colloidal and dissolved	Daily	Weekly	Depends on use of this water
	Resin analysis	Initial	6 months	

*TDS, total dissolved solids by conductivity
** May vary considerably depending on source and season.
*** Will vary depending on service cycle.
Artiss (1986); Courtesy, Marcell Dekker

different type of pump used? Was an RO unit added? Were substantial physical changes instituted? If so, these should be added to the P&ID list, and the system drawings should be updated. In particular, changes to the SOPs should be documented.

Routine data analysis should be performed on an ongoing basis by the QC laboratory to see whether or not the system continues to function satisfactorily. How are out-of-specification results explained? Was the sampling or the system at fault? What was the cause of the deviation? What action was taken to correct it? Deviations from the SOPs must be explained. Deviation reports are required. For example, if the SOP states that sanitizations are needed every 3 days, and such an action was taken only after 5 days, the reason for the deviation requires being set forth. Or with regard to UV lamps, were they cleaned or replaced in accordance with the standard maintenance schedule? Routine audits should, therefore, be made of the maintenance records (e.g., of the sanitization practices). The FDA inspector will certainly examine maintenance logs.

The data, particularly the microbiological, should be plotted, at least monthly. Identification should be made of organisms that are present. In particular, changes in the types and numbers of organisms should be looked for. The risk

Table 13-10
Sampling Program for Reverse Osmosis and Distillation Equipment

Location *Sample Point*	*Component*	*Frequency* *Validation*	*Operation*	*Comments*
Reverse osmosis equipment	Microbial	Daily	Daily	
	Cl_2 residual	Continuous	Continuous	Critical on some equipment
	Pyrogen	Daily	Daily	Depends on use
	Condustivity	Continuous	Continuous	
	Chemical USP	Daily	Daily	Depends on use
	Feedwater hardness	Daily	Daily	Critical on some equipment
Distillation equipment (assume USP water for injection)	Microbial	Multiple times in cycle	Daily	
	pH		Daily	
	Pyrogen		Daily	
	Conductivity	Continuous	Continuous	Inlet and outlet
	Chemical--USP	Multiple times in cycle	Daily	
	Blowdown-TDS		Weekly	
	Particulates		Weekly	

Notes: Check individual modules during validation period and weekly thereafter.
For RO and distillation equipment, establish repeatability and time for system stabilization
Artiss (1986); Courtesy, Marcel Dekker

assessment of such changes should be made.

These routine and periodic examinations constitute an internal audit of the water system. In addition, the FDA inspectors in their audits will look at the validation data compiled by the drug manufacturer and by vendors on his behalf. The pharmaceutical processor should also audit vendors' data.

Periodic checks should be made of the validation data, of the protocols and procedures (i.e., of the operational instructions), to see that they are being followed. The FDA investigators will, for their part, do so during their inspections.

The water system audit, whether performed by the FDA or self-performed by the drug manufacturer, is essentially an inquiry into the post-validation actions. The documentation will set forth the activities pertinent to the proper operation of the water system, and will establish what was factually performed in the actual exercise. The recorded test and operational data will be examined in the compliance audit for their adequacy to support the conclusions derived therefrom. The regulatory investigators will require explanation of the discrepancies between promise and performance. For example, the responses to bacterial excursions will be examined. What corrective actions were taken?

The audit will cover system design, calibration and maintenance, the moni-

Table 13-11
Sampling Program for Storage and Other LOcations

Location	*Component*	*Frequency*		*Comments*
Sample Point		*Validation*	*Operation*	
Storage	Microbial	Multiple	Daily	
	pH	times in	Daily	
	Pyrogen	cycle	Daily	If req. for WFI
	Chemical USP		Daily	
Distribution	Microbial	Daily	Weekly	On rotation
use points	Pyrogen	Daily	***	
	Chemical TDS*	Daily	Monthly	Fast, low-cost
	Chemical USP**	Weekly	***	
	Particulates	Daily	MOnthly	
	pH	Weekly	***	
Clean steam	Blowdown	Daily	Weekly	To prevent scale
generator	chemical TDS	Daily	Weekly	build-up

*TDS, total dissolved solids (by conductivity)
**TDS, total dissolved solids (by evaporation)
***Sample only when indicated by failure to satisfy other tests
Artiss (1986); Courtesy, Marcel Dekker

toring program, remedial actions to alert and action levels, and the qualifications of the water system in general. The system design will be examined. This will include the sampling ports before and after each of the purification units, such as carbon beds, softeners, DI beds, RO, UV lights, filters, stills, and the product-water holding tanks. The feedwater quality will be examined by way of its analytical data. The system design considerations as regards recirculation, constructions of stainless steel or polymeric materials, and the possibilities for heat sanitization and hot storage will be checked.

In particular, inspections will be made for sanitary fittings, pitched piping, the absence of threaded joints, the use of pressure-relief rupture discs and diaphragm valves, and the avoidance of dead legs. The absence of in-line filters is preferred. Heat exchangers will be inspected for their double-tube or sheet constructions, or for the ongoing monitoring of constant positive pressure to their thermal-fluid transference side.

With regard to the RO units, the auditors will ascertain that the pretreatment of the feedwaters is performed as specified, and that the RO unit is not followed by DI beds with their inevitable encouragements to organism growths. As in the case of the heat exchangers, the inspectors will make reference to the FDA's *Inspection Technical Guide.*

The use of ion-exchange resins will be audited. Where regeneration is performed in situ, purity specifications for the regenerant chemicals, and a testing protocol for their eventual removal will be sought. As regards DI resin for portable units, it should be remembered that dedicated resins and containers are preferred where individual or bulk regenerations are involved. The maintenance program for non-dedicated resins should include vendor certification of the industries serviced, to ensure the avoidance of resins used in electroplating shops with their concomitant heavy-metal impurities. Vendor assurances of such restricted uses will be looked for, as also the vendor's particulars and records on resin regeneration, storage, and delivery. Standby resin beds are to have time levels for the standby intervals, and also suitable storage and maintenance controls (such as recirculation and refrigeration) over organism growth. Inspections could be made for these.

In addition, auditing the maintenance programs will involve examining records for the backflushing, sanitizing, and periodic replacement of the activated carbon beds; as also the sanitization, whether by chemicals, hot water, or steam, of the water distribution and storage facilities. With regard to filters, whether for venting or water flow, the frequency of sanitizations and change, as prescribed in the maintenance procedures, will be examined. Regulatory investigators will inspect to see whether proper maintenance is being performed upon UV lamp installations. Periodic checks and recordings of lamp intensities are to be made. These will be compared with their operating requirements. Conformity with lamp cleaning and replacement schedules will be looked for.

Records will be examined to learn whether the correct flowrates through the UV units were complied with. It could be helpful to check microbiologically for the recovery of atypical organism morphologies consequent to UV irradiation.

The microbiological assays and procedures will be examined closely. Time levels and storage requirements indicated for microbiological samples should be obeyed. The frequency of testing at appropriate locations will be checked. It will be ascertained whether aseptic techniques and sterile utensils were used in the performance of the microbiological assays, along with the proper nutrient media, and incubation times and temperatures stipulated in the SOPs. The appropriateness of the supporting data to the claim of microbiological validation having been realized will be examined closely.

Documentation will be inspected to ensure the adequacy of record keeping. Inspection of the various qualification steps (e.g., Installation Qualification, Purification-unit Qualification, and Performance Qualification will be made. Data supporting claims of validation will be examined for the correctness of the conclusions being drawn.

The questions asked by FDA investigators do not necessarily reflect established regulations and practices, nor do they imply that satisfactory techniques or approaches are necessarily available to the industry. The obligation of the investigator is to establish an overall balanced judgment in complicated situations where contradictory factors may be at work. An extensive and even overreaching probing may be a useful device in such circumstances.

Opportunities abound for investigators, at times, to arrive at apparently contradictory conclusions. The different inspectors may each have a particular expertise and technique. Not every inspection is meant to cover the entire system. A given inspection may be intended for a particular investigative purpose. Therefore, an absence of adverse observations on the inspector's 483 form does not constitute an endorsement of any unremarked-upon operation, nor does it exempt the pharmaceutical processor from untoward consequences. The general intent, however, is clear: to safeguard the public safety while sorting out acceptable practices from those that require improvement and optimization.

The pharmaceutical water producer should be prepared, and should not hesitate, on the basis of documented experimental data, to dispute the FDA investigator's adverse judgments and observations where these seem to be erroneously derived. In the resolution of such contradictory points of view lies the potential for the ongoing developmental progress of pharmaceutical water systems.

Summary

The audit will examine the documented evidence upon which are based the multifaceted design and operation of the water system in all its complexity, to see whether the claims made for the system's adequacy and validation are justified.

derive from the now surfacing bioengineering needs to avoid transitional metal ions. Under this umbrella, however, a greater confidence will come to repose in the RO process in general. On-line air and vent filter integrity testing will become widespread, advanced by the certainty that this can now be done. A concomitant result will be the assessment of air filter hydrophobicity, a quality necessary in biofermentation operations.

To a growing extent it will become apparent that the raw water quality is perhaps the governing influence in pharmaceutical system design. Increasingly, therefore, attention will be paid to the choice and design of pretreatment units.

Choices will always be possible; whether the use of activated carbon or chemical (bisulfite) addition for the removal of chlorine, or the selection of ion exchange, reverse osmosis, or one of the electrodeionization processes for ion removal. Perhaps the real genius in water system design will become evident when the technical practitioners accept that the points of decision are not technical alone but that they become defined in technico-economic terms. However the water system future evolves, it will be a time of great progress and of significant advancement. We face it with confidence and with understanding.■

UNIGENE LABORATORIES, INC.
INSTALLATION QUALIFICATION PROTOCOL

TITLE: CHILLED WATER SYSTEM GENERATION, STORAGE AND DISTRIBUTION	PROTOCOL NO: VP039.IQ REV. NO: DRAFT EFF. DATE: NEW SUPERSEDES: PAGE 23 of 38

14. **FIELD VERIFICATION**

C. INSTRUMENTS/DEVICES

2.] Critical Instruments

Control Parameter: V-910 Level, Continued

Equipment Number: V-910 P/M Number:

Date of Last Calibration: Frequency:

Reference Drawings: FU-901

Devices in V-910 Level Loop:

Tag Number:	LALL-01				
Manufacturer:	Panalarm	Model:	w/ Ann-7	S/N:	
Function:	Low Low Level Alarm	Size:	NA	Range:	

Tag Number:	HS-04				
Manufacturer:	Allen Bradley	Model:	800T-J2A	S/N:	
Function:	HOA Switch for P-910	Size:	NA	Range:	NA

Comments:

Verified by: Date:

Reviewed by: Date:

UNIGENE LABORATORIES, INC.
INSTALLATION QUALIFICATION PROTOCOL

TITLE: CHILLED WATER SYSTEM GENERATION, STORAGE AND DISTRIBUTION	PROTOCOL NO: VP039.IQ REV. NO: DRAFT EFF. DATE: NEW SUPERSEDES: PAGE 24 of 38

14. **FIELD VERIFICATION**

C. INSTRUMENTS/DEVICES

2.] Critical Instruments

Control Parameter: Chilled Water Supply Pressure

Equipment Number: NA ____________ P/M Number: ____________

Date of Last Calibration: ____________ Frequency: ____________

Reference Drawings: FU-901

Devices Controlling Chilled Water Supply Pressure:

Tag Number:	PCV-09				
Manufacturer:	Fisher	Model:	63EG	S/N:	
Function:	Chilled Water Supply Pressure	Size:		Range:	Set @ 60 PSIG

Comments: ____

____

____

____

____

Verified by: ____________________ Date: ____________

Reviewed by: ____________________ Date: ____________

UNIGENE LABORATORIES, INC.
INSTALLATION QUALIFICATION PROTOCOL

TITLE: CHILLED WATER SYSTEM GENERATION, STORAGE AND DISTRIBUTION	PROTOCOL NO: VP039.IQ REV. NO: DRAFT EFF. DATE: NEW SUPERSEDES: PAGE 25 of 38

14. **FIELD VERIFICATION**

C. INSTRUMENTS/DEVICES

2.] Critical Instruments

Control Parameter:______________________________

Equipment Number:________________ P/M Number:____________

Date of Last Calibration:________________ Frequency:__________

Reference Drawings:______________________________

Tag Number:		
Manufacturer:	Model:	S/N:
Function:	Size:	Range:

Tag Number:		
Manufacturer:	Model:	S/N:
Function:	Size:	Range:

Tag Number:		
Manufacturer:	Model:	S/N:
Function:	Size:	Range:

Comments:______________________________

Verified by:____________________ Date:__________

Reviewed by:____________________ Date:__________

Attachment # 8a
Doc. # 23-2100-1
Edition:
Page 60 of 65

CRITICAL INSTRUMENT CHECKLIST

Company: ______________________ Date: ____________

Equipment: ______________________

Equipment: ____________	Function: ____________
Manufacturer: ____________	Model No: ____________
Serial No.: ____________	Calibration Date: ______
Range: ____________	Scale Division: ______
Equipment: ____________	Function: ____________
Manufacturer: ____________	Model No: ____________
Serial No.: ____________	Calibration Date: ______
Range: ____________	Scale Division:
Equipment: ____________	Function: ____________
Manufacturer: ____________	Model No: ____________
Serial No.: ____________	Calibration Date: ______
Range: ____________	Scale Division: ______
Equipment: ____________	Function: ____________
Manufacturer: ____________	Model No: ____________
Serial No.: ____________	Calibration Date: ______
Range: ____________	Scale Division: ______
Comments:	

Performed By: ______________________ Date: __________

Reviewed By: ______________________ Date: __________

Attachment # 9A
Doc. # 23-2100-1
Edition:
Page 61 of 65

REFERENCE INSTRUMENT CHECKLIST

Company:______________________ Date:__________

Equipment:______________________

Equipment:__________	Function:__________
Manufacturer:__________	Model No:__________
Serial No.:__________	Calibration Date:______
Range:__________	Scale Division:______
Equipment:__________	Function:__________
Manufacturer:__________	Model No:__________
Serial No.:__________	Calibration Date:______
Range:__________	Scale Division:
Equipment:__________	Function:__________
Manufacturer:__________	Model No:__________
Serial No.:__________	Calibration Date:______
Range:__________	Scale Division:______
Equipment:__________	Function:__________
Manufacturer:__________	Model No:__________
Serial No.:__________	Calibration Date:______
Range:__________	Scale Division:______

Comments:

Performed By:______________________ Date:__________

Reviewed By:______________________ Date:__________

RUTGERS UNIVERSITY
WAKSMAN INSTITUTE
CCPFF, PISCATAWAY, NJ

INSTALLATION QUALIFICATION
AUTOCLAVE #2
PROTOCOL NO. P10-IQ

13.2.2 VALVES

Listed below are the Valves found in the Autoclave.

DESCRIPTION								
Valve I.D.No.	Manufacturer	Model No.	Mat'l	Type	Location	Yes/No	Initialed by	Date

Comments: ______________________________

____

____

Compiled By: ____________________ Date: ______________

Reviewed By: ____________________ Date: ______________

OPERATIONAL QUALIFICATION
WATER FOR INJECTION SYSTEM

PROTOCOL NUMBER

FLOW VELOCITY - "NO LOAD" CONDITIONS

Study - Distribution Loop	1	2	3
[FR] = Flowrate (GPM)			
[D] = Pipe inner diameter (in)			
[FV] = Flow velocity (fps) $\frac{FR\,(.409)}{D^2}$			
[SV] = Specified flow velocity	≥ 5 fps	≥ 5 fps	≥ 5 fps
Pass/Fail			
Comments:			

Calculation derived:

NOTE: Area $(ft^2) = \pi \left(\left[\frac{D\ in}{2}\right] \left[\frac{ft}{12\ in}\right] \right)^2 = .00545D^2$

Flow Velocity (fps) =

$$\left(\frac{gal}{min}\right) \left(\frac{min}{60\ sec}\right) \left(\frac{ft^3}{7.48\ gal}\right) \left(\frac{1}{Area(ft)^2}\right) = \frac{GPM\ (.409)}{SV^2} = \frac{FR\ (.409)}{D^2}$$

Comments: ______________________________

Performed by: ____________________ Date: ____________________

Reviewed by: ____________________ Date: ____________________

ABBREVIATIONS AND ACRONYMS

ABS - acrylonitrile-butadiene-styrene (polymer)
ASME - American Society of Mechanical Engineers
ASTM - American Society for Testing and Materials
BET - bacterial endotoxin testing
BOD - biological oxygen demand
BPC - bulk pharmaceutical chemicals
Btu - British thermal units
BWFI - Bacteriostatic Water for Injection
CA - cellulose acetate
CDI - continuous deionization
CG - confluent growth
CGMP - current Good Manufacturing Practice
CH - chloral hydrate
CIP - clean in place
COD - chemical oxidation demand
CP - chloropicrin
CR - neoprene
CST - critical surface tension
CTFA--Cosmetic Toiletry and Fragrance Assoc.
DBP - disinfection by-products
DC - direct current
DCAA - dichloroacetic acid
DCAN - dichloroacetonitrile
DF - decontamination factor
DI - deionized, deionizing, deionization
DNA - deoxyribonucleic acid
DOC - dissolved oxidizable carbon
DQ - Design Qualification
DRAM - dynamic random access memory
DVB - divinylbenezene
DVC - direct viable count
E. coli - *Escherichia coli*
ECTFE - ethylene chlorotrifluoroethylene
ED - electrodialysis
EDR - electrodialysis reversal
EDTA - ethylenediaminetetraacetic acid
EFA - effective filtration area
EIR - Establishment Inspection Report
ELISA--enzyme-linked immunosorbent assays
EOL - end of lamp life
EPA - Environmental Protection Agency
EPR - ethylene propylene rubber
EPX - energy-dispersive X-ray
ES - effective size
ESCA - electron spectroscopy for chemical analysis
et al. - and others
ETFE - ethylenetetrafluoroethylene
EU - endotoxin units
EVP eliminator of volatile pollutants
fab - fabricating
FDA - Food and Drug Administration
FEP - fluorinated ethylene-propylene
FFR - fully fluorinated rubber
FRP - fiberglass-reinforced plastic
FTIR - Fourier transform infrared
GAC - granular activated carbon
GMPs/LVPs - Good Manufacturing Practices for Large-Volume Parenterals
GRP - fiberglass-reinforced plastic (European usage)
HCN - hydrogen cyanide
HEPA - high-efficiency particulate air filter
HIMA - Health Industries Manufacturing Association
HMS - harmonic mean size
HPC - heterotrophic plate count
HPLC - high-pressure liquid chromatography
HVAC - heating, ventilating, and air-conditioning
ICP/MS - inductively coupled plasma / mass spectrometry
i.d. - inner diameter
IQ - Installation Qualification
IV - intravenous
JTU - Jackson turbidity units
KHP - potassium hydrogen phthalate
LAL - limulus amoebocyte lysate
LED - light-emitting diodes
LPS - lipopolysaccharide
LRV - log reduction value
LSI - Langelier Saturation Index
LVPs - Large-Volume Parenterals
MCAA - monochloroacetic acid
MCL - maximum contamination level
MCLGs - Maximum Contaminant Level Goals
Md - mass of distillate produced
ME - multiple effects (still)
MIB - 2-methylisoborneol
Ms - mass of steam consumed
mTGE - Tryptone Glucose Broth
MTR - mill test reports
m.w. *(or MW)* - molecular weight
MWCO - molecular-weight cutoff
NAA - neutron activation analysis
NBR - nitrile butyl rubber
NCCLS - National Council Clinical Laboratory Standards
NDIR - nondispersive infrared analysis
NF - *National Formulary*
NIST - National Institute for Standards and Technology
NPDWR - National Primary Drinking Water Regulations
NPOC - nonpurgeable oxidizable carbon

NR - natural rubber, polyisoprene
N_{RE} - Reynolds number
NSDWR - National Secondary Drinking Water Regulations
NSF - National Sanitation Foundation
NTU - nephelometric turbidity units
o.d. - outer diameter
OQ - Operational Qualification
ORP - oxidation-reduction potential
OSHA - Occupational Safety and Health Adm.
PA - polyamide
PAA - polyacrylic acid
PCA - plate count agar
PCE - perchlorethylene
PEEK - polyetheretherketone
PEG - polyethylene glycol
PFA - polyfluoroallomer
PhRMA - Pharmaceutical Research and Manufacturing Association (formerly Pharmaceutical Manufacturers Association)
PMA - Pharmaceutical Manufacturers Association *(see WQC/PMA)*
POC - purgeable organic carbons
POU - point of use
PP - polypropylene
PQ - Process Qualification
PTFE - polytetrafluoroethylene
PVC - polyvinyl chloride
PVDF - polyvinylidene fluoride
PVF - polyvinyl fluoride
PVP - polyvinylpyrrolidone
PW - Purified Water
P&ID - Process Instrumentation Drawings
QC - quality control
RA - roughness average
RNA - ribonucleic acid
RO - reverse osmosis
ROOH - hydroperoxide
RTD - resistance temperature detector
SA - strongly acidic
SB - strongly basic
SCD - streaming-current detector
SDI - silt density index
SEM - scanning electron microscope
SMC - selective membrane conductivity
SMCLs - Secondary Maximum Contaminant Levels
SMP - standard maintenance procedure
SOP - standard operating procedure
SVPs - small-volume parenterals
TCAA - trichloroacetic acid
TCAN - trichloroacetonitrile
TCC - total coliform counts
TCE - trichloroethylene
TCP - 2,4,6-trichlorophenol
TDS - total dissolved solids
TFE - tetrafluoroethylene
TGA - triptoglucose agar
TGB - Tryptone Glucose Broth *(see also mTGE)*
THM - trihalomethane
TIG - tungsten inert gas
TMA - total mineral acidity
TNTC - too numerous to count
TOC - total organic carbon
TSA - tryptone soy agar
TSS - total suspended solids
TTHM - total trihalomethane
UC - uniformity coefficient
UF - ultrafilters, ultrafiltration
ULSI - ultra large scale integrations
USP - United States Pharmacopeia
USPC - United States Pharmacopeia Convention
UV - ultraviolet
VC - vapor compression (still)
VLSI - very large scale integrations
VOC - volatile organic carbons
WA - weakly acidic
WB - weakly basic
WFI - Water for Injection
WPIT - water pressure integrity test
WQC/PMA - Water Quality Committee of the Pharmaceutical Manufacturers Assoc.
w/w - weight-to-weight (ratio)
XPS - X-ray photoelectron spectroscopy

COMMON CHEMICAL SYMBOLS

Ag - silver
Al - aluminum
$AlCl_3$ - aluminum chloride
As - arsenic
Ba - barium
Br - bromine
C - carbon
$CHBr_3$ - bromoform
$CHBrCl_3$ - bromodichloromethane
$CHBr_2Cl$ - dibromochloromethane
$CHCl_3$ - chloroform
CO_2 - carbon dioxide
CO_3^{2-} - carbonate anion
Ca - calcium
Ca^{2+} - calcium cations
$CaCO_3$ - calcium carbonate
CaO - calcium oxide
Cd - cadmium
Cl_2 - chlorine
Cl^- - chlorate anion
ClO_2 - chlorine dioxide
Co - cobalt
Cr - chromium
Cu - copper

F_2 - flourine
Fe - iron
H - hydrogen
H^+ - hydrogen cation
HCO_3^- - bicarbonate anion
H_2CO_3 - carbonic acid
HCl - hydrochloric acid
H_2O - water
H_2O_2 - hydrogen peroxide
H_3O^+ - hydronium ion
HOBr (also HBrO) - hypobromous acid
HOCl - hypochlorous acid
H_2S - hydrogen sulfide
Hg - mercury
K - potassium
K^+ - potassium cation
K_2O - potassium oxide
Li - lithium
Mg - magnesium
Mg^{2+} - magnesium cation
MgO - magnesium oxide
$Mg(OH)_2$ - magnesium hydroxide
Mn - manganese
MnO_2 - manganese dioxide
N - nitrogen
NH_4^+ - ammonium
NH_3 - ammonia
NO_3^- - nitrate anion
Na - sodium
Na^+ - sodium cation
NaCl - sodium chloride
Na_2O - sodium oxide
NaOCl - sodium hypochlorite
Ni - nickel
O_2 - oxygen
OCl^- - hypochlorite anion
OH^- - hydroxide anion
P - phosphorus
PO_4^{3-} - phosphate anion
Pb - lead
S - sulfur
SO_2 - sulfur dioxide
SO_4 - sulfate
SO_4^{2-} - sulfate anion
Si - silicon
SiO_2 - silica
Sr - strontium
Zn - zinc

UNITS OF MEASURE
Btu - British thermal units
cfu/mL - colony-forming units per milliliter
cm/sec - centimeters per second
cm^2 - square centimeters
EU - endotoxin units
ft - feet
ft^2 - square feet
ft^3 - cubic feet
ft/sec - feet per second
g - grams
g - gravitational constant
gpd - gallons per day
gph - gallons per hour
gpm - gallons per minute
gpm/ft^3 - gallons per minute per cubic foot
gr - grains
gr/gal - grains per gallon
g/h - grams per hour
JTU - Jackson turbidity units
kcal - kilocalories
kg - kilograms
kHz - kilohertz
kJ/L - kilojoules per liter
kPa - kilopascals
kW - kilowatts
L - liter
Lpm *(or L/m)* - liters per minute
L/h *(or Lph)* - liters per hour
M - molar
meq/L - milliequivalents per liter
mg/L - milligrams per liter
mL - milliliters
mL/min - milliliters per minutes
mm - millimeters
mm^2 - square millimeters
mMHO/cm - micromhos per centimeter
mS/cm - microsiemens per centimeter
m^3/m - cubic meters per meter
nm - nanometer
NTU - nephelometric turbidity units
Pa - pascals
ppb - parts per billion
ppm - parts per million
psid - pounds per square inch differential
psig - pounds per square inch gauge
R - performance ratio
RA - roughness average
rms - root mean square
rpm - rotations per minute
SCFM - standard cubic feet per minute *(*
SDI - silt density index
sec - second
UC - uniformity coefficient
w/w - weight-to-weight (ratio)
µg/L - micrograms per liter
$\mu j/cm^2$ - microjoules per square centimeter
µm - micron
µS - microsiemens
µS/cm - microsiemens per centimeter
$\mu Ws/cm^2$ - microwatt-seconds per square centimeter
µΩ/cm - microohms per centimeter

BIBLIOGRAPHY

Abrams, I.M. "New Requirements for Ion-Exchange in Condenser Polishing", 37th Annual Meeting of the International Water Conference, Pittsburgh, PA (October 26-28, 1976).

Abrams, I.M. Personal Communications (1990).

Abshire, R.L. "Topical and Opthhalmic Products", *Proceedings of PMA Water Seminar Program,* pp. 143-146, Atlanta, GA (February 1982).

Abshire, R.L. "The Use of UV Radiation as a Method of Sterilization in the Pharmaceutical Industry", *Process Ozone + Ultra-Violet Water Treatment,* W.J. Masschelein, Coordination (Paris, France: International Ozone Association, European Committee pp, D.1.1.-D.1.19) (1986).

Abshire, R.L.; Dunton, H. "Resistance of Selected Strains of *Pseudomonas Aeruginosa* to Low-Intensity Ultraviolet Radiation", *Applied and Environmental Microbiology* (June 1981).

Abshire, R.L.; Schlech, B.L.; Dunton, H. "The Development of a Biological Indicator for Validating Ultraviolet Radiation Sterilization of Polyethylene Bottles", *Journal of Parenteral Science and Technology 37(5),* pp. 191-197 (1983).

Adair, F. "Uses of Water - Nasal and Oral Liquids", *Proceedings Pharmaceutical Manufacturers Association Meeting,* pp. 147-150, Atlanta, GA (February 1-2, 1982).

Adair, F.W.; Geffic, S.G.; Heymann, H. "Lytic Effects of DI or Tri Carboxylic Acids Plus Sodium Dodecyl Sulfate Against *Pseudomonas aeruginosa* ", *Antimicrobial Agents and Chemotherapy 16(3),* pp. 419-420 (1979).

Addiks, R. "Examining the Backwashing of Rapid Granular Filter Media", *Filtration and Separation 28(1),* pp. 38-41 (1991).

Adin, A.; Hatukai, S. "Optimisation of Multilayer Filter Beds", *Filtration and Separation 28(1),* pp. 33-36 (1991).

Agalloco, J.P. "Steam Sterilization-In-Place Technology", *Journal of Parenteral Science and Technology 44(5),* pp. 253-256 (1990-A).

Agalloco, J.P. "Steam in Place", PDA Short Course, Parenteral Drug Association, Philadelphia, PA (1990-B).

Aieta, E.M.; Reagan, K.M.; Lang, J.S.; McReynolds, L.; Kang, J.W.; Glaze, W.H. "Advanced Oxidation Processes for Treating Groundwater Contaminated with TCE and PCE: Pilot-Scale Evaluations", *Journal American Water Works Association 80(5),* pp. 64-72 (1988).

Alkan, M.H.; Groves, M.J. "The Measurement of Filter Pore-Size by a Gas Permeability Technique", *Drug Development and Industrial Pharmacy 4(3),* pp. 225-241 (1978).

Allen, T. *Particle Size Measurement,* Chapman and Hall Ltd., London, England (1975).

American Filtration Society, Symposium on "The Pore", Hershey, PA (May 20-23, 1991).

American Iron and Steel Institute, AIS-SS 601-477-25M-GP "Design Guidelines for the Selection and Use of Stainless Steels", American Iron and Steel Institute, Washington, DC (1977).

American Iron and Steel Institute, AIS-SS 803-479-25M-GP "Welding of Stainless Steels and Other Joining Methods", American Iron and Steel Institute, Washington, DC (1977).

American Society for Testing and Materials, ASTM-A380, "Standard Practice for Cleaning and Descaling Stainless Steel Parts, Equipment, and Systems", *Annual Book of ASTM Standards,* Vol. 10.05, Designation A-380, American Society for Testing and Materials, Philadelphia, PA (1980).

American Water Works Association, "Chapter 8: Filtration", *Water Treatment Plant Design,* pp. 117-147 American Water Works Association, New York, NY (1969).

Amjad, Z. "Advances in Scaling and Deposit Control for RO System", *Ultrapure Water 4(6),* pp. 34-38 (1987).

Amjad, Z. "Mechanistic Aspects of Reverse Osmosis Mineral Scale Formation and Inhibition", *Ultrapure Water 5(6),* pp. 23-28 (1988).

Ammerer, N.H. "Controlling TOC Effluent Levels from Newly Regenerated Resins", *Ultrapure Water 6(9),* pp. 34-40 (1989).

Ammerer, N.H.; Dahmen, G.B. "Curing Silica Problems with Double Pass Reverse Osmosis", *Ultrapure Water 7(4),* pp. 41-46 (1990).

Anderson, C.C. "A Comparison of High Purity Water TOC Measurements Using Commercially Available Equipment", *Transcripts of Fifth Annual Semiconductor Pure Water Conference,* pp. 195-218, San Francisco, CA (January 16-17, 1986).

Anderson, R.E. "Ion-Exchange Separations", Section 1-12, pp. 1-359 to 1-414, in *Handbook of Separation Techniques for Chemical Engineers,* P.W. Schweitzer, ed., McGraw-Hill Book Company, New York (1979).

Anderson, R.L.; Bland, L.A.; Favero, M.S.; McNeil, M.M.; Davis, B.J.; Mackel, D.C.; Gravelle, R.R. "Factors Associated with *Pseudomonas pickettii* Intrinsic Contamination of Commercial Respiratory Therapy Solutions Marketed as Sterile", *Applied and Environmental Microbiology 50(6),* pp. 1343-1348 (1985).

Angelucci III, L.A. *Documentary Relative to Pharmaceutical Water System Validations,* John Brown Company, Berkeley Heights, NJ

A.N.R.T., National Association for Technical Research (Paris). "Filtration Performance of Metal Fabrics", *Filtration and Separation,* pp. 500-502 (November/December 1966).

Antopol, S.C.; Ellner, P.D. "Susceptibility of *Legionella pneumophila* to Ultraviolet Radiation", *Applied and Environmental Microbiology 38(2),* pp. 347-348, (1979).

Anwar, H.; Das Gupta, M.K.; Costerton, W. "Testing the Susceptibility of Bacteria in Biofilms to Antibacterial Agents" *Antimicrobial Agents and Chemotherapy 34,* pp. 2043-2046 (1990).

Applebaum, S.B. "Chapter 3: Removal of the Major Ionic Dissolved Impuritites in Water", *Demineralization by Ion Exchange,* Academic Press, New York (1968).

Aranovitch, H.; Ford, R. "Weakly Acidic Cation Performance Treating Water Containing High Iron", *Ultrapure Water 12(4)* pp. 60-64 (1995).

Argo, D.G.; Ridgway, H.F. "Biological Fouling of Reverse Osmosis Membranes at Water Factory 21", *Proceedings of the Water Supply Improvement Association,* Vol. 1,

Honolulu, HI (1982).

Arseneaux, A.A.; Stoner, L.D.; Whipple, S.S; Moore, S.M. "A Reverse Osmosis System on High-Organic-Content Well Water", *Ultrapure Water 7(9),* pp. 18-26 (1990).

Artiss, D.H. "Materials, Surface Finishes and Components for Sanitary Applications", *Proceedings of PMA Water Seminar Program,* pp. 34-49, Atlanta, GA (February 1982a).

Artiss, D.H. "Welding Quality-Assurance of Total Control", *Proceedings of PMA Water Seminar Program,* pp. 73-91, Atlanta, GA (February 1982b).

Artiss, D.H. "Water System Validation", Chapter 9, *Validation of Aseptic Pharmaceutical Processes,* Carleton, F.J.; Agalloco, J.P., Eds., p. 212, Marcel Dekker, New York (1986).

Artiss, D.H. "PDA Course on Validation of Pharmaceutical Water Systems", Parenteral Drug Association, Bethesda, MD (1978).

Ashanti, Y.; Catravas, G.N. "Highly Reactive Impurities in Triton x-100 and Brij-35: Partial Characterization and Removal", *Analytical Biochemistry 109,* pp. 55-62 (1980).

Avallone, H.L. "High Purity Water", ISPE High Purity Water Seminar, Atlanta, GA (1985).

Avallone, H.L. "Microbiological Control of Topicals", 18th Annual FDA/ASQC-FDC Conference, Princeton, NJ (March 26, 1987).

Avallone, H.L., Personal Communications (1992)

Badenhop, C.T. *The Determination of the Pore Distribution and the Consideration of Methods Leading to the Prediction of Retention Characteristics of Membrane Filters,* Doctor of Engineering Thesis, Bibliotek, University of Dortmund, Germany (June 1983).

Badenhop, C.T.; Spann, A.T.; Meltzer, T.H. "A Consideration of Parameters Governing Membrane Filtration", *Membrane Science and Technology,* Flinn, J.E., Ed., pp. 120-138, Plenum Press, New York (1970).

Bader, H.; Hoign, J. "Determination of Ozone in Water by the Indigo Method: A Submitted Standard Method", *Ozone: Science & Engineering,* 4:169 (1982).

Baffi, R.; Dolch, G.; Garnick, R.; Huang, Y.F.; Mar, B.; Matsuhiro, D.; Niepelt, B.; Parra, C.; Stephan, M. "A Total Organic Carbon Analysis Method for Validating Cleaning Between Products in Biopharmaceutical Manufacturing", *Journal of Parenteral Science and Technology 45(1),* pp. 13-19 (1991).

Bahrani, K.S.; Martin, R.J. "Adsorption Studies Using Gas-Liquid Chromatography: Effect of Molecular Structure", *Water Research, 10,* pp. 731-736 (1976).

Balazs, M. K., Personal Communications 1987)

Balmer, K.B.; Larter, M. "Evaluation of Chelant, Acid and Electropolishing for Cleaning and Passivating 316L Stainless Steel (ss) Using Auger Spectroscopy", *Pharmaceutical Engineering 13(3),* pp. 20-28 (1993).

Banes, P.H. "Passivation: Understanding and Performing Procedures on Austenitic Stainless Steel Systems", *Pharmaceutical Engineering 10(6),* pp. 41-46 (1990).

Banes, P.H. "Passivation of Pharmaceutical Water Systems", Conference on Pharmaceutical Waters, Medical TechSources, Atlantic City, NJ (May 24-25, 1995).

Bates, W.T.; Coulter, B.L.; Thomas, J.D. "Pretreatment Guidelines for Reverse Osmosis", *Ultrapure Water 5(4),* pp. 34-41 (1988).

Baumann, H.; Stucki, S. "On Line Organic Removal in Ultrapure Water Systems with an Electrochemical Ozonizer", *Transcripts of Seventh Annual Semiconductor Pure Water Conference,* pp. 307-321, Santa Clara, CA (January 14-15, 1988).

Baumann, H.; Stucki, S. "Process Technologies for Water Treatment", Tenth Brown Boveri Symposium (1989).

Beardsley, S.S., Coker, S.D. and Whipple, S.S. "The Economics of Reverse Osmosis and Ion Exchange, *Ultrapure Water 12(2),* pp. 41-52 (1995).

Beasley, J.K. "The Evaluation and Selection of Polymeric Materials for Reverse Osmosis Membranes", *Desalination 22,* pp. 181-189 (1977).

Beckwith, T.D.; Moser, J.R. "Germicidal Effectiveness of Chlorine, Bromine, and Iodine", *Journal American Water Works Association 25,* pp. 367-374 (1933).

Benedek, A.; Johnston, L. "Considerations in Choosing RO Versus Ion Exchange for Demineralization", *Ultrapure Water 5(7),* pp. 57-62 (1988).

Berman, D.; Meyers, T.; Chrai, S. "Factors Involved in Cycle Development of a Steam-in-Place System", *Journal of Parenteral Science and Technology 40(4),* pp. 119-121 (1986).

Berkleman, R.L.; Anderson, R.L.; Davis, B.J.; Highsmith, A.K.; Peterson, W.J.; Bond, W.W.; Cook, E.H.; Mackel, D.C.; Favero, M.S.; Martone, W.J.; "Intrinsic Bacterial Contamination of a Commercial Iodophor Solution: Investigation of the Implemented Manufacturing Plant", *Applied and Environmental Microbiology 47(4),* pp. 752-756 (1984).

Bernatowicz, J.; Collins, B. "Producing Purified Water by Two Bed/Cation Polisher Deionization", *Pharmaceutical Engineering 6(1),* pp. 26-27, 38 (1986).

Blackmer, R.A. "Smith, Kline and French Laboratories, Philadelphia, PA, Sterile Operations Facility", *Journal of Parenteral Science and Technology 38(5),* pp. 183-189 (1984).

Blanden, P.D.; James, J.B; Krygier, V.; Howard, G., Jr, "Comparison of Bacterial and Endotoxin Retention by Charge-Modified Sterilizing Grade Filters During Intermittent Long Term Use", *Journal of Parenteral Science and Technology 45(5),* pp. 229-232 (1991).

Blatt, W.R.; David, A.; Michaels, A.S.; Nelsen, L.L. "Solute Polarization and Cake Formation in Membrane Ultrafiltration: Causes, Consequences and Control Techniques", *Membrane Science and Technology,* Flinn, J.E., Ed., pp. 47-97, Plenum Press, New York (1970).

Böddeker, K.W.; Hilgendorf, W.; Kaschemekat, J. "Reverse Osmosois — Concepts and Realization of the GKSS Plate System", *Proceedings Sixth International Symposium Fresh Water from the Sea 3,* pp. 271-276 (1978).

Bordner, R.H., U.S. Environmental Protection Agency. Private communications (1987).

Borgquist, J.; Brodie, D. "The Production of Low TOC Ion-Exchange Resins", *Ultrapure Water Expo '89-East Conference on High Purity Water, Proceedings,* pp. 43-47,

Philadelphia, PA (April 24-26, 1989).

Bowman, F.W.; Calhoun, M.P.; White, M. "Microbiological Methods for Quality Control of Membrane Filters", *Journal of Pharmaceutical Sciences 56(2),* pp. 453-459 (1967).

Bratby, J. "Coagulation and Flocculation Tests", Chapter 8 in *Coagulation and Flocculation,* p. 268, Uplands Press, Croyden, U.K. (1980).

Brock, T.D. "Membrane Filtration: A User's Guide and Reference Manual", *Science Technology,* pp. 55-58, Madison, WI (1983).

Brose, D.J., Hendricksen, G., "A Quanitative Analysis of Preservative Adsorption on Microfiltration membranes", *Pharmaceutical Technology, 18(3),* pp. 64-73 (1994).

Brown, P.W. "Storage and Distribution of Distilled Water, LVP's", *Proceedings of PMA Water Seminar Program,* pp. 111-115, Atlanta, GA (1982).

Brown, C.J. and Fletcher, C.J., "Water Deionization by Recoflo Short Bed Ion Exchange", *47th Annual Meeting International Water Conference*, Pittsburgh, PA, (1986).

Bukay, M., "Dead Legs: A Widespread Threat to DI Water Systems", *Ultrapure Water 4(3),* pp. 66-70 (1987)

Bulletin on Material Welds and Finishers (WF,890-1), DCI Inc., St Cloud, MN (

Burns, T.F.; Booth, C. "Ultrafiltration Pretreatment of Reverse Osmosis Make-Up Systems", *Ultrapure Water 5(9),* pp. 44-47 (1988).

Burris, Jr., M.K. "Boiler Water Treatment Principles, Part I", *Ultrapure Water 4(2),* pp. 60-63 (1987a).

Burris, Jr., M.K. "Boiler Water Treatment Principles, Part II", *Ultrapure Water 4(3),* pp. 61-65 (1987b).

Burris, Jr., M.K. "Oxygen Scavengers", *Ultrapure Water 4(4),* pp. 54-58 (1987c).

Cain, C.W. "Filter Aid Filtration—The Interaction of Filter Aid Pore Sizes and Turbidity Pore Sizes", American Institute of Chemical Engineers, Vancouver, BC (September 1973).

Calman, C.; Simon, G.P. "Behavior of Ion Exchangers in Ultrapure Water Systems", Conference on Ion Exchange, London, U.K. (1969).

Camper, A.K.; Hamilton, M.; Johnson, K. "Bacterial Colonization of Surfaces in Flowing Systems: Methods and Analyses", Ultrapure Water Expo '94, Philadelphia, PA (May 9-11, 1994).

Carazzone, M.; Arecio, D.; Fava, M.; Sancin, P. "A New Type of Positively Charged Filter: Preliminary Test Results", *Journal of Parenteral Science and Technology 39(2),* pp. 69-74 (1985).

Carling, J.B.; Roy, M. "Controlling Pretreatment Coagulants with Streaming Current Technology", *Ultrapure Water Expo '90-East Conference on High Purity Water, Proceedings,* pp. 111-115, Philadelphia, PA (April 24-26, 1989).

Carlson, S.; Hasselbarth, U.; Mecke, P. "Understanding The Disinfecting Action of Chlorinated Swimming Pool Waters Through Determination of Redox Potentials", *Arch. Fr. Hyg. 152,* pp. 306-319 (1968).

Carman, P.C. "Fluid Flow Through Granular Beds", Trans. Inst. Chem., London 15, pp. 150-155 (1937).

Carmody, J.C.; Martyak, J.E. "Controlling Bacterial Growth in an Ultrapure Water System", *Microcontamination 7(1),* pp. 28-35 (1989).

Carson, L.A.; Petersen, N.J. "Photoreactivation of *Pseudomonas cepacia* after Ultraviolet Exposure: A Potential Source of Contamination in Ultraviolet Treated Waters", *Journal of Clinical Microbiology* (May 1975).

Carter, J., "Evaluation of Recovery Filters for Use in Bacterial Retention Testing of Sterilizing-Grade Filters", *PDA Jour. Pharm. Sci. & Technology 50(3)*, pp. 147-154 (1996).

Carter, J.W. "Membrane Techniques (Reverse Osmosis and Ultrafiltration)", Towards Absolute Water, A Survey of Current Water Purification, *Proceedings of International Symposium,* pp. 103-114, Lane End, High Wycombe, Bucks, England (May 1976).

Cartwright, P.S. Private communication (1991).

Carvell, J.P. "Sterility and Containment Considerations in Valve Selection", *Pharm. Eng. 12(1),* pp. 31-35 (1992).

Celeste, "Operation of the FDA: A Summary, Chapter in *"Filtration in the Pharmaceutical Industry"*, 2nd. Ed., T.H. Meltzer and M.W. Jarnitz, Marcel Dekker, NY (In Press).

Chang, H.W.; Bock, E. "Pitfalls in the Use of Commercial Nonionic Detergents for the Solubilization of Integral Membrane Proteins: Sulfhydryl Oxidizing Contaminants and Their Elimination", *Biochemistry 104,* pp. 112-117 (1980).

Chapman, K.G.; Alegnani, W.C.; Heinze, G.E.; Flemming, C.W.; Kochling, J.; Croll, D.B.; Kladko, M.; Lehman, W.J.; Smith, D.C.; Adair, F.W.; Amos, R.L.; Enzinger, R.M.; Grant, D.E.; Soli, T.E. "Protection of Water Treatment Systems—Part I—The Problem", *Pharmaceutical Technology 7(5),* pp. 48-57 (1983a).

Chapman, K.G.; Alegnani, W.C.; Heinze, G.E.; Flemming, C.W.; Kochling, J.; Croll, D.B.; Fitch, M.W.; Kladko, M.; Lehman, W.J.; Smith, D.C.; Adair, F.W.; Amos, R.L.; Enzinger, R.M.; Soli, T.E. "Protection of Water Treatment Systems—Part IIB—Potential Solutions", *Pharmaceutical Technology 7(9),* pp. 38-49 (1983b).

Chapman, K.G.; Alegnani, W.C.; Heinze, G.E.; Flemming, C.W.; Kochling, J.; Croll, D.B.; Kladko, M.; Lehman, W.J.; Smith, D.C.; Adair, F.W.; Amos, R.L.; Enzinger, R.M.; Soli, T.E. "Protection of Water Treatment Systems—Part IIB—Potential Solutions", *Pharmaceutical Technology 7(9),* pp. 86-92 (1983c).

Chapman, K.G.; Alegnani, W.C.; Heinze, G.E.; Flemming, C.W.; Kochling, J.; Croll, D.B.; Kladko, M.; Lehman, W.J.; Smith, D.C.; Adair, F.W.; Amos, R.L.; Enzinger, R.M.; Frieben, W.R.; Soli, T.E. "Protecton of Water Treatment Systems—Part III—Validation and Control", *Pharmaceutical Technology 8(9),* pp. 54-69 (1984).

Characklis, W. "Attached Microbial Growths—II. Frictional Resistance Due to Microbial Slimes", *Water Research 7,* pp. 1249-1258 (1973).

Characklis, W. "Fouling Biofilm Development: A Process Analysis", *Biotechnology & Bioengineering 23,* pp. 1923-1940 (1981).

Chawla, G.L.; Varma, M.M.; Balram, A.; Murali, M.M. "Trihalomethane Removal and

Formation Mechanism in Water", *Chemical Engineering Report,* District of Columbia University (1983).

Chesney, D.L., The FDA-483: Its History and Present Use", *Pharm. Tech*, 20(4), pp. 88-97 (1996).

Chet, J.; Asketh, P.; Mitchell, R. "Repulsion of Bacteria from Marine Surfaces", *Applied and Environmental Microbiology 15,* pp. 1043-1045 (1975).

Christian, D.A.; Meltzer, T.H. "The Penetration of Membranes by Organism Grow-Through and Its Related Problems", *Ultrapure Water 3(3),* pp. 39-44 (1986).

Chu, T.S. "Trihalomethanes Can Cause RO/DI System Problems", *Transcripts of Eighth Annual Semiconductor Pure Water Conference,* pp. 229-255, Santa Clara, CA (January 18-20, 1989a).

Chu, T.S. "Investigating THMs As a Cause of RO/DI System Problems: The Summertime Blues Revisited", *Microcontamination 7(7),* pp. 35-38, 104, 105, (1989b).

Chu, T.S.; Houskova, J. "Ionic Concentrations Found in Pure Water Used by the Semiconductor Industry", *Transcripts of Fourth Annual Semiconductor Pure Water Conference,* pp. 180-196, San Francisco, CA (January 10-11, 1985).

Clancy, J.L.; Cimini, L. "Improved Methods for Recovering Bacteria from Water", *Ultrapure Water Expo '91-East Conference on High Purity Water, Proceedings,* pp. 118-125, Philadelphia, PA (April 29 - May 1, 1991).

Coates, J.L.; Dover, F.N.; Ruley, W.B. "The Water for Injection System at the Upjohn Company", *Journal of Parenteral Science and Technology 37(4),* pp. 113-116 (1983).

Code of Federal Regulations. "Human and Veterinary Drugs", 21CFR, Parts 201, 207, 210, 211, 212 (1976).

Cohen, N. "Pretreatment Strategies for TOC Reduction in WFI and USP Purified Water", *Pharmaceutical Technology 19(6),* pp. 96-104 (1995).

Coin, L.; Gomella, C.; Hannoun, C.; Trimoreau, J.C. "Ozone Inactivation of Poliomyelitis Virus in Water", *La Presse Medicale 72(37),* pp. 1883-1884 (1967a).

Coin, L.; Hannoun, C.; Gomella, C. "Inactivation of Poliomyelitis Virus in the Presence of Water", *La Presse Medicale 72(37),* pp. 2153-2156 (1967b).

Cole, J.C. "Considerations in Application of Bacteria-Retentive Air-Vent Filters", *Pharmaceutical Technology 1(1),* pp. 49-53 (1977).

Coleman, D.C. Private communication (1991).

Coleman, D.C.; Evans, R.W. "Fundamentals of Passivation and Passivity in the Pharmaceutical Industry", *Pharmaceutical Engineering 10(2),* pp. 43-49 (1990).

Coleman, D.C.; Evans, R.W. "Investigation of the Corrosion of 316L Stainless Steel Pharmaceutical Water for Injection Systems", *Pharmaceutical Engineering 11(4),* pp. 9-13 (1991).

Collentro, W.V. "Pretreatment Part 1: Activated Carbon Filtration", *Ultrapure Water 2(5),* pp. 24-33 (1985a).

Collentro, W.V. "Pretreatment Part 2: Activated Carbon Filtration", *Ultrapure Water 2(6),* pp. 45-48 (1985b).

Collentro, W.V. "Treatment of Water With Ultraviolet Light-Part II", *Ultrapure Water 3(6)*, pp. 49-51 (1986).

Collentro, W.V. "A New Approach to the Production of Ultra High Purity, Low TOC Water", *Ultrapure Water 4(9)*, pp. 40-43 (1987).

Collentro, W.V. "An Overview of USP Purified Water - Part II", *Ultrapure Water 9(9)*, pp. 28-38 (1992).

Collentro, W.V. "An Overview of USP Purified Water - Part III", *Ultrapure Water 10(2)*, pp. 27-34 (March 1993).

Collentro, W.V. "Microbiological Control in Purified Water Systems—Case Histories", Ultrapure Water Expo '94, Philadelphia, PA (May 9-11, 1994).

Colwell, R.R. "Viable but Non-Culturable Bacteria and Their Implications for Water Purification", Ultrapure Water Expo '94, Philadelphia, PA (May 9-11, 1994).

Colwell, R.R.; Huq, A. "Viable but Non-Culturable Bacteria and Their Implications for Water Purification", *Ultrapure Water* 12(3), pp. 67-74 (1995).

Comb, L. Private communication (1991).

Comb, L.; Fulford, K. "CA/PA Two-Pass Reverse Osmosis — A Case History", *Ultrapure Water 8(7)*, pp. 44-49 (1991).

Comb, L.; Schneekloth, P. "High Purity Water Using Two-Pass Reverse Osmosis", *Ultrapure Water 7(3)*, pp. 49-53 (1989).

Combs, R.F.; Veloz, T.M. "Fabrication of Stainless Steel for High Purity Water Systems", *Ultrapure Water 7(3)*, pp. 54-57 (1990).

Conley, J.D.; Puzig, E.H. "Bromine Chemistry, An Alternative to Dechlorination", *Proceedings of the Condenser Technology Symposium of the Electric Power Research Institute* (1987).

Conway, R.S. "State of the Art in Fermentation Air Filtration", *Biotechnology & Bioengineering 26*, pp. 844-847 (1984).

Cooper, M.S. "A Review of the ASM Seminar on Microbiological Consideration for Purified Water", *Microbiological Update 2(2)* (May 1984).

Cooper, M.S. "Review of Microbiological Test Methods Compendium", *Microbiological Update 2(3)* (June 1984).

Cooper, M.S. "Pharmaceutical and Cosmetics Process Water", *Microbiological Update 5(4)* (July 1987).

Cooper, M.S. "Water", *Microbiological Update 6(3)* (June 1988).

Citation not found.

Cooper, M.S. "Water for Pharmaceutical and Cosmetic Manufacture", *Microbiological Update 6(11)* (February 1989).

Cooper, M.S. "Microbial Limit Testing of Non-Sterile Products", *Microbiological Update 6(12)* (March 1989).

Cooper, M.S. "Filtration of Gases and Vent Filters", *Microbiological Update 7(2)* (May 1989).

Cooper, M.S. "Sterilization Topics", *Microbiological Update 7(7)* (October 1989).

Cooper, M.S. "Purified Pharmaceutical Water", *Microbiological Update 13(11)* (January 1996).

Cooper, M.S. "Private Communications (1996).

Costerton, J.W. "The Role of Polysaccharides in Nature and Disease", National Meeting of the American Society for Microbiology (March 1984-A).

Costerton, J.W. "Mechanisms of Microbial Adhesion to Surfaces", *Current Perspectives in Microbial Ecology,* Klug, M.J.; Reddy, C.A., Eds., pp. 115-123 American Society for Microbiology, Washington, DC (1984-B).

Costerton, J.W.; Boivin, J., Jr. "Chapter 3: Microbial Influenced Corrosion", *Biological Fouling of Industrial Water Systems: A Problem Solving Approach,* Mittelman, M.W.; Geesey, G.G., Eds., Water Micro Associates, Long Beach, CA (1987).

Costerton, J.W.; Geesey, G.G. "Microbial Contamination of Surfaces", *Surface Contamination,* Vol. 1, Mittal, K.L., Ed. Plenum Press, New York, NY (1979).

Costerton, J.W.; Geesey G.G.; Cheng, K.J. "How Bacteria Stick", *Scientific American 238,* pp. 86-95 (1978).

Cotton, S.H. "Optimize Oxygen Control in Your Boiler-Feed Systems", *Power 124(10),* pp. 52-56 (1980).

Coulter, B.L.; Thomas, D.J. "The History, Development, and Present Application of Mixed-Bed Ion Exchange for the Production of High Purity Demineralized Water", *Ultrapure Water 4(8),* pp. 40-46 (1987).

Crane, G.A. "A Replacement for the Oxidizable Substances Test", *Pharmacopeial Forum 15,* pp. 5554-5555 (1989).

Crane, G.A.; Mittelman, M.W.; Stephan, M. "Total Organic Carbon Measurement as a Substitute for the USP Oxidizable Substances Test", *Journal of Parenteral Science and Technology 45(1),* pp. 20-28 (1991).

Crits, G.J. "Pretreatment Methods for Ion Exchange and Reverse Osmosis", *Ultrapure Water 6(6),* pp. 48-57 (1989).

Cruver, J.E. "Water Disinfection—A Comparison of Chlorine, Ozone, UV Light, and Membrane Filtration", Eighth Annual Membrane Technoglogy/Planning Conference & First High-Tech Separations Symposium, Newton, MA (October 15-17, 1990).

Curcie, W. "Investigations into the Fouling of Hollow Fiber Polyamide RO Membranes", *Ultrapure Water 6(8),* pp. 13-23 (1989).

Cutler, F.M. "Evaluation and Selection of Ion Exchange Resins for Producing High Purity Water", *Transcripts of Sixth Annual Semiconductor Pure Water Conference,* pp. 90-109, Santa Clara, CA, (January 15-16, 1987).

Cutler, F.M. Private communications (1991).

Cutler, R.M.; Nykanen, J.F. "High Purity Water Production, Storage, and Distribution", *Pharmaceutical Engineering 8(5),* pp. 29-34 (1988).

D'Angelo, P. Private communications (1991).

Davies, C.M. *Air Filtration,* p. 123, Academic Press, London, U.K. (1973).

Dawson, M.D. Private communications (1991).

Dawson, M.D.; Novitsky, T.J.; Gould M.J. "Microbes, Endotoxins and Water", *Pharmaceutical Engineering 8(2),* pp. 9-12 (1988).

Dean, D.A. "Sources of Particulate Contamination in Sterile Packaging", *Pharmaceutical Technology 9(8),* pp. 33-36 (1985).

Decedue, C.J.; Unruh, W.P. "Detection and Measurement of Particles in Water Prepared for HPLC", *Biotechnics 2(2),* pp. 78-81 (1984).

Del Ciello, R. "Astra's WFI System — An Overview", *Proceedings of PMA Water Seminar Program,* pp. 66-72, Atlanta, GA (February 1982).

DeLuca, P.P. "Microcontamination Control: A Summary of an Approach to Training", *Journal of Parenteral Science and Technology 37(6),* pp. 218-224 (1983).

De Rudder, D.; De Muynck, C.; Remon, J.P.; Bawim R.; Gyselinck, P. "Validation Technique for the Filling Operation of Oxygen Sensitive Injectables", *Journal of Parenteral Science and Technology 43(5),* pp. 225-226 (1989).

Desaulniers, C. and Fey, T, "The Product-Bubble Point and Its Use in Filter Integrity Testing", *Pharm. Tech. 42(10)*, pp. 42-52 (1990).

Dietrich, J.A. "Principles of Operating Vacuum Degasifiers", *Ultrapure Water 9(5),* pp. 43-47 (1992).

DiSessa, P.A. "The Generation of Pharmaceutical Grade Water by Distillation", *Pharmaceutical Technology 4(11),* pp. 102-112 (1980).

DiSessa, P.A. "Treatise on Pharmaceutical and Institutional Water Systems", Barnstead Company, Boston, MA (1981).

Disi, S.A. "Distillation for WFI Systems", Conference on Pharmaceutical Waters, Medical Tech Sources, Atlantic City, NJ (May 24-25, 1995).

Dobiasch, P.H.S. "Principles of Combined U.V. and Ozone Generation", *Process Ozone + Ultra-Violet Water Treatment,* W.J. Masschelein, Coordination (Paris, France: Int'l Ozone Association, European Committee pp. B.E.1-B.3.7) (1986).

Dosmar, M.; Wolber, P. "Design Considerations for the Integration of Crossflow Processes in Biopharmaceutical Applications", *Pharmaceutical Engineering 11(3),* pp. 15-18 (1991).

Dosmar, M.; Wolber, P.; Bracht, K.; Tröger, H.; Waibel, P. "The Water Intrusion Integrity Test for Hydrophobic Membrane Filters", *Journal of Parenteral Science and Technology 46(4),* pp. 102-106 (1992).

Driscoll, Jr., C.T.; Letterman, R.D.; Fitch, D.E. "Residual Aluminum in Filtered Water", *American Water Works Association Research Foundation Bulletin 90530,* AWWA Research Foundation, Denver, CO (1987).

Dunleavy, M.J. "Membrane Technologies In the Power Industry", The Ninth Annual Membrane Technology/Planning Conference & Second High-Tech Separations Symposium, Newton, MA (November 4-6, 1991).

Dunning, D.; Hanselka, R. "DI System Cleaning/Sanitation", *Transcripts of Eighth*

Annual Semiconductor Pure Water Conference, pp. 137-155, Santa Clara, CA (January 18-20, 1989).

Durham, L. "Qualifying Colloidal Fouling in RO Systems", *Ultrapure Water 8(7),* pp. 65-68 (1991).

Dvorin, R.; Pasqua, T. "Dissolved Solids, Carbon Dioxide, and Silica Reductions by Electrodialysis Reversal", *Ultrapure Water 5(9),* pp. 18-23 (1988).

Dvorin, R.; Zahn, J. "Organic and Inorganic Removal by Ultrafiltration", *Ultrapure Water 4(9),* pp. 44-46 (1987).

Dwyer, J.L. "Chapter 10: Control of Contaminants in Liquids", *Contamination Analysis and Control,* pp. 234-237, Reinhold Publishing Company, New York, NY (1966).

Elford, W.J. "The Principles of Ultrafiltration as Applied in Biological Studies", *Proceedings of the Royal Society, 112B,* pp. 384-406, London, U.K. (1933).

Ellner, P.D.; Ellner, S. "A Biological Method for Measuring the Actual Dosage Delivered by Ultraviolet Water Purifiers", Private Communication (1986).

Elstad, N.L. "Practical Aspects of Silt Density Index Testing", *Fluid Particle Separation Journal 5(1),* pp. 6-9 (1992).

Elyanow, D.; Sievka, E.; Mahoney, J. "The Determination of Supersaturation Limits in an EDR Unit with Aliphatic Anion Membranes", *Technical Proceedings Water Supply Improvements Association 9th Annual Conference,* Washington, DC (1981).

Emery, A.P.; Girard, J.E.; Jandik, P. "The Analysis and Identification of Ion Exchange Degradation Products in Ultrapure Water", *Transcripts of Seventh Annual Semiconductor Pure Water Conference,* pp. 170-193, Santa Clara, CA (January 14-15, 1988).

Emory, S.F.; Koga, Y.; Azuma, N.; Matsumoto, K. "The Effects of Surfactant Type and Latex-Particle Feed Concentration on Membrane Retention", *Ultrapure Water 10(2),* pp. 41-44 (1993).

Environmental Protection Agency, EPA 543-9-82-026, Pesticide Assessment Guidelines Subdivision G. Product Performance, "Efficacy of Antimicrobial Agents: Public Health Uses" (October 1982).

Environmental Protection Agency. *The Safe Drinking Water Act, A Pocket Guide to the Requirements for the Operators of Small Water Systems,* EPA Regional Office of the Safe Drinking Water Hotline 800-426-4791. Published by EPA, Region 9, W-6-1, San Francisco, CA (1990).

Erbe, F. "Die Bestimmung der Porenvertenung Nach Ihrer Grosse", *Filtern and Ultra-Filtern, Kolloid Z 63(3),* pp. 277-285 (1933).

Evans-Strickfaden, T.T., Ashima, K.H., Highsmith, A.K. and Ades, E.W., "Endotoxin Removal Using 6,000 Molegular Weight Cut-off Polyacrylonitrile (PAN) and Polysulfone (PS) Hollow Fiber Ultrafiltration", *PDA Jour. Pharm. Sci. & Tech. 50(3)*, pp. 154-158 (1996).

Everett, N.A. "Cost Considerations in the Selection of a Water Purification System", *Bulletin of the Parenteral Drug Association 30(4),* pp. 196-200 (1976).

Exner, M.; Tuschewetski, G.J.; Scharnagel, J. "Influence of Biofilms by Chemical Disinfectants and Mechanical Cleaning", *Zbl. Bakt. Hyg. B 183,* pp. 549-563 (1987).

Farina, L. "Inspection of Deionized Water Systems", U.S. Food and Drug Administration, Hicksville, NY, Office, 183 South Broadway, Room 212, Hicksville, NY 11801.

Farrington, J.K. "Use of Reverse Osmosis (RO) Water Treatment Systems in Pharmaceutical Manufacturing", The Proprietary Association (now the Non-Prescription Drug Manufacturers, Washington, DC) Manufacturing Control Seminar, Philadelphia, PA (October 10-12, 1984).

Federal Register 4(31), 6878-6894, Human Drugs — "CGMP for LVP's and SVP's", 21CFR, Part 212 Proposed Regulations.

Federal Register, Volume 54 (124): 27566, "Total Coliform Rule" (June 29, 1989).

Fernandez, F.; Calderon, R.L.; Hauser, P.H. "Colonization of GAC Water Filters by Water Distribution Bacteria", *Abstracts of the Annual Meeting of the American Society for Microbiology,* Washington, DC (1986).

Fiore, J.V.; Babineau, R.A. "Filtration, an Old Process with a New Look", *Food Technology 33,* pp. 67-72 (1979).

Fiore, J.V.; Olson, W.P.; Holst, S.L. "Depth Filtration", *Methods of Plasma Protein Fractionation,* Curling, J.M., Ed., Academic Press, New York, NY (1980).

Fisher, S.; Otten, G. "Giving the Resin Its Annual Health Check", *Ultrapure Water 2(6),* pp. 30-34 (1985).

Flemming, H.C. "Peressigsaure als Desinfectionsmittel", *Krankenhaushyg, Arbeitshyg, Praev. Medicin 179(2),* pp. 97-111 (1984).

Flemming, H-C. "Microbes on Ion-Exchangers" in *Ion Exchange for Industry,* Streat, M., Ed., Ellis Harwood Ltd., Chichester, U.K. (1988).

Fletcher, C.J. and Pace, V., "New Performance Standards for Demineralizers Set By Recoflo Technology", *American Power Conference*, Chicago, Il (1995).

Food and Drug Administration, "Guideline on Sterile Drug Products Produced by Aseptic Processing", Division of Manufacturing and Product Quality, Office of Compliance Center for Drugs and Biologics, Rockville, MD (1988).

Food and Drug Administration, "Mid-Atlantic Region Guideline To Inspection of Bulk Pharmaceutical Chemicals" Rockville, MD (March 1991).

Food and Drug Administration, "Guide to Inspections of High Purity Water Systems", The Division of Field Investigations, Office of Regional Operations, Office of Regulatory Affairs, FDA, Rockville, MD (July 1993).

Foster, F. Private communications (1991).

Forster, H.A. "Clean-Steam — An Overview of the Pharmaceutical Manufacturing Industry", *Proceedings of the PMA Water Seminar,* pp. 50-65, Atlanta, GA (1982).

Francis, P.D. "The Use of Ultraviolet Light and Ozone to Remove Organic Contaminants in Ultrapure Water", presented at Integrated Circuit Manufacturers Consortium Conference, Coventry, U.K. (February 9-10, 1987).

Frank, J.F.; Kaffi, R.A. "Surface-Adherent Growth of *Listeria monocytogenes* Is Associated with Increased Resistance to Surface Sanitizers and Heat", *J. Food Prot. 53,* pp. 550-554 (1990).

Frederick, K.H. "Design of High Purity Water Systems", *Ultrapure Water 4(6),* pp. 54-58 (1987-A).

Frederick, K.H.; Cartwright, P. *Beyond the Basics: An Advanced Course in High Purity Water Systems*, Tall Oaks Publishing, Littleton, CO.

Fry, E. "The FDA Perspective: Drugs", PDA/PMA International Conference on Sterilization in the 1990s, Washington, DC (August 27-29, 1990).

Futatsuki, T.; Urai, N.; Shindo, I. "Waste Water Reclamation Systems and Closed Water Systems", *Proceedings of Tenth Annual Semiconductor Pure Water Conference,* pp. 42-68, Santa Clara, CA (February 26-28, 1991).

Gabler, F.R. "Chapter 11: Principles of Tangential Flow Filtration: Applications to Biological Processing", *Filtration In the Pharmaceutical Industry,* Meltzer, T.H. Ed., Marcel Dekker, New York (1987).

Gagnon, S.; Cheney, J.; Drake, H. "Low TDS, High TOC and Their Effect on High Purity Water Production in New England", *Ultrapure Water Expo '91-East Conference on High Purity Water, Proceedings,* pp. 53-62, Philadelphia, PA (April 29 - May 1, 1991).

Gagnon, S.; Plank, E.; Kling, A. "Case Study — Reverse Osmosis Problem", *Ultrapure Water 10(7),* pp. 33-43 (1993).

Gagnon, S.R. and Lesiczka, R. "AT&T Technologies--RO System Case Study", *Ultrapure Water 11(4),* pp. 45-53 (1994).

Gagnon, S.R. and Rodriguez, J.. "Applying Quality Assurance Concepts to Ensure the Performance of Pharmaceutical High-Purity Water Treatment Systems", *Microcontamination 12(1),* pp. 43-50 (1994).

Ganzi, G.C. Personal communications (1991).

Ganzi, G.C.; Egozy, Y.; Giuffrida, A.J.; Jha, A.D. "High Purity Water by Electrodeionization; Performance of the Ionpure (TM) Continuous Deionization System", *Ultrapure Water 4(3),* pp. 75-79 (1987).

Ganzi, G.C.; Parise, P.L. "The Production of Pharmaceutical Grades of Water Using Continuous Deionization Post-Reverse Osmosis", *Journal of Parenteral Science and Technology 44(4),* pp. 231-241 (1990).

Garvan, J.M.; Gunner, B.W. "Particulate Contamination of Intravenous Solutions," *British Journal of Clinical Practice 25,* pp. 119-121 (1971).

Geesey, G.G. "Survival of Microorganisms in Low Nutrient Waters", *Biological Fouling of Industrial Water Systems: A Problem Solving Approach,* Mittelman, M.W.; Geesey, G.G., Ed., Water Micro Associates, San Diego, CA (1988).

Geldreich, E.E.; Taylor, R.H.; Blanson, J.C.; Reasoner, D.J. "Bacterial Colonization of Point-of-Use Water Treatment Devices", *Journal American Water Works Association 77,* pp. 72-80 (1985).

Gelzhäuser, P. "Application and Design of UV Units", *Proceedings Ozone + Ultra-Violet Water Treatment,* Masschelein, W.J., Coordination, (Paris, France: International Ozone Association, European Committee, 1986), pp. B.2.1.-B.2.19 (1986).

Ghosh, K.; Schnitzer, H. "UV and Visible Absorption Spectroscopic Investigations in Relation to Macromolecular Characteristics of Humic Substances", *Journal of Soil*

Science 30, pp. 735 (1979).

Giorgio, R.J. "Considerations in the Design of Hot Circulating Water-for-Injection Systems", *Pharmaceutical Technology 2,* pp. 19-24 (1978).

Giusti, D.M.; Conway, R.A.; Lawson, C.T. "Activated Carbon Adsorption of Petrochemicals", *Journal Water Pollution Control Federation 46(5),* pp. 947-965 (1974).

Glaze, W.H. "Drinking Water Treatment with Ozone", *Environmental Science and Technology 21(3),* pp. 224-230 (1987).

Glaze, W.H.; Kang, J.W. "Advanced Oxidation Processes for Treating Groundwater Contaminated with TCE and PCE: Laboratory Studies", *Journal American Water Works Association 80(5),* pp. 57-63 (1988).

Glaze, W.H.; Kang, J.W.; Aieta, E.M. "Ozone-Hydrogen Peroxide Systems for Control of Organics in Municipal Water Supplies", *The Role of Ozone in Water and Wastewater Treatment,* Smith, D.W.; Finch, G.R., Eds., pp. 233-244 TekTran International Ltd., Kitchener, Ontario, Canada (1987b).

Glaze, W.H.; Kang, J.W.; Chapin, D.H. "The Chemistry of Water Treatment Processes Involving Ozone, Hydrogen Peroxide and Ultraviolet Radiation", *Ozone: Science & Engineering, Volume 9,* pp. 335-352, Internationl Ozone Association (1987-A).

Glaze, W.H.; Koga, H.; Cancilla, D.; Wang, K.; McGuire, J.J.; Liang, S.; Davis, M.K.; Tate, C.H.; Aieta, E.M. "Evaluation of Ozonization By-Products from Two California Surface Waters", *Journal American Water Works Association 81(8),* pp. 66-73 (1989).

Goddard, J.L. "Address to the Parenteral Drug Association", Bulletin of the Parenteral Drug Association 20, pp. 183-188 (1966).

Godec, R,; O'Neill, K.; Hutte, R. "New Technology for TOC Analysis in Water", *Ultrapure Water 9(9),* pp. 17-22 (1992).

Goeminne, H.; Bruye, H.; Roos, J.; Aernoudt, E. "The Geometrical and Filtration Characteristics of Metal-Fibre Filters—A Comparative Study", *Filtration and Separation,* pp. 351-355 (July/August 1974).

Goodlett, R.; Comstock, D. "Filtration Study Results: Pilot Study at 7-UP Corp.", *Ultrapure Water 12(4),* pp. 55-59 (1995).

Goozner, R.; Gotlinsky, G. "Field Results for the Reduction of SDI by Pre-RO Filters", *Ultrapure Water 7(2),* pp. 20-30 (1990).

Gordon, G.; Pacey, G.E. "An Introduction to the Chemical Reactions of Ozone Pertinent to Its Analysis", *Analytical Aspects of Ozone Treatment of Water and Wastewater Treatment,* Rice, R.G.; Bollyky, L.J.; Lacy, W.J., Eds., pp. 41-52, Lewis Publishers, Inc., Chelsea, MI (1986).

Gould, M.J., Private communications (1990).

Gould, M.J. "Evaluation of Microbial/Endotoxin Contamination Using the LAL Test", *Ultrapure Water 10(6),* pp. 43-47 (1993).

Gould, M.J.; Dawson, M.E.; Novitsky, T.J. "LAL Applications", *Transcripts of Ninth Annual Semiconductor Pure Water Conference,* pp. 192-199, Santa Clara, CA (January 17-18, 1990).

Gould, M.J.; Dawson, M.D.; Novitsky, T.J. "Particulates as Measured by the Limulus Amebocyte Test", Fine Particle Society Twenty-First Annual Meeting, Session On Membrane Filter Applications, San Diego, CA (August 21-25, 1990).

Governal, R.A.; Shadman, F. "Oxidation and Removal of Organic Particles in High-Purity Water Systems Using Ozone and UV", *Ultrapure Water 9(4),* pp. 44-50.

Grant, D.C.; Peacock, S.L.; Accomazzo, M.A. "A Comparison of Particle Shedding Characteristics of High Purity Water Filtration Cartridges", *Transcripts of Fifth Annual Semiconductor Pure Water Conference,* pp. 252-277 (January 1986).

Gray, D.M. "On-Line Conductivity and Resistivity Measurement", *Ultrapure Water 5(5),* pp. 43-48 (1988).

Gray, D.M. "Continuous pH Measurement in High Purity Water", *Ultrapure Water 6(5),* pp. 38-44 (1989).

Greenbank, M. and Spotts, S., "Effects of Starting Material on Activated Carbon Characteristics and Performance", *Industrial Water 27(1),* pp. 19-31(1995).

Gressett; G, and Korcyl, M. Private Communications (1994).

Griffin, C.; Fournier, C.; Pacek, M.; Dunleavy, M.J. "Regeneration Without Chemicals", Condensate Polishing Workshop, Scottsdale, AZ (June 20, 1991).

Griffin, C. "Advancement in the Use of Continuous Deionization in the Production of High-Purity Water", *Ultrapure Water 8(8),* pp.52-60 (1991).

Grimes, T.L.; Fonner, D.E.; Griffin, J.C.; Pauli, W.A.; Schadewald, F.H. "An Automated Method for Cleaning Tanks and Parts Used in the Processing of Pharmaceuticals", *Bulletin of the Parenteral Drug Association 31(4),* pp. 179-186 (1977).

Gsell, G.V.; Disi, S.A. "Distillation Theory and Practice for the Production of USP Water for Injection", *Medical Manufacturing TechSource,* Pharmaceutical Waters '94 Symposium, pp. 132-172, Atlantic City, NJ (May 25-26, 1994).

Guiliford, J., "Stainless Steels and their Finishes", Chapter in *Filtration for the Pharmaceutical Industry, 2nd. ed.*, T.H. Meltzer and M.W. Jarnitz, Marcel Dekker, New York, NY (In Press)

Guillet, J. "Chapter 1: Fundamental Processes in the Photodegradation of Polyolefins" in *Stabilization and Degradation of Polymers,* Allars, D.L.; Hawkins, W.L., Eds., Advances in Chemistry Series, American Chemistry Society, Washington, DC (1978).

Gupta, H.B. "Classification of Commercially Available RO Membranes", *Ultrapure Water 3(2),* pp. 26-34 (1986a).

Gupta, H.B. "Part II: Design Concepts in Reverse Osmosis for Industrial Applications", *Ultrapure Water 3(3),* pp. 46-50 (1986b).

Gurley, B. "Ozone: Pharmaceutical Sterilant of the Future", *Journal of Parenteral Science and Technology 39(6),* pp. 256-261 (1985).

Haas, C.N.; Karra, S.B. "Kinetics off Microbial Inactivation by Chlorine: Review of Results in Demand-Free Systems", *Water Research 18,* pp. 1443-1449 (1984).

Hagar, D.G.; Loven, C.G.; Giggy, C.L. "On-Site Chemical Oxidation of Organic Contaminants in Groundwater Using UV Catalyzed Hydrogen Peroxide", Annual American Water Works Association Conference, Orlando, FL (June 19-23, 1988).

Hall, D. "A Study of Particulate Contamination in High Purity Water for Integrated Circuit Manufacture", *Transcripts of Third Annual Semiconductor Pure Water Conference,* pp. 105-126, San Jose, CA (January, 1984a).

Hall, D. "Variations in Particulate Contamination in High Purity Water", *European Semiconductor Design and Production 5(2),* pp. 182-186 (1984b).

Hango, R.A. "Membranes in the Electronic Industry for High Purity Water Production", Membrane Technology Planning Conference, Cambridge, MA (November 5-7, 1986).

Hango, R.A. "DI Water Polishing Experience and System Performance", Semicon/West '86, San Mateo, CA (May 19, 1986).

Hango, R.A. Private communications (1989).

Hango, R.A. "Practical Solutions to Ultrapure Water Contamination Problems", *Proceedings of International Conference on Particle Detection, Metrology and Control,* pp. 683-707, Arlington, VA (February 5-7, 1990).

Hango, R.A.; Doane, F.; Bollyky, L.J. "Wastewater Treatment for Reuse in Integrated Circuit Manufacturing", *Wasser/Berlin '81d*; Colloquium Verlag, Otto H. Hess, pp. 303-313, Berlin, Federal Republic of Germany (1981).

Hango, R.A.; Pettengill, N.E. "A Cost Effective Approach to DI Distribution System Upgrade", *Transcripts of Sixth Annual Semiconductor Pure Water Conference,* pp. 3-20, Santa Clara, CA (January 15-16, 1987).

Hango, R.A.; Syverson, W.A.; Miller, M.A.; Fleming, Jr., M.J. "DI Water Point of Use Filter Program For 1-MB DRAM Semiconductor Manufacture", *Transcripts of Eighth Annual Semiconductor Pure Water Conference,* pp. 73-94, Santa Clara, CA (January 18-20, 1989).

Hango, R.A.; White, J.L. "Semiconductor Pure Water Contamination Problems", *Proceedings of International Conference on Particle Detection, Metrology and Control,* pp. 683-707, Arlington, VA (February 5-7, 1990).

Hanselka, R. "Contamination Sources in Deionized-Water Vessels and High-Purity Valving", *Microcontamination 2,* 54-57 (1984).

Hanselka, R. "Material Selection and Proper Installation Procedures for Ultrapure Water Systems", Seminar on Fine Tuning Your Pure Water System for Maximum Efficiency from Balazs Analytical Seminars on Advanced Concepts for Ultrapure Water Systems, Santa Clara, CA, (1991).

Hanselka, R.; Putzier, C. "Material Selection and Proper Installation Procedures for High Purity Water Systems", *Transcripts of Ninth Annual Semiconductor Pure Water Conference,* pp. 26-35, Santa Clara, CA (January 17-18, 1990).

Hanselka, R.; Williams, M.; Bukay, M. "Materials of Construction for Water Systems. Part I: Physical and Chemical Properties of Plastics", *Ultrapure Water 4(5),* pp. 46-50 (1987a).

Hanselka, R.; Williams, R.; Bukay, M. "Materials of Construction For Water Systems, Part 3: Proper Selection of Elastomers", *Ultrapure Water 4(8),* 52-59 (1987b).

Haraguchi, Y.; Imaoka, T.; Takano, S. "A New Ultrapure Water System for Megabit Semiconductor Chip Production", *Transcripts of Sixth Annual Semiconductor Pure Water Conference,* pp. 32-35, Santa Clara, CA (January 15-16, 1987).

Harm, W. "Biological Effects of Ultraviolet Radiation", Cambridge University Press Cambridge, U.K. (1980).

Health Industries Manufacturing Association, "Microbiological Evaluation of Filters for Sterilizing Liquids", Document No. 3, Volume 4, HIMA, Washington, DC (1982).

Helenius, A.; Simons, K. "Solubilization of Membranes by Detergents", *Biochimica et Biophysica Acta 415,* pp. 29-79 (1975).

Henley, M. "Electronics and Pharmaceuticals Are Important UF Markets", *Ultrapure Water 8(4),* pp. 14-17 (1991).

Hiatt, W.C.; Vitzthum, G.H.; Wagener, K.B.; Gerlach, K.; Josefiak, C. "Microporous Membranes Via Upper Critical Temperature Phase Separation", *Material Science of Synthetic Membranes,* Lloyd, D.R., Ed., American Chemical Society, Washington, DC (1984).

Hill, R.; Lorch, W. "Ion Exchange", *Handbook of Water Purification,* Lorch, W., Ed., pp. 191-284, McGraw-Hill Publishing Company, London, New York (1981).

Hoffman, B.J. "A Chemical Approach to Understanding Ion Exchange Performance", *Transcripts of Fourth Annual Semiconductor Pure Water Conference,* pp. 3-21, San Francisco, CA (January 10-11, 1985).

Hoffman, B.J.; Kasahara, M.; Gavaghan, M. "The Effects of Chlorine on Mixed Beds in Ultrapure Water Systems", *Transcripts of Sixth Annual Semiconductor Pure Water Conference,* pp. 59-74 (January 15-16, 1987).

Holton, J.; Seiler, D.; Fulford, K.; Cargo, J.T. "Extractable Analysis of Modified Polyvinylidene Fluoride Polymers Utilized in Deionized Water Applications", *Ultrapure Water 10(4),* pp. 47-52 (1993).

Hou, K.C.; Gerba, C.P.; Gayel, S.M.; Zerda, K.S. "Capture of Latex Beads, Bacteria, Endotoxin and Viruses by Charge Modified Filters", *Applied and Environmental Microbiology 40,* pp. 892-896 (1980).

Hou, K.C.; Zaniewski, R. "Depyrogenation by Endotoxin Removal with Positively Charged Depth Filter Cartridge", *Journal of Parenteral Science and Technology 44(4),* pp. 204-209 (1990).

Howard, G., Jr.; Duberstein, R. "A Case of Penetration of 0.2 μm-Rated Membrane Filters by Bacteria", *Journal of the Parenteral Drug Association, 34(2),* pp. 95-102 (1980).

Hudack, D.A.; Terribile, P.D. "Sampling Plans and Sampling Methods Used for Water Testing in the Pharmaceutical Industry", *Ultrapure Water 6(8),* pp. 61-66 (1989).

Hunt, J.R. "Particle Dynamics in Sea Water: Implications for Predicting the Fate of Discharged Particles", *Environmental Science and Technology, 16,* pp. 303-309 (1982).

Husted, G., Private Communications (1994)

Husted, G.; Rutkowski, A. "Control of Microorganisms in Mixed Bed Resin Polishers by Thermal Sanitization", *Watertech '91 Proceedings,* pp. 43-51, San Jose, CA (November 20-22, 1991).

IAMFEs-USPHS and DIC "3-A Accepted Practices for Permanently Installed Sanitary Product Pipelines and Cleaning Systems", *Journal of Milk and Food Technology 29(3),*

Iler, R.K. *The Chemistry of Silica: Solubility, Polymerization, Colloids and Surface Properties, and Biochemistry,* John Wiley and Sons, New York, NY (1979).

Imaoka, T.; Yagi, Y.; Kasama, Y.; Sugiama, I.; Isagawa, T.; Ohmi, T. "Advanced Ultrapure Water Systems For ULSI Processing", *Proceedings of Tenth Annual Semiconductor Pure Water Conference,* pp. 128-146, Santa Clara, CA (February 26-28, 1991).

Imbalzano, J.F.; Kratzer, D.J. "Inertness of Polymers Containing Fluorine to High Purity Water", *Ultrapure Water 3(3),* pp. 51-58 (1986).

Jabblar, A.H. "Research Study of Stainless Steel Tube Samples Surfaces Using Scanning Electron Microscopy and Auger Electron Spectroscopy Techniques", Technical Report 53908, Structure Probe, Metuchen, NJ (1989).

Jackman, D.L. "Troubleshooting Pharmaceutical Water Systems", Course notes for Parenteral Drug Association periodic presentations (March 1989).

Jackman, D.L. Private communication to T.H. Meltzer (1991).

Jackman, D.L.; Sneed, L.C. "Using Stills for USP Purified Water Production", *Ultrapure Water 7(8),* pp. 58-70 (1990).

Jackson, K.F. "Module Design", Eighth Annual Membrane Technology/Planning Conference and First High-Tech Separations Symposium, Newton, MA (October 15-17, 1990).

Jacobs, S. "The Distribution of Pore Diameters in Graded Ultrafilter Membranes", *Filtration and Separation, 9(5),* pp. 525-530 (1972).

Joel, A.R. "Sorbozon: Ozone Generation With Internal Oxygen Recycle", in *The Role of Ozone in Water and Wastewater Treatment,* Smith, D.W.; Finch, G.R., Eds., pp. 83-88, TekTran International Ltd. Kitchener, Ontario, Canada (1987).

Johnson, W.M. "Ozone Process Water Systems", TechSource Symposium on Current Compliance and Validation Issues, Morristown, NJ (August 28-29, 1990).

Johnston, P.R. "Submicron Filtration", *Chemical Engineering Progress 71,* pp. 70-73 (1975).

Johnston, P.R. "The Most Probable Pore-Size Distribution in Fluid Filter Media, Parts I and II," *Journal of Testing and Evaluation 11(2),* pp. 117-125 (1983).

Johnston, P.R. "Chapter 3: Particles In Fluids", *Fundamentals of Fluid Filtration, A Technical Primer,* Tall Oaks Publishing Company, Littleton, CO (1990).

Johnston, P.R.; Lukaszewicz, R.C.; Meltzer, T.H. "Certain

"Imprecisions in the Bubble Point Measurement", *Journal of Parenteral Science and Technology 35(1),* pp. 36-39 (1981).

Johnston, P.R.; Meltzer, T.H. "Comments on Organism Challenge Levels in Sterilizing Filter Efficiency Testing", *Pharmaceutical Technology 3(11),* pp. 66-70, 110 (1979).

Jonas, A.M. "Potentially Hazardous Effects of Introducing Particulate Matter into the Vascular System of Man and Animals", *Proceedings of FDA Symposium on Safety of Large-Volume Parenteral Solutions,* pp. 23-27, Washington, DC (1966).

Jornitz, M. W. Private communications (1991).

Juberg, D.L.; Pauli, W.A.; Artiss, D.H. "Application of Reverse Osmosis for the

Generation of Water for Injection", *Bulletin of the Parenteral Drug Association 31(2)*, pp. 70-78 (1977).

Juran, J.M. *Quality Control Handbook,* 3rd ed., McGraw-Hill, New York, NY, pp. 22-29, App. 2, p. 2 (1974).

Kaakinen, J.W., Moody, C., FRanklin, J. and Amerlaan A.C.F., "SDI Instrumentation to Estimate the Fouling Potential of RO Feedwater", *Ultrapure Water 11(2)*, pp. 42-54(1994).

Kamiyama, Y.; Lesan, R.; Shintani, T.; Tomaschke, J. "A Comparison of Different Classes of Spiral-Wound Membrane Elements at Low Concentration Feeds", *Ultrapure Water 7(3),* pp. 18-24 (1990).

Katz, M.G. "Measurment of Pore-Size Distribution in Microporous Filters and Membranes", *Proceedings of World Filtration Congress III,* pp. 508-512, Downington, PA, (1982).

Katz, W.E.; Clay, F.G. "Triple-Membrane Demineralizers", *Ultrapure Water 3(5),* pp. 38-44 (1986).

Keer, D. "Gathering Validation Documentation for Pharmaceutical Water Systems-Paer 2", Ultrapure Water 13(3), pp. 32-42 (1995).

Kemmer, I. "Chapter 8: Coagulation and Flocculation" *The Nalco Water Handbook,* 2nd ed., Kemmer, I., Ed., McGraw-Hill, New York (1988).

Kemp, A.R. "Counter-Current Ion Exchange", 22nd Annual Liberty Bell Corrosion Course, Philadelphia, PA (September 24-26, 1984).

Kenley, R.A.; Koberda, M.; DeMond, W.; Hammond, R.B.; Hines, J.; Ashline, K.; Vincent, M.; Sriram, R.; Martinez, A.; Raghavan, N.; Knight, C. "Eliminating Interferences in a Compendial Test for Oxidizable Substances in Water", *Journal of Parenteral Science and Technology 44(5),* pp. 264-271 (1990).

Kesting, R.E. *Synthetic Polymeric Membranes,* McGraw-Hill, Inc., New York, NY, pp. 142-152 (1971).

Kesting, R.E.; Murray, A.S.; Jackson, K.; Newman, J.M. "Highly Anisotropic Microfiltration Membranes", *Pharmaceutical Technology 5(5),* pp. 52-60 (1981).

Kladko, M. "Designing a Cost-Effective USP Purified Water System", *Proceedings of PMA Water Seminar Program,* pp. 123-137, Atlanta, GA (1982).

Kogure, K.; Simidu, U.; Taga, N. "A Tentative Direct Microscopic Method for Counting Live Marine Bacteria", *Canadian Journal of Microbiology 25*, pp. 415-420 (1979).

Komorita, J.D.; Snoeyink, V.L. "Technical Note: Monochloramine Removal from Water by Activated Carbon", *Journal American Water Works Association, 71(1)*, pp.62-65 (1985).

Korin, A. "Economic Considerations of Cross Flow Filtation", Eighth Annual Membrane Technology/Planning Conference & First High-Tech Separation Symposium, Newton, MA (October 15-17, 1990).

Kosaka, K.; Yokoyama, F.; Koike, K.; Urai, N. "Operation Results of Large Scale UPW Plants with New Technologies", *Ultrapure Water 5(1),* pp. 14-25 (1988).

scripts of Eighth Annual Semiconductor Pure Water Conference, pp. 58-72, Santa Clara, CA (January 18-19, 1989).

Lilly, L. "Using a Three-Pronged Synergistic Approach to Maintain DI Water Purity at Point of Use", *Microcontamination 8(6),* pp. 35-38, 108 (1990).

Loeb, S.; Sourirajan, S. "Sea Water Demineralization by Means of an Osmotic Membrane", *Advances in Chemistry Series 38,* pp. 117-132 (1962).

Lukaszewicz, R.C.; Johnston, P.R.; Meltzer, T.H. "Prefilter/Final Filters: A Matter of Particle/Pore Size Distributions", *Journal of Parenteral Science and Technology 35(1),* pp. 40-47 (1981).

Lukaszewicz, R.C.; Meltzer, T.H.; Davis, R.; Bilicich, L. "Fluocarbon Filter Materials: Characteristics, Distinctions and Uses", *Fluid Filtration: Liquid, Vol. II,* ASTM STP 975, Johnston, P.R.; Schroeder, H.G., Eds., American Society for Testing and Materials, Philadelphia, PA (1984).

Luttinger, L.B. "The Use of Polyelectrolytes in Filtration Processes", *Polyelectrolytes for Water and Wastewater Treatment,* Schwoyer, W.L.K., Ed., pp. 211-242, CRC Press, Cleveland, OH, (1981).

Mafu, A.A.; Roy, D.; Goulet, J.; Magny, P. "Attachment of *Listeria monocytogenes* to Stainless Steel, Glass, Polypropylene, and Rubber Surfaces after Short Contact Times", *J. Food Prot. 53,* pp. 742-746 (1990).

Mahoney, R.F. "Unique Energy-Savings Vapor Compression Methodology for Producing Pharmaceutical Grade Water", *Proceedings of PMA Water Seminar Program,* pp. 5-11, Atlanta, GA (1982).

Maier, K.; Scheuermann, E.A. "Formation of Semipermeable Membranes", *Kolloid Z. 171,* pp. 122-135 (1960).

Majumdar, S.B.; Cechler, W.; Sproul, O.J. "Inactivation of Poliovirus in Water by Ozonation", *Journal Water Pollution Control Federation 46,* pp. 2048-2053 (1974).

Majumdar, S.B.; Glassman, S.J. "A Viable Treatment for Circulating Cooling Water Systems", presented at 36th American Power Conference, Illinois (1974).

Maltais, J.B.; Stern, T. "An Evaluation of Various Biocides for Disinfection of Reverse Osmosis Membranes and Water Distribution Systems", *Ultrapure Water 7(3),* pp. 37-40 (1990).

Manfredi, J. Private communications (1991).

Manfredi, J.J. "Distribution System Design and Equipment", Medical Manufacturing TechSource(is that a publication?), Pharmaceutical Waters '94 Symposium, Atlantic City, NJ, pp. 50-115 (May 25-26, 1994).

Manfredi, J.J. "Trouble Shooting Pharmaceutical Water Systems", Medical Manufacturing TechSource(is that a publication?), Pharmaceutical Waters '94 Symposium, Atlantic City, NJ, pp. 173-204 (May 25-26, 1994).

Mangan, D. "Metallurgical, Manufacturing and Surface Finish Requirements for High Purity Stainless Steel System Components", *Journal of Parenteral Science and Technology 45(4),* pp. 170-176 (1991).

Mangravite, F. "Overview of the Use of Polymeric Flocculants and Inorganic Coagulants in Filtration", *Fluid/Particle Separation Journal 2(2),* pp. 95-99 (1989).

Maquet, N. "A Comparison of Fluorinated Polymer Pipeworks for Semiconductor High Purity Water Applications", *Transcripts of Seventh Annual Semiconductor Pure Water Conference,* pp. 5-14, Santa Clara, CA (January 14-15, 1988).

Marquardt, K.; Dengler, H.; Hoffman, H. "Ten-Year Experience in Producing High Purity Water by Reverse Osmosis, Part II—Operating and Performance Data", *Ultrapure Water 4(8),* pp. 31-39 (1987).

Marshall, J.C.; Meltzer, T.H. "Certain Porosity Aspects of Membrane Filters, Their Pore Distributions and Anisotropy", *Bulletin of the Parenteral Drug Association 30(5),* pp. 214-225 (1976).

Marshall, K.C. "Biofilms: An Overview of Bacterial Adhesion, Activity, and Control at Surfaces", *American Society for Microbiology News 58(4),* pp. 202-207 (1992).

Martin, J.M. *Water Microbiology*, Pall Corp., Glen Cove, NY.

Martin, J.M. "Charge Modified Filters for Pharmaceutical Water", Conference on Pharmaceutical Waters, Medical TechSources(Publication?), Atlantic City, NJ (May 24-25, 1995).

Martyak, J.E. "Reverse Osmosis/Deionized Water Bacterial Control at the Central Production Facility", *Microcontamination 6(1),* pp. 34-37, 55 (1988).

Martyak, J.E.; Carmody, J.C.; Lindahl, A.R. "Reviewing Analytical Techniques for the Characterization of Deionized Water", *Microcontamination 9(2),* pp. 19-26 (1991a).

Martyak, J.E.; Carmody, J.C.; Lindahl, A.R. "Reviewing Four Case Studies Where Analytical Characterization Techniques for Deionized Water Were Employed", *Microcontamination 9(4),* pp. 37-40 (1991b).

Matsaoka, T.; Kubota, Y.; Namiuchi, S.; Takubo, T.; Veda, T.; Shibata, H.; Nakamura, H.; Yoshitake, J.; Yamayoshi, T.; Dai, H.; Kamiki, T., "Ozone Decontamination of Bioclean Rooms", *Applied and Environmental Microbiology 43,* pp. 509-513 (1982).

Matsuo, I. "Novel Ultrafiltration Module", *Proceedings of Tenth Annual Semiconductor Pure Water Conference,* pp. 108-127, Santa Clara, CA (February 26-28, 1991).

McAfee, A.L.; Nowlin, B.; Beardsley, S. "Pretreatment of an Ion Exchange Demineralizer with Reverse Osmosis", *Ultrapure Water 7(7),* pp. 54-62 (1990).

McAfee, A.L.; McCormack, A. "Retrofitting and Enlarging Makeup Demineralizer System for Peaking Plant at Texas Utilities Electric Company", *Ultrapure Water 5(8),* pp. 50-53 (1988).

McCoy, W.F. "Chapter 9: Strategies for the Treatment of Biological Fouling", *Biological Fouling of Industrial Water Systems: A Problem Solving Approach,* Mittelman, M.W.; Geesey, G.G., Eds., Water Micro Associates, Long Beach, CA (1987).

McCoy, W.F.; Bryers, J.D., Robbins, J.; Costerton, J.W. "Observations of Fouling Biofilm Formation", *Canadian Journal of Microbiology 27,* pp. 910-917 (1981).

McCoy, W.F.; Costerton, J.W. "Fouling Biofilm Development in Tubular Flow Systems", *Developments in Industrial Microbiology 23,* pp. 551-558 (1982).

McGarvey, F.X. "Factors Related to the Design and Operation of Mixed-Bed Ion-

Exchange Units", *Transcripts of Ninth Annual Semiconductor Pure Water Conference,* pp. 77-89, Santa Clara, CA (January 17-18, 1990a).

McGarvey, F.X. Private communications (1990b).

McGarvey, F.X.; Tamaki, D. "Selection of Ion Exchange Resins for Semiconductor Plants", *Ultrapure Water 6(4),* pp. 32-36 (1989).

McGuire, M.J.; Davis, M.K. "Treating Water with Peroxone, A Revolution in the Making", *Water Engineering & Management,* pp. 42-49 (May 1988).

McNutt, J.L.; Sinisgalli, P.; Chaffee, W. "Ultrapure Water System Hydraulics", *Transcripts of Fifth Annual Semiconductor Pure Water Conference,* pp. 18-32, San Francisco, CA (January 16-17, 1986).

McWilliam, A.J. "The Design of High Purity Water Distribution Systems", *Pharmaceutical Engoneering 15(5),* pp. 54-71 (1995).

Meade, E.H.; Song, P. "Bacteria Recovery in High Purity Water Systems", *Ultrapure Water 2(6)* pp. 35-39 (1985).

Meltzer, T.H. "The Advantages of Asymmetric Filter Morphology", *Ultrapure Water 3(6),* pp. 43-48 (1986).

Meltzer, T.H. "Chapter 1: Depth-Filters, Particles and Filter Ratings", *Filtration in the Pharmaceutical Industry,* pp. 3-60, Marcel Dekker, New York (1987a).

Meltzer, T.H. "Chapter 3: Filter Porosity Characteristics", *Filtration in the Pharmaceutical Industry,* pp. 100-122, Marcel Dekker, New York (1987b).

Meltzer, T.H. "Chapter 7: The Integrity Tests", *Filtration in the Pharmaceutical Industry,* pp. 263-278, Marcel Dekker, New York (1987-C).

Meltzer, T.H. "An Investigation of Membrane Cartridge Shedding: A Quantative Comparison of Four Competitive Filters", *Transcripts of Sixth Annual Semiconductor Pure Water Conference,* pp. 221-239, Santa Clara, CA (January 15-16, 1987-F)(?1987c?).

Meltzer, T.H. "The Utilitarian Significance of Membrane Pore-Size Distributions", *Ultrapure Water 4(2),* pp. 16-24 (1987-H)(1987e?).

Meltzer, T.H. "The Pore Structures of Microporous Filters", *Ultrapure Water 5(5),* pp. 49-55 (1988).

Meltzer, T.H. "A Critical Review of Filter Integrity Testing, Part 1 — The Bubble Point Method; Assesing Filter Compatibility; Initial and Final Testing", *Ultrapure Water 6(4),* pp. 40-51 (1989a).

Meltzer, T.H. "Membrane Filters in Semiconductor Usage: Extractables and Testing for Ozone Compatibility", *Transcripts of Eighth Annual Semiconductor Pure Water Conference,* pp. 256-257, Santa Clara, CA (January 18-19, 1989b).

Meltzer, T.H. "A Critical Review of Filter Integrity Testing, Part II—The Diffusive Air Flow and Pressure-Hold Methods: Initial and Final Testing", *Ultrapure Water 6(5),* pp. 45-56 (1989c).

Meltzer, T.H. "Chapter 6: Pharmaceutical Water: Generations, Storage, Distribution and Quality Testing", *Sterile Pharmaceutical Manufacturing,* Vol. I, Groves, M.J.; Olson, W.P.; Anisfeld, M.H., Eds., Interpharm Press, Buffalo Grove, IL (1991a).

Meltzer, T.H. "Maximizing Particle Removals", *Proceedings of Tenth Annual Semiconductor Pure Water Conference,* Santa Clara, CA (February 26-28, 1991b).

Meltzer, T.H. "The Insufficiency of Single Point Diffusive Air Flow Integrity Testing", *Journal of Parenteral Science and Technology 46(1),* pp. 19-24 (1992).

Meltzer, T.H.; Jornitz, M.W.; Waibel, P.J. "The Hydrophobic Air Filter and the Water Intrusion Test", *Pharmaceutical Technology 18(9),* pp. 76-87 (1994).

Meltzer, T.H.; Rice, R.G. "Chapter 5: Ultraviolet and Ozone Systems", *Biological Fouling of Industrial Water Systems: A Problem Solving Approach,* Geesey, G.G.; Mittelman, M.W., Eds., Water Micro Associates, San Diego, CA (1987).

Merrill, D.T.; Drago, J.A. "Evaluation of Ozone Treatment in Air-Conditioning Cooling Towers", *Condenser Biofouling Control,* Carey, J.F.; Jorden, R.M.; Aitken, A.H.; Burton, D.T.; Grays, R.H., Eds., Ann Arbor Science, Ann Arbor, MI (1980).

Meulemans, C.C.E. "The Basic Principles of UV Sterilization of Water", *Proc. Ozone + Ultra-Violet Water Treatment,* Masschelein, W.J., Coordination, pp. B.1.1-B.1.13, Paris, France: Intl. Ozone Assoc., European Committee, (1986).

Meyer, A.E.H.; Seitz, E.O. *Ultraviolette Strahlen,* W. de Ruyter, Publishers(location?) (1949).

Meyers, P.S. "Destruction of TOC Using Ultraviolet Light", 18th Annual Meeting International Water Conference, Pittsburgh, PA (November 2-4, 1987).

Michaud, D. "Granulated Activated Carbon", A Series of Three Papers, *Water Conditioning and Purification,* June pp. 20-26, July pp.38-50, and August pp. 36-41 (1988).

Michels, D.L. "Letter to the Pharmaceutical Industry Re: Validation and Control of Deionized Water Systems", FDA, Rockville, MD., Bureau of Drugs, Assoc. Dir. of Compliance (1981).

Mittelman, M.W. "Biological Fouling of Purified Water Systems, Part 1", *Microcontamination 3(10),* pp. 51-55, 70 (1985).

Mittelman, M.W. "Biological Fouling of Purified Water Systems, Part 3, Treatment", *Microcontamination 4(1),* pp. 30-40, 70 (1986).

Mittelman, M.W. "Chapter 7: Biological Fouling of Purified Water Systems", *Biological Fouling of Industrial Water Systems, A Problem Solving Approach,* Mittelman, M.W.; Geesey, G.G. Eds., Water Micro Associates, San Diego, CA (1987).

Mittelman, M.W. Private communications (1989).

Mittelman, M.W. "Bacterial Growth and Biofouling Control in Purified Water Systems" in *Biofouling and Biocorrosion in Industrial Systems: Proceedings of the International Workshop on Industrial Biofouling and Biocorrosion,*(??) Stuttgart (September 13-14, 1990) Flemming, H.C.; Geesey, G.G., Eds., Springer-Verlag (1990).

Mittleman, M.W.; Geesey, G.G. "Copper-Binding Characteristics of Expolymers from a Fresh-Water Sediment Bacterium", *Applied and Environmental Microbiology 49,* pp. 846-851 (1985).

Mittleman, M.W.; Geesey, G.G. "Chapter 10: Sampling and Enumeration of Fouling Organisms", *Biological Fouling of Industrial Water Systems: A Problem Solving Approach,* Mittleman, M.W.; Geesey, G.G. Eds., Water Micro Associates, Long Beach,

CA (1987).

Montgomery, G.; Bradley, R. "A New Solution to Produce High Quality Water: Double-Pass RO", *Ultrapure Water 2(5),* pp. 18-19 (1985).

Morris, J.C. "Aspects of the Quantitative Assessment of Germicidal Efficiency", *Disinfection: Water and Wastewater,* Johnson, J.D., Ed., pp. 1-10, Ann Arbor Science Publishers, Inc., Ann Arbor, MI (1975).

Morris, J.C.; Wei, I.W. "Chlorine Ammonia Breakpoint Reactions: Model Mechanisms and Computer Simulation", Meeting of American Chemical Society, Division of Water, Air and Waste Chemicals, Minneapolis, MN (April 15, 1969).

Motomura, Y.; Yabe, K. "Piping Materials and Distribution Systems for Advanced Ultrapure Water", *Proceedings of Tenth Annual Semiconductor Pure Water Conference,* pp. 1-22, Santa Clara, CA (February 26-28, 1991).

Mouwen, H.C.; Meltzer, T.H. "Sterlizing Filters; Pore-Size Distribution and the 1 X 10^7/ cm^2 Challenge", *Pharmaceutical Technology 17(7),* pp. 28-35 (1993).

Mücke, H. "Untersuchungen Über Einflusse auf die Zersetzung von Verdünnter Peressigsäure", *Pharmazie 32,* pp. 613-619 (1977).

Munson, T. Private communications (1987).

Munson, T. *F.D.A. Views on Pharmaceutical Water,* Food and Drug Administration, Rockville, MD (1993).

Muraca, P.W.; Yu, V.L.; Goetz, A. "Disinfection of Water Distribution Systems for Legionella: Review of Application Procedures and Methodologies", *Infection Control and Hospital Epidemiology 11(2),* pp. 79-88 (1990).

Myers, J.A. "Interim Report on the Clinical Trial of the Millipore Infusion Filter Unit", *Pharmaceutical Journal 208,* pp. 547-549 (1972).

Nakamura, M.; Kosaka, K.; Shimizu, H. "Process for the Removal of Silica in High Purity Water Systems", *Ultrapure Water 5(9),* pp. 31-37 (1988).

Nakayama, S.; Tanaka, M.; Yamauchi, S.; Tabata, N. "An Antibiofouling Ozone System for Cooling Water Circuits, I., Application to Fresh Water Circuits", *Ozone: Science & Engineering 2(4),* pp. 327-336 (1980).

Nakayama, S.; Tanaka, M.; Yamauchi, S.; Tabata, N. "Antibiofouling Ozone System for Cooling Water Circuits, II., An Application to Seawater", *Ozone: Science & Engineering 7(1),* pp. 31-45 (1985).

Nalco, *The Nalco Water Handbook*, Eds., M.E. Crawford and R.T. Margolies, Nalco Chemical Co., McGraw-Hill Inc.(1988).

National Sanitation Foundation, "Ultraviolet Microbiological Water Treatment Systems", Standard Number 55 (1989).

Nebel, C. "Ozone", in *Kirk Othmer Encyclopedia of Chemical Technology, Vol. 16,* pp. 683-713, John Wiley & Sons, Inc., New York (1981).

Nebel, C. "Ozone in High Purity Water Systems", *Sixth Ozone World Congress Proceedings,* pp. 139, International Ozone Assoc., Norwalk, CT (1983).

Nebel, C.; Gottschling, R.D.; Hutchinson, R.L.; McBride, T.J.; Taylor, D.M.; Pavoni,

J.L.; Tittlebaum, M.E.; Spencer, H.E.; Fleischman, M. "Ozone Disinfection of Industrial-Municipal Secondary Effluents", *Journal Water Pollution Control Federation 45,* pp. 2493-2507 (1973).

Nebel, C.; Nebel, T. "Ozone: The Process Water Sterilant", *Pharmaceutical Manufacturing 1(2),* pp. 16-22 (1984).

Nebel, C.; Nezgod, W.W. "Purification of Deionized Water by Oxidation with Ozone", *Solid State Technology,* pp. 185-193 (October 1984).

Nebel, C.; Unangst, P. "An Evaluation of Various Mixing Devices for Dispensing Ozone in Water", *Water and Sewage Works,* Ref. No. 1973, p. R-6 (1973).

Nickel, J.C.; Ruseska, I.; Costerton, J.W. "Tobramycin Resistance of Cells of *Pseudomonas aeruginosa* Growing as Biofilm on Urinary Catheter Material", *Antimicrobial Agents and Chemotherapy 27,* pp. 619-624 (1985).

Nickerson, G.T. "Pump and Energy Efficiency Survey for Deionized Water Systems", *Ultrapure Water 2(1),* pp. 16-18 (1985).

Nickerson, G.T. "A Continuous High Purity Water Improvement Program for Submicron Device Manufacturing", *Ultrapure Water 7(2),* pp. 71-74 (1990).

Nishimura, R.; Judo, K. "Pitting Corrosion of AISI 304 and 316 Austenitic Stainless Steel Covered with Anodic Oxide Films", *Corrosion Journal 44(1),* pp. 29-35 (1988).

Noble, P.T., "Transport Considerations for Microbiological Control in Piping", *J. Pharm Sci. & Tech. 48(2)*, pp. 76-85 (1994).

Novitsky T.J. "Monitoring and Validation of High Purity Water Systems with the Limulus Amebocyte Test for Pyrogens", *Pharmaceutical Engineering 4*, pp. 21-33 (1984).

Nykanen, J.F.; Cutler, R.M. "Designing and Operating a Pharmaceutical Ultrapure Water System", *Microcontamination 8(5),* pp. 51-54, 102-103 (1990).

O'Brien, M.J. "Applicable Processes for Organic Removal in Makeup and High Purity Water Systems", *Ultrapure Water 4(9),* pp. 16-23 (1987).

Ogedengbe, O. "Characterization and Specification of Local Sands for Filters", *Filtration and Separation 21(4),* pp. 331-334 (1984).

Olefjord, J. "The Passive State of Stainless Steel", *Materials Science and Engineering 42,* pp. 161-171, Elsevier Sequoia S.A. Lausanne (1980).

O'Melia, C.R. "Aquasols: The Behavior of Small Particles in Aquatic Systems", *Environmental Science and Technology 14,* pp. 1052-1060 (1980).

Ong, H.L.; Bisque, R.E. "Coagulation of Humic Colloids by Metal Ions", *Soil Science 106(3),* pp. 220 (1966).

Orwin, L.W.; Gong, A.L. "Computer Simulation of DI Water Distribution Loops", *Transcripts of Fifth Annual Semiconductor Pure Water Conference,* pp. 33-44, San Francisco, CA (January 16-17, 1986).

Otten, G. "Thermocompression Water Stills", *Bulletin of the Parenteral Drug Association 30,* pp. 21-25 (1976).

Outschoorn, A.S. Private communications (1990).

Owens, D.L. *Pracical Principles of Ion Exchange Water Treatment,* Tall Oaks Publishing Co., Littleton, CO (1985).

Paerl, H.W. "Influence of Attachment on Microbial Metabolism and Growth in Aquatic Ecosystems", *Bacterial Adhesion, Mechanisms and Physiological Significance,* Savage, D.C.; Fletcher, M. Eds., pp. 363-400, Plenum Press, New York, (1985).

Pall, D.B.; Kirnbauer, E.A. "Bacteria Removal Prediction in Membrane Filters" 52nd Colloid and Surface Symposium, Univ. of Tennessee, Knoxville, TN (1978).

Pall, D.B.; Kirnbauer, E.A.; Allen, B.T. "Particulate Retention by Bacteria Retentive Membrane Filters", *Colloids and Surfaces 1,* pp. 235-256 (1980).

Pall, "Guide to Extractables in Effluents from Pall P-Rated Ultipor N-66 Filter Cartridges", Pall Corporation, East Hills, New York, NY (1996).

Parekh, B.; Vakhshoari, K.; Zakha, J. "Filtration of High-Purity Water for Semiconductor Manufacturing", *Ultrapure Water 10(4),* pp. 53-59 (1993).

Parenteral Drug Association, "Fundamentals of a Microbiological Environmental Monitoring Program", Technical Report No. 13, PDA Environmental Task Force (1990).

Parise, P.L.; Allegrezza, A.E., Jr.; Parekh, B.S. "Chlorine-Resistant Polysulfone Reverse Osmosis Membrane and Module", *Ultrapure Water 4(7),* pp. 54-65 (1987).

Parise, P.L.; Parekh, B.S.; Waddington, G. "The Use of Ionpure Continuous Deionization for the Production of Pharmaceutical and Semiconductor Grades of Water", *Ultrapure Water 7(8),* pp. 14-28 (1990).

Parker, J.H. "Establishment and Use of Minimum Product Bubble Point in Filter Integrity Testing", *Pharmaceutical Manufacturing, 3,* pp. 13-15 (1986).

Parks, G.A. "Equilibria Concepts in Natural Water Systems", *Advances in Chemistry Series 67,* American Chemical Society, Washington, DC (1967).

Partridge, N.A.; Regnier, F.E.; White, J.L.; Hem, S.L. "Influence of Dietary Constituents on Intestinal Absorption of Aluminum", *Kidney International 35,* pp. 1413-1417 (1989).

Pate, K.T. "Ozone Compatibility Study of DI Water Filters", *Ultrapure Water 7(6),* pp. 42-50 (1990).

Pate, K.T. "DI Water Ultrafilters Filtration Efficiency and Ozone Compatability Study", *Ultrapure Water Expo '91-East Conference on High Purity Water, Proceedings,* pp. 100-109, Philadelphia, PA (April 29 - May 1, 1991a).

Pate, K.T. "Measurement and Control of Dissolved Silica in High Purity Water Systems", *Proceedings of Watertech Conference,* pp. 52-61, San Jose, CA (November 20-22, 1991b).

Pate, K.T.; McIntosh, R.; Hanselka, R. "Degradation by High Intensity UV Light", *Ultrapure Water 7(5),* pp. 49-54 (1990).

Patterson, M.K.; Husted, G.R.; Rutkowski, A.; Mayette, D.C. "Isolation, Identification, and Microscopic Properities of Biofilms in High-Purity Water Distribution Systems", *Ultrapure Water 8(4),* pp. 18-24 (1991).

Paul, D.H.; Rahman, A.M. "Membrane Fouling—The Final Frontier?", *Ultrapure Water 7(3),* pp. 25-36 (1990).

Paulson, D.J. "An Overview of and Definitions for Membrane Fouling", Fifth Annual Membrane Technology & Planning Conference, Cambridge, MA (October 22, 1987).

Paulson, D.J.; Bertelson, R.A. "Evaluating Spiral Wound Sepralator Performance", Eighth Annual Membrane Technology/Planning Conference and First High-Tech Separations Symposium, Newton, MA (October 15-17, 1990).

Paulson, D.J.; Phelps, B.W.; Gach, G.J. "Design Innovations for Processing High-Fouling Solutions", Third Chemical Congress of North America, Symposium in Reverse Osmosis and Ultrafiltration (June 6-10, 1988).

Pavoni, J. "Virus Removal from Wastewater Using Ozone", *Water Sewage Works 119,* p. 59 (1972).

Pearson, F.C., III. *Pyrogens,* pp. 28-29, Marcel Dekker, New York (1985).

Perry, R.H.; Chilton, C.H. *Chemical Engineering Handbook,* 5th Ed., McGraw-Hill, New York, NY (1973).

Peters, C.R. "Water Treatment for Industrial Boilers", *Ultrapure Water 4(6),* pp. 17-26 (1987).

Petersen, R.J. "Reverse Osmosis Membranes", Filmtec Corporation, Minneapolis, MN.

Pharmaceutical Manufacturers Association, Action and Alert Levels Committee. "Use of Alert and Action Levels in Pharmaceutical Manufacturing", *Pharmaceutical Manufacturing* (October 24-26, 1984).

Piekaar, H.W.; Clarenburg, L.A. "Aerosol Filters: Pore Size Distribution in Fibrous Filters", *Chemical Engineering Science 22,* pp. 1399-1408 (1967).

Pittner, G. "Reverse Osmosis Systems", U.S. Patent 4,574,049, Assigned to Arrowhead Industrial Water, Inc. (Applied for June 4, 1984; Granted March 4, 1986).

Pittner, G.A.; Bertler, G. "Point-Of-Use Contamination Control of Ultrapure Water Through Continuous Ozonization", *Ultrapure Water 5(4),* pp. 16-23 (1988).

Pittner, G.A.; Levander, R.R.; Bossler, J.F. "Unique Double-Pass Reverse Osmosis System Eliminates Ion Exchange for Many Deionization Applications", *Ultrapure Water 3(5),* pp. 23-27 (1986).

Plumer, A.L. *Principles and Practices of Intravenous Therapy,* 2nd ed., Little Brown, Boston, MA (1970).

Pohland, H.W. "Reverse Osmosis", Chapter 8, *Handbook of Water Purification,* Lorch, W., Ed., McGraw-Hill, London, U.K. (1981).

Pohland, H.W.; Bettinger, G.E. "Successful Operation of a Permasep Permeator Reverse Osmosis System on Biologically Active Feed Water", *Synthetic Membranes, Vol. I: Desalination,* Turbak, A.F., Ed., American Chemical Society Symposium Series No. 153, ASC, Washington, DC (1981).

Poirier, S.J.; Kantor, K.J. "Progress Report on TOC Reduction Technologies Being Studied by the Semiconductor and Power Industries", *Ultrapure Water 4(5),* pp. 40-45 (1987).

Pope, R.J.; Federici, N.J. "Effective Odor Control Technology at Wastewater Treatment Plants", *Waterworld News,* pp. 12-13 (September-October 1989).

Powitz, R.W.; Hunter, J. "Design and Performance of Single-Lamp, High Flow Ultraviolet Disinfectors", *Ultrapure Water 2(1),* pp. 32-34 (1985).

Presswood, W.G.; Meltzer, T.H. "Membrane Filters for the Bacterial Assay of Waters", Gelman Sciences Water Microbiology Symposium, Ann Arbor, MI (1980).

Probstein, R.F.; Chan, K.K.; Cohen, R.; Rubenstein, I. "Model and Preliminary Experiments on Membrane Fouling in Reverse Osmosis", *Synthetic Membranes, Vol. 1: Desalination,* Turbak, A.F., Ed., pp 131-145, American Chemical Society, Washington, DC (1981).

Pryor, A.; Bukay, M. "Water Conservation Through Cooling Tower Ozonation", *Ultrapure Water 7(4),* pp. 24-30 (1990).

Puckorius, P.R. and also Bukay, M.; Pryor, A. "Letters from Our Readers", *Ultrapure Water 7(6),* pp. 19-20 (1990).

Purchas, D. "Chapter 5: Removal of Insoluble Particles", *Handbook of Water Purification,* Lorch, W., Ed., McGraw Hill Book Co., London, New York (1981).

Quinn, R.M. "Optimization of Reverse Osmosis/Ion Exchange System", *Ultrapure Water 6(2),* pp. 18-23 (1989).

Raistrick, J.H. "The Revelance of Zeta Potential to the Filtration of Small Particles from Potable Liquids", *World Filtration Congress III,* Vol. I, pp. 310-316, Downingtown, PA (1982).

Reasoner, D.J.; Geldreich, E.E. "New Medium for the Enumeration and Subculture of Bacteria from Potable Water", *Applied and Environmental Microbiology 49(1),* pp. 1-7 (1985).

Rechen, H.C. "The Role of Ultrafiltration in the Production of Pyrogen-Free Purified Water", *Pharmaceutical Manufacturing 1(7),* pp. 28, 31, 55 (1984).

Reif, O.W., Solkern, P. and Rupp, J., "A Standard Approach for the Analysis of Extractables", *PDA Jour. of Pharm Sci and Tech. 57* (In Press).

Reti, A.R. "An Assessment of Test Criteria in Evaluating the Performance and Integrity of Sterilizing Filters", *Bulletin of the Parenteral Drug Association 31(4),* pp. 187-194 (1977).

Reti, A.R.; Leahy, T.J.; Meier, P.M. "The Retention Mechanism of Sterilizing and Other Submicron High Efficiency Filter Structures", *Proceedings of the Second World Filtration Congress,* pp. 427-436, London, NY (1979).

Rice, R.G. "Ozone for Point of Use/Point Of Applications Part III", *Water Technology,* pp. 27-32 (August 1987).

Rice, R.G.; Bollyky, L.J. "Fundamental Aspects of Ozone Technology for Cooling Tower Water Treatment", *Ozone Treatment of Water for Cooling Applications,* pp. 1-19, Rice, R.G., Ed., Int'l Ozone Assoc., Norwalk, CT (1981)

Rice, R.G.; Bollyky, L.J.; Lacy, W.J. *Analytical Aspects of Ozone Treatment of Water and Wastewater,* Lewis Publishers, Inc., Chelsea, MI (1986).

Ridgway, H.F.. "Microbiological Fouling of Reverse Osmosis Membranes: Genesis and Control", Chapter 6, *Biological Fouling of Industrial Water Systems: A Problem Solving Approach,* Mittelman, M.W.; Geesey, G.G., Eds., Water Micro Associates, San Diego,

CA (1987).

Ridgway, H.F.; Argo, D.G.; Olson, B.H. "Factors Influencing Biofouling of Reverse Osmosis Membranes at Water Factory 21: Chemical, Microbiological, and Ultrastructural Characterization of the Fouling Layer", Vol III B, U.S. Dept. of Interior, Office of Water Res. and Technol., Washington, DC (1981).

Ridgway, H.F.; Olson, B.H. "Chlorine Resistance Patterns of Bacteria From Two Drinking Water Distribution Systems", *Applied and Environmental Microbiology, 44,* pp. 72-987 (1982).

Ridgway, H.F.; Rigby, M.G.; Argo, D.G. "Adhesion of a Mycobacterium to Cellulose Diacetate Membranes Used in Reverse Osmosis", *Applied and Environmental Microbiology 47,* pp. 61-67 (1984a).

Ridgway, H.F.; Rigby, M.G.; Argo, D.G. "Biological Fouling of Reverse Osmosis Membranes: The Mechanism of Bacterial Adhesion", *Proceedings of the Water Reuse Symposium III: The Future of Water Reuse, Vol. III,* pp. 1314-1350, San Diego, CA (1984b).

Ridgway, H.F.; Rigby, M.G.; Argo, D.G. "Bacterial Adhesion and Fouling of Reverse Osmosis Membranes", *Journal American Water Works Association 77,* pp. 97-106 (1985).

Ridgway, H.F.; Rogers, D.M.; Argo, D.G. "Effects of Surfactants on the Adhesion of Mycobacteria to Reverse Osmosis Membranes" *Transcripts of Fifth Annual Semiconductor Pure Water Conference,* San Francisco, CA (January 16-17, 1986).

Riley, C.D. "Synergetic Design of Ultrapure Water Systems for Microelectronic Applications", *Microelectronic Manufacturing & Testing,* pp. 21-23 (July, 1983).

Roberson, C.E.; Hem, J.D. "Solubility of Aluminum in the Presence of Hydroxide, Fluoride and Sulfate", Geological Survey Water-Supply Paper 1927-C, U.S. Government Printing Office, Washington, DC (1969).

Rollins, D.M.; Colwell, R.R. "Viable But Non-Culturable Stage of *Campilobacter leluni* and Its Role in the Aquatic Environment", *Applied and Environmental Microbiology 52,* p. 531 (1986).

Rootare, H.M. "A Short Literature Review of Mercury Porosimetry and a Discussion of Possible Sources of Error", Aminco Reprint 439, American Instrument Co., Silver Spring, MD (1970).

Rossitto, J. Letter to *Liquid Filtration Newsletter No. 50,* The McIlvaine Company, Northbrook, IL (October 10, 1983).

Roszak, D.B.; Grimes, D.J.; Colwell, R.R. "Viable but Non-recoverable Stage of *Salmonella enteritidis* in Aquatic Systems", *Canadian Journal of Microbiology 30,* pp. 334-338 (1984).

Rubow, K.L. *Submicron Aerosol Filtration Characteristics of Membrane Filters,* PhD Thesis, University of Minnesota, Minneapolis, MN (1981).

Rudie, B.J.; Torgrimson, T.A.; Spatz, D.D. "Reverse Osmosis and Ultrafiltration Membrane Compaction Studies Using Ultrafiltration Pretreatment, Reverse Osmosis and Ultrafiltration," *American Chemical Society Symposium Series 281,* Sourirajan, S.; Matsuuka, T., Eds. (1985).

Saari, R.; Suomela, H.; Haahti, E.; Raaska, E. "Production of Pyrogen-Free Distilled Water for Pharmaceutical Purposes", *Bulletin of the Parenteral Drug Association 31(5)*, pp. 248-253 (1977).

Sakamoto, T.; Miyasaka, T. "Study Confirming the Accuracy of a Method for Measuring TOC by Wet Oxidation", *Ultrapure Water 4(9)*, pp. 24-31 (1987).

Saleem, M. ; Schlitzer, R.L. "Comparative Recovery of Bacteria from Purified Water by the Membrane Filtration Technique and the Standard Plate Count Method", *Abstracts of the Annual Meeting of the American Society for Microbiology*, New Orleans, LA (March 1983).

Sanders, T.M.; Furne, T.J. "High Purity Water Systems Material Selection", *Transcripts of Fifth Annual Semiconductor Pure Water Conference*, pp. 3-16, San Francisco, CA (January 16-17, 1986).

Sato, H.; Hashimoto, N.; Shinoda, T.; Takino, K. "Dissolved Oxygen Removal in Ultrapure Water for Semiconductor Manufacturing", *Proceedings of the Tenth Semiconductor Pure Water Conference*, pp. 147-164, Santa Clara, CA (February 19-21, 1991).

Saunders, L. "Chapter 6: Distillation", *Handbook of Water Purification*, Lorch, W., Ed., McGraw Hill Book Co., London, U.K. (1981).

Saunier, B.M.; Selleck, R.E. "The Kinetics of Breakpoint Chlorination in Continuous Flow Systems", *Journal American Water Works Association 71(3)*, pp. 164-172 (1979).

Scaramelli, A.B.; DiGiano, F.A. "Effect of Sorbed Organisms on the Efficiency of Ammonia Removal by Chloramine-Carbon Surface Reactions", *Journal Water Pollution Control Federation*, pp. 693-705 (April 1977).

Scheer, L.A.; Steere, W.C.; Geisz, C.M. "Temperature and Volume Effects on Filter Integrity Tests", *Pharmaceutical Technology 17(2)*, pp. 22-23.

Schenck, G.O. "Chapter 10: Ultraviolet Sterilization", *Handbook of Water Purification*, Lorch, W., Ed., McGraw Hill Book Co., London, U.K. (1981).

Schmauss, L.R.; Aiken, J.W. "Economics of the Electrodialysis Reversal Process in Conjunction with Ion Exchange", *Ultrapure Water 1(3)*, pp. 32-35 (1984).

Schneider, W.K.G.; Rump, H.H. "Use of Ozone in the Technology of Bottled Waters", *Ozone: Science & Engineering 5*, pp. 95-101 (1983).

Schnitzer, M.; Kodama, H. "Montmorillonite: Effect on pH on Its Adsorption of a Soil Humic Compound", *Science 153*, p. 70 (1966).

Schroeder, H.G.; DeLuca, P.P. "Theoretical Aspects of Sterile Filtration and Integrity Testing", *Pharmaceutical Technology 4(11)* pp. 80-85 (1980).

Schroeder, H.G.; DeLuca, P.P. "The Pressure Hold Test: An Aspect of Integrity Testing", Society of Manufacturing Engineers Conference on Filtration in Pharmaceutical Manufacturing, Philadelphia, PA (March 26-28, 1985).

Scruton, S.H. "Upgrading Water Purity for Manufacturing Nonsterile Pharmaceutical Products", *Pharmaceutical Technology 4*, pp. 39-42 (1980).

Seiler, D.A.; Barber, L. "Handling of High Purity Fluids with New, Flexible PVDF", *Ultrapure Water 6(4)* pp. 37-38 (1989).

Sergent, R.H. "Enhanced Water Management Using Bromine Chemistry", Paper No. TP-86-9, Cooling Tower Institute, Houston, TX (1986).

Seyfried, P.L.; Fraser, D.J. "Persistence of *Pseudomonas aeruginosa* in Chlorinated Swimming Pools", *Canadian Journal of Microbiology 26,* pp. 350-355 (1980).

Sharpe, A.D. "Recent Experience with the Application of Ultrafiltration in the Power Utility Industry", *Ultrapure Water 2(2),* pp. 38-41 (1985).

Shaw, K.R. "Overpressure Safety Relief with Rupture Discs in the Pharmaceutical Industry", *Pharmaceutical Engineering 12(1)*, pp. 22-29 (1992).

Shelton, J.R. "Chapter 18: Stabilization Fundamentals in Thermal Autoxidation of Polymers", *Stabilization and Degradation of Polymers,* Allars, D.L.; Hawkins, W.L., Eds., Advances in Chemistry Series, American Chemical Society, Washington, DC (1978).

Shin-Ho-Lee; Frank, J.F. "Inactivation of Surface-Adherent *Listeria monocytogenes* by Sodium Hypochlorite and Heat", *J. Food Prot. 54,* pp. 4-6 (1991).

Short, J.L. "Extension of Spiral Wound Module Technology from Reverse Osmosis to Ultra & Microfiltration ABCOR/KMS Experience Over the Last 15 Years", Eighth Annual Membrane Technology/Planning Conference and First High-Tech Separations Symposium, Newton, MA (October 15-17, 1990).

Simonetti, J.A.; Schroeder, H.G. "The Effect of Various Analytical Membranes on the Modified Silt Density Index Test", *Ultrapure Water 2(3),* pp. 14-20 (1985).

Simonetti, J.A.; Schroeder, H.G.; Meltzer, T.H. "A Review of Latex Sphere Retention Work: Its Application to Membrane Pore Size Rating", *Ultrapure Water 3(4),* pp. 46-51 (1986).

Singer, D.C. "An Approach to Microbiological Trending of Pharmaceutical Water Systems", *Proceedings, Ultrapure Water Expo '94,* pp. 6-7, Philadelphia, PA (May 9-11, 1994).

Singer, P.C. "Formation and Control of Trihalomethanes, Disinfection By-Products: Current Perspectives", *Journal American Water Works Association 81,* pp. 219-237 (1989).

Singer, P.C.; Chang, S.D. "Correlations Between Trihalomethanes and Total Organic Halides Formed During Water Treatment", *Journal American Water Works Association 81(8),* pp. 61-65 (1989).

Sinha, D. "Pretreatment Process Considerations for the Semiconductor Industry", *Ultrapure Water 7(6),* pp. 21-30 (1990).

Sinha, D. "Controlling Ultrapure-Water Contamination from Air and Process Gas", *Microcontamination 9(8),* pp. 29-33 (1991).

Sinha, D.; Van Winkle, J. "PVC Pipe for High-Purity DI Water Systems", *Ultrapure Water 10(9),* pp. 33-39 (1993).

Sixsmith, T. Private communications (1991).

Sixsmith, T.; Hanselka, R. "An Evaluation of Currently Available Joining Methodologies for DI Water Piping", *Ultrapure Water 6(4),* pp. 52-54 (1989).

Sladek, F.J.; Suslavich, R.V.; John, B.I.; Dawson, F.W. "Optimum Membrane Structures for Growth of Coliform and Fecal Coliform Organisms", *Applied Microbiology 30,* pp. 685-691 (1975).

Sloane, P.; Hernon, B.P. "Catalytic Hydrogen Deoxygenation and Triple Membrane Demineralization at North Anna Nuclear Station", 51st Annual Meeting International Water Conference, Pittsburgh, PA (1990).

Smith, P.J. "Design of Clean Steam Distribution Systems", *Pharm. Eng. 15(2),* pp. 72-79 (1995).

Smith, V.C. "Problems in the Production and Handling of Ultra Pure Water", International Water Conference, Engineers Society of Western Pennsylvania, Pittsburgh, PA (November 1968).

Smith, V.C. "The Design of Distillation Equipment for the Production of Ultra Pure Water", American Association for Contamination Control, Eighth Annual Technical Meeting, New York, NY (May 1969).

Smith, V.C. "Can Reverse Osmosis Replace Distillation as a Process for Producing Pure Water", R3 Symposium, Gothenburg, Sweden (April 1975).

Smith, V.C. "Distillation System and Processes", U.S. Patent 4,344,826, Assigned to Vaponics, Inc. (Issued August 17, 1982).

Smith, V.C. "Requirements for and Types of Feedwater Systems for Water Stills", *Ultrapure Water 5(8),* pp. 35-39 (1988).

Smith, V.C. Private communications (1991).

Smolders, C.A. "Morphology of Skinned Membranes: A Rationale From Phase Separation Phenomena", *Ultrafiltration Membranes and Applications,* Polymer Science and Technology Series, Vol. 13, Cooper, A.R., Ed., Plenum Press, New York (1979).

Sourirajan, S. "The Mechanism of Demineralization of Aqueous Sodium Chloride Solutions by Flow, Under Pressure, Through Porous Membranes", *Industrial and Engineering Chemistry Fundamentals 2(1),* pp. 51-55 (1963).

Sourirajan, S. "Separation of Some Inorganic Salts in Aqueous Solution by Flow, Under Pressure, Through Porous Cellulose Acetate Membranes", *Industrial and Engineering Chemistry Fundamentals 3(3),* pp. 206-210 (1964).

Speaker, L.M. "Modifying Membrane Surfaces with Oriented Monolayers of Amphiphilic Compounds", U.S. Patent 4,554,076, Assigned to Georgia Tech. Research Institute, Atlanta, GA (November 19, 1985).

Standard Methods for the Examination of Water and Wastewater, Seventeenth Edition 1989, Amer. Public Health Assoc., Washington, DC; Thirteenth Edition, 1971; Fifteenth Edition, 1981; Sixteenth edition, 1985.

Standard Methods for the Examination of Water and Wastewater, American Public Health Association, Washington, DC (13th ed., 1971; 15th ed., 1981; 16th ed., 1985; 17th ed., 1989).

Stevens, A.A.; Moore, L.A.; Miltner, R.J. "Formation and Control of Non-Trihalomethane Disinfection By-Products", *Journal American Water Works Association 81(8),* pp. 54-60 (1989).

Stewart, D. "Validating The Performance and Rating of Absolute Filters", Integrated Circuit Manufacturers Consortium Conference, Coventry, U.K. (February 9-10, 1987).

Stoecker, J.G.; Pope, D.H. "Study of Biochemical Corrosion in High Temperature Demineralized Water", Paper No. 126, *Proceedings of the National Association of Corrosion Engineers,* Annual Meeting NACE Publications, Houston, TX (1986).

Stone, T.E., Goel, V. and Leszczak, J., "Methodology for Analysis of Filter Extractables: A Model Stream Approach", *Pharm. Tech. 18(10)*, pp. 116-130 (1994).

Stopka, K. "Our Experiences with 14 Ozone-Treated Cooling Towers", *Ozone Treatment of Water for Cooling Applications,* Rice, R.G., Ed., pp. 55-61, Int'l Ozone Assoc., Norwalk, CT (1981).

Strauss, S.D. "Removing Oxygen Prevents Corrosion", *Power 117(6),* pp. 16 (1973).

Strauss, S.D.; Kunin, R. "Ion Exchange — Key to Ultrapure Water for High-Pressure Fossil and Nuclear Steam Generations", *Power 124(9),* pp. S1-S16 (1980).

Stucki, S.; Theis, G.; Kötz, R.; Devantay, H.; Christen, H.J. "In-Situ Production of Ozone in Water Using a Membrel Electrolyzer", *Journal of the Electrochemical Society 132(2),* (1985).

Sugam, R.; Guera, C.R. "Comparison of Chlorine and Ozone for Power Plant Cooling Water Treatment", *Ozone Treatment of Water and for Cooling Applications,* Rice, R.G., Ed., pp. 63-73, Int'l. Ozone Association, Norwalk, CT (1981).

Sugisawa, M.; Kajiama, Y.; Ushikoshi, K.; Hotetsu, A.; Ohmi, T. "Oxygen Passivated Stainless Steel for High-Temperature and Ozone-Injected Ultrapure Water", *Water Proceedings Semiconductor Pure Water and Chemicals Conference,* (oral presentation), pp. 108-127, Santa Clara, CA (February 11-13, 1992).

Sullivan, D.L. "Lilly's Process Water System", *Proceedings of PMA Water Seminar Program,* pp. 92-95, Atlanta, GA (February 1982).

Sweadner, K.J.; Forte, J.; Nelsen, L.L. "Filtration Removal of Endotoxin (Pyrogens) in Solution in Different States of Aggregation", *Applied and Environmental Microbiology 34,* pp. 382-385 (1977).

Takahashi, H.; Goto, S.; Takata, S.; Shibata, M.; Hata, T. "Method for Treating the Surface of Stainless Steel by High Temperature Oxidation", U.S. Patent 4,776,897, Assigned to Shinko-Pfaudler Co., Chuo, Japan (October 11, 1988).

Tanaka, T.; Sato, T.; Suzuki, T. "Disinfection of *Escherichia coli* by Using Water Dissociation Effect on Ion-Exchange Membranes", *Membranes and Membrane Processes, Proceedings of the European-Japan Congress on Membranes and Membrane Processes,* Drioli, E.; Nakagaki, M., Eds., Stresa, Italy (June 18-22, 1984).

Tanford, C. *The Hydrophobic Effect: Formation of Micelles and Biological Membranes,* 2nd ed., Wiley, New York, NY (1980).

Tankha, A.; Williford, H. "GMP Considerations in the Design and Validation of a Deionized Water System", *Pharmaceutical Engineering 7(4),* pp. 17-20 (1987).

Tanny, G.B.; Strong, D.K.; Presswood, W.G.; Meltzer, T.H. "The Adsorptive Retention of *Pseudomonas diminuta* by Membrane Filters", *Journal of the Parenteral Drug Association 33(1),* pp. 40-51 (1979).

Water Quality Committee - Pharmaceutical Manufacturers Association, "Updating Requirements for Pharmaceutical Grades of Water: Conductivity", *Pharmacopeial Forum 17(6),* pp. 2669-2675 (1991).

Water Quality Committee - Pharmaceutical Manufacturers Association, "Updating Requirements for Pharmaceutical Grades of Water: Microbial Considerations", *Pharmacopeial Forum 18(6),* pp. 4397-43399 (1992a).

Water Quality Committee - Pharmaceutical Manufacturers Association, "Updating Requirements for Pharmaceutical Grades of Water: Heavy Metals", *Pharmacopeial Forum 18(6),* pp. 4395-4396 (1992b).

Water Quality Committee - Pharmaceutical Manufacturers Association, "Updating Requirements for Pharmaceutical Grades of Water: Aluminum", *Pharmacopeial Forum 18(6),* pp. 4392-4394 (1992c).

Water Quality Committee - Pharmaceutical Manufacturers Association, "Updating Requirements for Pharmaceutical Grades of Water: Validation and Technology Selection", *Pharmacopeial Forum 19(6),* pp. 6633-6645 (1993a).

Water Quality Committee - Pharmaceutical Manufacturers Association, "Updating Requirements for Pharmaceutical Grades of Water: Total Solids", *Pharmacopeial Forum 19(4),* pp. 2669-2675 (1993b).

Water Quality Committee - Pharmaceutical Manufacturers Association, "Updating Requirements for Pharmaceutical Grades of Water: Total Organic Carbon", *Pharmacopeial Forum 19(4),* pp. 5858-5862 (1993c).

Water Quality Committee - Pharmaceutical Manufacturers Association, (1994).

Water Quality Committee - Pharmaceutical Research and Manufacturers Association, (1996).

Water Supply Research, Office of Res. & Development, USEPA "Ozone, Chlorine Dioxide and Chloramines as Alternatives to Chlorine for Disinfection of Drinking Water", Second Conference on Water Chlorinates, Gatlinburg, TN (October 31 - November 4, 1977).

Watson, W.W.; Novitsky, T.J.; Quinby, H.L. "Determination of Bacterial Number and Biomass in the Marine Environment", *Applied and Environmental Microbiology 33,* pp. 940-946 (1977).

Weber, W.H.; Voice, T.C.; Jodellah, A. "Adsorption of Humic Substances: The Effects of Heterogeneity and System Characteristics", *Journal American Water Works Association,* pp. 612-619 (December 1983).

Wei, J.W.; Morris, J.C. "Dynamics of Breakpoint Chlorination", *Chemistry of Water Supply Treatment and Distribution,* Rubin, A.J., Ed., Ann Arbor Science Press, Ann Arbor, MI (1974).

Weissman, B. "Pall Septa Optimization Studies", EPRI Condensate Polishing Workshop on Powdered Resin Technology, Philadelphia, PA (January 27-29, 1988).

Weitnauer, A.K., "A Practical Approach to Controlling Growth in USP Purified Water", Ultrapure Water 13(3), pp. 26-30 (1996).

Weitnauer, A.K.; Comb, L.F. "Two-Pass RO for Pharmaceutical Grade Purified Water",

Ultrapure Water 13(2), pp. 42-45 (1996).

Westinghouse Electric Corporation, "Water Sterilization by Ultraviolet Radiation", Research Report BL-R-6-1059-3023-1.

Wheeler, W.W. "A Simplified Application of Chlorine For Biological Control", Paper No. TP-187-A, Cooling Tower Institute, Houston, TX (1978).

Whipple, S.S.; Ebach, E.A.; Beardsley, S.S. "The Economics of Reverse Osmosis and Ion Exchange", *Ultrapure Water 4(7),* pp. 28-43 (1987).

White, G.C. *Handbook of Chlorination,* Van Nostrand Reinhold Co., New York, NY (1985).

White, J.L.; Parise, P.L; Parekh, B.S. "Demineralization by Continuous Deionization - Performance and Applications", *Ultrapure Water 6(7),* pp. 46-51 (1989).

Whittaker, C.; Ridgway, H.F.; Olson, B.H. "Evaluation of Cleaning Strategies for Removal of Biofilms from Reverse Osmosis Membranes", *Applied and Environmental Microbiology 48,* pp. 395-403 (1984).

Whittet, T.D. "Sterile and Apyrogenic Water", Chapter 13, *Handbook of Water Purification,* Lorch, W., Ed., McGraw Hill Book Co., London, U.K. (1981).

Wickert, K. "Validation of Positively Charged Filters Used for Endotoxin Control", *Pharmaceutical Engineering 13(1),* pp. 41-45 (1993).

Wickramanayake, G.B.; Rubin, A.J.; Sproul, O.J. "Effects of Ozone and Storage Temperature on *Giardia* Cysts", *Journal American Water Works Association 77(8),* pp. 74-77 (1985).

Wiegler, N.; Anderson, C.C. "Removing Trihalomethanes from DI Water: A Consideration of the Alternatives", *Microcontamination 8(10),* pp. 37-42, 108-112 (1990).

Wiegler, N.; Anderson, C.C.. "Removal of Trihalomethanes By Means of Active Carbon Bed and UV Light", *Transcripts of Ninth Annual Semiconductor Pure Water Conference,* pp. 121-149, Santa Clara, CA (January 17-18, 1990).

Williams, R.; Hanselka, R.; Kennedy, R.; Castro, S.; Rusconi, S.J. *Transcripts of Seventh Annual Semiconductor Pure Water Conference,* pp. 145-169, Santa Clara, CA (January 14-15, 1988).

Williams, R.E.; Meltzer, T.H. "Membrane Structure: The Bubble Point and Particle Retention: A New Theory", *Pharmaceutical Technology 7(5),* pp. 36-42 (1983).

William, W., Webb, G. and Paul, D., "Surface Water RO System Biofouling", *Ultrapure Water 11(8),* pp. 36-41 (1994).

Wrasidlo, W.; Hofmann, R. "Hochasymmetriche Polysulfonmembranen in Neue Sterifiltergeneration", Brunswick Technetics Ausgabe No. MFP 001 (1982).

Wrasidlo, W.; Hofmann, F.; Simonetti, J.A.; Schroeder, H.G. "Effect of Vehicle Properties on the Retention Characteristics of Various Membrane Filters", PDA Spring Meeting, San Juan, PR (1983).

Wrasidlo, W.; Mysels, K.J. "The Structure and Some Properties of Graded Highly Asymmetric Porous Membranes", *Journal of Parenteral Science and Technology 38(1),* pp. 24-31 (1984).

Yabe, K.; Motomura, Y.; Ishikawa, H.; Mizuniwa, T.; Ohmi, T. "Responding to the Future Quality Demands of Ultrapure Water", *Microcontamination 7(2),* pp. 37-46, 68 (1989).

Yagi, Y.; Shinoda, T.; Saito, M. "Analysis and Behavior Evaluation of Bacteria in Ultrapure Water", *Proceedings of Semiconductor Pure Water and Chemicals Conference,* Water Proceedings, pp. 148-163, Santa Clara, CA (February 11-13, 1992).

Yarnell, P.; Kato, M.; Hoffman, B. "The Effects of Ozone on Ion Exchange Mixed Beds in Ultrapure Water", *Transcripts of Eighth Annual Semiconductor Pure Water Conference,* pp. 195-228, Santa Clara, CA (January 18-20, 1989).

Yasuda, H.; Tsai, J.T. "Pore-Size Microporous Polymer Membranes", *Journal of Applied Polymer Science 18,* pp. 805-819 (1974).

Young, L.Y.; Mitchell, R. "The Role of Chemotactic Responses in Primary Microbial Film Formation", *Proceedings of the Third International Congress on Marine Corrosion and Fouling,* pp. 617-623, National Bureau of Standards, Gaithersburg, MD (1972).

Young, L.Y.; Mitchell, R. "Negative Chemotaxis of Marine Bacteria to Toxic Chemicals", *Applied Microbiology 25,* pp. 972-975 (1973).

Young, J.H., Ferko, B.L. and Gaber, R.P., "Parameters Covering Steam Sterilization of Deadlegs", *J. Pharm Sci & Tech 48(3)*, pp. 140-147 (1994).

Youngberg, D.A. "Sterilizing Storage Tanks in a Pure Water System", *Ultrapure Water 2(4),* pp. 45 (1985).

Zahka, J.; Smith, P.T. "Ozone Compatibility of Membrane Filters for DI Water", *Transcripts of Seventh Annual Semiconductor Pure Water Conference,* pp. 322-340, Santa Clara, CA (January 14-15, 1988).

Zahka, J.; Vakhshoori, K. "Ozone Compatibility of an All-PVDF DI Water Ultrafilter", *Ultrapure Water 7(6),* pp. 32-40 (1990).

Zeff, J.D.; Leitis, E.; Nguyen, D. "UV-Oxidation Case Studies on the Removal of Toxic Organic Compounds in Ground, Waste and Leachate Waters", PACHEC Conference, Acapulco, Mexico (October 19-23, 1988).

Zeiher, E.H.K.; Pierce, C.C.; Woods, D. "Biofouling of Reverse Osmosis Systems: Three Case Studies", *Ultrapure Water 8(7),* pp. 50-64 (1991).

Zinnbauer, F.E. "Ultraviolet Water Disinfection Comes of Age", *Ultrapure Water 2(1),* pp. 27-29 (1985).

Zobell, C.E. "The Effect of Solid Surfaces Upon Bacterial Activity", *Journal of Bacteriology 46,* pp. 39-59 (1943).

Zoccolante, G.V. "Innovations in Water Purification", *Semiconductor International 10(2),* pp. 86-89 (1987).

Zoccolante, G.V. "USP Purified Water System Design", Johnson & Johnson Sterilization Sciences Group, Penfield, Inc., Plantsville, CT, Presentation (June 5-6, 1989).

Zoccolante, G.V. "Nontraditional Water for Injection Systems: Methods of Production and Validation Issues", Medical Manufacturing TechSource, Pharmaceutical Waters '94 Symposium, Atlantic City, NJ, pp. 12-31 (May 25-26, 1994).

Zoccolante, G.V. Private communications (1991).

AUTHOR INDEX

T

U, V

SUBJECT INDEX